Advances in
Myocardiology
Volume 4

Advances in Myocardiology
Series Editors: N. S. Dhalla and G. Rona

Volume 1   Edited by M. Tajuddin, P. K. Das, M. Tariq, and N. S. Dhalla

Volume 2   Edited by M. Tajuddin, B. Bhatia, H. H. Siddiqui, and G. Rona

Volume 3   Edited by E. Chazov, V. Smirnov, and N. S. Dhalla

Volume 4   Edited by E. Chazov, V. Saks, and G. Rona

A Continuation Order Plan is available for this series. A continuation order will bring delivery of each new volume immediately upon publication. Volumes are billed only upon actual shipment. For further information please contact the publisher. Volumes 1 and 2 of this series were published by University Park Press, Baltimore.

Advances in Myocardiology
Volume 4

Edited by

E. Chazov, M.D., and V. Saks, M.D.

*Cardiology Research Center
Academy of Medical Sciences
Moscow, USSR*

and

G. Rona, M.D.

*Institute of Pathology
McGill University
Montreal, Quebec, Canada*

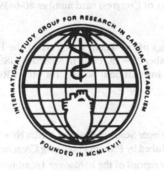

Springer Science+Business Media, LLC

ISBN 978-1-4757-4443-9   ISBN 978-1-4757-4441-5 (eBook)
DOI 10.1007/978-1-4757-4441-5

Library of Congress card number 80-643989

Derived from the proceedings of the Tenth Congress of the International Society for Heart Research, held September 23 – 29, 1980, in Moscow, USSR, and organized by the Soviet Section of the International Society for Heart Research, Moscow.

This volume is dedicated to

DR. ALBERT WOLLENBERGER, Berlin–Buch, and
DR. TACHIO KOBAYASHI, Tokyo

for their untiring efforts in promoting the cellular and
molecular aspects of cardiology in the pursuit of
understanding heart function in health and disease.

Preface

This volume of Advances in Myocardiology is derived from a part of the proceedings of the 10th Congress of the International Society for Heart Research, which was held in Moscow on September 23–29, 1980. This book contains selected papers which have been arranged in two sections, Cardiac Hypertrophy, Adaptation, and Pathophysiology and Cardiac Hypoxia, Ischemia, and Infarction. The first section, on the pathophysiology of heart hypertrophy and failure, contains 24 chapters that focus on the derangement of biochemical, physiological, and immunological processes during the development of heart disease due to a wide variety of pathogenic factors. Some of the recent developments in understanding the myocardial synthetic machinery in heart hypertrophy are also described in these papers, and we believe that the contents of this section will stimulate further research in the area of heart disease. The second section, which mainly deals with myocardial ischemia, contains 35 chapters providing the necessary background for the diagnosis of ischemic heart disease and some possible therapeutic approaches.

It hardly needs to be emphasized that ischemic heart disease is a major cause of death in highly industrialized countries, but unfortunately the exact mechanism by which ischemic insult leads to the development of heart cell damage is far from understood. We are hopeful that the articles in this section will provide valuable information in this field and thus will help in improving the treatment of ischemic heart disease. It should be pointed out that the interaction between the eastern and western experimental cardiologists was not only stimulating in terms of understanding the scientific problems being pursued in different parts of the world but was also a rewarding experience for those who participated in the Moscow meeting. Furthermore, we believe that the papers in this book, when considered as a whole, will bridge the gap between basic heart research and the practice of cardiology.

E. Chazov
V. Saks
G. Rona

Contents

CARDIAC HYPOXIA, ISCHEMIA, AND INFARCTION

CARDIAC HYPERTROPHY, ADAPTATION, AND PATHOPHYSIOLOGY

Pathogenesis and Prophylaxis of Cardiac Lesions in Stress

F. Z. Meerson

Institute of General Pathology and Pathologic Physiology
USSR Academy of Medical Sciences
Moscow, USSR

Abstract. Emotional or painful stress excites the brain centers which trigger stress reactions, this excitement being followed by an increase in catecholamine concentration. The following chain of events is thought to occur under the influence of the catecholamine excess: activation of lipid peroxidation in the membranes; labilization of lysosomes; damage to sarcolemmal membranes which are responsible for calcium transport; increased calcium concentration in the heart sarcoplasm. The contraction of myofibrils, the decrease in efficiency of ATP resynthesis in the mitochondria, and the activation of phosphorylase and proteases all arise from the calcium excess. This results in necrotic foci and alterations of heart function. The damages can be effectively prevented by suppression of stress-responding centers with γ-aminobutyric acid, blockade of β receptors with propranolol, inhibition of lipid peroxidation by antioxidants, inhibition of proteolytic lysosomal enzymes with trasilol, or blocking of calcium entry into the myocytes with verapamil. The possible application to clinical practice of chemical prophylaxis of stress damage in the heart is discussed.

The important role of stressful situations and of emotional stress in cardiac pathology is indisputable. Stress has a direct damaging effect on the heart and potentiates that of hypoxia on the myocardium (13). However, the molecular mechanism by which high concentrations of catecholamines and glucocorticoids affect myocardial cells in stress still remains unclear, and this essentially limits the development of prophylactic methods of cardiac stress affections. Nevertheless, it is obvious that such prophylaxis is one of the important problems of current cardiology.

It is the purpose of this chapter to demonstrate, on the basis of new experimental data, the main links of the pathogenetic chain of stress-induced injury to the heart and the possibilities of prophylaxis of such injury by selective chemical blockade of definite links in this chain.

PATHOGENESIS OF THE STRESS-INDUCED INJURY TO THE HEART

Emotional and painful stress has been induced in the form of the so-called neurosis of anxiety by the well-known method of Desiderato et al. (2). The main feature of this model is that an animal waits intensely for

3

painful electric shocks for 6 hr and actually receives them at occasional intervals.

As a result, a standard stress syndrome develops which involves activation of adrenergic and hypophyseal–adrenal systems, weight loss, thymus involution, development of ulcerations of the stomach (17), and damage to cardiac metabolism, structure, and function (8), the last being the main object of the research. For these investigations, hearts of animals were taken at various periods following termination of stress induction, from 2 hr to 4 days.

The findings that substantial doses of exogenous catecholamines activated peroxidation of lipids (POL) in the myocardium (6) and that products of this process—hydroperoxides of lipids—destroyed membranes of sarcoplasmic reticulum in vitro (5) became the focus of our investigations. It permitted the suggestion that POL activation induced by the excess of catecholamines could be an important link in heart stress damage.

On the basis of this view, the influence of emotional/painful stress (EPS) on POL in myocardium has been studied (15). We have determined primary molecular products of POL—hydroperoxides of polyenic lipids—and terminal products of POL—fluorescent Schiff bases—in the heart, skeletal muscle, and brain of rats exposed to stress. Lipids were extracted from these organs by the method of Folch (4). Accumulation of hydroperoxides in polyenic lipids has been evaluated using the UV spectrum of absorption of the lipid solution (in methanol–hexane, 5:1) characteristic of the diene conjugates by setting the coefficient of molar extinction at λ_{max} 232 nm equal to 2.1×10^4 $M^{-1}cm^{-1}$. The spectra were recorded with a Shimadzu spectrophotometer. Terminal products of POL—products of interaction of short-chain dialdehydes with aminophospholipids—were determined by the spectra of fluorescence of the lipid solution in chloroform with maximum excitation of the fluorescence at 360 nm and maximum emission in the 420- to 440-mm region using an Aminco–Bowman spectrophotometer.

Figure 1 shows typical UV absorption spectra (panel A) and emission spectra of lipid solutions extracted from the myocardium of controls and stress-exposed animals (panel B). It can be seen (Figure 1A) that the lipids extracted from the hearts of animals exposed to EPS have an absorption spectrum characteristic of hydroperoxides of polyenic lipids with maxima at 230–235 nm and 270–280 nm which were virtually absent in controls. Further, it is obvious that intensities of fluorescence of Schiff bases, which are the terminal products of POL, are significantly higher for lipids of animals exposed to EPS than those of the controls (Figure 1B).

The hatched zones in Figure 1 reflect accumulation of the intermediate and terminal products of peroxide oxidation of lipids in EPS.

As shown in Table 1, the content of hydroperoxides in lipids of myocardium is augmented threefold under the action of EPS, and the intensity of fluorescence of the terminal products of POL (Schiff bases) was increased fivefold; the respective values for skeletal muscle are 2.0 and 2.7 and for

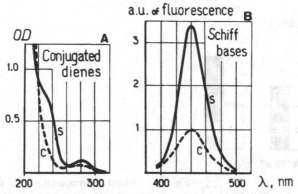

Figure 1.   Effect of emotional/painful stress (EPS) on the UV absorption (A) and emission (B) spectra of lipids extracted from the myocardium: dashed line, control; solid line, EPS.

the brain, 1.7 and 2.1. Thus, activation of the process of POL occurring in the organism after exposure to EPS is more pronounced in the heart than in other organs.

Since lipid peroxides are able to disturb membrane structures of cells, further investigations have been carried out with two purposes. First, the state of the lysosomes whose labilization under the action of lipid peroxides might form a link in the pathogenetic chain of stress-induced injury to the myocardium has been studied. Second, the activity of enzymes in blood plasma has been measured, since the passage of these enzymes from the cells into blood may be the immediate result of damage to the cell membranes (18).

The diagram in Figure 2 shows that stress leads to reduced activity of acid cathepsins in the lysosomal and mitochondrial fractions of the myocardium by 25% and simultaneously increases the activity of these ferments in the supernatant by 45%. This shift apparently shows that labilization of lysosomal membranes occurs under the action of EPS, leading to the lysosomal release of the proteolytic enzymes. This concept is consistent with the data presented in the same figure showing that stress leads to a twofold increase in activity of cathepsins in the blood plasma.

Table 1.   Accumulation of Products of Lipid Peroxidation in EPS

Parameters	Groups of animals	Tissue		
		Myocardium	Skeletal muscle	Brain
Hydroperoxides of lipids (unit	Control ($N = 10$)	0.35 ± 0.05	0.40 ± 0.05	0.15 ± 0.05
of optic density)	EPS ($N = 11$)	0.9 ± 0.05	0.80 ± 0.01	0.25 ± 0.05
Significance (P)		0.001	0.01	0.1
Fluorescence of Schiff bases	Control	19.1 ± 2.9	13.0 ± 1.7	9.3 ± 0.1
(relative unit of fluorescence)	EPS	95.5 ± 20.8	35.3 ± 7.3	20.0 ± 1.5

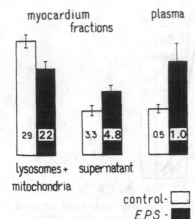

myocardium plasma
fractions

lysosomes + supernatant
mitochondria

control- □
EPS - ■

Figure 2.   Effect of emotional/painful stress (EPS) on activity of acid cathepsins (g tyrosine/mg protein per hr) in heart and plasma.

Figure 3 shows that 2 hr following stress the enzymic activity of aspartate transaminase, alanine transaminase, lactate dehydrogenase, and malate dehydrogenase in blood plasma was increased about twofold.

Thus, after the endured stress, simultaneously with activation of POL, and probably under the influence of POL products, lysosome membranes are labilized, and lysosome proteolytic enzymes are released into the cytoplasm and blood plasma. Simultaneously, more extensive damage occurs to cellular membranes, which becomes the cause of the pronounced fermentemia which appears in the organism.

In the next stage of our investigations, we sought to obtain a quantitative estimate of the breakdown of structures, i.e., of proteins and nucleic acids in heart and other organs, caused by a hard stress syndrome.

During the study of the effect of stress syndrome on RNA breakdown, 35 rats were twice injected intraabdominally at intervals of 24 hr with 50 μCi ^{14}C-labeled orotic acid. Two days following the first injection, the initial radioactivity of RNA was measured in heart and other organs in some animals. Then, half of the remaining animals were exposed to stress, and the other animals served as controls. Further determination of the specific radioactivity of rRNA in the tissues of these animals was carried out 1, 3, and 7 days following injections of the isotope.

Table 2 shows that in the heart and brain stress resulted in a significant

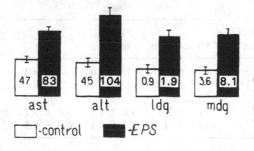

ast   alt   ldg   mdg

□ -control   ■ -EPS

Figure 3.   Effect of emotional/painful stress (EPS) on activity of plasma enzymes: content of aspartate (ast) and alanine (alt) transaminases (mol/ml per hr); activity of lactate dehydrogenase (ldg) and malate dehydrogenase (mdg), (mol/min per mg protein).

Table 2.   Effect of Emotional/Painful Stress on the Dynamics of rRNA
Degradation

	Half-life (1/2 days)		Time of turnover (days)		Replacement (% per day)	
	Control	EPS	Control	EPS	Control	EPS
Heart	6.9	5.2	9.95	7.5	10.04	13.32
Brain	9.3	8	13.4	11.54	7.45	8.66
Liver	5.3	3.8	7.65	5.48	13	18

reduction in half-life and turnover of rRNA and in a significant increase in
the percentage of rRNA replaced per day. This complex of alterations directly demonstrates that the increase in the disintegration of rRNA is markedly pronounced in the myocardium. The half-life and rate of turnover are
reduced by about one-fourth, and the percentage of replacement in RNA
is increased 1.4-fold.

During the study of protein degradation, 45 rats were twice injected
intraabdominally with 50 μCi of ^{35}S-labeled methionine per 100 g of body
weight at an interval of 24 hr. Two days following the second injection of
the label, the initial radioactivity of the proteins in the heart and other organs
was measured in some animals. Then, half of the remaining animals were
exposed to EPS, and the rest of them served as controls. Further determination of specific radioactivity of the protein in tissues of these groups
of animals was carried out 1, 3, 5, and 7 days following introduction of the
isotope.

The data in Table 3 show the result of this experiment and indicate that
stress produced a decrease of over one-fourth in the half-life and turnover
time and an increase of over one-third in the percentage of replacement in
myocardium. In other words, EPS caused a significant increase in the disintegration of the protein in myocardium.

Thus, under the influence of stress, a significant increase in the rate of
disintegration of RNA and protein occurs in myocardium together with
accumulation of hydroperoxides of lipids and labilization of lysosomes. In
the course of further experiments, it was important to find out in which
myocardial cells the disintegration of proteins occurred and the damage from
emotional/painful stress developed.

During the morphological investigations carried out for this purpose
(16), serial topographical sections 5–7 μm in thickness were stained with
picrofuchsin according to Van Gieson, with colloidal iron according to Hill,
and by the Selye method; the reaction of Perls was carried out with subsequent staining with hematoxylin–eosin. The PAS reaction and the reaction
according to Brachet were also carried out. Polarization microscopy was
used to evaluate the state of the contractile apparatus of muscle cells in the
myocardium and the character of myofibrillary changes (23). The main fact
established in the microscopic studies is that during the earliest hours fol-

Table 3.   Effect of Emotional/Painful Stress on the Dynamics of Protein Degradation

	Half-life (1/2 days)		Time of turnover (days)		Replacement (% per day)	
	Control	EPS	Control	EPS	Control	EPS
Heart	12.5	9.3	18.03	13.41	5.54	7.45
Brain	15.5	10.2	22.36	14.71	4.47	6.79

lowing stress focal changes of the contracture type are developed in muscle cells of the heart; these developments progress until the changes reach their maximum, that is, they lead to a complete contracture of muscle cells within 39–45 hr. In some cases, the contracture is accompanied by pronounced necrotic changes and leads to the death of muscle cells with their subsequent degeneration and formation of fibroblastic granulomas; in other cases, the development of the contracture is reversed, and recovery of cellular structures occurs.

Figure 4 shows the myocardium 45 hr following stress, that is, at the phase of maximum morphological change. Figure 4A shows the result of polarization microscopy and demonstrates a deep contracture with fusion of A disks of myofibrils, forming continuous anisotropic conglomerates in single fibers. Figure 4B, at lower magnification, illustrates a great number of such muscle fibers changed by contracture and showing considerable anisotropy. Figure 4C demonstrates the results of Perls's reaction; groups of necrobiotically changed muscle fibers with a positive reaction to iron are seen. Finally, Figure 4D shows formation of the cellular infiltrate around necrotized muscle fibers. In the necrobiotic focus, nuclei are changed by pyknosis, homogenization, and fragmentation of muscle fibers.

In evaluating the fact that changed muscle cells of the heart appear under the influence of stress-induced focal contracture, it should be taken into account that the concentration of ATP in the myocardium of an animal after stress is not different from that in a control, both in the state of rest and in maximum loading of the heart. Therefore, focal contractures of the muscle cells may hardly be explained by a hypoxic or other deficiency of high-energy phosphates. The most probable reason for these kinds of contractures is disturbance of membranous transport of Ca^{2+}; since active removal of this cation from myofibrils to the sarcolemma and sarcoplasmatic reticulum constitutes the basis of normal relaxation, focal disturbances of relaxation are the basis of focal contractures after stress. This fact allowed us to suggest that the peroxides of lipids and proteolytic lysosomal enzymes in stress affect the membrane Ca^{2+} transport apparatus, and, as a result, focal contracture damage to the myocardium occurs.

To verify this hypothesis I, in collaboration with U. V. Arhipenko and I. I. Rozitskaja, studied the effect of emotional/painful stress on the Ca^{2+}-transport system. In this investigation, animals were decapitated 2 hr fol-

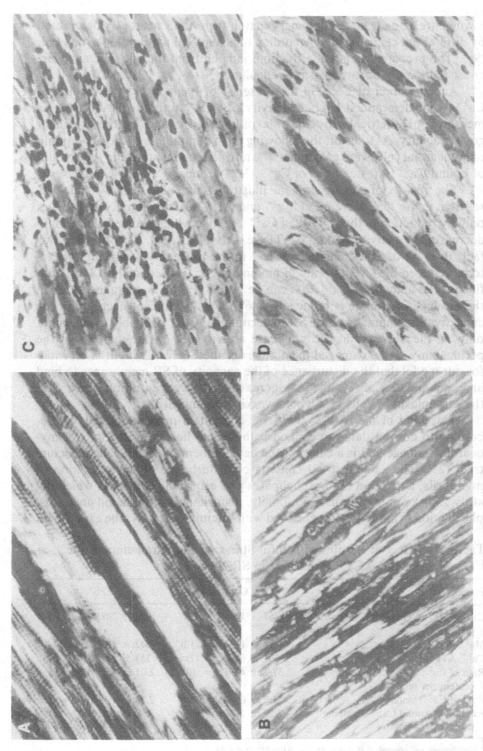

Figure 4. Damage to the rat myocardium 45 hr following emotional/painful stress: A, photographed in polarized light (×197); B, the same (×49); C, reaction of Perls (×126); D, stained with hematoxylin–eosin (×49).

lowing stress, and the microsomal fraction from their hearts was extracted by differential centrifugation according to a standard method Meerson et al. (9a). The prepared membrane fraction, judging from the enzymic analysis, consisted mainly of sarcoplasmic reticulum.

Accumulation of Ca^{2+} in the presence of oxalate and the binding of Ca^{2+} were determined by radioactivity of ^{45}Ca. Activity of ATPase was measured pH-metrically by the rate of hydrolysis and by the attendant greater acidity. As a result, the following main parameters of the Ca^{2+} pump of myocardial cells were calculated: the rate of accumulation and the amount of bound Ca^{2+}, the activities of Ca^{2+}, Mg^{2+}, and $Mg^{2+}-Ca^{2+}$ ATPases.

The results of the experiment illustrated in Table 4 show that EPS resulted in the 15% decrease in Mg^{2+} and Ca^{2+} ATPase activity and occurs only by reduction in the activity of Ca^{2+} ATPase which showed almost 30% decrease; the activity of Mg^{2+} ATPase did not change. According to this fact, the rate of accumulation of Ca^{2+} in the presence of oxalate appears to be reduced by 38%; the rate of binding of Ca^{2+} is reduced by 41%; and, finally, the amount of Ca^{2+} that can be bound by the membranes of SR in the absence of oxalate is reduced by 46%. This significant decrease in the capacity of membranes of the SR to accumulate Ca^{2+} probably depends not only on the decrease in Ca^{2+} ATPase activity but on the increase in the permeability of the damaged membranes of the SR for Ca^{2+}. It is essential for our model that the disturbance of the capacity of SR membranes to bind and accumulate Ca^{2+} lead to an increase in the concentration of Ca^{2+} in the sarcoplasm of cells of a whole working organism.

This kind of increase in the Ca^{2+} content in myocardial cells is, according to current data, a common pathological link in most forms of myocardial damage and is a cause of the development of the so-called calcium triad (21). The calcium triad consists of disturbance of the relaxation of myofibrils, activation of phospholipases and especially proteases which destroy Z-disks of myofibrils, and, finally, disturbance of oxidation and phosphorylation in mitochondria enriched with calcium. Actually, the experiment

Table 4.   Effect of Emotional/Painful Stress on the Parameters of the Enzymic System of Ca^{2+} Transport in SR Vesicles

Parameters	Control	EPS[a]
$Ca^{2+}-Mg^{2+}$ ATPase (nmol/mg protein per min)	$1267 \pm 163 (N = 12)$	$1026 \pm 249^* (N = 11)$
Mg^{2+} ATPase	$694 \pm 113 (N = 12)$	$642 \pm 153 (N = 10)$
Ca^{2+} ATPase	$502 \pm 68 (N = 12)$	$359 \pm 127^{**} (N = 10)$
Rate of Ca^{2+} accumulation (nmol/mg protein per min)	$37.2 \pm 4.0 (N = 10)$	$23.1 \pm 4.2^{***} (N = 8)$
Rate of Ca^{2+} binding	$3.8 \pm 0.42 (N = 10)$	$2.23 \pm 1.14^* (N = 8)$
Amount of bound Ca^{2+} (nmol/mg protein per 5 min)	$7.20 \pm 2.78 (N = 10)$	$3.90 \pm 1.22^* (N = 7)$

[a] Significance vs. control. * $P < 0.1$; ** $P < 0.05$; *** $P < 0.05$.

carried out by V. V. Malyshev, V. I. Lifantyev, and me (unpublished data) showed that after stress and simultaneously with the decrease in the activity of the Ca^{2+} transport system in SR, disturbances of oxidation and phosphorylation develop in mitochondria of the myocardium. The results of the polarographic investigation represented in Table 5 show the changes in the main parameters of oxidation and phosphorylation in mitochondria isolated from myocardium at various times following the stress. It is seen that during the oxidation of the NAD-dependent substrates glutamate and malate by mitochondria, the disturbances of oxidation and phosphorylation appear by 2 hr following the stress; they intensify and reach their maximum in a day or two. In 2 days, the rate of respiration activated by ADP and the index of respiratory control were decreased by 40%; the ADP/O_2 ratio that is the index of effectiveness of phosphorylation was reduced almost one-third.

This complex of shifts clearly shows that after stress, the coupling between oxidation and phosphorylation in mitochondria was damaged. Further, it is seen that after complete uncoupling of oxidation and phosphorylation by dinitrophenol, the consumption of oxygen by animals exposed to stress was reduced twofold. This means that the changes developing in mitochondria in stress not only lead to the disturbance of coupling but limit the oxidation itself, that is, the transport of electrons in the dissociated respiratory chain.

During the oxidation of the NAD-dependent substrate succinate in animals exposed to stress, analogous but quantitatively less pronounced changes of respiration and phosphorylation have been observed.

Thus, there are reasons to suggest that in EPS hydroperoxides of lipids and proteolytic ferments lead to alteration of the membrane Ca^{2+} transport apparatus, and the excess of Ca^{2+} induces the disturbance of relaxation of myofibrils and can damage mitochondria through the activation of phospholipases. It is obvious that in a whole organism the development of such a complex of changes must inevitably lead to disturbances of the contractive function the rhythmic maintainance of which is known to be controlled by the transport of Ca^{2+}.

Actually, the investigations carried out in our laboratory [Meerson et al. (19)] on isolated papillary muscle by the method of Sonnenblick (24), on isolated working heart by Neely et al. (22), on isolated isovolumic heart by Fallen et al. (3), and finally, on the heart in situ showed that the amplitude of contraction, the rates of contraction and relaxation of the myocardium, the developing pressure, and the relative volume of hearts of animals exposed to stress were significantly decreased by 30–50% (11–13).

The aortic pressure curve is shown in Figure 5. It is seen in the upper part of the figure that the systolic pressure in the control was reduced by about 20 mm Hg 3 min after the twofold decrease in Ca^{2+} concentration. It is seen in the lower part of the figure that the heart of an animal after stress responded to a similar decrease in the Ca^{2+} concentration by an enormous depression of the systolic pressure.

Table 5.   Oxidative and Phosphorylative Functions of Mitochondria of Hearts of Rats in the Course of EPS[a]

	V_3	V_4	V_3/V_4	ADP/0	ADP/±	V_{DNP}
Glutamate + malate						
Control	173.2 ± 12.3	47.6 ± 5.9	3.95 ± 0.3	2.9 ± 0.2	469.2 ± 19.5	134.8 ± 5.5
2 hr	123.3 ± 5.2**	38.3 ± 1.1	3.2 ± 0.1*	2.4 ± 0.15	300.9 ± 30.1***	69.0 ± 4.2***
24 hr	133.4 ± 9.2*	54.6 ± 3.0	2.45 ± 0.1***	2.0 ± 0.1**	275.2 ± 29.2***	87.2 ± 3.3***
45 hr	104.3 ± 5.5***	41.7 ± 4.2	2.4 ± 0.15***	2.0 ± 0.1**	233.9 ± 11.3***	78.9 ± 8.0***
72 hr	154.2 ± 6.1	58.2 ± 4.6	2.7 ± 0.2**	2.55 ± 0.2	434.0 ± 43.8	96.8 ± 7.4**
96 hr	170.6 ± 7.8	38.9 ± 2.6	4.0 ± 0.3	2.4 ± 0.15	421.7 ± 48.0	98.9 ± 6.2***
Succinate						
Control	250.5 ± 17.2	87.9 ± 5.7	2.85 ± 0.2	1.95 ± 0.15	524.2 ± 37.5	199.8 ± 11.2
2 hr	225.7 ± 7.8	75.4 ± 4.8	2.9 ± 0.2	1.7 ± 0.1	412.6 ± 26.7*	162.7 ± 14.6
24 hr	215.4 ± 19.6	117.6 ± 9.6*	1.85 ± 0.15**	1.4 ± 0.15*	322.6 ± 26.8**	119.8 ± 18.4**
45 hr	189.2 ± 12.9**	102.3 ± 9.8	1.8 ± 0.1***	1.3 ± 0.15*	279.7 ± 24.4***	127.9 ± 7.7**
72 hr	240.5 ± 14.7	106.8 ± 11.1	2.0 ± 0.15**	1.85 ± 0.2	468.6 ± 31.7	214.8 ± 13.6
96 hr	271.8 ± 19.2	98.4 ± 5.1	2.6 ± 0.15	1.7 ± 0.1	439.4 ± 32.2	161.5 ± 16.5

[a] Significance of difference from control: * $P < 0.05$; ** $P < 0.01$; *** $P < 0.001$.

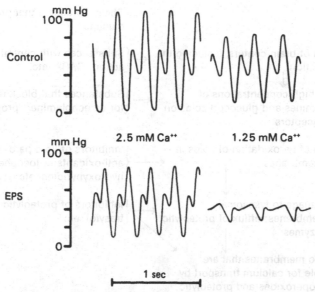

Figure 5.   Effect of reduction in calcium concentration in the perfusate on the aortic pressure developed by the isolated working hearts of animals exposed to EPS.

This fact directly demonstrates that the capacity of the membrane mechanism of myocardial cells in animals exposed to stress is significantly reduced. This phenomenon, observed in a whole working heart, is explained by the abovementioned data which show stress deeply disturbs the functioning of the membrane Ca^{2+} transport system in myocardial cells.

On the whole, the data obtained allow the following scheme to be proposed as a working hypothesis of pathogenesis of stress-induced damage to the heart.

It is shown in the scheme of Figure 6 that excitation of the higher vegetative centers which determine the stress reaction leads to a manyfold increase in the concentration of catecholamines in the blood. As result of the action of catecholamines on the adrenoreceptors located in the sarcolemma, besides the known effect of activation of the adenylate cyclase system, a most important phenomenon develops—the activation of lipid peroxidation which forms, as our experiments showed, a key link in the pathogenesis of the stress damage. Further, under the action of POL products—hydroperoxides of lipids—labilization of lysosomes and the release of protolytic ferments which are able to damage cell structures occur into blood and sarcoplasm. In consequence of the simultaneous action of the hydroperoxides of lipids and proteolytic ferments, damage occurs to the membranes of sarcoplasmic reticulum and sarcolemma responsible for Ca^{2+} transport, its opportune removal, and the relaxation of myofibrils. As a result, the next link of the pathogenetic chain is realized: the content of Ca^{2+} increases in the sarcoplasm of myocardial cells. The excess of Ca^{2+}

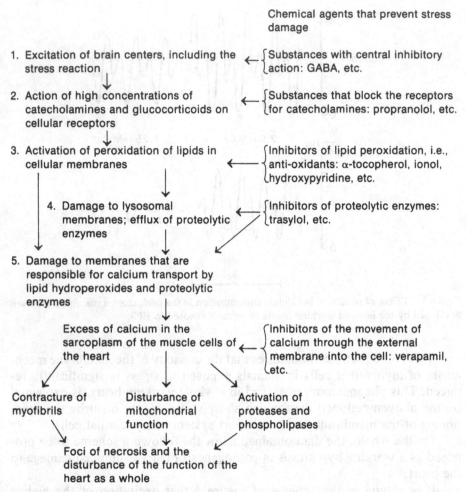

Figure 6.   Scheme of the pathogenesis of myocardial lesions in stress and (right) methods of experimental prophylaxis.

induces a complex of shifts referred to as the calcium triad and consisting of the contracture of myofibrils, damage to mitochondria in which oxidation–phosphorylation coupling is broken, and activation of phospholipases and proteases. As a result of the development of the triad, irreversible contracture and necrobiosis of separate groups of cells and pronounced disturbances of the contractile function of heart on the whole appear.

It is essential that the focal damage to the structure and the total disturbance of heart function be distinctly pronounced when the stress situation is over; they represent not a simple reaction to a stressor but lasting results of the insult. This fact, together with the vast clinical evidence on the role of emotional stress in the etiology of circulatory diseases, suggests that just such relatively persistent disturbances of metabolism and function maintained after the termination of stress and accumulated from one stress episode to another may play a role in the gradual development of those forms of so-called primary noncoronarogenic cardiosclerosis and chronic cardiac insufficiency that often arise in people who earlier had not suffered from circulatory diseases. It is very likely at the same time that the complex of stress disturbances described above may be superimposed on changes arising in the heart as a result of basic circulatory diseases and therefore potentiate the disturbance of compensation and development of cardiac insufficiency in ischemia, cardiac defects, and hypertension.

Thus, the stress damage, the pathogenesis of which is roughly reflected in the scheme of Figure 6, obviously plays an important role in the development of the major forms of cardiac insufficiency.

CHEMOPROPHYLAXIS OF STRESS INSULT TO THE HEART

The scheme presented roughly characterizes not only the main links of the pathogenesis of stress but also the main possibilities of prophylaxis of such damages. There are factors shown in the right side of the scheme (Figure 6) by which selective inhibition of each individual link of the pathogenetic chain of stress damage to the heart has been produced in our laboratory.

It has been established that inhibiting the excitation of the brain centers that control the stress system with the inhibitory metabolite γ-hydroxybutyrate, blocking the cardiac adrenoreceptors through which the effect of catecholamines is realized by propranolol, suppressing lipid peroxidation with natural and synthetic antioxidants, inhibiting lysosomal enzymes with trasylol, and, finally, blocking Ca^{2+} inflow into cells with verapamil all, to various degrees but always with demonstrable effectiveness, prevent the stress-induced injury to the organism (8,13,14,20).

Indeed, the pronounced prophylactic effect of the factors listed in Figure 6 is convincing evidence of the validity of the proposed model for stress insult.

As a concrete example of an effective chemoprophylaxis, it is useful to examine the action of synthetic antioxidants. This example is of interest because the prophylactic effect of antioxidants confirms the involvement of lipids in the pathogenesis of stress injury and because a historical perspective on the application of antioxidants in the cardiologic clinic, not only in stress but also in ischemic myopathy, is well established (7,9,10).

Taking this fact into consideration, we used the powerful and nontoxic antioxidant 2,6-di-*tert*-butyl-1,4-methylphenol, commonly known as ionol. In our experiment, ionol was injected intraabdominally in a dose of 120 mg/kg daily within 3 days before the stress action.

Table 6 shows that the increase in the hydroperoxides of Schiff bases in myocardium observed after stress was significantly blocked by the introduction of ionol.

Figure 7 shows that ionol pretreatment completely prevents the pronounced fermentemia that usually develops in animals in stress, thereby significantly preventing the stress damage to cellular membranes. Further investigations showed that ionol blockade of peroxidation prevents the labilization of lysosomes, development of focal damage in the myocardium, and disturbances of the contractile function of heart usually seen in animals exposed to stress.

To give a final assessment of the prophylactic effect of ionol blockade of peroxidation on stress injury to the heart, besides these criteria, the isolated isovolumic heart preparation of Fallen et al. (3) was used. In an experiment on the isovolumic heart, in parallel with the recording of contractile function, samples of perfusate passed through the coronary bed were taken, and the activity of the enzyme creatine phosphokinase (CPK) was measured according to the method of Bergmeyer (1). The release of CPK from myocardium is known to be one of the most reliable indicators of myocardial cell death, and in hypoxia it generally increases in proportion to the increase in the concentration of ATP in the myocardium (25). Consequently, the experiments provided a hypoxic test during which the standard perfusing solution 96% saturated with oxygen and containing glucose was replaced for 20 min with a solution only 20% saturated with oxygen and deprived of substrates.

The data on the release of CPK from the isolated heart into the perfusate are presented in Table 7. The top line of the table shows that the control heart at first released much enzyme into the perfusate but then, because of adequate oxidation, less ferment was excreted; its output increased again during the special hypoxic test. The next three lines show that, in principle, the same changes in rate of release of ferment obtains in all series of experiments in isolated hearts, although the absolute quantities of creatine phosphokinase released into the perfusate under the action of stress and

Table 6. Effect of Ionol on Activation of Lipid Peroxidation in Myocardium in Emotional/Painful Stress

	Accumulation of hydroperoxides of lipids (mol/mg lipid)	Intensity of fluorescence of Schiff bases (relative units)
Control ($N = 5$)	16.7 ± 1.4	10.5 ± 3.5
Stress ($N = 7$)	47.6 ± 2.4	27.6 ± 4.2
	$P < 0.001$ vs. control	$P < 0.01$ vs. control
Ionol ($N = 7$)	16.7 ± 0.5	10.6 ± 2.2
Ionol + stress ($N = 7$)	28.6 ± 2.4	13.2 ± 1.8
	$P < 0.001$ vs. stress	$P < 0.01$ vs. stress

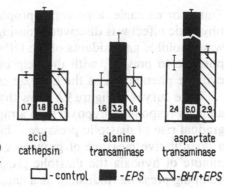

Figure 7.   Effect of the antioxidant ionol (BHT) on the fermentemia of animals exposed to emotional/painful stress (EPS).

acid cathepsin   alanine transaminase   aspartate transaminase

□ - control   ■ - EPS   ◪ - BHT+EPS

antioxidant are significantly changed. On the whole, two statements follow from Table 7.

First, in all stages of the experiment, hearts of animals exposed to stress release into the perfusate more enzymes than those of controls by 50–70%. This correlates with the data of our laboratory that stress potentiates hypoxic injury to the heart.

Second, introduction of antioxidant in control animals and animals exposed to stress reduces the loss of enzyme two- to threefold. In other words, the antioxidant prevented both the damaging effect of hypoxia and the potentiating effect of stress on this damage. This protecting effect of ionol was also present with respect to the contractile function of heart.

The curves in Figure 8 show the reaction of isolated hearts to the hypoxic test. The most significant result is that hypoxic depression of contractile function was most acute in animals that had endured stress, and reestablishment of contractile function occurred slowly and not completely. Ionol pretreatment abolished this effect of stress and caused a still more important phenomenon: the reestablishment of myocardial contractile function in control animals during oxygenation under the action of ionol appears to be significantly more rapid and complete than that without ionol.

It should be pointed out that ionol is not a unique factor: not identical but similar results have been obtained with other synthetic antioxidants.

Table 7.   Activity of Creatine Phosphokinase in the Perfusate of the Isolated Rat Heart

	35 min of perfusion	95 min of perfusion	20 min of hypoxia
1. Control ($N = 8$)	46.87 ± 6.7	19.65 ± 2.15	31.64 ± 3.78
2. Stress ($N = 8$)	86.55 ± 10.52	29.56 ± 1.89	47.26 ± 5.25
P_{1-2}	0.01	0.01	0.05
3. Ionol ($N = 8$)	16.11 ± 4.31	8.80 ± 2.59	10.02 ± 3.62
P_{1-3}	0.01	0.01	0.01
4. Ionol + stress ($N = 7$)	18.44 ± 4.85	10.57 ± 1.27	18.70 ± 1.96
P_{2-4}	0.01	0.01	0.02
P_{3-4}	0.05	0.05	0.05

Thus, for example, a powerful prophylactic antistress and, especially, antihypoxic effect was discovered during the examination of the rapidly acting water-soluble antioxidants of the OP-6 class of oxypyridines. It is regularly possible to prevent, with the help of this antioxidant, such otherwise inevitable phenomena as the hypoxic contracture of the heart.

The curves in Figure 9A show that isolated isovolumic hearts of control animals respond to hypoxia with a rapid fall of systolic pressure and a slow gradual rise of diastolic pressure. This rise of diastolic pressure represents a quantitative measure of growing contracture. It is seen that at the 20th minute of hypoxia the diastolic pressure reached 40 mm Hg, and the developing pressure (indicated as a hatched zone) appears to be reduced from 100 to 20 mm Hg.

Figure 9B illustrates the response to the same hypoxia of isolated hearts of animals that received the antioxidant for 3 days before the experiment. In the animals exposed to stress, the hypoxic contracture, like all other manifestations of hypoxic damage, is more pronounced than that in controls (Figure 9C). Nevertheless, the protecting anticontractural effect of OP-6 is quite convincingly apparent (Figure 9D).

It is seen that introduction of an inhibitor of lipid peroxidation did not influence the primary hypoxic depression of systolic pressure but almost completely prevented the development of a rise in diastolic pressure and the development of contracture.

On the whole, the developing pressure was twofold greater than that in the hearts of unprotected animals.

Thus, the antioxidants first prevent the depression of contractile function and the loss of CPK induced by stress damage; second, they remove the potentiating effect of stress on the development of hypoxic damage;

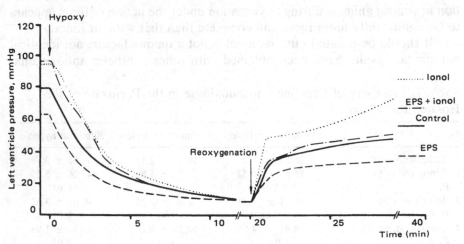

Figure 8.   Disturbances of the contractile function of the isolated heart caused by emotional/painful stress (EPS) and hypoxia and the prevention of these disturbances with ionol.

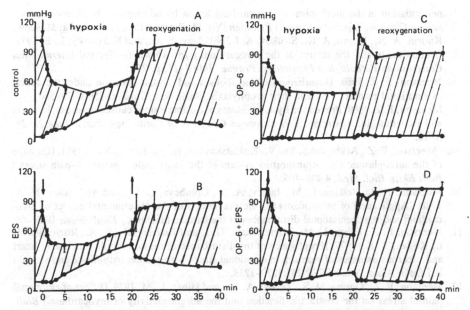

Figure 9.   Prevention with the water-soluble antioxidant OP-6 of the hypoxic contracture of isolated working hearts from control animals and animals exposed to emotional/painful stress. Upper curves, systolic; lower curve, diastolic pressure in the left ventricle; hatched zones, developing pressure.

third, they are able to protect the heart from the injury caused by hypoxia itself by preventing the hypoxic contracture.

Stress, hypoxia, and especially their combination form the leading pathogenetic complex in the major diseases of human heart. Therefore, there are reasons to believe that the data on experimental prophylaxis of stress- and hypoxia-induced heart damage presented here will find an application in the cardiology clinic of the future.

REFERENCES

1. Bergmeyer, H. U. 1970. *Methode der Enzymatische Analyse.* Verlag Chemie, Weinheim.
2. Desiderato, O., MacKinnon, J. R., and Nisson, H. 1974. Development of gastric ulcers in rats following stress termination. *J. Comp. Physiol. Psychol.* 87:208–214.
3. Fallen, E. J., Elliot, W., and Gorlin, R. 1967. Apparatus for study of ventricular function and metabolism in the isolated perfused rat heart. *J. Appl. Physiol.* 22:836.
4. Folch, J., Lee, M., and Stanley, G. H. S. 1957. A simple method for the isolation and purification of total lipids from animal tissues. *J. Biol. Chem.* 226:497–509.
5. Kagan, V. J., Churakova, T. D., Karagodin, V. P., Arkhipenko, Y. V., Bilenko, M. V., and Kozlov, Y. P. 1979. [Disturbances of the fermentative systems of calcium transport in the membranes of sarcoplasmic reticulum under the action of the hydroperoxides, phospholipid, and the hydroperoxides of the fatty acids.] *Biull. Eksp. Biol. Med.* 2:145–149.
6. Kogan, A. K., Kudrin, A. N., and Nikolaev, S. M. 1976. [On the role of free radical lipid

20   F. Z. Meerson

peroxidation in the mechanism of myocardium lesion by adrenaline.] In: *Svobodnoradikalnoe Okislenie Lipidov v Norme i Patologii* (Yu. M. Petrusevitch, ed.), Nauka, Moscow.

7. Kudrin, A. N., Kogan, A. K., Strukov, A. I., Nikolaev, S. M., and Kaktursky, L. B. 1975. [Antioxidants and the infarct of the myocardium.] In: *Abstracts, Second International Congress on Pathological Physiology, Prague, July 8–11*, p. 216.

8. Meerson, F. Z. 1980. Disturbances of metabolism and cardiac function under the action of emotional painful stress and their prophylaxis. *Basic Res. Cardiol.* 75(4):479–500.

9. Meerson, F. Z. 1980. Prevention by antioxidants of cardiac lesions caused by stress, hypoxia and ischemia. In: *Abstracts, VIII European Congress of Cardiology. Paris, June 22–26*, p. 18.

9a. Meerson, F. Z., Arkhipenko, Yu. V., Kozhitskaya, I. I., and Kagan, V. E. 1981. [Damage of the sarcoplasmic Ca^{2+}-transporting system of the heart under emotional–pain stress.] *Bull. Eksp. Biol. Med.* 4:406–406.

10. Meerson, F. Z., Belkina, L. M., Igolev, A. A., Golubeva, L. U., and Abdikaliev, N. A. 1980. [Application of antioxidants for the prevention of the experimental infarct of myocardium and reoxigenisational disturbances of the cardiac functions.] *Kardiologiia* 10:81–86.

11. Meerson, F. Z., Giber, L. M., Markovskaja, G. I. and Radzievskiy, S. A., Rozitskaja, I. I., Kogan, A. K., 1977. [Prophylaxis of the disturbance of the contractile function of heart and ulcerous damages of stomach in emotional stress with sodium oxibutirate and vitamin E.] *Dokl. Akad. Nauk SSSR* 237:1230–1233.

12. Meerson, F. Z., Gorina, M. S., Zeland, A. M., and Giber, L. M. 1979. [Effect of emotional painful stress on the contractile function and the adrenoeactivity of myocardium.] *Biull. Eksp. Biol. Med.* 11:528–530.

13. Meerson, F. Z., Kagan, V. E., Golubeva, L. U., Ugolev, A. A., Snimkovich, M. V., Giber, L. M., and Rozitskaja, J. J. 1979. [Prevention of stress and hypoxic affections of the heart with antioxidant ionol.] *Kardiologiia* 8:108–111.

14. Meerson, F. Z., Kagan, V. E., Prilipko, L. L., and Rozitskaja, J. J. 1981. [Inhibition of the activation of the peroxide oxidation of lipids in emotional painful stress by ionol and gamoxibutirate.] *Biull. Eksp. Biol. Med.* 12:661–663.

15. Meerson, F. Z., Kagan, V. E., Prilipko, L. L., Rozitskaja, I. I., Giber, L. M., and Kozlov, Tu. P. 1979. [Activation of the peroxide oxidation of lipids in emotional painful stress.] *Biull. Eksp. Biol. Med.* 10:404–406.

16. Meerson, F. Z., Malyshev, V. V., Kagan, V. E., Treshuk, L. I., and Rozitskaja, I. I. 1980. [Activation of the peroxide oxidation of lipids and focal contractural lesions in myocardium in emotional painful stress.] *Arch. Pathol.* 42(2):9–12.

17. Meerson, F. Z., Malyshev, V. V., Popova, N. S., and Markovskaja, G. I. 1979. [Decrease in stress reaction and ulcerous damages of stomach under the action of GABA.] *Biull. Eksp. Biol. Med.* 12:659–661.

18. Meerson, F. Z., Pavlova, V. I., Kamilov, F. K., and Yakushev, V. S. 1979. [Application of sodium gamoxybutyrate for the prophylaxis of lesions caused by emotional painful stress.] *Patol. Fiziol. Eksp. Ter.* 3:26–31.

19. Meerson, F. Z., Shimkovich, M. V., and Horunzji, V. A. 1980. [Effect of emotional painful stress on the reactivity of myocardium to the changes in calcium concentration.] *Biull. Eksp. Biol. Med.* 3:272–274.

20. Meerson, F. Z., and Trihpoeva, A. M. 1981. [Prevention of disturbances of the contractile function of myocardium appearing after emotional painful stress by gamoxybutyrate and antioxidant ionol.] *Biull. Eksp. Biol. Med.* 11:531–533.

21. Meerson, F. Z., and Ugolev, A. A. 1980. [Disturbance of the membrane transport of calcium as a common link in the pathogenesis of the different forms of cardiac insufficiency.] *Kardiologiia* 1:68–75.

22. Neely, J. R., Libermeister, H., Battersby, E. J., and Morgan, H. E. 1967. Effect of pressure development on oxygen consumption by isolated rat heart. *Am. J. Physiol.* 212:804–814.

23. Semenova, L. A., and Tsellarius, U. G. 1978. [*Ultrastructure of Heart Muscle Cells in Focal Metabolitic Lesions.*] Nauka, Novosibirsk.

24. Sonnenblick, E. H. 1962. Force–velocity relation in mammalian heart muscle. *Am. J. Physiol.* 202:931–939.
25. Spikerman, P. G., Gobhard, M. M., and Nordbac, H. 1975. Myocardial high energy phosphates and enzyme release during anaerobiosis in the isolated perfused dog heart. In: *Abstract. International Study Group for Research in Cardiac Metabolism, Brussels.* p. 41.

Energy Metabolism of the Heart in Catecholamine-Induced Myocardial Injury

Concentration-Dependent Effects of Epinephrine on Enzyme Release, Mechanical Function, and "Oxygen Wastage"

A. R. Horak and L. H. Opie

MRC Ischaemic Heart Disease Research Unit
Department of Medicine
University of Cape Town and Groote Schuur Hospital
Cape Town, South Africa

Abstract. Epinephrine caused a dose-related release of lactate dehydrogenase (LDH) from the isolated perfused working rat heart. Thus, epinephrine, at 10^{-8} M, did not increase release of LDH, but at 10^{-6} M, it gave a peak release of 712 ± 48 mU/g fresh wt. per min ($N = 41$) 10 min after addition (control: 17 ± 2 mU/g per min, $N = 36$). The effects of 10^{-7} M epinephrine (peak release: 159 ± 28 mU/g per min, $N = 29$) were mimicked by theophylline, 10^{-3} M. Increased release of LDH was also achieved by dibutyryl cAMP, 5×10^{-4} M (399 ± 67 mU/g per min, $N = 6$), but not by cAMP, 5×10^{-4} M. Increased tissue cAMP could be related to the extent of enzyme loss induced by epinephrine or by theophylline. Both tissue cAMP and LDH decreased when propranolol, 10^{-5} M, was added to epinephrine 10^{-6} M. Epinephrine-induced enzyme loss was also decreased by halving the perfusate Ca^{2+} or doubling the perfusate Mg^{2+} or by verapamil, 2×10^{-7} M, thereby showing a role for Ca^{2+} entry. However, there was no evidence for excess excitation-coupling with major ATP depletion. Although decreased efficiency of pressure work ("oxygen wastage") was a graded phenomenon, it was apparent even with epinephrine, 10^{-8} M. As the epinephrine concentration rose, so did heart rate, coronary flow, oxygen uptake, the degree of "oxygen wastage," the level of tissue cAMP, and the extent of enzyme release. At 10^{-7} M epinephrine, the efficiency of pressure work was only 68% of control, but there was no depletion of high-energy phosphate compounds despite marked enzyme loss. Rather, there was a small loss of ATP only at the highest epinephrine concentration (10^{-6} M) with an increase of phosphocreatine, suggesting that intracellular transfer of energy was impaired. Epinephrine-induced enzyme release and "oxygen wastage" could occur at concentrations below 10^{-6} M which did not cause detectable depletion of the tissue content of ATP.

Numerous workers, led by Rona et al. (25), have shown that catecholamines in high concentrations can have toxic effects on the myocardium. The mechanism of such damage is still not fully elucidated, but Fleckenstein et al. (6–8) showed that (1) cardiotoxic doses of β agonists could break down ATP and phosphocreatine and that (2) this phenomenon was mediated by Ca^{2+} because it was accompanied by increased uptake of Ca^{2+} by the myocardium and was counteracted by Ca^{2+}-antagonist drugs such as verapamil. However, the doses of catecholamines used to obtain these effects were high

23

(e.g., 30 mg/kg), and the expected circulating concentration far exceeded the physiological circulating catecholamine levels which are in the order of 10^{-9} M (28,33), or lower according to recent data.

We, and Waldenström et al. before us (29), have already shown that catecholamines in supraphysiological concentrations (epinephrine, 10^{-6} M, or norepinephrine, 10^{-7} M to 10^{-4} M) can release substantial amounts of enzyme from the isolated perfused rat heart; such release of enzyme at these very high catecholamine concentrations is accompanied by a decrease in the myocardial content of ATP but not of phosphocreatine (23). We have also shown that both $[Ca^{2+}]$ and lipolysis are concerned in the mechanisms underlying release of enzyme (23). The purpose of this chapter is to establish further the concentrations of catecholamines required to produce "toxic" effects on the heart, including enzyme release, and to examine the possible role of high-energy phosphate compounds in such effects of catecholamines.

METHODS

The hearts of male Long–Evans rats (220–230 g, fed ad libitum) were perfused via the left atrium (18,21) with Krebs–Henseleit solution (14), pH 7.4, 37°C, equilibrated with $O_2:CO_2$ 95%:5%, at an atrial filling pressure of 10 cm H_2O and an aortic hydrostatic pressure of 100 cm H_2O. A recirculating volume of about 100 ml was used. Glucose, 11.1 mM, was the usual substrate.

Time Sequence of the Perfusion

After mounting, all hearts were perfused retrogradely (15) for an initial 15-min nonrecirculating washout period at 65 cm H_2O, and then left atrial perfusion was commenced. Aortic output and coronary flow were measured at 15-min intervals by collecting the perfusate in a graduated tube. Aliquots of this collection were immediately assayed for lactate dehydrogenase (LDH) activity. The LDH in both the arterial and venous effluent was determined by the method of Wroblewski and La Due (32), and LDH release from the hearts was expressed as mU/g per min at 25°C, where the wet weight was calculated from the body weight by a nomogram. In a few experiments, creatine kinase activity was assayed with the Boehringer Monotest® kit, Code 15873.

After 35 min of left atrial perfusion, epinephrine or various other drugs were added to the recirculating fluid to give the desired circulating concentration of that drug. Concentrations of epinephrine of 10^{-8} M, 10^{-7} M, and 10^{-6} M, theophylline, 10^{-3} M, and dibutyryl cAMP, 10^{-4} M and 5×10^{-4} M, were used. Propranolol, 10^{-5} M, was added 10 min before the epinephrine in some experiments. In some experiments (propranolol plus epinephrine), the heart rate was kept at 360 beats/min by means of atrial pacing with an electronic stimulator (Grass Model S88, 5-V square wave, duration 4 msec).

Mechanical Performance

Cardiac output was the sum of the aortic output and coronary flow. Heart rate was taken from the ECG recorded from the aortic and atrial perfusion cannulae. The aortic pressure was measured with a Statham P23 dB pressure transducer and monitored on a Devices twin-channel recorder (MX2P-148).

In some experiments, efficiency of the heart was measured. The mechanical efficiency of the heart, expressed as Joules of work per milliliter of oxygen uptake, was calculated from (1) the oxygen uptake, measured from the arteriovenous oxygen difference measured by a Radiometer macroelectrode (type PHMM1), and (2) the work of the heart, calculated as pressure power production derived from measurements of the cardiac output, the peak aortic pressure, the ejection period, and the mechanical characteristics of the system (13). However, kinetic work was not taken into account, and only the efficiency of pressure work was monitored.

Analytical Methods

In experiments for the analysis of tissue metabolites, the hearts were freeze-clamped by the Wollenberger (31) technique by aluminium tongs cooled to the temperature of liquid nitrogen. Hearts were usually clamped 10 min after epinephrine. The atria were removed, and frozen perfusate around the edges of the samples was chipped off with chilled forceps. The samples were stored in liquid nitrogen. The frozen stored tissue was extracted and analyzed for glycogen, tissue ATP, and phosphocreatine (21). Tissue cAMP was measured by the Radiochemical Centre cAMP assay kit, Code TRK 432. Tissue metabolites were expressed in terms of fresh weight (dry wt. × 5, ref. 21).

Materials

Epinephrine, donated by Petersen Laboratories, Cape Town, South Africa, was freshly prepared each day from powder which had been stored in a deep freeze under liquid nitrogen and kept in the dark until use. Solutions of the following were also freshly prepared each day. DL-Propranolol hydrochloride was obtained from I.C.I. (South Africa, Ltd). Theophylline (1,3-dimethylxanthine) was obtained as the pure crystalline salt from Merck AG (Darmstadt, Federal Republic of Germany). N^6,2'-O-dibutyryl adenosine 3',5'-monophosphate (dbcAMP) (98% purity) and cyclic 3',5'-adenosine monophosphate (cAMP) as the sodium salt (98% purity) were obtained from the Sigma Chemical Company (St. Louis, MO). Verapamil HCl was obtained as Isoptin® from Knoll Pharmaceuticals, Ludwigshafen, Federal Republic of Germany. All other substrates, chemicals, and enzymes were of purest commercially available chemical grade and obtained from the Boehringer Corporation, Miles Seravac, Analar, British Drug Houses, or Maybaker Laboratories.

Statistical Procedures

All results were expressed as mean values ± the standard error of the mean. P values were derived from the conventional Student's t-test using two-tailed values and allowing for unequal variances when applicable (3).

RESULTS

Effect of Epinephrine on Enzyme Release

Cumulative Release of Lactate Dehydrogenase. Epinephrine in concentrations of 10^{-7} M and 10^{-6} M, but not 10^{-8} M, caused greatly increased myocardial release of lactate dehydrogenase (LDH). The release occurred rapidly and was concentration related. Cumulative release values of LDH in ten control hearts and seven hearts perfused with epinephrine, 10^{-8} M (added after 35 min of perfusion), were identical by coincidence, being 1556 ± 127 mU/g at 75 min of perfusion. But epinephrine 10^{-7} M, also added after 35 min of perfusion, caused an almost fivefold increase in the cumulative LDH release to 4770 ± 876 mU/g at 75 min ($N = 9$; $P < 0.01$). Hearts perfused with 10^{-6} M epinephrine had a 20-fold increase in enzyme release to 19,667 ± 1984 mU/g at 75 min ($N = 15$; P vs. control <0.001, vs. 10^{-7} M <0.001).

Rate of Release. The rate of release of LDH (Figure 1) reached a peak at 10 min after epinephrine addition and then rapidly diminished (23). Thus, epinephrine, 10^{-8} M, had a rate of release (20 ± 2 mU/g per min) similar to that of control hearts (17 ± 2 mU/g per min) 10 min after the addition of epinephrine; 40 min after addition of epinephrine, the rate fell to 10 ± 1 mU/g per min (controls: 13 ± 2 mU/g per min). Epinephrine, 10^{-7} M, gave a peak value of 159 ± 28 mU/g per min ($N = 29$; $P < 0.001$ vs. controls), falling to 35 ± 12 mU/g per min 30 min later ($N = 9$; NS from controls). Epinephrine, 10^{-6} M, caused a marked peak release of 712 ± 48 mU/g per min at 10 min ($N = 41$; $P < 0.001$ vs. 10^{-7} M), falling to 189 ± 38 mU/g per min 30 min later ($P < 0.001$ vs. controls; $P < 0.01$ vs. 10^{-7} M).

Release of Creatine Kinase. The release of creatine kinase (CK) was measured in one series after 10^{-6} M epinephrine; the pattern of release was very similar to that of LDH. Values at 30 min of perfusion were 3.1 ± 1.9 mU/g per min and increased to 672.2 ± 181.8 mU/g per min at 45 min (10

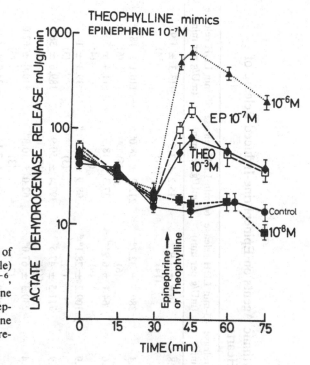

Figure 1. Patterns of release of lactate dehydrogenase (log scale) after addition of epinephrine (10^{-6}, 10^{-7}, or 10^{-8} M) or theophylline (10^{-3}). Note similar effects of epinephrine 10^{-7} M and theophylline 10^{-3} M and absence of enzyme release with epinephrine 10^{-8} M.

min after 10^{-6} M epinephrine was added) and 293.0 ± 83.2 mU/g per min ($N = 4$) at 60 min.

Role of β Receptor in Epinephrine-Induced Release of LDH

When propranolol (10^{-5} M) was added 10 min before epinephrine, the release of LDH by 10^{-7} M epinephrine was nearly completely prevented, and the release produced by 10^{-6} M epinephrine was markedly reduced (Table 1). Because propranolol markedly slowed the heart rate, all propranolol-treated hearts were paced at 360 beats/min.

Phosphodiesterase inhibition and LDH Release

Theophylline (10^{-3} M), also added after 35 min of left atrial perfusion, increased LDH release with a pattern very similar to that found with 10^{-7} M epinephrine (Figure 1).

Dibutyryl Cyclic AMP and LDH Release

To further support the possibility that LDH release could be related to intracellular formation of cAMP, hearts were perfused with the addition of dbcAMP (10^{-4} M or 5×10^{-4} M) which considerably increased release of LDH (see Figure 1 of ref. 12); the effect of dbcAMP (5×10^{-4} M) was still

Table 1. Effects of Perfusate Ionic Changes and of Antiarrhythmic Agents on Epinephrine-Induced Release of Lactate Dehydrogenase from Isolated Perfused Working Rat Heart

	15-min LDH release (mU/g per min)	30-min LDH release (mU/g per min)	45-min LDH release (mU/g per min)	60-min LDH release (mU/g per min)	75-min LDH release (mU/g per min)
1. Control, no additions Ca^{2+} = 2.5 mM Mg^{2+} = 1.19 mM	33.6 ± 2.1 (14)	24.2 ± 1.8 (14)	16.6 ± 1.9 (14)	15.2 ± 3.5 (14)	13.3 ± 1.9 (14)
2. Epinephrine 10^{-6} M[e] (first series)	34.5 ± 2.1 (16)	23.3 ± 3.4 (16)	380.3 ± 32.7[a] (6)	212.2 ± 28.0[a] (6)	110.1 ± 18.0[a] (6)
3. Epinephrine 10^{-6} M[e] ½ × Ca^{2+}[f]	33.9 ± 4.6 (9)	14.9 ± 2.6 (9)	64.1 ± 6.9[a,d] (9)	37.3 ± 18.9[c] (4)	11.4 ± 5.9[c] (4)
4. Epinephrine 10^{-6} M[e] 2 × Mg^{2+}[f]	18.7 ± 4.0 (7)	16.1 ± 5.9 (7)	109.2 ± 28.1[a,d] (7)	98.9 ± 32.5[a,b] (3)	39.3 ± 14.4[b] (3)
5. Epinephrine 10^{-6} M[e] (second series)	32.3 ± 2.3 (41)	28.5 ± 2.9 (41)	711.5 ± 47.5 (41)	397.4 ± 50.9 (17)	189.6 ± 38.9 (17)
6. Epinephrine 10^{-6} M[e] verapamil 2 × 10^{-7} M[e]	30.6 ± 6.5 (3)	27.5 ± 6.4 (3)	230.3 ± 67.0[d] (3)	62.0 ± 10.8[d] (3)	110.0 ± 62.0 (3)
7. Epinephrine 10^{-6} M[e] verapamil 1 × 10^{-6} M[e]	29.0 ± 3.5 (7)	—	49.0 ± 5.9[d] (7)	32.0 ± 7.1[d] (7)	24.0 ± 4.3[d] (7)
8. Epinephrine 10^{-6} M[e] propranolol 10^{-5} M[e]	44.9 ± 6.2 (6)	29.5 ± 2.4 (6)	75.7 ± 8.4[d] (6)	29.3 ± 2.8[d] (6)	23.5 ± 6.2[d] (6)

[a] $P < 0.001$ vs. group 1.
[b] $P < 0.05$ vs. group 2 or 5.
[c] $P < 0.005$ vs. group 2 or 5.
[d] $P < 0.001$ vs. group 2 or 5.
[e] Drug added at 35 min of perfusion.
[f] Altered ionic composition present throughout perfusion.

present (albeit diminished) in the presence of β blockade by propranolol, 10^{-5} M (data not shown). Release of LDH with equimolar butyric acid or cAMP was much lower than that with dbcAMP and propranolol (12). All of these experiments were conducted over a total of 120 min to follow more accurately the delayed LDH release achieved with the dibutyryl compound (peak effect 10–55 min after addition of dbcAMP).

Propranolol versus Verapamil

Each agent substantially reduced LDH release, with verapamil (10^{-6} M) reducing peak enzyme release more than propranolol (10^{-5} M) (Table 1).

Calcium Antagonist Procedures: Verapamil or Changes in Extracellular Ca^{2+} and Mg^{2+}

Doubling the extracellular Mg^{2+} concentration from 1.19 to 2.38 mM reduced release of LDH with 10^{-6} M epinephrine to about one-third. Halving the extracellular Ca^{2+} concentrations from 2.5 mM to 1.25 mM greatly reduced LDH release to values similar to those found with propranolol plus 10^{-6} M epinephrine (Table 1).

Substrates and LDH Release

The LDH release from either the nonligated isolated heart or the ligated heart is substrate related, the highest rates being achieved with perfusates containing free fatty acids (4) and rates being decreased by increasing glucose concentrations (20). Similarly, rates of LDH release, achieved by 10^{-6} M epinephrine, were decreased by increasing the circulating glucose concentration from 5.5 to 22 mM, from 45-min values of 603 ± 99 ($N = 10$) to 233 ± 42 ($N = 6$; $P < 0.005$). Rates were increased by the addition of physiological concentrations of palmitate (0.6 mM palmitate bound to albumin, 3 g per 100 ml) to glucose, 11 mM, from 380 ± 33 ($N = 6$) to 744 ± 143 ($N = 9$; $P < 0.05$). All units were mU/g per min.

Effects on Myocardial Performance

Heart Rate. Epinephrine caused a concentration-dependent increase in heart rate, the peak occurring at 10 min (Table 2). The rate increased from 235 ± 5 beats/min (controls) to 275 ± 6 (10^{-8} M), 319 ± 6 (10^{-7} M), and 351 ± 5 (10^{-6} M), all being different from controls and from one another with $P < 0.001$. The pattern of response in heart rate was similar to that found with enzyme release; i.e., a peak response was reached within 10 min, with a gradual return towards normal. The effect of heart rate on enzyme release was tested. Hearts were paced atrially at 360 beats/min from the same moment that epinephrine would have been added. However, there

Table 2. Effect of Increasing Concentrations of Epinephrine on Mechanical Performance and Oxygen Uptake of Isolated Perfused Working Rat Heart

	Heart rate (beats/min)		Coronary flow (beats/min)		Aortic output (ml/min)		Cardiac output (ml/min)		Oxygen uptake (µl/g per min)		Peak aortic pressure (mm Hg)		Efficiency of work (joules/ml O$_2$)	
	Before	After	Before	After	Before	After	Before	After	Before	After	Before	After	Before	After
1. Control	236 ± 5 (30)	235 ± 5 (30)	16.1 ± 0.5 (32)	16.8 ± 1.1 (32)	29.5 ± 1.0 (32)	28.9 ± 1.2 (32)	45.1 ± 1.1 (32)	45.4 ± 1.1 (32)	172 ± 11 (10)	172 ± 14 (10)	116 ± 3 (7)	115 ± 2 (7)	4.43 ± 0.16 (6)	4.39 ± 0.17 (6)
2. Epinephrine 10^{-8} M	242 ± 7 (16)	275*** ± 6 (16)	15.6 ± 0.7 (19)	19.8*** ± 0.9 (19)	26.1 ± 1.2 (19)	23.8** ± 1.5 (19)	41.7 ± 1.3 (19)	43.0** ± 1.8 (19)	159 ± 8 (6)	199*** ± 12 (6)	121 ± 5 (6)	114** ± 4 (6)	4.15 ± 0.36 (6)	3.44** ± 0.31 (6)
3. Epinephrine 10^{-7} M	241 ± 6 (8)	319*** ± 6 (8)	15.6 ± 0.6 (29)	22.3*** ± 0.6 (29)	26.4 ± 1.1 (29)	16.8*** ± 1.1 (29)	42.0 ± 1.2 (29)	39.1*** ± 1.5 (29)	165 ± 4 (5)	287*** ± 19 (7)	109 ± 3 (5)	129** ± 2 (7)	3.85 ± 0.33 (5)	2.63** ± 0.15 (7)
4. Epinephrine 10^{-6} M	240 ± 5 (38)	351*** ± 5 (38)	15.8 ± 0.3 (66)	21.8*** ± 0.3 (66)	28.2 ± 0.7 (66)	14.1*** ± 0.8 (66)	44.1 ± 0.8 (66)	35.4*** ± 0.9 (66)	166 ± 5 (11)	293*** ± 11 (12)	109 ± 3 (10)	124** ± 3 (10)	4.08 ± 0.24 (10)	1.96*** ± 0.12 (10)
5. Theophylline 10^{-3} M	225 ± 8 (14)	345*** ± 13 (14)	15.7 ± 0.5 (13)	19.8*** ± 0.5 (14)	27.8 ± 2.0 (13)	16.8*** ± 1.5 (14)	43.4 ± 1.9 (13)	37.3*** ± 1.6 (13)	—	—	—	—	—	—
6. Dibutyryl cAMP 10^{-4} M	266 ± 9 (5)	256 ± 7 (5)	16.1 ± 0.6 (11)	22.5*** ± 0.5 (11)	28.1 ± 1.6 (11)	19.9** ± 2.1 (11)	44.1 ± 1.6 (11)	41.9* ± 2.1 (11)	163 ± 8 (4)	208*** ± 14 (4)	106 ± 1 (4)	106 ± 3 (4)	3.69 ± 0.09 (4)	2.83*** ± 0.07 (4)
7. Dibutyryl cAMP 5 × 10^{-4} M	273 ± 22 (5)	314 ± 16 (5)	15.0 ± 0.7 (5)	22.3*** ± 0.5 (5)	31.8 ± 2.0 (5)	20.4*** ± 0.7 (5)	46.8 ± 1.4 (5)	42.7† ± 1.0 (5)	161 ± 6 (5)	238** ± 12 (5)	109 ± 3 (5)	131* ± 3 (5)	3.96 ± 0.45 (5)	2.83† ± 0.23 (5)
8. Paced at 360 beats/min	236 ± 5 (5)	360 (5)	16.7 ± 2.0 (5)	19.0† ± 1.7 (5)	29.9 ± 2.2 (5)	27.5† ± 1.8 (5)	46.6 ± 3.9 (5)	46.5 ± 3.5 (5)	182 ± 25 (4)	199 ± 18 (4)	—	—	—	—

^{a} Drug was added at 35 min of perfusion. "Before" values were taken at 30 min. "After" values were taken at 45 min of perfusion. Significance of difference between Before and After: †$P < 0.05$; *$P < 0.025$; **$P < 0.01$; ***$P < 0.001$. Number of measurements in parentheses.

was no increase in enzyme release above control levels, and cardiac output stayed constant. The oxygen uptake rose slightly from 182 ± 12 to 199 ± 16 μl/g per min ($P < 0.05$, paired t-test).

Coronary Flow. Epinephrine caused an increase in coronary flow (Table 2). The increase occurred rapidly, reached a peak in 10 min, and followed a similar pattern to the other parameters. There was, however, no difference between 10^{-7} M and 10^{-6} M epinephrine at peak levels (22.3 ± 0.6 and 22.0 ± 0.7 ml/g per min; P vs. control <0.001 for both). Even the effect of 10^{-8} M epinephrine was significantly different from control values (19.8 ± 1 vs. 16.8 ± 1 ml/g per min; $P < 0.003$).

Aortic Output. In all concentrations, epinephrine caused a decrease in aortic output with a maximal effect slightly earlier than 10 min. Thus, aortic output fell from 28.9 ± 1.2 ml (controls at 45 min) to 23.8 ± 1.5 ml with 10^{-8} M epinephrine ($P < 0.005$) to 16.8 ± 1.1 ml with 10^{-7} M epinephrine ($P < 0.001$) and 14.2 ± 1.5 ml with 10^{-6} M epinephrine ($P < 0.001$).

Cardiac Output. Epinephrine, 10^{-8} M, caused a small but significant ($P < 0.002$) rise in cardiac output, whereas 10^{-7} M epinephrine caused a small fall in cardiac output. Epinephrine, 10^{-6} M, had a major effect on the cardiac output which fell from 44 to 35 ml/min. The decrease in cardiac output did not recover even 40 min after addition of 10^{-6} M epinephrine (Table 2).

Effects of Epinephrine or Pacing on Oxygen Uptake

Epinephrine, 10^{-8} M, produced a transient increase in the oxygen uptake by the heart, similar in magnitude to that produced by pacing (both values 199 μl/g per min), although the peak heart rate (275 ± 7 beats/min) was much lower than pacing at 360 beats/min and despite a higher cardiac output during pacing (46.1 ml/min) than with 10^{-8} M epinephrine (43.7 ml/min) (Table 2).

Epinephrine, both 10^{-7} M and 10^{-6} M, increased myocardial oxygen consumption even more, with the oxygen consumption reaching a similar peak of about 290 μl/g per min for both concentrations 10 min after addition of the drug. With 10^{-6} M epinephrine, the oxygen consumption remained elevated at this level until the end of the experiment, after 75 min of perfusion time, but with 10^{-7} M epinephrine, the oxygen consumption fell after the peak increase so that at 60 min of perfusion (25 min post-epinephrine), the oxygen uptake was 254 ± 8 μl/g per min, which was lower ($P < 0.05$) than the value found with 10^{-6} M epinephrine at the same time (297 ± 13 μl/g per min).

Efficiency of Pressure Work

In these experiments, kinetic power was ignored. Hence, efficiency of total power production was underestimated. Nevertheless, the results (Table

2) are of interest as they indicate the direction of the change found. Thus, increasing doses of epinephrine led to increasing degrees of myocardial inefficiency. Epinephrine 10^{-8} M, only led to about a 17% loss of efficiency (Table 2), but at 10^{-6} M, it produced a loss of 52%. Dibutyryl cAMP (10^{-4} M and 5×10^{-4} M) decreased myocardial efficiency by about 25%. There was a greater loss of efficiency with 10^{-6} M than with 10^{-7} M epinephrine, although the peak oxygen uptake reached with both was similar; this greater decrease of efficiency reflected the greater depression of cardiac output with 10^{-6} M epinephrine.

Decreased Heart Work

To assess whether decreased heart work by itself could decrease enzyme release and thereby explain the decreased release of enzyme with 10^{-6} M epinephrine plus propranolol, hearts were perfused in the Langendorff (15) (nonworking) mode (without performing external mechanical work) throughout the time sequence of the protocol. The enzyme release produced by 10^{-6} M epinephrine was reduced, and the time of peak release was delayed (255 ± 100 mU/g per min, 25 min after addition); the release was lower than the peak release in working hearts (712 ± 48 mU/g per min). The value in the Langendorff hearts was still, however, higher than that in working hearts with 10^{-6} M epinephrine plus propranolol (peak release, 72 ± 13 mU/g per min). Hence, decreased external work did decrease peak enzyme release achieved by 10^{-6} M epinephrine, but decreased work was not the only factor explaining the protective effect of propranolol.

Tissue Contents of High-Energy Phosphate Compounds and Glycogen

With 10^{-6} M epinephrine, the content of ATP fell only slightly, and phosphocreatine rose at 45 min of perfusion (i.e., 10 min after epinephrine; Table 3, Figure 2), suggesting that (1) enzyme release could not be related to overall loss of ATP and that (2) there was a block of energy transfer between phosphocreatine and ATP. But with 10^{-7} M epinephrine, the tissue content of ATP did not fall at all at 45 min (i.e., 10 min after adding the epinephrine, at the time of peak release of LDH). However, phosphocreatine rose substantially, again suggesting interference with energy transfer. Thus, a dose of epinephrine (10^{-7} M) increasing cumulative LDH release by 960% acted without a decrease in the tissue content of ATP.

Increasing doses of epinephrine produced increasing glycogen depletion which was β blocked (data not shown); dbcAMP (5×10^{-4} M) also caused glycogen depletion (0.46 ± 0.08 μmol C_6/g, $N = 4$) when compared with cAMP, 5×10^{-4} M (5.89 ± 0.81, $N = 5$; $P < 0.005$), both values at 120 min of perfusion. But theophylline (10^{-3} M), which caused as much LDH release as did epinephrine (10^{-7} M), caused no glycogen depletion (control:

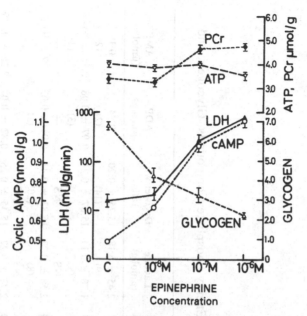

Figure 2.   Effect of progressive increase of concentration of added epinephrine on release of lactate dehydrogenase (LDH), on tissue cAMP, tissue glycogen, and tissue contents of ATP and of phosphocreatine (PCr). All values 10 min after addition of epinephrine, i.e., after 35 min of perfusion time (see Figure 1). Note: (1) with epinephrine 10^{-7} M, LDH release is increased but ATP and PCr do not fall; (2) general concordance between pattern of rise of cAMP (ref. 11) and release of LDH (the latter on a log scale). Glycogen unit = μmol glucose equivalent/ g fresh wt.; C = control (no addition of epinephrine).

6.77 ± 0.67, N = 16; epinephrine, 10^{-7} M: 3.34 ± 0.39, N = 19; theophylline, 10^{-3} M: 6.20 ± 0.75, N = 7; all values at 45 min; units, μmol C_6/ g).

Tissue Cyclic AMP

As already reported in detail elsewhere (12), increasing doses of epinephrine to 10^{-6} M caused a progressive rise in tissue cAMP from 0.494 ± 0.019 nmol/g (N = 12) in controls to 1.129 ± 0.041 nmol/g (N = 14); theophylline (10^{-3} M) also increased tissue cAMP to 0.816 ± 0.027 (N = 8; $P < 0.001$). Values with 10^{-6} M epinephrine were not changed by changing the external glucose concentration. Thus, the effects of epinephrine or theophylline could have been mediated by the β receptor and formation of cAMP, but the modifying effects of glucose were not directly related to changes in tissue cAMP; changes in external Mg^{2+} could also be related to a decreased cAMP (0.845 ± 0.042 nmol/g; N = 5; $P < 0.005$), but in the case of halving the external Ca^{2+}, peak enzyme release dropped very substantially from 711 ± 48 (N = 41) mU/g per min to 64 ± 7 (N = 9) mU/g per min, whereas cAMP only fell from 1.129 ± 0.041 to 0.942 ± 0.049 (N = 5) nmol/g (NS).

Table 3. Effects of Epinephrine and Dibutyryl Cyclic AMP on High-Energy Phosphate Compounds, Glycogen, and Lactate Contents of Isolated Working Rat Heart

Condition	ATP (μmol/g)	Phospho-creatine (μmol/g)	Total (ATP + PCr) (μmol/g)	Glycogen (μmol C_6/g)	Lactate (μmol/g)	Dry/wet wt. ratio	ADP (μmol/g)	AMP (μmol/g)
1. Control working heart	4.04 ± 0.09 (16)	3.47 ± 0.11 (16)	7.51 ± 0.14 (16)	6.77 ± 0.67 (16)	2.45 ± 0.18 (9)	15.25 ± 0.20 (14)	0.94 (2)	0.19 (2)
2. Epinephrine 10^{-8} M	3.86 ± 0.12 (14)	3.29 ± 0.12 (14)	7.15 ± 0.17 (14)	4.32 ± 0.44 (13)	1.70 ± 0.14 (8)	15.87 ± 0.21 (13)	0.97 ± 0.08 (3)	0.18 ± 0.008 (3)
P vs. 1	NS	NS	NS	<0.01	NS	NS		
3. Epinephrine 10^{-7} M	3.95 ± 0.15 (20)	4.67 ± 0.26 (20)	8.62 ± 0.30 (20)	3.40 ± 0.39 (19)	2.58 ± 0.23 (8)	15.83 ± 0.41 (20)	0.94 ± 0.09 (3)	0.17 ± 0.019 (3)
P vs. 1	NS	<0.001	<0.005	<0.001	NS	NS	—	—
4. Epinephrine 10^{-6} M	3.45 ± 0.11 (37)	4.80 ± 0.16 (37)	8.25 ± 0.19 (37)	2.60 ± 0.19 (36)	2.73 ± 0.27 (8)	15.45 ± 0.25 (32)	0.82 ± 0.07 (3)	0.22 ± 0.019 (3)
P vs. 1	<0.001	<0.001	<0.005	<0.001	NS	NS	—	—
5. Epinephrine 10^{-6} M; ½ Ca^{2+}	3.83 ± 0.13 (6)	5.25 ± 0.13 (6)	9.08 ± 0.18 (6)	2.81 ± 0.44 (5)	—	15.11 ± 0.52 (6)	—	—
P vs. 1	NS	<0.001	<0.001	<0.001		NS		

6. Epinephrine 10^{-6} M; $2 \times Mg^{2+}$	3.96 ± 0.10 (5)	5.43 ± 0.10 (5)	9.39 ± 0.14 (5)	3.60 ± 0.64 (5)	—	15.04 ± 0.30 (5)
P vs. 1	NS	<0.001	<0.001			NS
7. Epinephrine 10^{-6} M + propranolol 10^{-5} M	3.80 ± 0.13 (6)	5.48 ± 0.27 (7)	9.28 ± 0.30 (7)	6.58 ± 0.75 (7)	—	14.81 ± 8.29 (7)
P vs. 1	NS	<0.001	<0.001	NS		NS
8. Epinephrine 10^{-6} M + verapamil 2×10^{-7} M	3.56 ± 0.16 (4)	5.40 ± 0.40 (4)	8.96 ± 0.43 (4)	2.11 ± 0.61 (4)	—	14.16 ± 1.08 (4)
P vs. 1	<0.05	<0.001	<0.001	NS		NS
9. Theophylline 10^{-3} M	3.72 ± 0.14 (8)	2.82 ± 0.10 (8)	6.54 ± 0.17 (8)	6.39 ± 1.29 (6)	—	14.26 ± 0.43 (8)
P vs. 1	NS	<0.005	<0.001	NS		<0.05
10. Dibutyryl cAMP 10^{-4} M	3.58 ± 0.19 (6)	4.15 ± 0.32 (6)	7.73 ± 0.37 (6)	1.70 ± 0.56 (4)	—	14.29 ± 0.76 (6)
P vs. 1	<0.025	NS	NS	NS		NS
11. Initial value before working heart (Langendorff system)	3.98 ± 0.12 (6)	6.10 ± 0.31 (6)	10.08 ± 0.32 (6)	15.62 ± 1.95 (6)	—	15.90 ± 0.31 (6)
P vs. 1	NS	<0.001	<0.001	<0.001		<0.001

[a] All measurements (except group 7) made at 45 min of perfusion, i.e., 10 min after addition of epinephrine or other intervention. Dash indicates the absence of data.

DISCUSSION

Critique of Model

The isolated perfused working rat heart model is a standard well-described physiological preparation (18,21). It responds to an increase in heart work (work jump) by a decrease in the cardiac content of high-energy phosphates (21,30). Hence, the failure of low concentrations of epinephrine to decrease the cardiac stores of high-energy phosphates in this study at the same time that enzyme release was increased is evidence that catecholamines do not act via excess breakdown of ATP as proposed by Fleckenstein and his group in another model (8).

The basal release of enzymes from this preparation is abnormal but can be related to the initial excision, and by 90 min post-ligation, the rate of release of LDH in the present preparation was extremely low and only just measurable. Arguments for the adequacy of oxygenation of this preparation have already been given (4). In particular, increased heart work achieved by isoproterenol is accompanied by autofluorescence changes in the direction of NAD^+ and away from NADH (17). Such autofluorescent changes probably reflect those in the mitochondrial redox state and are the opposite to those expected in hypoxia (22).

An important question is whether the changes induced are those of epinephrine or those of toxic epinephrine metabolites (5). We used the same procedure to study fresh, unoxidized epinephrine as Dhalla et al. (5) used to study fresh isoproterenol: the drug was dissolved freshly in small volumes of perfusion medium just prior to use. But the major enzyme release occurred within the early minutes after addition of epinephrine, not later on as would have occurred with progressive oxidation. Furthermore, Dhalla et al. caused isoproterenol to undergo spontaneous oxidation by gassing the perfusion medium with 95% O_2 and 5% CO_2 at room temperature for 11–12 hr prior to use, and the solutions that were maximally effective had a pink to bright red color; in our case, the solutions were clear. In addition, the epinephrine powder itself was kept under nitrogen in the deep freeze; discolored powder was discarded. Oxidized isoproterenol as used by Dhalla et al. (5) had a major effect in decreasing the contractile force of the heart (assessed by force displacement), whereas in our experiments, epinephrine in the two lowest concentrations had no such effect on the cardiac output (Table 2). Thus, our results very probably reflect the effects of epinephrine and not those of its oxidized products.

β Stimulation and High-Energy Phosphates of the Heart

We found that epinephrine caused a dose-related loss of enzyme lactate dehydrogenase (LDH) from the isolated rat heart. An important advantage of using the isolated heart model was the avoidance of catecholamine effects on circulating free fatty acids which in turn could have harmful effects such as increased enzyme release even in normal isolated hearts (4). The release of LDH was β blocked and stimulated by theophylline and by external dibutyryl cAMP. The release was decreased by measures designed to decrease calcium effects such as adding verapamil, decreasing the external calcium, or increasing the external magnesium. Thus, according to the proposals of Fleckenstein (6–8), the mechanisms should involve excess excitation–contraction coupling and, hence, breakdown of high-energy phosphate compounds. Depletion of the ATP content of the heart was also invoked by Waldenström et al. (29) to explain the harmful effects of norepinephrine on the perfused heart. But with an epinephrine dose (10^{-7} M) that caused substantial loss of LDH, there was no loss of myocardial ATP, whereas the content of phosphocreatine increased. With 10^{-6} M epinephrine, ATP fell, but phosphocreatine rose, so that the content of total high-energy phosphate compounds was unchanged. There is thus no simple relationship between epinephrine-induced enzyme release and depletion of high-energy phosphate compounds.

One explanation for our findings is altered intracellular transfer of energy. The increase of phosphocreatine could be explained by impaired transfer of high-energy phosphates between phosphocreatine and ATP. The latter proposal would suppose compartmentation of ATP (10). There was considerable loss of cellular creatine kinase from the heart during addition of epinephrine. We cannot exclude that sufficient creatine kinase isoenzyme was lost from a specific subcellular site to impair transfer of energy from cytoplasmic phosphocreatine to cytoplasmic ATP.

A second explanation resides in the concept of a small pool of ATP, produced chiefly by glycolysis, which could play a role in the maintenance of membrane integrity (2,20). Thus, increasing rates of glycolysis, as presumably achieved by increasing external glucose concentrations, could protect against enzyme release, whereas decreasing rates of glycolysis, as presumably achieved by addition of FFA to the medium, exaggerated enzyme release. Our data are compatible with but do not specifically prove or disprove this postulated mechanism, because glycolysis was not measured.

Both of the above explanations depend on the existence of compartmentalized ATP in the cytoplasm. Of interest is the effect of agents or procedures that caused a major decrease in release of LDH (propranolol, ½ Ca^{2+}, 2 × Mg^{2+}) which all reversed the small fall of tissue ATP caused by 10^{-6} M epinephrine by itself. None decreased phosphocreatine. Thus, impaired energy transfer from phosphocreatine to ATP is unlikely to be a basic defect in epinephrine-mediated myocardial damage.

β Stimulation and Cyclic AMP

The effects of epinephrine and theophylline in causing LDH release and those of propranolol in decreasing epinephrine-induced release could be related to alterations in tissue cAMP (12). The criteria of Sutherland et al. (26) required to show that cAMP mediated any given effect of catecholamines could be satisfied (12). Hence, accumulation of intracellular cAMP could be linked to the effect of epinephrine in increasing LDH release from the heart (12), acting at least in part by a Ca^{2+}-dependent mechanism (23,24).

Concentrations of Epinephrine, Oxygen Wastage, and Other Effects on Mechanical and Metabolic Parameters

Epinephrine in increasing concentrations caused a tachycardia, an increase in coronary flow, a decrease in aortic output, first a small rise and then a fall in cardiac output, an increase in oxygen uptake, an increase in peak aortic pressure, a fall of effciency of work, a fall of glycogen, and an increase of tissue cAMP (Table 4). At the highest concentrations of epinephrine (10^{-6} M), there were large increases in release of lactate dehydrogenase but only a small fall of tissue ATP. Even low concentrations of epinephrine (10^{-8} M), which caused only a modest rise in heart rate and cAMP and no change in cumulative enzyme release, caused decreased efficiency of work, i.e., oxygen wastage. Interestingly, the increased cardiac output with 10^{-8} M epinephrine resulted from an increased coronary flow which more than compensated for the small decrease of aortic output. There was no inotropic effect as judged by peak aortic pressure, yet oxygen uptake and coronary flow rose. Thus, the oxygen wastage was found even in the absence of an inotropic effect. Very substantial oxygen wastage took place with 10^{-7} M epinephrine when hearts were functioning at two-thirds of normal efficiency; there was an inotropic effect as judged by an increase of the peak aortic pressure. At the highest epinephrine concentration, 10^{-6} M, hearts functioned at less than half normal efficiency, and only at this concentration was overall tissue ATP decreased.

Oxygen wastage caused by an increasing concentration of epinephrine was associated with a marked and increasing fall of aortic output, but the peak aortic pressure rose at 10^{-7} M and 10^{-6} M epinephrine. Hence, the decreased cardiac output must have resulted from impaired relaxation and not impaired contraction of the heart. It should be noted that cardiac output fell less than aortic output because the fall in aortic output was partially compensated by the rise in coronary flow. T. D. Noakes in this laboratory (unpublished data) has presented evidence that the rate of relaxation determines the cardiac output of this preparation. Excess entry of Ca^{2+} could explain impaired relaxation; Opie et al. (23) found that the addition of verapamil (2×10^{-7} M) or halving the perfusate $[Ca^{2+}]$ allowed cardiac output to rise rather than fall after the addition of 10^{-6} M epinephrine. Because the $[Ca^{2+}]$ used in control experiments was 2.5 mM and, therefore, twice the normal ionized value, we must emphasize that the normal expected effect of epinephrine in increasing cardiac output is found when the medium Ca^{2+} is normal, i.e., 1.25 mM.

Table 4. Comparative Effects of Epinephrine and Dibutyryl Cyclic AMP on Mechanical and Metabolic Parameters of Isolated Perfused Working Rat Heart[a]

Condition	Heart rate (beats/min)	Coronary flow (ml/min)	Aortic output (ml/min)	Cardiac output (ml/min)	O$_2$ uptake (μl/g per min)	Peak aortic pressure (mm Hg)	Efficiency of pressure work (joules/ml O$_2$)	Peak LDH release (mU/g per min)	Tissue glycogen (μmol C$_6$/g)	Tissue AMP (nmol/g)	Tissue ATP (μmol/g)	Tissue PCr (μmol/g)
1. Control value	236	16.1	29.5	45.1	172	116	4.43	16.6	6.77	0.494[b]	4.04	3.47
2. Control % change at 35 min	100%[c]	104%[c]	98%[c]	100%[c]	100%[c]	100%[c]	99%[c]	100%[d]	100%[d]	100%[d]	100%[d]	100%[d]
3. Epinephrine 10^{-8} M	114%	128%	92%	103%	125%	94%	83%	120%[e]	64%	137%	96%	95%
4. Epinephrine 10^{-7} M	132%	143%	64%	93%	174%	118%	68%	960%	49%	199%	98%	135%
4. Epinephrine 10^{-6} M	147%	144%	49%	80%	177%	114%	? ↓↑	4285%	34%	229%	85%	138%
6. Theophylline 10^{-3} M	153%	124%	60%	84%	? ↑↓	100%	77%	508%	92%	165%	92%	81%
7. Dibutyryl cAMP 10^{-4} M	96%	140%	68%	96%	128%	100%	—	196%	—	—	89%	120%
8. Dibutyryl cAMP 5 × 10^{-4} M	115%	149%	64%	91%	148%	120%	71%	1030%	—	—	—	—

[a] See Figure 2 for experimental design. Drugs were added at 35 min of perfusion, and percentage changes at 35 min of perfusion.
[b] Dashes indicate absence of data.
[c] Data from Horak et al. (12).
[c] Compared with value at 30 min of perfusion.
[d] Values at 45 min in control hearts are taken as 100%.
[e] Cumulative values at 75 min same as in control. See Figure 1.
[f] See discussion in text.

Epinephrine versus Theophylline versus Dibutyryl Cyclic AMP

These agents had dissimilar effects on the heart. Theophylline resembled epinephrine in increasing heart rate, coronary flow, tissue cAMP, and glycogen and in decreasing aortic and cardiac outputs, but tissue phosphocreatine fell rather than rose, and tissue glycogen was maintained. Theophylline has complex effects on the heart, and its chronotropic effect includes local catecholamine release and a vagolytic effect (27) besides its generally accepted role in inhibition of phosphodiesterase. We did not measure oxygen uptake with theophylline, but the decreased aortic output suggests a negative inotropic effect, whereas the increased coronary flow suggests an increased oxygen uptake (there is a close correlation between oxygen uptake and coronary flow in the perfused rat heart, 19). Thus, theophylline probably caused oxygen wastage with a very modest fall of tissue ATP.

Dibutyryl cAMP resembled epinephrine in causing an increase in coronary flow, a fall in aortic output, an increased oxygen uptake, decreased efficiency of work, increased LDH release, glycogen breakdown, a slight fall of ATP, and a rise of phosphocreatine. But dbcAMP failed to increase the heart rate. Gartner and Vahouny (9) have already argued that there might be different receptors for the inotropic and the chronotropic effects of β stimulation; they also found that epinephrine (10^{-5} M) increased heart rate whereas dbcAMP (10^{-3} M) did not. They also showed that 10 min of exposure of the heart to dbcAMP was adequate to obtain an intracellular metabolic effect (glycogen breakdown) and hence showed intracellular penetration. Further support for a differential effect of dbcAMP on heart rate and inotropism comes from studies with N^6-alkyl-8-substituted cAMP derivatives which increase contractile activity but not the heart rate of the dog (16).

Recently, Higgins et al. (11) have shown that increasing medium Ca^{2+} concentrations led to increased loss of lactate dehydrogenase from anoxic heart cell cultures.

CONCLUSIONS

Depletion of high-energy phosphate compounds caused by epinephrine was not directly related to the extent of enzyme loss from normal isolated working rat hearts. Rather, oxygen wastage, as shown by a decreased efficiency of pressure work, was found even with low concentrations of epinephrine (10^{-8} M) which caused only a minimal change in the pattern of release of lactate dehydrogenase. With increasing epinephrine concentrations, accumulation of tissue cAMP could be linked to enzyme release. Involvement of Ca^{2+} was shown by the reduction of enzyme loss in hearts perfused with verapamil or during ionic variations. Furthermore, reduction of the perfusate Ca^{2+} by half eliminated the effect of epinephrine in causing oxygen wastage (23). Thus, Ca^{2+} can be related to both aspects of myocardial cell injury: oxygen wastage and enzyme release. These observations could explain why cAMP, presumably acting via Ca^{2+}, can cause cardiac necrosis (1).

There are two important reservations to our conclusions. First, the $[Ca^{2+}]$ of the Krebs–Henseleit perfusion fluid corresponded to the total $[Ca^{2+}]$ of blood and was in reality twice the normal ionized value. Perfusate $[Mg^{2+}]$ was similarly high. The high perfusate $[Ca^{2+}]$ used markedly potentiated the pathological effects of epinephrine. Second, the degree of oxygen wastage was determined by measurements of the efficiency of pressure work only, ignoring kinetic work. Furthermore, the number of observations was small. Notwithstanding these reservations, it was not possible to separate the pathological from the physiological effects of increasing concentrations of epinephrine, and both were associated with a rise of tissue cAMP. A further conclusion is that pathological effects were found in the absence of a fall of tissue high-energy phosphate compounds; rather, there appeared to be a separate effect whereby epinephrine impaired intracellular transfer of energy.

ACKNOWLEDGMENTS

This work forms part of the program of the Medical Research Council of South Africa who are thanked for their support. The Chris Barnard Fund generously provided support for A. Horak. We thank Dr. C. Hamm for assistance with verapamil perfusions and Dr. T. Podzuweit for measurements of cAMP (see 12).

REFERENCES

1. Bhagat, B., Sullivan, J. M., Fischer, V. W., Nadel, E. M., and Dhalla, N. S. 1978. cAMP activity and isoproterenol-induced myocardial injury in rats. In: T. Kobayashi, Y. Ito, and G. Rona (eds.), Recent Advances in Studies on Cardiac Structure and Metabolism. Vol. 12: Cardiac Adaptation, pp. 465–470. University Park Press, Baltimore.
2. Bricknell, O. L., and Opie, L. H. 1978. Effects of substrates on tissue metabolic changes in the isolated rat heart during underperfusion and on release of lactate dehydrogenase and arrhythmias during reperfusion. Circ. Res. 43:102–115.
3. Ciba–Geigy. 1970. Statistical Methods in Scientific Tables, pp. 172–173. Ciba–Geigy, Basel.
4. de Leiris, J., and Opie, L. H. 1978. Effect of substrates and of coronary artery ligation on mechanical performance and on release of lactate dehydrogenase and creatine phosphokinase in isolated working rat hearts. Cardiovasc. Res. 12:585–596.
5. Dhalla, N. S., Yates, J. C., Lee, S. L., and Singh, A. 1978. Functional and subcellular changes in the isolated rat heart perfused with oxidized isoproterenol. J. Mol. Cell Cardiol. 10:31–41.
6. Fleckenstein, A. 1971. Specific inhibitors and promoters of calcium action in the excitation–contraction coupling of heart muscle and their role in the prevention or production of myocardial lesions. In: P. Harris and L. H. Opie (eds.), Calcium and the Heart, pp. 135–188. Academic Press, London, New York.
7. Fleckenstein, A., Janke, J., Döring, H. J., and Leder, O. 1974. Myocardial fiber necrosis

due to intracellular Ca overload—a new principle in cardiac pathophysiology. In: N. S. Dhalla (ed.), *Recent Advances in Studies on Cardiac Structure and Metabolism*. Vol. 4. *Myocardial Biology*, pp. 563–580. University Park Press, Baltimore.

8. Fleckenstein, A., Janke, J., Döring, H. J., and Leder, O. 1975. Key role of Ca in the production of noncoronarogenic myocardial necroses. In: A. Fleckenstein and G. Rona (eds.), *Recent Advances in Studies on Cardiac Structure and Metabolism*. Vol. 6: *Pathophysiology and Morphology of Myocardial Cell Alteration*, pp. 21–32. University Park Press, Baltimore.

9. Gartner, S. L., and Vahouny, G. V. 1972. Effects of epinephrine and cyclic 3',5'-AMP on perfused rat hearts. *Am. J. Physiol.* 222:1121–1124.

10. Gudbjarnason, S., Mathes, P., and Ravens, K. G. 1970. Functional compartmentation of ATP and creatine phosphate in heart muscle. *J. Mol. Cell Cardiol.* 1:325–339.

11. Higgins, T. J., Allsopp, D., Bailey, P. J. 1980. The effect of extracellular calcium concentrations and Ca-antagonist drugs on enzyme release and lactate production by anoxic heart cell cultures. *J. Mol. Cell. Cardiol.* 12:909–927.

12. Horak, A. R., Podzuweit, T., and Opie, L. H. 1980. Cyclic AMP as mediator of catecholamine-induced enzyme release from isolated perfused working rat heart. In: M. Tajuddin, P. K. Das, M. Tariq, and N. S. Dhalla (eds.), *Advances in Myocardiology*, Vol. 1, pp. 367–373. University Park Press, Baltimore.

13. Kannengiesser, G. J., Opie, L. H., and van der Werff, T. J. 1979. Impaired cardiac work and oxygen uptake after reperfusion of regional ischaemic myocardium. *J. Mol. Cell. Cardiol.* 11:197–207.

14. Krebs, H. A., and Henseleit, K. 1932. Untersuchungen über die Harnstoffbildung im Tierkörper. *Hoppe Seylers Z. Physiol. Chem.* 210:33–66.

15. Langendorff, O. 1895. Untersuchungen am überlebenden Saügertierherzen. *Pfluegers Arch.* 61:291–332.

16. Miller, J. P., Boswell, K. H., Meyer, R. B., Christensen, L. F., and Robins, R. K. 1980. Synthesis and enzymatic and inotropic activity of some new 8-substituted and 6,8-disubstituted derivatives of adenosine cyclic 3',5'-monophosphate. *J. Med. Chem.* 23:242–251.

17. Moravec, J., Corsin, A., Owen, P., and Opie, L. H. 1974. Effect of increased aortic perfusion pressure on autofluorescent emission of the isolated rat heart. *J. Mol. Cell. Cardiol.* 6:187–200.

18. Neely, J. R., Liebermeister, H., and Morgan, H. E. 1967. Effect of pressure development on membrane transport of glucose in isolated rat heart. *Am. J. Physiol.* 212:815–822.

19. Opie, L. H. 1965. Coronary flow rate and perfusion pressure as determinants of mechanical function and oxidative metabolism of isolated perfused rat heart. *J. Physiol. (Lond.)* 180:529–541.

20. Opie, L. H., and Bricknell, O. L. 1979. Role of glycolytic flux in effect of glucose in decreasing fatty-acid-induced release of lactate dehydrogenase from isolated coronary-ligated rat heart. *Cardiovasc. Res.* 13:693–702.

21. Opie, L. H., Mansford, K. R. L., and Owen, P. 1971. Effects of increased heart work on glycolysis and adenine nucleotides in the perfused heart of normal and diabetic rats. *Biochem. J.* 124:475–490.

22. Opie, L. H., and Owen, P. 1975. Assessment of mitochondrial free NAD^+/NADH ratios and oxaloacetate concentrations during increased mechanical work in isolated perfused rat heart during production or uptake of ketone bodies. *Biochem. J.* 148:403–415.

23. Opie, L. H., Thandroyen, F. T., Muller, C., and Bricknell, O. L. 1979. Adrenaline-induced "oxygen-wastage" and enzyme release from working rat heart. Effects of calcium antagonism, β-blockade, nicotinic acid, and coronary artery ligation. *J. Mol. Cell. Cardiol.* 11:1073–1094.

24. Reuter, H. 1974. Localization of β-adrenergic receptors, and effects of noradrenaline and cyclic nucleotides on action potentials, ionic currents and tension in mammalian cardiac muscle. *J. Physiol. (Lond.)* 242:429–451.

25. Rona, G., Chappel, C. I., Balazs, T., and Gaundry, R. 1959. An infarct-like myocardial

lesion and other toxic manifestations produced by isoproterenol in the rat. *Arch. Pathol.* (*Chicago*) 67:443–445.

26. Sutherland, E. W., Robison, G. A., and Butcher, R. W. 1968. Some aspects of the biological role of adenosine-3',5'-monophosphate. *Circulation* 37:279–306.

27. Urthaler, F., and James, T. N. 1976. Both direct and neurally mediated components of the chronotropic actions of aminophylline. *Chest* 70:24–32.

28. Vetter, N. J., Strange, R. C., Adams, W., and Oliver, M. F. 1974. Initial metabolic and hormonal response to acute myocardial infarction. *Lancet* 1:284–288.

29. Waldenström, A. P., Hjalmarson, A. C., and Thornell, L. T. 1978. A possible role of noradrenaline in the development of myocardial infarction. An experimental study in the isolated rat heart. *Am. Heart J.* 95:43–51.

30. Williamson, J. R., Ford, C., Illingworth, J., and Safer, B. 1976. Coordination of citric acid cycle activity with electron transport flux. *Circ. Res.* 38(Suppl. 1):39–48.

31. Wollenberger, A., Ristau, O., and Schoffa, G. 1960. Eine einfache Technik der extrem schnellen abkühling grösserer Gewebestücke. *Pfluegers Arch.* 270:399–412.

32. Wroblewski, F., and La Due, J. S. 1955. Lactic dehydrogenase activity in blood. *Proc. Soc. Exp. Biol. Med.* 90:210–213.

33. Young, R. C., Thomas, M., Evans, M. E., and Opie, L. H. 1972. Catecholamines and myocardial infarction. In: E. Bajusz and G. Rona (eds.), *Recent Advances in Studies on Cardiac Structure and Metabolism.* Vol. 1: *Myocardiology,* pp. 163–168. University Park Press, Baltimore.

The Permissive Role of Catecholamines in the Pathogenesis of Hamster Cardiomyopathy

G. Jasmin and L. Proschek

Department of Pathology
Faculty of Medicine
University of Montreal
Montreal, Quebec H3C 3J7, Canada

Abstract. It was previously shown that β-adrenergic blockers exert a protective action on the development of heart necrotic changes in cardiomyopathic hamsters. To further investigate the possible role of catecholamines in the pathogenesis of the hamster hereditary cardiomyopathy, the ventricular adrenergic nerve terminals were visualized by fluorescence histochemistry, and NE uptake and turnover were determined after i.v. injection of labeled NE. It was found that the fluorescent nerve endings strongly proliferate with the occurrence of heart necrotic changes. With healing of the myocardial lesions, the difference between control and myopathic hearts is less apparent, and NE nerve endings are literally absent in the terminal stage of the disease. There was a marked increase in NE uptake during the necrotic stage and, at the same time, a considerable rise in elimination rate constant with a maximum level at terminal stage, suggesting that the NE turnover is related to the progression of the disease. In light of the present findings, it can be surmised that NE plays a permissive role in the genesis of the hamster disease by promoting the heart necrotic changes.

The cardioprotection afforded by verapamil and propranolol during early stages of hamster hereditary cardiomyopathy (7,9,11) has prompted us to investigate further the possible role of catecholamines in the genesis of the heart necrotic changes. Although it is generally agreed that the protective mechanism of verapamil consists in the selective prevention of an excessive calcium influx into critically altered cardiocytes (4,24), propranolol would act mainly as a membrane stabilizer of heart muscle cells (19) subjected to an elevated adrenergic tone during the course of the hamster cardiomyopathy. These two somewhat differently acting pharmacological agents proved to be equally efficient in preventing the mitochondrial oxidative phosphorylation defect related to the severity of the heart necrotic changes (9). For these and other considerations outlined elsewhere (11), we undertook to investigate: (1) the configuration of adrenergic nerve terminals in heart muscle at different stages of the disease and (2) the uptake and turnover index of labeled norepinephrine ([³H]-NE) following in vivo administration of the radioactive amine.

45

MATERIAL AND METHODS

Male and female Syrian hamsters, 28 to 260 days of age, from the UM-X7.1 myopathic line and sex-matched random-bred healthy controls (supplied by Canadian Breeding Farm and Laboratories, St.-Constant, Quebec) were used. They were maintained under controlled housing conditions with free access to Purina Laboratory Chow and tap water. Animals were divided into three groups according to representative stages in the course of the cardiomyopathy as outlined in Table 1. In the third group, animals with failing hearts were evaluated separately.

Fluorescent Histochemistry

Histochemical demonstration of heart sympathetic nerve terminals was made in pentobarbital-anesthetized animals (4–5 mg/100 g body wt. i.p.). The left ventricle was punctured with a 21-gauge needle and infused with a freshly prepared 4% paraformaldehyde phosphate-buffered solution, pH 7.2 (14), the left auricle being sectioned to let the fixative out. After a 10-min infusion, hearts were excised, and the septum was dissected, placed on a cryostat chuck, and quenched in isopentane cooled with liquid nitrogen. Ten-micrometer sections mounted on glass cover slips were exposed to formaldehyde vapors for 2 hr at 80°C. The cover slips were placed on clean glass slides using Eukitt® as a mounting medium. The preparations were examined in a fluorescence microscope equipped with an Osram HPO 200 mercury lamp and lights filtered by appropriate Leitz filter (type IKP).

Kinetics of [³H]Norepinephrine in Vivo

Cardiomyopathic and control hamsters of 20–24 animals in each representative stage were divided into five subgroups. Under ether anesthesia, each hamster was injected intravenously with 8–10 µCi/100 g body wt. of [7-³H]-dl-NE (10 Ci/mmol; 49 µCi/g, Amersham Corp., Oakville) in 0.150 or 0.300 ml of 0.9% NaCl according to age. The retention of [³H]-NE radioactivity in hearts was determined from 0 to 24 hr. At appropriate times (5 min, 2, 6, 12, and 24 hr) after the injection, the hamsters were killed by decapitation, and their hearts were removed, rinsed, and cooled in ice; then the ventricles were dissected free of atria, blotted, and weighed. The tissue was homogenized by using a Polytron® homogenizer in 5 volumes of ice-cold 0.4 N perchloric acid (13) containing 1% ascorbic acid. The homogenate was centrifuged at 23,000 g for 20 min. The radioactivity of a 1-ml aliquot of the supernatant was measured in toluene–Triton X-100 (2:1 v/v) scintillation cocktail supplemented by a nonionic detergent on a Packard-Tri-Carb® liquid scintillation spectrometer, Model 3320. The counting efficiency was calculated in disintegrations per minute (dpm) after background substraction

Table 1. Changes of Norepinephrine (NE) Uptake at Zero Time and Elimination Rate Constant in the Ventricles during the Development of Cardiomyopathy[a]

Disease stage (days)	[3H]-NE uptake at zero time				[3H]-NE elimination rate constant (K) (hr^{-1})	
	(dpm × 10^3/g w.w.)		(dpm × 10^3/ventricle)			
	Control	Myopathic	Control	Myopathic	Control	Myopathic
Prenecrotic (28–30)	942 ± 91	944 ± 55 (N.S.)	197 ± 18	176 ± 12 (N.S.)	0.0789 ± 0.0011	0.0837 ± 0.0029 (N.S.)
Necrotic (90–100)	1335 ± 134	2402 ± 132 ($P < 0.005$)	527 ± 7	745 ± 74 ($P < 0.025$)	0.0776 ± 0.0061	0.1224 ± 0.0153 ($P < 0.01$)
Terminal (230–260) Nonfailing	1705 ± 67	1931 ± 183 (N.S.)	785 ± 16	715 ± 62 (N.S.)	0.0762 ± 0.0023	0.1332 ± 0.0286 ($P < 0.01$)
Heart failure		1463 ± 299 (N.S.)		544 ± 47 ($P < 0.05$)		0.2955 ± 0.0341 ($P < 0.001$)

[a] A minimum of 40 cardiomyopathic hamsters in each age group were used in two independent experiments. All values represent the mean ± S.E.

by using [^{3}H]hexadecane as an internal standard. The final results were expressed in dpm per gram of ventricle wet weight or per total mass.

Since the measured decline of the logarithm of residual radioactivity vs. time fulfilled first-order kinetics over a 24-hr period for control and diseased hearts (failing hearts, up to 12 hr), linear regression analysis (3) was used to calculate the NE elimination rate constant K and NE uptake at zero time. The NE half-life ($T_{1/2}$) as an index of heart NE turnover and/or heart hyperactivity was calculated from the NE elimination rate constant K as $T_{1/2}$ = 0.693/K for each age group of control and cardiomyopathic hamsters. The Student's t-test was used to determine the statistical significance of the results. Differences were considered significant if $P < 0.05$.

RESULTS

Myocardial Nerve Endings

Fluorescent nerve endings are rather sparse in normal and myopathic hamsters prior 40 days of age. The nerve terminals became more prominent with the occurrence of myolytic foci in 50-day-old hamsters. With progression of necrotic changes, the pattern of fluorescent fibers was more dendritic, in association with numerous yellow coarse granules reminiscent of residual bodies (Figure 1a,b). With subsidence of necrotic changes, the difference between normal and myopathic hearts became less apparent except for the density of yellow fluorescent granules. In the terminal stage, the nerve endings, especially in failing hearts, were literally absent (Figure 1c,d).

Norepinephrine Uptake and Elimination Rate Constant

As shown in Table 1, there was no appreciable difference in [^{3}H]-NE uptake and elimination rate between normal and myopathic hearts at the prenecrotic stage of the disease. With the occurrence of necrotic changes, the uptake values increased by 80% and 40% per gram of ventricle and per total mass, respectively, and at the same time, the elimination rate constant was equally increased by 70%. During the terminal stage, the uptake values in nonfailing hearts were close to that of the controls, although the elimination rate constant remained unchanged. In failing hearts, there was a relative decrease in uptake values but a considerable increase, by almost 400%, in the elimination rate constant.

Norepinephrine Half-Life

The [^{3}H]-NE half-life as a quantitative assessment of NE turnover rate was determined through kinetic measurements at different stages of the disease as outlined in the section on material and methods. Figure 2 illus-

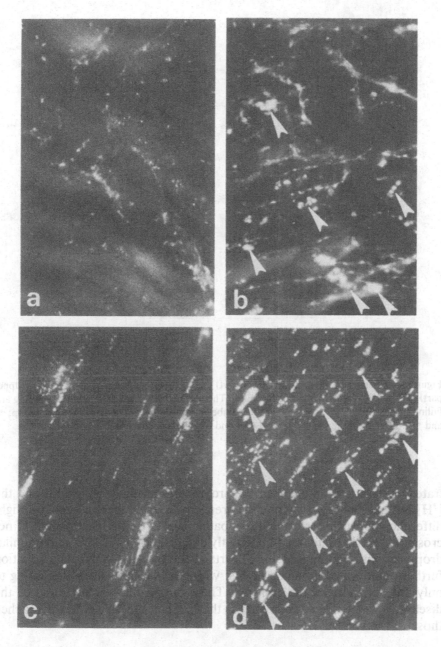

Figure 1.   Fluorescent adrenergic nerve terminals in the interventricular septum after exposure of cryostat sections to paraformaldehyde gas: (a) innervation observed in a 70-day-old normal hamster; (b) highly developed network in a necrotic focus of a cardiomyopathic animal of the same age; yellow fluorescent residual bodies are already visible (arrowheads); (c) slender innervation in normal hamsters at 250 days of age; (d) failing heart in an animal of the same age loaded with yellow fluorescent residual bodies (arrowheads). ×200.

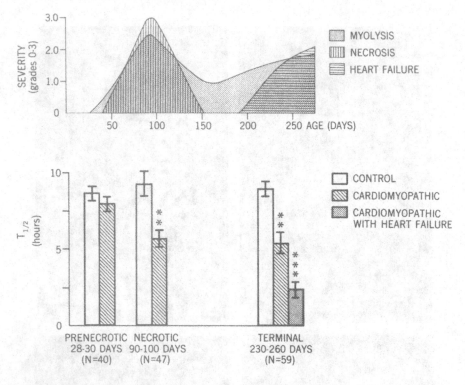

Figure 2.   Changes in NE half-life (lower part) during the progression of heart lesions (upper part) in UM-X7.1 cardiomyopathic hamsters. The terminal stage values relate to nonfailing and failing hearts (means ± S.E.). N = the number of cardiomyopathic hamsters per group; ** and *** differ from the control at $P < 0.01$ and 0.001, respectively.

trates the relationship between the progression of the heart lesions and the [^{3}H]-NE half-life ($T_{1/2}$). During the prenecrotic stage, there was only a slight difference between normal and myopathic hearts. With development of necrosis, the NE half-life was significantly diminished by 40–45%, and a similar drop was observed in nonfailing hearts at the terminal stage. The situation further deteriorated in failing hearts, with NE half-life values amounting to only 26% of those of the controls. Thus, during the whole course of the disease, it can only be inferred that the NE half-life values never reached those of the controls.

DISCUSSION

The pathomechanism of the hamster hereditary polymyopathy is still unknown. Myocardial necrotic changes are not apparent prior to 30 days of age, show increasing severity until 100 days, and subside thereafter (7,10).

Histogenic studies reveal that the cardiocytes disintegrate either by myofibrillar dissolution, leaving sarcolemmal remnants and occasional few nuclei, or by coagulation of the sarcoplasm which becomes highly granular and calcified (2,8). These pathological changes bear a great deal of resemblance to those resulting from an overtreatment with isoproterenol, methoxamine, and metaraminol (5,6,25). One additional common feature with catecholamine-induced heart lesions is the disturbance in myocardial calcium metabolism (15). The severity of both pathological processes relates to an abnormal movement of calcium across the cell membrane with mitochondrial calcium loading, depletion of high-energy phosphates, and eventual calcium precipitation within the mitochondrial matrix (8,18). Hence, verapamil as a calcium antagonist and propranolol as a β blocker are efficient in preventing the heart necrotic lesions; these pharmacologically different drugs prolong the viability of cardiocytes mainly by depressing calcium influx which invariably leads to irreversible cellular pathological changes. It should be pointed out, however, that the rise in urinary NE during early development of the hamster cardiomyopathy is not prevented by verapamil treatment (11,12), and we can only surmise that the myocytolytic changes in the heart derive mainly from a catecholamine overproduction.

Some investigators (21,22) have suggested that the pathomechanism of hamster cardiomyopathy is closely related to plasma membrane permeability changes as evidenced by the presence of horseradish peroxidase, a macromolecular tracer which penetrates into the damaged cardiac muscle cells (16). It is noteworthy that the horseradish peroxidase uptake coincides with the presence of contraction band lesions ultrastructurally demonstrable prior to any other evident cell necrotic changes. Such contraction bands lead to typical dislocation of intercalated disks with collapse of myofilaments and eventual myocytolysis (8). Essentially similar pathological changes have been reported in catecholamine-induced cardiac lesions (20).

As suggested by Sole et al., the pathological process may possibly result from an increase in adrenergic tone leading to an eventual depletion of NE stores and a concomitant rise of dopamine during congestive heart failure (23). It is noteworthy that the increase in the fluorescence intensity of nerve endings coincides with the development of heart necrotic changes. It is nonetheless relevant that NE uptake is singularly elevated during this critical stage, with a significant rise of the elimination rate constant during the progression of the disease, more specifically in animals with failing hearts. Within the same line of thinking, Angelakos et al. suggested that the hamster hereditary heart disease should be classified as an adrenergic cardiomyopathy (1). There findings are based mainly on the elevation of myocardial amine reserve conducive to heart failure. Our histochemical and biochemical findings well emphasize the proliferation of adrenergic nerve endings during the necrotic stage of the disease and demonstrate that these nerve terminals become depleted with the occurrence of heart failure. A lower amine concentration in failing hearts may simply reflect a higher turnover rate, as shown by the NE half-life values. In light of the present studies, we can only infer that norepinephrine plays a "permissive" role in promoting heart lesions during the necrotic stage. The term noradrenosis was proposed many years ago to characterize sympathetic nerve proliferation in human cardiomyopathies (17), and we believe that this concept well applies to the pathology of the hereditary hamster cardiomyopathy.

ACKNOWLEDGMENTS

This study was supported by grants from Medical Research Council of Canada (MA-1827) and the Muscular Dystrophy Association of Canada. The authors wish to thank Mr. Simeon Sokoloff, Department of Biochemistry, for the counting of radioactivity.

REFERENCES

1. Angelakos, E. T., King, M. P., and Carballo, L. 1973. Cardiac adrenergic innervation in hamsters with hereditary myocardiopathy: Chemical and histochemical studies. In: E. Bajusz and G. Rona (eds.), *Recent Advances in Studies on Cardiac Structure and Metabolism*. Vol. 2: *Cardiomyopathies*, pp. 519–531. University Park Press, Baltimore.
2. Büchner, F., Onishi, S., and Wada, A. 1978. *Cardiomyopathy Associated with Systemic Myopathy*, pp. 46–91. Urban & Schwarzenberg, Baltimore, Munich.
3. Ferguson, G. A., 1971. *Statistical Analysis in Psychology and Education*, 3rd ed., pp. 96–119. McGraw-Hill, New York.
4. Fleckenstein, A. 1971. Specific inhibitors and promoters of calcium action in the excitation–contraction coupling of heart muscle and their role in the prevention or production of myocardial lesions. In: P. Harris and L. Opie (eds.), *Calcium and the Heart*, pp. 135–188. Academic Press, London.
5. Jasmin, G. 1966. Morphologic effects of vasoactive drugs. *Can. J. Physiol. Pharmacol.* 44:367–372.
6. Jasmin, G. 1969. Factors influencing the production of cardiomyopathies by methoxamine and metaraminol. *Ann. N.Y. Acad. Sci.* 156:333–343.
7. Jasmin, G., and Bajusz, E. 1973. Polymyopathie et cardiomyopathie héréditaire chez le hamster de Syrie. Inhibition sélective des lésions du myocarde. *Ann. Anat. Pathol. (Paris)* 18:49–66.
8. Jasmin, G., and Eu, H. Y. 1979. Cardiomyopathy of hamster dystrophy. *Ann. N.Y. Acad. Sci.* 317:46–58.
9. Jasmin, G., and Proschek, L. 1980. Prevention of myocardial degeneration in hamsters with hereditary cardiomyopathy. In: A. Fleckenstein and H. Roskamm (eds.), *Calcium-Antagonismus*, pp. 144–150. Springer-Verlag, Berlin, Heidelberg.
10. Jasmin, G., and Proschek, L. 1982. Hereditary polymyopathy and cardiomyopathy in the Syrian hamster. I. Progression of heart and skeletal muscle lesions in the UM-X7.1 line. *Muscle Nerve* 5:20–25.
11. Jasmin, G., Solymoss, B., and Proschek, L. 1979. Therapeutic trials in hamster dystrophy. *Ann. N.Y. Acad. Sci.* 317:338–348.
12. Kabara, J. J., Riggin, R. M., and Kissinger, P. T. 1976. Abnormal levels of urinary catecholamines in dystrophic mice and hamsters. *Proc. Soc. Exp. Biol. Med.* 151:168–172.
13. Landsberg, L., and Axelrod, J. 1968. Influence of pituitary, thyroid and adrenal hormones on norepinephrine turnover and metabolism in the rat heart. *Circ. Res.* 22:559–571.
14. Laties, A. M., Lund, R., and Jacobowitz, D. 1967. A simplified method for the histochemical

localization of cardiac catecholamine-containing nerve fibers. *J. Histochem. Cytochem.* 15:535–541.

15. Lossnitzer, K., Morh, W., Konrad, A., and Guggenmoos, R. 1978. Hereditary cardiomyopathy in the Syrian golden hamsters. Influence of verapamil as calcium antagonist. In: M. Kaltenbach, F. Loogen, and E. G. J. Olsen (eds.), *Cardiomyopathy and Myocardial Biopsy*, pp. 27–37. Springer-Verlag, Berlin, Heidelberg.

16. Mendell, J. R., Higgins, R., Sahek, Z., and Cosmos, E. 1979. Relevance of genetic animal models of muscular dystrophy to human muscular dystrophies. *Ann. N.Y. Acad. Sci.* 317:409–430.

17. Pearse, A. G. E. 1964. The histochemistry and electron microscopy of obstructive cardiomyopathy. In: G. E. W. Wolstenholme and M. O'Connor (eds.), *Cardiomyopathies*, pp. 132–171. Churchill, London.

18. Proschek, L., and Jasmin, G. 1982. Hereditary polymyopathy and cardiomyopathy in the Syrian hamster. II. Development of heart necrotic changes in relation to defective mitochondrial function. *Muscle Nerve* 5:26–32.

19. Reimer, K. A., Rasmussen, M. M., and Jennings, R. B. 1976. On the nature of protection by propranolol against myocardial necrosis after temporary coronary occlusion in dogs. *Am. J. Cardiol.* 37:520–527.

20. Rona, G., Hüttner, I., and Boutet, M. 1977. Microcirculatory changes in myocardium with particular reference to catecholamine-induced cardiac muscle cell injury. In: H. Meessen (ed.), *Handbuch der Allegemeinen Pathologie III/7. Mikrozirkulation/Microcirculation*, pp. 791–888. Springer-Verlag, Berlin, Heidelberg.

21. Singh, J. N., Dhalla, N. S., McNamara, D. B., Bajusz, E., and Jasmin, G. 1975. Membrane alteration in failing hearts of cardiomyopathic hamsters. In: A. Fleckenstein and G. Rona (eds.), *Recent Advances in Studies on Cardiac Structure and Metabolism. Vol. 6: Pathophysiology and Morphology of Myocardial Cell Alteration*, pp. 259–268. University Park Press, Baltimore.

22. Slack, B. E., Boegman, R. J., Downie, J. W., and Jasmin, G. 1980. Cardiac membrane cholesterol in dystrophic and verapamil-treated hamsters. *J. Mol. Cell. Cardiol.* 12:179–185.

23. Sole, M. J., Kamble, A. B., and Hussain, M. N. 1977. A possible change in the rate-limiting step for cardiac norepinephrine synthesis in the cardiomyopathic Syrian hamster. *Circ. Res.* 41:814–817.

24. Sperelakis, N., and Schneider, J. A. 1976. A metabolic control mechanism for calcium ion influx that may protect the ventricular myocardial cell. *Am. J. Cardiol.* 37:1079–1085.

25. Todd, G. L., Cullan, G. E., and Cullan, G. M. 1980. Isoproterenol-induced myocardial necrosis and membrane permeability alterations in isolated perfused rabbit heart. *Exp. Mol. Pathol.* 33:43–54.

Adaptive and Pathological Alterations in Experimental Cardiac Hypertrophy

R. Jacob, G. Kissling, G. Ebrecht, C. Holubarsch,
I. Medugorac, and H. Rupp

Physiological Institute (II)
University of Tübingen
Tübingen, Federal Republic of Germany

Abstract. Based on investigations of various models of experimental cardiac hypertrophy (renal hypertension, spontaneous hypertension, aortic stenosis, swimming training, thyrotoxicosis), an attempt has been made to characterize adaptive and pathological alterations that are inherent to or accompany the process of hypertrophy. In principle, the designation of a process as adaptive is rooted in a teleological point of view and implies that the basic tendency of the respective structural and functional alterations is appropriate for coping with the altered functional requirements. This does not mean, however, that such alterations are favorable under all conditions and in all stages of hypertrophy. Since organisms generally reveal relatively stereotypic reaction patterns, the terms "adaptive" and "pathological" are not mutually exclusive in the final analysis. In the chronically pressure-loaded ventricle, nearly all alterations are ambiguous (myocardial mass increase, prolongation of the action potential, overproportional increase of intracellular contractile material, decrease of myofibrillar ATPase activity). The altered ATPase activity, which is based on a shift in the isoenzyme pattern of myosin in the direction of isoenzyme V_3, is accompanied by a decrease in unloaded shortening velocity but an increase in the efficiency of tension development, as is reflected in reduced oxygen consumption (per wall stress and heart rate) of the whole heart under isovolumetric conditions. This change in the elementary contractile process and the myofibrillar ATPase activity need not be interpreted a priori as negative. However, the ability to adapt to other types of loading, e.g., physical exertion with corresponding increase in heart rate, is limited by the specialization for coping with enhanced pressure load. The term "overadaptation" should be reserved for stages and degrees of hypertrophy in which the negative effects of double-faced alterations predominate. Rapid, excessive increase in pressure loading, as well as long-term hemodynamic overloading, leads to degenerative alterations of the myocardium. At the level of the whole ventricle, structural dilatation results in a decreased cardiac efficiency. Fibrosis of the ventricular wall, the pathogenesis of which is not always unequivocal, is also a negative factor for mechanical performance. Since there are pronounced degrees of hypertrophy without connective tissue increase, e.g., in thyrotoxicosis, fibrosis and accompanying decreased distensibility of the myocardium apparently are not necessarily involved in the development of hypertrophy. Ischemically induced alterations stemming from vasculopathy should be distinguished from hypertrophy-induced changes. The adaptive alteration of the heart in swim-trained rats, which involves an increase in myofibrillar ATPase activity and a shift in the myosin isoenzyme pattern in the direction of V_1, leads to an increase in functional capacity at all levels and is in agreement with the generally accepted concept of contractility.

Chronically increased hemodynamic loading of the heart leads to structural and functional alterations that include a variably pronounced increase in myocardial mass. As a rule, heart enlargement reflects the growth of individual cells (37). Hypertrophy permits enhancement of the absolute performance of the organ in accordance with the altered requirements. A period of compensation, however, is often followed by contractile failure. Thus, the question of the extent to which the hypertrophy process itself comprises the cause of cardiac insufficiency has been a continuous source of discussion in the literature (1,3,6,8–10,16,25,30,38,44–46,56,58,59). Recently, attempts have been made to distinguish "physiological" from "pathological" forms of hypertrophy (62) or from overadaptation (46) as early as the compensatory stage. The criteria of such discrimination, however, seem to require further reflection.

The aim of the present study has been to attempt to characterize adaptive and pathological phenomena inherent to or accompanying the process of cardiac hypertrophy on the basis of our own investigations of several experimental animal models during the stabilized stage of hypertrophy and the stage of preinsufficiency. The study is based on investigations by our group in recent years (14,20,23,26–29,31,32,34–36,42,43,51,52,61) as well as some newer unpublished results. With the above goal in mind, we analyzed results obtained from cardiac hypertrophy induced by Goldblatt hypertension, spontaneous hypertension, experimental aortic stenosis, swimming training, and experimental thyrotoxicosis. In view of the large number of alterations reported in the detailed studies of other authors (1,6,8,17,33,40,44,45,54), we have to restrict our comments to a few selected examples at the whole-ventricular, tissue, single-cell, and biochemical levels. The discussion of the findings will necessarily include some fundamental considerations concerning the definition and characterization of adaptive and pathological phenomena.

MATERIALS AND METHODS

Models of Hypertrophy

Most of the investigations dealt with the pressure-hypertrophied myocardium of Goldblatt rats. In young male Wistar rats (body weight 140–170 g), arterial hypertension (180–200 mm Hg) leading to left ventricular hypertrophy was induced by constricting the left renal artery under ether narcosis (Goldblatt II). Measurements were performed 4, 6, 8, 12–13, and 24 weeks after the operation. Details of the operation technique and plethysmographic measurement of arterial blood pressure have been reported (31,35). A further group of Wistar rats of the same body weight was subjected to coarctation of the ascending aorta directly distal to the aortic valve. The inner vessel diameter was reduced with a silk thread to 50–60% of the original value. The rats were sacrificed 5–7 weeks or 20 weeks after operation for measurement of mechanical and biochemical parameters.

Spontaneously hypertensive rats were used primarily for measurements of myocardial distensibility at the ages of 40 and 80 weeks. Systolic blood pressure was 150–170 mm Hg.

Several groups of Sprague–Dawley and Wistar rats (body weight 140–360 g) were subjected to long-term physical training. Swimming training lasted 6–8 or 12–13 weeks, 2 hr daily; one group of Wistar rats was trained 1.5 hr twice daily.

In order to produce cardiac hypertrophy caused by thyrotoxicosis, male Wistar rats (initial weight 110–160 g) were treated with L-thyroxine by daily injections over a period of 2 weeks (0.1 mg/100 g body weight in the first and 1 mg/100 g body weight in the second week).

All animals were provided with a standard dry meal (ssniff®, Intermast GmbH, Soest, FRG) and tap water ad libitum.

Measurement of Left Ventricular Dynamics in Situ

After the chest was opened under urethane anesthesia (1.2 g/kg body weight), an electromagnetic flow probe was placed around the aortic trunk. Central systemic pressure was measured using a cannula in the left carotid artery, and the left ventricle was pierced at the apex with a double-barreled cannula for pressure and volume measurements. One bore was connected to a Statham P23 Db pressure transducer; the other was attached to a syringe, the piston of which was coupled to a potentiometer for recording volume changes; left ventricular end-diastolic volume was measured using a modified method of Ullrich et al. (60) as described previously (20,29,35). Individual volume values were read from the end-diastolic pressure–volume relationships measured at the end of each experiment. Isovolumetric contractions were obtained by brief occlusions of the ascending aorta in order to permit construction of the active isovolumetric pressure–volume curves. The end-diastolic volume of the left ventricle was varied by gradual obstruction of the inferior vena cava. Systolic left ventricular pressure (P), the rate of left ventricular pressure rise (dP/dt), diastolic left ventricular pressure (EDP; high sensitivity), aortic flow, and volume changes (ΔV) were simultaneously recorded (seven-channel recorder, Hellige).

Assuming a thick-walled sphere, wall stress (σ) was calculated as average stress using the following formula with intraventricular pressure (P), intraventricular volume (V), and ventricular weight (W) (20):

$$\bar{\sigma} = P/\{[(V + W)V]^{2/3} - 1\}$$

and as midwall stress:

$$\sigma_R = (VP/W) \{1 + 4(V + W)/[V^{1/3} + (V + W)^{1/3}]^3\}$$

The elastic tangent modulus of the midwall region was calculated according to the formula:

$$E_R = 3\left\{\frac{VP}{W} - \sigma_R + \left[\frac{\sigma_R}{V} + \frac{W\sigma_R - VP}{W(V + W)} + \frac{\sigma_R}{P}\frac{dP}{dV}\right]\frac{V^{1/3} + (V + W)^{1/3}}{V^{-2/3} + (V + W)^{-2/3}}\right\}$$

Oxygen consumption was measured in a recently developed in situ heart preparation under substantially isovolumetric conditions after clamping of the ascending aorta by using the arteriovenous oxygen difference (Lex O_2 Con) and pulmonary flow which corresponds to coronary flow in this preparation (34).

Measurement of Myocardial Mechanics in the Isolated Strip Preparation

These experiments were carried out on trabecular preparations from the rear wall of the left ventricle. The muscle strips were fixed in a measuring apparatus described previously (14). A temperature-controlled Tyrode solution was used for perfusion (concentration in mM: glucose 25, NaCl 130.5, KCl 4.9, $CaCl_2$ 2.2, NaH_2PO_4 0.8, $NaHCO_3$ 20.0). The solution was constantly bubbled with 95% O_2 and 5% CO_2 (pH 7.4). The temperature was set at 25°C or 32°C depending on the subject of the experiment.

Length–tension relationship were recorded by shortening the muscle strip by 0.1 mm every 30 sec beginning at l_{max}, the muscle length at which developed tension is maximum. Stress (σ) was calculated (F/A) and related to strain (ϵ) which was evaluated by $(l - l_0)/l_0$. The muscle length at zero stress is l_0, which was measured after recording of the third length–tension relationship in each experiment. The tangent elastic modulus ($\Delta\sigma/\Delta\epsilon$) was also calculated for each measured point of the length–tension relationship and related to stress, σ or $[\epsilon = b\cdot(\sigma - c)]$.

Under steady-state conditions, the isometric length–tension relationships were recorded, and the force–velocity relationships were determined from afterloaded contractions as well as from isometric and isotonic quick-release experiments (14,31,32).

Furthermore, trabecular preparations were glycerinated for at least 30 min. Quick-release experiments were performed after activation using solutions with defined Ca^{2+} concentrations at 6.5°C. The shortening velocity was plotted as a function of sarcomere length which was measured as an average of 10 sarcomeres using a light microscope (5,26).

Biochemical Investigations

Tissue weight and content of basic constituents were determined, and proteins were fractionated. The hydroxyproline concentration was measured in samples of 1–50 mg dry weight (42). The actomyosin solution was extracted from single left ventricles and purified by the dilution technique. Myofibrillar ATPase activity and Ca^{2+} ATPase activity of myosin were determined by measuring the liberation of inorganic phosphate (43,52).

Polyacrylamide gel electrophoresis in pyrophosphate was carried out at 2°C at 10 $V \cdot cm^{-1}$ for approximately 20 hr. The gel contained 3.8% acrylamide and 0.12% N,N'-methylene-bis-acrylamide. The electrophoresis buffer was 20 mM $Na_4P_2O_7$ (pH 8.8) in the presence of 10% glyercol (21). Myosin for the electrophoresis was extracted from small pieces of ventricles with 40 mM $Na_4P_2O_7$ (pH 8.8), 1 mM 1,4-dithioerythritol, 5 mM EGTA.

Morphological and Electrophysiological Investigations

The morphological and electrophysiological findings discussed in the present study have been reported by Wendt-Gallitelli et al. (61) and Gülch et al. (12,13).

The degree of hypertrophy is defined as the ratio of left ventricular weight of the hypertrophied heart to left ventricular weight of age-matched controls at a given body weight (13).

RESULTS AND DISCUSSION

Alterations at the Whole-Heart Level: Ventricular Configuration, Pressure–Volume Relations, Wall Stress

The characteristics of ventricular mass and configuration (inset silhouette sketches) and typical isovolumetric pressure–volume relationships are presented in Figure 1 for different forms of chronic loading. Pressure-induced left ventricular mass increase is manifested as the concentric form of hypertrophy in experimental aortic stenosis (Figure 1A) and in the 8-week stage of Goldblatt hypertension (Figure 1C). The "athletic heart" from swimming training reveals signs of harmonic growth corresponding more to the volume type of hypertrophy (Figure 1B). The anatomic configuration is reflected in the end-diastolic pressure–volume diagrams. The pressure-loaded ventricles of Goldblatt rats in the 8-week stage after operation as well as of rats subjected to aortic stenosis (Figures 1C, 1A) show a slight steepening of the resting tension curves. The 4-week stage of Goldblatt hypertension, however, involves a mixed pressure- and volume-induced form of hypertrophy with increased diastolic ventricular capacity (see Figure 4A), correlating well with the temporarily increased circulating blood volume (29,35). Swim-trained rats—with less pronounced myocardial mass increase—also have a significantly flatter resting tension curve (Figure 1C).

With the exception of the 24-week stage of Goldblatt hypertension (Figure 1D), the curves of total pressure are shifted significantly upwards in all models and stages. Thus, the distance between end-diastolic and sys-

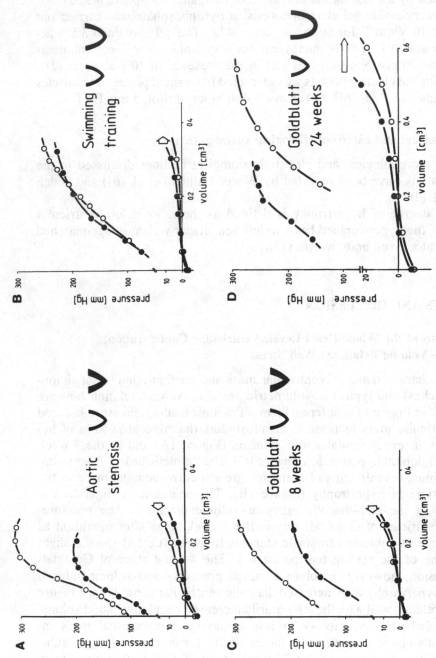

Figure 1. Isovolumetric pressure–volume relationships and schematic configuration of the hypertrophied left ventricle of the rat. Averaged data of 10–20 hypertrophic ventricles (○), and the same number of age-matched controls (●). A. Experimental aortic stenosis 7 weeks after operation; degree of left ventricular hypertrophy 20%. B. Swimming training for 13 weeks; degree of hypertrophy 15%. C. Goldblatt hypertension 8 weeks after operation; degree of hypertrophy 45%. D. Goldblatt hypertension 24 weeks; degree of hypertrophy 55%.

tolic pressure–volume curves is increased, reflecting enhanced working capacity of the whole ventricle during the stabilized stage of hypertrophy.

As shown by the pressure–volume loops (Figure 2) the pressure-loaded heart pumps a stroke volume that corresponds approximately to control values despite increased afterload on the whole ventricle. Stroke work and power are increased, as is the rate of pressure rise (*dP/dt*), the maximum rate of ejection being normal at this stage.

Thus, geometric configuration and pressure–volume relationships simply and convincingly show that the heart adapts structurally and functionally to the altered loading conditions. The concentric hypertrophy of the left ventricle is of advantage in transforming developed wall stress into pressure, as can be derived from the equation of Laplace. In contrast, the eccentric form of the left ventricle in swim-trained rats complies with the necessity of being able to expel a temporarily increased stroke volume and cardiac output.

Negative effects of mass increase per se were not detectable in examination of cardiac dynamics at the degrees of hypertrophy (maximally 100%) observed in our animals.

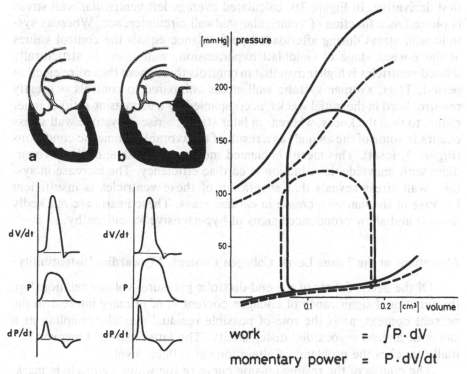

Figure 2.   Cardiac dynamics in pressure-induced left ventricular hypertrophy. The semischematic presentation is based on findings from the 8-week stage of Goldblatt hypertension (b) and age-matched controls (a). Pressure–volume loops are constructed with the aid of systolic volume values derived from (electromagnetic) flow measurements.

In particular, remarkable loss of mechanical energy due to interfascicular frictional or deformational resistances could be substantially excluded on the basis of the plot of the isovolumetric pressure–volume curve and the end-systolic pressure–volume coordinates. If ischemia or energy deficit play a role in the genesis of fibrosis in Goldblatt rat myocardium (see the following section) these factors hardly result from myocardial mass increase per se. However, danger to subendocardial muscle layers from inadequate growth of the vascular bed must be considered, even in cases of moderately increased muscle mass and particularly under physical exercise (22,57).

The situation is quite different in the 24-week stage of Goldblatt hypertension when some of the animals reveal pronounced augmentation of left ventricular inner diameter with, however, inadequate increase in myocardial mass (Figure 1D). Strictly speaking, the term "ventricular dilatation" is reserved by us for this type of configuration. Accordingly, the corresponding pressure–volume relations are shifted significantly to the right, both in diastole and systole. Although indications of congestive heart failure are not present, and end-diastolic pressure is still in the normal range, end-diastolic and end-systolic volumes are increased, the ejection fraction being significantly reduced (Figure 3A), as are maximum flow rate and its first derivative. In Figure 3B, calculated average left ventricular wall stress is plotted as a function of ventricular midwall circumference. Whereas systolic wall stress during afterloaded performance equals the control values at the 8-week stage of Goldblatt hypertension, wall stress in structurally dilated ventricles is higher than that in controls throughout the entire ejection period. Thus, average systolic wall stress compared to controls is greatly renormalized in the initial weeks, accompanied by a decreasing ratio of inner radius to wall thickness, whereas in later stages, a rise in systolic wall stress occurs in some of the animals as a result of unfavorable geometric conditions (Figure 3, inset). This means enhanced mechanical loading of the myocardium with unavoidable reduction in cardiac efficiency. The increase in systolic wall stress reveals that adaptation of these ventricles is insufficient because of the limited increase in cardiac mass. These hearts are markedly fibrotic and show pronounced signs of hypertensive vasculopathy.

Alterations at the Tissue Level: Collagen Content, Myocardial Distensibility

Of the determinants of the end-diastolic pressure–volume relationship, the functional significance of collagen content is of primary interest in the present context, as is the role of possible residual diastolic coupling as a cause of altered myocardial distensibility. The latter aspect, however, actually touches the problems of alterations at cellular level.

The course of the resting tension curve of the whole ventricle is markedly influenced by anatomic size, form, and wall thickness. Thus, only limited conclusions about the passive properties of myocardial tissue can be made on the basis of end-diastolic pressure–volume relationships alone.

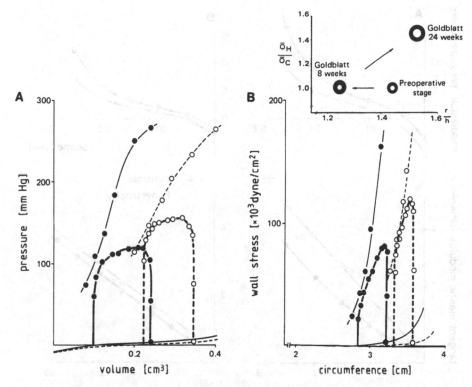

Figure 3. Unfavorable geometric conditions in the state of preinsufficiency. (A) Left ventricular isovolumetric pressure–volume relationships and pressure–volume loops of a Goldblatt heart in the 24-week stage with ventricular dilatation and an age-matched control. Pressure–volume loops were constructed with the aid of systolic volume values derived from (electromagnetic) flow measurements. (B) Mean wall stress calculated from the data of A, assuming a thick-walled spherical shell, is plotted as a function of the circumference at the middle of the ventricular wall. Inset: Wall stress (as related to age-matched controls) as a function of the radius/wall thickness ratio in various stages. (●) Control animal: body weight 450 g; left ventricular weight 0.872 g. (○) Goldblatt rat: body weight 400 g; left ventricular weight 1.119 g.

Figure 4 shows typical left ventricular diastolic pressure–volume diagrams of the swimming rat and the Goldblatt rat at the 4-week stage. In both cases, the resting tension curve is flatter than the curve of age-matched controls. However, when the calculated tangent elastic modulus is related to wall stress, it becomes apparent that the distensibility of ventricular wall tissue is not increased in either model. In fact, the elastic modulus is even increased in renal hypertension, whereas there is no significant change in the athletic heart.

With regard to the passive tissue properties, investigation of isolated linear muscle preparations is much more informative. In principle, reduced myocardial distensibility can be attributed to distinctly different causes as

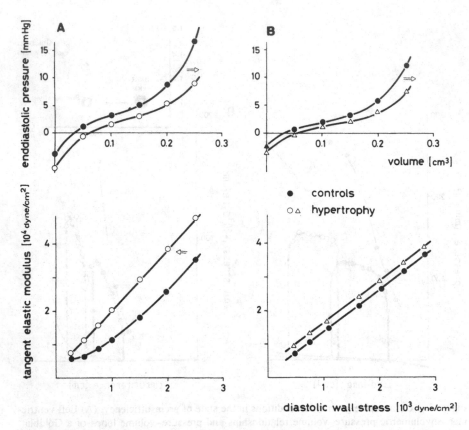

Figure 4.   End-diastolic pressure–volume relationships and calculated (midwall) elastic modulus/wall stress relations in two models of cardiac hypertrophy. Each curve is based on averaged data of ten hypertrophic ventricles and ten controls. (A) Goldblatt rats, 4-week stage; degree of hypertrophy 40%. (B) Swimming rats after a training period of 7 weeks; degree of hypertrophy 15%.

shown by our preparatory work with experimental models (23). The "fibrosis type" is characterized by a steep slope of the relationship between stress and tangent elastic modulus. The "contracture type" is observed, for example, in caffeine–Ca^{2+} contracture or in hypoxic contracture. In this case, with residual diastolic coupling, apparently every additionally recruited interaction site leads to a proportional increase in stress and elastic modulus, and thus the elastic modulus–stress plot under contracture cannot be separated from the control curve.

In Figure 5, the resting-tension curve, elastic modulus–stress relationship, and hydroxyproline concentration in different models of experimental hypertrophy are presented. Neither parameter reveals significant alterations in swimming rats or in experimental hyperthyroidism. Thus, both whole-ventricular determination (Figure 4) and direct measurements on native linear muscle preparations reveal that the increase in diastolic ventricular volume of the athletic heart can be exclusively attributed to muscle fiber growth and cannot be caused by decreased myocardial tone.

Apparently, increased stiffness is primarily a result of augmented connective tissue content. Although the cause may ultimately be the same, we can distinguish between two pathways of development in agreement with the observations of Hatt et al. in other models (16).

In Goldblatt hypertension, cell degeneration, necrosis, and fibrotic alterations are often manifested at an early stage because of the quick and excessive increase in pressure loading and, at least in part, hypertensive vasculopathy. In this connection, it is important to note that the most pronounced increase in connective tissue has been reported under long-term adaption to simulated altitude (4). Perivascular edema could also play a role in connective tissue formation (U. Helmchen, personal communication, 1980). In a portion of our Goldblatt animals primarily perivascular—yet frequently also diffuse—connective tissue augmentation, enhanced vascular

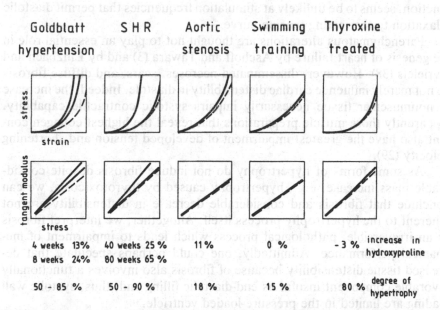

Figure 5.   Stress–strain relationships, tangent modulus–stress relationships, and hydroxyproline concentrations in various models of cardiac hypertrophy. The individual graphs and data are based on the mean values of myocardium from ten hypertrophied ventricles and ten age-matched controls. Hydroxyproline concentration was determined in the corresponding left ventricles (S.D. *ca.* 10% of the mean values). Concentration of hydroxyproline of the control ventricle corresponds to 100%. Goldblatt hypertension: In early stages diastolic distensibility can be unchanged or already decreased. Spontaneous hypertension: Controls were provided by normal Sprague–Dawley rats at the same age (SuT: SDT strain, Süddeutsche Versuchstierfarm, Tuttlingen, FRG). Aortic stenosis: 7 weeks after operation. Swimming training: 2 hr daily for 10 weeks. Thyrotoxicosis: Injections of L-thyroxine over a period of 2 weeks; for doses see Methods.

wall thickness, and correspondingly increased hydroxyproline concentration occurred as early as 4–8 weeks after operation (Figure 5). In such cases, the slope of the elastic modulus–stress relation (y) correlated reasonably well with the hydroxyproline concentration (x); e.g., in a group of 12 Goldblatt rats at the 8-week stage and 12 age-matched controls: $y = 7.65 x - 2.58$; $r = 0.69$.

Relatively pronounced scattering is not surprising when one considers that the hydroxyproline content was determined from tissue samples of the corresponding ventricle and not from the actual strip preparation used for mechanical investigations. In the 24-week stage, fibrosis is usually marked and myocardial distensibility considerably reduced.

In contrast to Goldblatt rats, cardiosclerosis in spontaneously hypertensive rats occurs much later without comparable vascular alterations and may be assigned to the onset of Meerson's stage 3 (44).

A functional component of decreased distensibility was substantially ruled out by the type of elastic modulus–stress relationship and by experiments designed to lower myoplasmic Ca^{2+} concentration (26). Thus, diastolic residual coupling, as results from impairment of sarcoplasmic reticulum function, seems to be unlikely at stimulation frequencies that permit diastolic relaxation to the resting tension curve.

Parenchymatous alterations are thought not to play an essential role in the genesis of heart failure by Aschoff and Tawara (3) and by Linzbach and Kyrieleis (38). However, disseminated necroses, scars, and diffuse fibrosis do not merely influence cardiac distensibility in diastole. Indeed, the increase in nonmuscular tissue necessarily impairs systolic contractile capability. Apparently those muscle preparations that reveal the highest collagen content also have the greatest impairment of developed tension and shortening velocity (29).

As some forms of hypertrophy do not induce fibrosis despite considerable mass increase, e.g., hypertrophy caused by thyrotoxicosis, we can conclude that fibrosis and considerable decrease in distensibility are not inherent to the hypertrophy process itself. Altogether, we interpret fibrosis as an irreversible, pathological process which leads to impairment of mechanical performance. Admittedly, one could perhaps speculate that decreased tissue distensibility because of fibrosis also involves a functionally favorable component insofar as end-diastolic filling and, thus, systolic wall loading are limited in the pressure-loaded ventricle.

Alterations at the Cellular Level: Action Potential, Excitation–Contraction Coupling, Proportion of Cell Constituents

Alterations in hypertrophied cardiac muscle fibers are not restricted merely to cell dimensions (61). There are qualitative and quantitative changes in nearly all functionally relevant parts of the cell.

Functional alterations of the surface membrane and sarcoplasmic reticulum membranes influence the action potential and excitation–contraction coupling. In contrast to swimming rat hearts, the myocardium of pressure-loaded ventricles shows marked prolongation of the action potential and the so-called Ca^{2+} action potential (13). There are corresponding differences in action potential shape within the normal nonhypertrophic heart which apparently depend on regional wall load (12). The prolonged action potential causes longer activation with corresponding lengthening of time to peak tension and probably increased Ca^{2+} influx. Thus, the action potential contributes to those characteristic features of contraction in the pressure-hypertrophied myocardium that we tend to view as adaptive. As with other phenomena inherent to hypertrophy, however, prolongation of the action potential can have a negative effect under certain conditions. For example, in isolated Goldblatt myocardium, incomplete relaxation appears at high stimulation frequencies, more because of a prolonged time to peak than a reduction in the rate of relaxation (29).

Inner membranes are also involved in the process of hypertrophy. In agreement with measurements of Page et al. (47), our findings in Goldblatt rat myocardium suggest that the quantitative increase in the T-tubule membranes may compensate for the relative decrease of surface membrane area. Indications of altered Ca^{2+} transport function of sarcoplasmic reticulum ensue from the change in the shape of the isometric mechanogram, e.g., more rapid relaxation of the swim-trained-rat myocardium, delayed initial tension rise, and slight tendency towards slower relaxation in Goldblatt myocardium (31,32). This interpretation agrees with reports on determination of Ca^{2+} transport ATPase of the sarcoplasmic reticulum (8,18,44,48). However, even in barely fibrotic preparations of Goldblatt myocardium at the 24-week stage, experimental improvement of electromechanical coupling (increase in Ca^{2+} and decrease in Na^+ concentration) does not increase the reduced mechanical parameters to the same level attained by correspondingly treated controls (27,29). This suggests that impairment of Ca^{2+} activation because of disturbances of excitation–contraction coupling is not the decisive detrimental factor in the Goldblatt model of cardiac hypertrophy.

Alterations of intracellular proportions are especially relevant to the topic of the present chapter. The proportion of myofibrillar volume to total cell volume was increased in the pressure-hypertrophied myocardium of Goldblatt rats (with the exception of the immediately postoperative stage), e.g., from 59% to 63% in the 4-week stage and to 71% after 24 weeks (61). Accordingly, the relative proportion of mitochondria is reduced (50,61) although this reduction may be compensated for by an increased mitochondrial number according to Hatt et al. (16). In addition to the prolonged activation and presumably altered cross-bridge kinetics (see following section), the relative increase in contractile material per unit area contributes to the increased isometric tension development in nonfibrotic Goldblatt myocardium during the early compensatory stage.

The adequacy of classifying such alterations in intracellular proportions as "overadaptation" will be discussed in the concluding section.

Regressive mitochondrial alterations were generally observed only in Goldblatt rats in which cell necroses and marked fibrosis were also present. As shown by investigations of other authors, regressive alterations of various cell organelles are not necessarily the result of hypertensive vasculopathy in hypertrophic myocardium, particularly in rapidly induced and excessive or long-lasting overload (16,44).

Alterations at the Level of Biochemical Structures: Myofibrillar ATPase Activity and Isoenzyme Pattern of Myosin, Unloaded Shortening Velocity and Elementary Isometric Force, Efficiency of Force Development

A current example of hypertrophy-induced alterations at the molecular level and their consequences for myocardial mechanics is provided by changes in myosin structure.

In renal hypertension and aortic stenosis, cardiac myofibrillar ATPase activity is decreased by approximately 30% (Figure 6) in contrast to the approximately 10% increase in swimming rat myocardium. Maximum unloaded shortening velocity changes in the same direction as, and to an extent comparably to, myofibrillar enzyme activity in both cases.

Figure 6 indicates that the causes of reduced maximum shortening velocity in pressure-hypertrophied myocardium can definitely be found in the contractile apparatus itself. Investigations on glycerinated, nonfibrotic fibers permitted the exclusion of membrane effects. Unloaded shortening velocity was estimated both under full activation and using another methodological approach which considers an internal load by extrapolating the shortening–length plots of different Ca^{2+} concentrations to the starting length (5). According to both methods, mechanical V_{max} is reduced by approximately 30%, which corresponds to the decrease in myofibrillar ATPase activity.

Apparently, enzyme activity of contractile proteins is related to changes in the myosin isoenzyme pattern. According to Hoh et al. (21), myosin from rat ventricular myocardium can be separated into three isoenzymes by gel electrophoresis in the presence of pyrophosphate. As shown in Figure 7, during Goldblatt hypertension, the isoenzyme pattern is shifted towards V_3, the isoenzyme of lowest mobility. This is in accordance with the findings of Lompre et al. in several other models of pressure-induced hypertrophy (39). An opposite redistribution was found following swimming training, in which V_1 predominated (52). A redistribution in the direction of V_3 (and V_2) results in decreased ATPase activity. In contrast, relative increase in V_1 enhances ATPase activity.

The existing isoenzyme pattern may explain the relatively slight capacity for increasing myofibrillar ATPase activity and mechanical V_{max} in the rat under swimming training on the one hand and the marked capacity for decreasing both parameters under chronic pressure load on the other

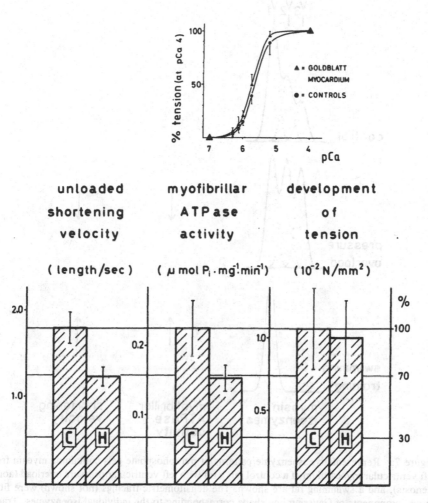

Figure 6.   Mechanical parameters and myofibrillar ATPase activity of Goldblatt rat myocardium 6 weeks after operation (degree of hypertrophy, 57%) in comparison with data of age-matched control ventricles (mean $\pm$ S.D.; C: N = 8; H: N = 8). Maximum unloaded shortening velocity of the glycerinated preparations was obtained by extrapolating the length–velocity relationships at different pCa values to the starting length of the respective quick releases (5) (mean sarcomere length: 2.15 μm). Tension was measured in the steady-state of force development of the glycerinated trabeculae at saturating free [Ca^{2+}]. Myofibrillar ATPase activity was determined in the same ventricles from which the trabeculae were dissected. Inset: Developed tension as a function of pCa in the bathing solution. Each point and vertical bar represent the mean and the standard deviation of eight different experiments. The Ca^{2+} for half-maximum activation as well as the coefficient n (C = 2.0; H = 2.2) of the Hill equation do not differ significantly between groups. Length and cross-sectional area of the preparations in both groups were: C = control, 1.80 $\pm$ 0.50 mm, 0.0642 $\pm$ 0.0010 mm^2; H = Goldblatt myocardium, 1.75 $\pm$ 0.41 mm; 0.0650 $\pm$ 0.0031 mm^2.

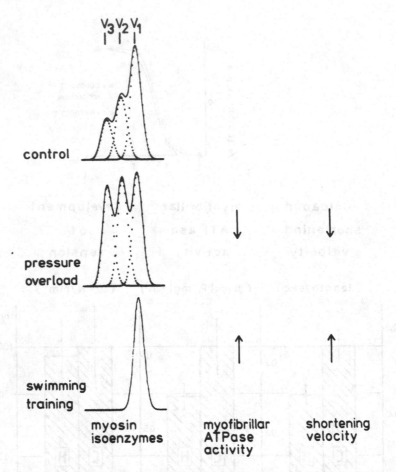

Figure 7.   Representative isoenzyme patterns of pyrophosphate gels containing myosin from left ventricular myocardium of a control rat, a rat with left ventricular pressure overload (aortic stenosis), and a swimming rat are shown. The densitometric tracings (not shown) were fit to three components of Gaussian line shape corresponding to the individual isoenzymes. Traces of V_2 and V_3 were detectable in more concentrated samples from swimming rat myocardium but are not shown in the simulated isoenzyme pattern. The degree of hypertrophy was 25% in aortic stenosis measured 20 weeks after operation and 28% in the swimming rat myocardium (190 hr training over 13 weeks).

hand. The capacity for increasing is limited because the existing isoenzyme pattern in the rat under control conditions already causes high values of both parameters. Thus, the isoenzyme pattern, which depends on species, age, and individual case history, apparently determines the potential adaptive range of contractile proteins under chronically altered loading or altered endocrine status (thyroxine).

In contrast to unloaded shortening velocity, isometric tension corresponds to control values in aortic stenosis and is even significantly increased in Goldblatt myocardium at the 4-week and 8-week stages, and thus, the force–velocity relationship, plotted on the basis of afterloaded contractions, reveals intersection of Goldblatt and control curves. Both shortening velocity and tension development show a decrease during the 24-week observation period (27,29,31).

Our original explanation for the deviating behavior of isometric tension was based on the prolongation of activation and on the relative increase of contractile material and thereby the number of interaction sites in nonfibrotic preparations (13,27,61). This explanation requires, however, that elementary tension development not decrease in accordance with the reduced myofibrillar ATPase activity.

Of particular interest in this regard, and with regard to the central topic of this chapter, is the behavior of mechanical tension when membrane effects have been eliminated. Under maximum Ca^{2+} activation, the alteration of tension development in nonfibrotic preparations is not significant at the 6-week stage of Goldblatt hypertension (Figure 6) (even considering a slight increase in myofibrillar content), as also shown by Henry et al. (19) and Maughan et al. (41) for other models of pressure-induced hypertrophy. The shape of the activation curve (Figure 6, inset) and the plot of myofibrillar ATPase activity as a function of $[Ca^{2+}]$ (51) suggest the lack of a change in Ca^{2+} sensitivity and cooperativity.

The discrepancy between the behavior of V_{max} and developed tension (Figure 6) may be explained by an alteration of cross-bridge kinetics as a result of the altered isoenzyme pattern. Measurements of oxygen consumption in the isovolumetrically beating whole ventricle are consistent with Alpert's (2) interpretation of improved efficiency of tension development. In aortic stenosis, oxygen consumption for any given calculated wall tension, heart rate, and muscle mass was found to be significantly lower than in age-matched controls (Figure 8). The same tendency is suggested in Goldblatt rat myocardium, although the difference was not statistically significant (34).

With one exception (11), primarily normal or increased values for oxygen consumption of the pressure-loaded heart are reported in the literature (7,15,53,57). Aside from substantial scattering of the data obtained under clinical conditions, the discrepancy between other authors and the results of Figure 8 may be explained by the following points: (a) Oxygen consumption is related to different parameters (pressure, stress, etc.). (b) It is conceivable that the decrease in oxygen consumption may only be detectable under isovolumetric conditions. (c) In view of the species-dependent isoenzyme pattern of myosin, the decrease in the rat is probably more pronounced than in other animals. (d) Other factors, e.g., at the level of mitochondria (15,53), could be superimposed on alterations at the myofibrillar level.

Thus, the functional importance of alterations of myofibrillar ATPase

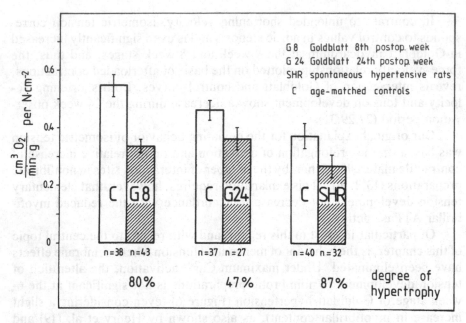

Figure 8. Oxygen consumption of the normal and pressure-hypertrophied rat heart in situ (with isometrically beating left ventricle) as related to averaged developed wall stress and heart rate.

activity and the elementary contractile process in pressure-hypertrophied hearts is equivocal. In any case, however, a decrease in shortening velocity should not be interpreted a priori as a sign of damage as would be suggested by the generally accepted concept of contractility (24,25). Although my-ocardial power decreases with reduction in V_{max}, and the isoenzyme pattern resembles that of aged rats, the underlying energy-saving alteration of cross-bridge kinetics is not incompatible with the concept of an adaptive process. Quick shortening under conditions of low loading would not be of any ad-vantage to chronically pressure-loaded myocardium. Furthermore, when considered from the viewpoint of comparative physiology, slow muscle is not inferior to fast muscle in principle. Experiments designed to transform fast skeletal muscle into slow muscle by altering the stimulation pattern (49) reveal that adaptation involving reduction of myofibrillar ATPase and me-chanical V_{max} need not be interpreted exclusively as the consequence of pathological disorder of protein turnover. Apparently new functional de-mands lead to an activation of genes that are not expressed to the same extent in the normal animal.

Reduction in ATPase activity and shortening velocity, however, are definitely unfavorable when high heart rates appear under physical exertion or emotional stress. Considerable reduction of both parameters may also be predominantly unfavorable in late stages of chronic loading.

CONCLUSIONS

As has become apparent in the preceding considerations, classification of alterations as adaptive implies an interpretation and an evaluation that are ultimately rooted in a teleological viewpoint. The suitability for coping with the altered functional requirements should be recognizable, at least in principle. Another possible criterion, reversibility, should be considered with caution, e.g., with regard to connective tissue reactions. Important insight may be forthcoming from comparative physiology and morphology (ontogenesis, regeneration, phylogenesis, adaptive and hypertrophic alterations of other organs, particularly skeletal muscle, including comparison of different species).

Problems do not arise in the interpretation of adaptive alterations resulting from physical training, because increased capacity of performance results at every level without contradicting the generally accepted concept of "contractility" (24,55). Evaluation of various alterations in chronic pressure loading is much more difficult, however. Increased pressure load of the heart leads to reactions of which mass increase of myocardium leading to renormalization of systolic wall stress represents the most obvious component. Even the consequences of regular compensatory hypertrophy, however, are ambivalent. Specilization for one type of loading, e.g., increased systemic pressure, necessarily narrows the capacity for adaptation to other requirements such as increased heart rate under physical exertion.

Furthermore, an alteration which is advantageous for mechanical performance may be unfavorable from the viewpoint of energetics, and vice versa, as pointed out in Table 1. This dilemma is extreme in overadaptation (table 2) a term which we do not apply to every hypertrophy-induced change in the proportion of cell constituents but rather reserve for those stages in

Table 1. Ambiguity of Adaptive Alterations in the Compensated Stage

Alterations	Consequences	
	Positive	Negative

Ventricular level
  Mass increase, alteration in
  configuration
	Increase in ventricular work
	and power, normalization
	of wall stress
		Reduction in coronary
		reserve, endangering of
		subendocardial layers in
		particular

Cellular level
  Prolongation of action
  potential, relative increase
  in contractile material
	(Relative) Improvement of
	developed tension
		Incomplete relaxation at
		high frequencies,
		endangering of energy
		production

Level of biochemical structures
  Alteration in cross-bridge
  kinetics, decrease in
  myofibrillar ATPase activity
	Increase in efficiency of
	tension development
		Decrease in unloaded
		shortening velocity and
		myofibrillar power

Table 2.   Hypertrophy in Chronic Pressure Load

Regular course of adaptation	Ambivalent, predominantly positive consequences
Overadaptation	Predominantly negative consequences
Disordered adaptation	Malformations, e.g., dislocation of contractile material
Inadequate adaptation and regressive alterations	Primary: Protein deficiency, incretory imbalance, (toxic) damage to genetic apparatus
	Secondary: Exhaustion of protein and nucleic acid synthesis: Energy deficiency

which the negative consequences predominate and clear functional disadvantages are present.

In addition, the process of adaptation can be disordered, leading, for example, to dislocated contractile material; or the process can be inadequate from the onset or—typically—in later stages. Under long-term or excessive overload, inadequate adaptation but also genuinely degenerative alterations may be interpreted as resulting from exhaustion of the genetic apparatus and from energy deficiency without or with vascular damage. Such alterations naturally have negative effects; the same applies to marked fibrosis, although its pathogenesis is not always unequivocal. Consequences of vasculopathy per se are not inherent to myocardial hypertrophy and should be regarded as accompanying alterations.

In sum, it is hardly possible to distinguish between "physiological" and "pathological" hypertrophy, particularly when considering only a single biochemical parameter such as myofibrillar ATPase activity or a certain pattern of isoenzymes of myosin. Since adaptive alterations may reveal negative effects in certain situations and stages of hypertrophy, "adaptive" and "pathological" reactions need not be mutually exclusive. It is also apparent that a teleological view is of limited value, although it may be stimulating. Real progress, however, requires careful analysis of the causal relationships.

ACKNOWLEDGMENT

This research was supported by the Deutsche Forschungsgemeinschaft (Ja 172/11).

REFERENCES

1. Alpert, N. R. 1973. Myosin ATPase-activity and mechanical performance in normal and hypertrophied hearts. In: H. Roskamm and H. Reindell (eds.), *Das Chronisch Kranke Herz*, pp. 130–136. Schattauer, Stuttgart, New York.

2. Alpert, N. R., and Mulieri, L. A. 1981. The utilization of energy by the myocardium hypertrophied secondary to pressure overload. In: B. Strauer (ed.), *The Heart in Hypertension*, pp. 153–163. Springer, Berlin, Heidelberg, New York.
3. Aschoff, L., and Tawara, S. 1906. *Die Heutige Lehre von den Pathologisch-Anatomischen Grundlagen der Herzschwache*. G. Fischer, Jena.
4. Bartosova, D., Chvapil, M., Korecky, B., Poupa, O., Rakusan, K., Turek, Z., and Vizek, M. 1969. The growth of the muscular and collagenous parts of the rat heart in various forms of cardiomegaly. *J. Physiol. (Lond.)* 200:285–295.
5. Brenner, B., and Jacob, R. 1980. Calcium activation and maximum unloaded shortening velocity. Investigations on glycerinated skeletal and heart muscle preparations. *Basic Res. Cardiol.* 75:40–46.
6. Buchner, F., and Onishi, S. H. 1970. *Herzhypertrophie und Herzinsuffizienz in der Sicht der Elektronenmikroskopie*. Urban & Schwarzenberg, Munich.
7. Cooper, G., Puga, F. J., Zujko, K. J., Harrison, C. E., and Coleman, H. N. 1973. Normal myocardial function and energetics in volume-overload hypertrophy in the cat. *Circ. Res.* 32:140–148.
8. Dhalla, N. S., Das, P. K., and Sharma, G. P. 1978. Subcellular basis of cardiac contractile failure. *J. Mol. Cell. Cardiol.* 10:363–385.
9. Eppinger, H. 1931. Zur Pathologie der Kreislaufkorrelation. In: A. Bethe (ed.), *Handbuch der Normalen und Pathologischen Physiologie*, Vol. 16/2, pp. 1289–1402. Springer, Berlin.
10. Fleckenstein, A. 1968. Experimentelle Pathologie der akuten und chronischen Herzinsuffizienz. *Verh. Dtsch. Ges. Kreislaufforsch.* 34:15–34.
11. Gamble, W. J., Phornphutkul, C., Jumar, A. E., Sanders, G. L., Manasek, F. J., and Monroe, R. G. 1973. Ventricular performance coronary flow, and MV_{O_2} in aortic coarctation hypertrophy. *Am. J. Physiol.* 224:877–883.
12. Gülch, R. W. 1980. The effect of elevated chronic loading on the action potential of mammalian myocardium. *J. Mol. Cell. Cardiol.* 12:415–420.
13. Gülch, R. W., Baumann, R., and Jacob, R. 1979. Analysis of myocardial action potential in left ventricular hypertrophy of Goldblatt rats. *Basic Res. Cardiol.* 74:69–82.
14. Gülch, R. W., and Jacob, R. 1975. Length–tension diagram and force–velocity relations of mammalian cardiac muscle under steady-state conditions. *Pfluegers Arch.* 355:331–346.
15. Gunning, J. F., and Coleman, H. N. 1973. Myocardial oxygen consumption during experimental hypertrophy and congestive heart failure. *J. Mol. Cell. Cardiol.* 5:25–38.
16. Hatt, P. Y., Jouannot, P., Moravec, J., and Swynghedauw, B. 1974. Current trends in heart hypertrophy. *Basic Res. Cardiol.* 69:479–483.
17. Hatt, P. Y., and Swynghedauw, B. 1968. Electron microscopic study of myocardium in experimental heart insufficiency. In: H. Reindell, J. Keul, and E. Doll (eds.), *Herzinsuffizienz, Pathophysiologie und Klinik*, pp. 19–23. Georg Thieme, Stuttgart.
18. Heilmann, C., Lindl, T., Muller, W., and Pette, D. 1980. Characterization of cardiac microsomes from spontaneously hypertonic rats. *Basic Res. Cardiol.* 75:92–96.
19. Henry, P. D., Ahumada, G. G., Friedman, W. F., and Sobel, B. E. 1972. Simultaneously measured isometric tension and ATP hydrolysis in glycerinated fibers from normal and hypertrophied rabbit heart. *Circ. Res.* 31:740–749.
20. Hepp, A., Hansis, M., Gülch, R., and Jacob, R. 1974. Left ventricular isovolumetric pressure–volume relations, "diastolic tone," and contractility in the rat heart after physical training. *Basic Res. Cardiol.* 69:516–532.
21. Hoh, J. F. Y., McGrath, P. A., and Hale, P. T. 1978. Electrophoretic analysis of multiple forms of rat cardiac myosin: Effects of hypophysectomy and thyroxine replacement. *J. Mol. Cell. Cardiol.* 10:1053–1076.
22. Holtz, J., von Restorff, W., Bard, P., and Bassenge, E. 1977. Transmural distribution of myocardial blood flow and of coronary reserve in canine left ventricular hypertrophy. *Basic Res. Cardiol.* 72:286–292.
23. Holubarsch, C., and Jacob, R. 1979. Evaluation of elastic properties of myocardium. Experimental models of fibrosis and contracture in heart muscle strips. *Z. Kardiol.* 68:123–127.
24. Hugenholtz, P. G., Ellison, R. C., Urschel, C. W., Mirsky, I., and Sonnenblick, E. H.

1970. Myocardial force–velocity relationships in clinical heart disease. *Circulation* 41:191–202.

25. Jacob, R. 1976. Pathophysiologie der Herzmuskelinsuffizienz. In: W. Frommhold (ed.), *Erkrankungen des Herzmuskels*, Vol. 5, *Tubinger Klinisch-Radiologie Seminar*, pp. 25–36. Georg Thieme, Stuttgart.

26. Jacob, R., Brenner, B., Ebrecht, G., Holubarsch, C., and Medugorac, I. 1980. Elastic and contractile properties of the myocardium in experimental cardiac hypertrophy of the rat. Methodological and pathophysiological considerations. *Basic Res. Cardiol.* 75:253–261.

27. Jacob, R., Ebrecht, G., Kämmereit, A., Medugorac, I., and Wendt-Gallitelli, M. F. 1977. Myocardial function in different models of cardiac hypertrophy. An attempt at correlating mechanical, biochemical and morphological parameters. *Basic Res. Cardiol.* 72:160–169.

28. Jacob, R., Kämmereit, A., Medugorac, I., and Wendt-Gallitelli, M. F. 1976. Maximalgeschwindigkeit der lastfreien Verkurzung (V_{max}), myokardiale Lesitungsfahigkeit und "Kontraktilitatsindizes" beim hypertrophierten Myokard. *Z. Kardiol.* 65:392–400.

29. Jacob, R., and Kissling, G. 1981. Left ventricular dynamics and myocardial function in Goldblatt hypertension of the rat. Biochemical, morphological and electrophysiological correlates. In: B. E. Strauer (ed.), *The Heart in Hypertension*, pp. 89–107. Springer, Berlin, Heidelberg, New York.

30. Jacob, R., and Nägle, S. 1969. Pathophysiologie des insuffizienten Herzens. *Hippokrates* 40:817–850.

31. Kämmereit, A., and Jacob, R. 1979. Alterations in rat myocardial mechanics under Goldblatt hypertension and experimental aortic stenosis. *Basic Res. Cardiol.* 74:389–405.

32. Kämmereit, A., Medugorac, I., Steil, E., and Jacob, R. 1975. Mechanics of the isolated ventricular myocardium of rats conditioned by physical training. *Basic Res. Cardiol.* 70:495–507.

33. Katz, A. M. 1970. Contractile proteins of the heart. *Physiol. Rev.* 50:63–158.

34. Kissling, G. 1980. Oxygen consumption and substrate uptake of the hypertrophied rat heart in situ. *Basic Res. Cardiol.* 75:185–192.

35. Kissling, G., Gassenmaier, T., Wendt-Gallitelli, M. F., and Jacob, R. 1977. Pressure–volume relations, elastic modulus, and contractile behavior of the hypertrophied left ventricle of rats with Goldblatt II hypertension. *Pfluegers Arch.* 369:213–221.

36. Kissling, G., and Wendt-Gallitelli, M. F. 1977. Dynamics of the hypertrophied left ventricle in the rat. Effects of physical training and chronic pressure load. *Basic Res. Cardiol.* 72:178–183.

37. Linzbach, A. J. 1948. Herzhypertrophie und kritisches Herzgewicht. *Klin. Wochenschr.* 26:459–463.

38. Linzbach, A. J., and Kyrieleis, C. 1968. Strukturelle Analyse chronisch insuffizienter menschlicher Herzen. In: H. Reindell, J. Keul, and E. Doll (eds.), *Herzinsuffizienz, Pathophysiologie und Klinik*, pp. 11–19. Georg Thieme, Stuttgart.

39. Lompre, A.-M., Schwartz, K., d'Albis, A., Lacombe, G., van Thiem, N., and Swynghedauw, B. 1979. Myosin isoenzyme redistribution in chronic heart overload. *Nature* 282:105–107.

40. Maron, B. J., Ferrans, V. J., and Roberts, W. C. 1975. Ultrastructural features of degenerated cardiac muscle cells in patients with cardiac hypertrophy. *Am. J. Pathol.* 79:387–434.

41. Maughan, D., Low, E., Litten, R., Brayden, J., and Alpert, N. R. 1979. Calcium-activated muscle from hypertrophied rabbit hearts. *Circ. Res.* 44:279–287.

42. Medugorac, I. 1980. Collagen content in different areas of normal and hypertrophied rat myocardium. *Cardiovasc. Res.* 14:551–554.

43. Medugorac, I., and Jacob, R. 1976. Concentration and adenosinetrophosphatase activity of left ventricular actomyosin in Goldblatt rats during the compensatory stage of hypertrophy. *Z. Physiol. Chem.* 357:1495–1503.

44. Meerson, F.Z. 1969. *Hyperfunktion, Hypertrophie and Insuffizienz des Herzens*. VEB Volk und Gesundheit, Berlin.

45. Meerson, F. Z. 1976. Insufficiency of hypertrophied heart. *Basic Res. Cardiol.* 71:343–354.

46. Meerson, F. Z., and Breger, A. M. 1977. The common mechanism of the heart's adaptation and deadaptation: Hypertrophy and atrophy of the heart muscle. *Basic Res. Cardiol.* 72:228–234.
47. Page, E., McCallister, L. P., and Power, B. 1971. Stereological measurements of cardiac ultrastructures implicated in excitaton–contraction coupling (sarcotubulus and T-system). *Proc. Natl. Acad. Sci. U.S.A.* 68:1465–1466.
48. Penpargkul, S., Malhotra, A., Schaible, T., and Scheuer, J. 1980. Cardiac contractile proteins and sarcoplasmic reticulum in hearts of rats trained by running. *J. Appl. Physiol.* 48:409–413.
49. Pette, D., and Heilmann, C. 1977. Transformation of morphological, functional and metabolic properties of fast-twitch muscle as induced by long-term electrical stimulation. *Basic Res. Cardiol.* 72:247–253.
50. Rabinowitz, M., and Zak, R. 1975. Mitochondria and cardiac hypertrophy. *Circ. Res.* 36:367–376.
51. Rupp, H. 1980. Cooperative effects of calcium on myofibrillar ATPase of normal and hypertrophied heart. *Basic Res. Cardiol.* 75:157–162.
52. Rupp, H. 1982. Calcium-dependent activation of cardiac myofibrils: The mechanisms that modulate myofibrillar ATPase and tension and their significance for heart function. In: E. Chazov, V. Smirnov, and N. S. Dhalla (eds.), *Advances in Myocardiology*, Volume 3, pp. 455–466. Plenum Medical Book Company, New York.
53. Sack, D. W., Cooper, G., and Harrison, C. E. 1977. The role of Ca^{2+} ions in the hypertrophied myocardium. *Basic Res. Cardiol.* 72:268–273.
54. Scheuer, J., and Bhan, A. K. 1979. Cardiac contractile proteins. *Circ. Res.* 45:1–12.
55. Sonnenblick, E. H. 1970. Contractility of cardiac muscle. *Circ. Res.* 27:479–481.
56. Spann, J. F., Jr., Buccino, R. A., Sonnenblick, E. H., and Braunwald, E. 1967. Contractile state of cardiac muscle obtained from cats with experimentally produced ventricular hypertrophy and heart failure. *Circ. Res.* 21:341–354.
57. Strauer, B. E. 1980. *Hypertensive Heart Disease.* Springer, Berlin Heidelberg, New York.
58. Swynghedauw, B., and Leger, J. J. 1975. A new myosin molecule in heart overloading. A stimulating working hypothesis. In: *Abstract Volume, International Study Group for Research in Cardiac Metabolism European Section, Brussels*, p. 69.
59. Swynghedauw, B., Schwartz, K., and Leger, J. J. 1977. Cardiac myosin. Phylogenic and pathological changes. *Basic Res. Cardiol.* 72:254–260.
60. Ullrich, K. J., Riecker, G., and Kramer, K. 1954. Das Druckvolumendiagramm des Warmbluterherzens. *Pfluegers. Arch.* 259:481–498.
61. Wendt-Gallitelli, M. F., Ebrecht, G., and Jacob, R. 1979. Morphological alterations and their functional interpretation in the hypertrophied myocardium of Goldblatt hypertensive rats. *J. Mol. Cell. Cardiol.* 11:275–287.
62. Wikman-Coffelt, J., Parmley, W. W., and Mason, D. T. 1979. The cardiac hypertrophy process: Analyses of factors determining pathological vs. physiological development. *Circ. Res.* 45:697–707.

Reflections on What Makes the Heart Grow

F. Kölbel, V. Schreiber, J. Štěpán, T. Přibyl, and I. Gregorová

Third Medical Department and Laboratory for Endocrinology and Metabolism,
Faculty of Medicine
Charles University
Prague, Czechoslovakia

Abstract. Under conditions of experimental cardiac overload and hypertrophy in rats, a digoxinlike immunoreactivity appears in their serum which is correlated with cardiac growth. It is hypothesized that this is caused by the presence of an endogenous cardiotropic factor displaying cross immunoreactivity with digoxin. Additional evidence of the existence of the putative cardiotropic factor is provided by the finding that the sera of rats with cardiac overload displaying digoxinlike immunoreactivity stimulate the multiplication of rat cardiac myocytes in the tissue culture. This factor may be an adrenal steroid different from corticosterone and aldosterone. The name *endocardin* or *endocardiotonin* for this substance is suggested.

The mechanisms of induction of myocardial growth in cardiac overload are still not completely known. The protein synthesis of the cardiac muscle and its changes resulting in cardiac hypertrophy are influenced, among other things, by hormones, with the strongest link existing between experimental cardiac hypertrophy and the thyroid gland and adrenals (5,6,8,10,12,14,19). The classical studies of Margaret Beznak demonstrated the minor role of growth hormone for the induction of experimental cardiac hypertrophy together with the indispensability of thyroid hormones (1).

With regard to the adrenals, a decreased content of ribosomes was demonstrated in the heart muscle of adrenalectomized animals (9) as was the indispensability of the presence of the adrenals for the induction of isoproterenol cardiomegaly (7). Among hormones that could rapidly increase the protein synthesis of the heart muscle, norepinephrine should be mentioned (2). This chapter deals with the problem of the possible existence of another endogenous cardioactive factor participating in the regulation of cardiac growth.

Our hypothesis is based on the general pharmacologic rule that receptors for exogenous drugs primarily evolved as receptors for endogenous factors. The well-known examples are curare–acetylcholine and morphine–endogenous euphorigens (endorphins). We wonder whether this rule could not also apply for digitalis.

MATERIALS AND METHODS

All experiments were performed on male Wistar albino rats of initial body weight 200 g. Cardiac hypertrophy was induced in two different ways: by constriction of the subdiaphragmatic portion of the abdominal aorta (20), and by feeding the animals a standardized desiccated thyroid preparation (Thyroidin®, Spofa, Czechoslovakia) with an average daily intake of 150 mg of desiccated thyroid per animal. Short-term stress was induced in different groups of animals, by 3 hr of swimming, by exposing the animals to 3 hr of hypoxia in a closed vessel, and by laparotomy performed under ether anesthesia. Digitoxin (Digitoxin®, Spofa, Czechoslovakia) was administered in a dose of 0.1 mg/rat per day in the standard laboratory (Larsen) diet.

At the end of each experiment, the animals were decapitated, and blood samples for further analyses were obtained at that time. The relative weights of isolated organs were calculated from their absolute weights and the body weight of each animal. The "apparent" serum digoxin concentration was determined by homogeneous enzymoimmunoassay (EMIT® Syva, U.S.A.) (13). As this method was used at the limit of its sensitivity, the results of these determinations are expressed in ΔA (absorbance changes) and not as the interpolated values of the "apparent" digoxin concentration. The serum corticosterone determinations were performed in a routine way using chromatographic methods (11,17). The results obtained were statistically evaluated using the analysis of variance and Duncan's test (4).

The tissue cultures of rat cardiac myocytes were grown in Eagle's medium. The sera tested were added as a 10% admixture to the cultivation media. The numbers of myocytes per dish were counted using the Celloscope Medata® 202 counter. The serum aldosterone levels were determined by radioimmunoanalysis using the Aldok kit (CEA, Sorin).

RESULTS

In the serum of rats with cardiac overload produced by stenosis of the abdominal aorta, we found digoxinlike immunoreactivity which correlated positively with both total heart and left ventricular weights (Figure 1) observed at different time intervals after the surgery.

The addition of the "digoxin-positive" sera of animals with aortic stenosis to the tissue culture of rat cardiac myocytes resulted in a more than twofold increase in the number of myocytes per dish when compared with the effect of control rat serum that exhibited no digoxinlike immunoreactivity (Figure 2).

The apparent digoxin immunoreactivity was never observed in the blood of acutely stressed animals with normal heart weights, in which the blood corticosterone levels were significantly increased in all experimental groups (Figure 3). In the group of animals with stenosis of the abdominal aorta and

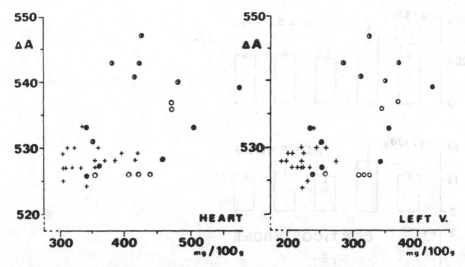

Figure 1.   Correlations between the relative total heart weights and left ventricular weights and the apparent serum digoxin immunoreactivity. Crosses, controls; empty circles, 1 week after stenosis of the abdominal aorta; half-filled circles, 2 weeks after stenosis; filled circles, 3 weeks after stenosis. Left: relative weight of the heart vs. serum apparent digitoxin: $y = 0.0460x + 513.31$, $r = 0.505$ $(P < 0.01)$. Right: relative weight of the left ventricle vs. serum apparent digitoxin: $y = 0.0585x + 517.18$, $r = 0.6043$ $(P < 0.01)$. Reproduced, with permission of the *Journal of Molecular and Cellular Cardiology*, from Schreiber et al. (16).

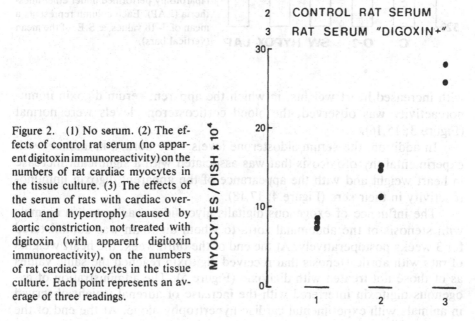

Figure 2.   (1) No serum. (2) The effects of control rat serum (no apparent digitoxin immunoreactivity) on the numbers of rat cardiac myocytes in the tissue culture. (3) The effects of the serum of rats with cardiac overload and hypertrophy caused by aortic constriction, not treated with digitoxin (with apparent digitoxin immunoreactivity), on the numbers of rat cardiac myocytes in the tissue culture. Each point represents an average of three readings.

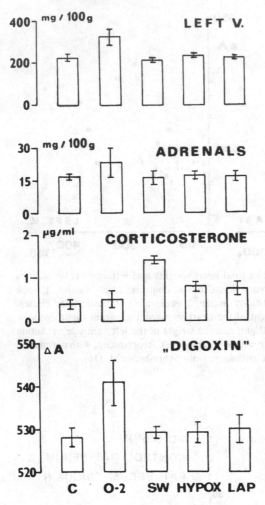

Figure 3.   Left ventricular and adrenal weights, serum corticosterone levels, and apparent digitoxin immunoreactivity in control rats (C), in rats 2 weeks after stenosis of the abdominal aorta (0–2), in rats following 3 hr swimming (SW), 3 hr hypoxia (HYPOX), and 3 hr after simple laparotomy performed under ether anesthesia (LAP). Each column represents a mean of 7–18 values ± S.E. of the mean (vertical bars).

with increased heart weights, in which the apparent serum digoxin immunoreactivity was observed, the blood corticosterone levels were normal (Figure 3; 15,16).

In addition, the serum aldosterone levels were normal in animals with experimental thyrotoxicosis that was associated with a significant increase in heart weight and with the appearance of the apparent digoxin immunoreactivity in their sera (Figure 4; 17,18).

The influence of exogenous digitalis glycosides was tested in animals with stenosis of the abdominal aorta to whom digitoxin was administered for 3 weeks postoperatively. At the end of the third week, the heart weights of rats with aortic stenosis that received digitoxin reached the same values as of those not treated with digitoxin (Figure 5). The administration of exogenous digitoxin interfered with the increase of adrenal weight observed in animals with experimental cardiac hypertrophy alone. At the end of the

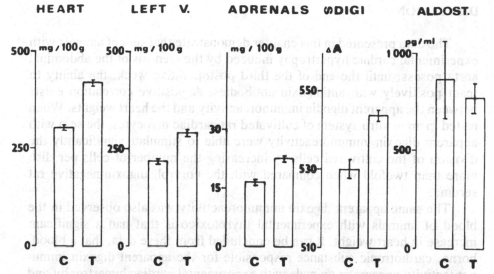

Figure 4.   Total heart and left ventricular (LEFT V.) weights, weights of the adrenals, serum apparent digitoxin immunoreactivity, and serum aldosterone levels in male rats with experimental thyrotoxicosis. Each column represents a mean of 7–12 values ± S.E. of the mean (vertical bars).

first postoperative week, the weight of the adrenals of animals with aortic stenosis given digitoxin was insignificantly lower than that in animals with aortic stenosis not treated with digitoxin. At the end of the third postoperative week, their adrenal weight dropped significantly below the adrenal weight found in animals with aortic stenosis alone (Figure 5).

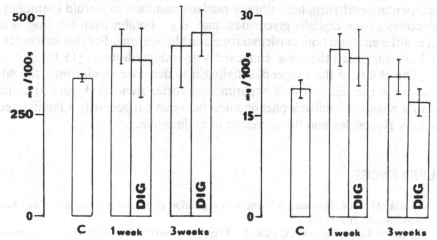

Figure 5.   Total heart and adrenal weights in control rats (C) and in rats 1 and 3 weeks following stenosis of the abdominal aorta not treated with digitoxin (empty columns), and in animals receiving digitoxin (DIG). Each column represents a mean of 6–20 values ± S.E. of the mean (vertical bars).

DISCUSSION

The data presented in this chapter demonstrate that sera of animals with experimental cardiac hypertrophy induced by the stenosis of the abdominal aorta posess, until the end of the third postoperative week, the ability to react positively with antidigoxin antibodies. A positive correlation exists between the apparent digoxin immunoreactivity and the heart weights. When tested in an in vitro system of cultivated rat cardiac myocytes, the sera with apparent digoxin immunoreactivity were able to stimulate significantly the division of the cultivated cells by increasing the number of cells per dish more than twofold when compared with the control, digoxin-negative rat serum.

The same apparent digoxin immunoreactivity was also observed in the blood of animals with experimental thyrotoxicosis that had a significant increase in heart weight. It can be concluded from these data, that a blood-borne, cardiotropic substance responsible for the apparent digoxin immunoreactivity appears in animals with experimental cardiac hypertrophy and is able to stimulate the division of cells in tissue culture. The apparent digitoxin immunoreactivity has been known for some time (3) in blood from the umbilical vein. However, it was interpreted as a nonspecific phenomenon without any connection with, e.g., peripartum hypoxia and the necessary adaptive changes in the myocardium of the left ventricle during the peri- and postpartum period.

In both models of experimental cardiac hypertrophy, the apparent digoxin immunoreactivity was connected with an increase in adrenal weight (Figures 4 and 5). However, it did not correlate with increased serum corticosterone and/or aldosterone levels. Consequently, it is most probable that the adrenals are producing a cardiotropic substance that is based on the cyclopentanoperhydrophenanthrene nucleus common to steroid hormones, aglycones of the digitalis glycosides, and, e.g., bufalin from the frog skin but is different from both corticosterone and aldosterone. For this substance, we have suggested the name endocardin or endocardiotonin (15,16).

The ability of the exogenous digitoxin to decrease significantly the adrenal weight in animals with experimental aortic stenosis (Figure 5) could mean a negative feedback phenomenon between exogenously administered digitalis glycosides and the secretion of endocardin.

REFERENCES

1. Beznak, M. 1964. Hormonal influences in regulation of cardiac performance. *Circ. Res.* 14–15(Suppl. 2):141–152.
2. Caldarera, C. M., Guarnieri, C., Clo, C., Ferrari, R., and Casti, A. 1979. Early biochemical events of myocardial hypertrophy In: P. Padieu and J.-P. Didier (eds.), *3eme Reunion de la Section Europeenne De l'ISHR*, pp. 125–138. Faculté de Medecine de Dijon, Dijon.
3. Drost, R. H., Plomp, T. A., Teunissen, A. J., Maas, A. H. J., and Maes, R. A. A. 1977.

A comparative study of the homogenous enzyme immunoassay (EMIT) and two radioimmunoassays (RIA's) for digoxin. *Clin. Chim. Acta* 79:557–567.

4. Duncan, D. B. 1955. Multiple range and multiple *F* tests. *Biometrics* 11:1–42.

5. Fízel, A., and Fízelová, A. 1972. Participation of catecholamines and cortical hormones in the myocardial metabolic adaptation to mechanical overload of the heart. In: E. Bajusz, and G. Rona (eds.) *Myocardiology* Vol. 1, pp. 814–827. Urban & Schwarzenberg, Munich, Berlin, Vienna.

6. Kölbel, F. 1978. Biochemické mechanismy vzniku hypertrofie levé srdeční komory [Biochemical mechanisms of the induction of left ventricular hypertrophy.] *Cesk. Fysiol.* 27:523–530.

7. Kölbel, F., Kapitola, J., Schreiberová, O., and Kölblová, V. 1970. Influence of adrenalectomy on the effects of isoproterenol in the rat. *Physiol. Bohemoslov.* 19:281–289.

8. Kölbel, F., Kapitola, J., Šonka, J., and Schreiberová, O. 1972. Hormonal and humoral modulation of the effects of isoproterenol. In: P.-Y. Hatt (ed.), *Les Surcharges Cardiaques*, pp. 39–47. INSERM, Paris.

9. Kölbel, F., Mommaerts, W. F. H. M., Kölblová, V., and Vančura, P. 1970. Cardiac muscle and liver ribosomes of the rat: The influence of laparotomy and laparotomy combined with adrenalectomy. *Experientia* 26:361–362.

10. Limas, C. J., and Chan-Stier, C. 1978. Myocardial chromatin activation in experimental hyperthyroidism in rats. *Circ. Shock* 42:311–322.

11. Mattingly, D. 1962. A simple fluorometric method for the estimation of free 11-hydroxycorticoids in human plasma. *J. Clin. Pathol.* 15:374–385.

12. Morris, B. J., Davis, J. O., Zatzman, M. L., and Williams, G. M. 1977. The renin angiotension aldosterone system in rabbits with congestive heart failure produced by aortic constriction. *Circ. Res.* 40:275–286.

13. Rubenstein, K. E., Schneider, R. S., and Ullman, E. F. 1972. *Biochem. Biophys. Res. Commun.* 47:846–851.

14. Schreiber, V., Kölbel, F., Horký, K., and Štěpán, J. 1980. Hormonální faktory v růstových reakcích srdečního svalu [Hormonal factors in growth reactions of heart muscle] *Cesk. Fysiol.* 29:489–500.

15. Schreiber, V., Kölbel, F., and Štěpán, J. 1980. Zdánlivá (?) imunoreaktivita digoxinu v séru krys se srdečním přetížením. K otázce endogenního kardiotonika (endokardinu) [Apparent (?) immunoreactivity of digoxin in the sera of rats with cardiac overload—on the problem of endogenous cardiotonic (endocardin)]. *Cas. Lek. Cesk.* 119:768–770.

16. Schreiber, V., Kölbel, F., Štěpán, J., Gregorová, I., and Přibyl, T. 1980. Digoxin-like immunoreactivity in the serum of rats with cardiac overload. *J. Mol. Cell. Cardiol.* 13:107–110.

17. Schreiber, V., Štěpán, J., Gregorová, I., Kölbel, F., Přibyl, T., Jahodová, J., and Janovská, J. 1980. Digoxinu podobná imunoreaktivita v seru hyperthyreoidních krys se srdeční hypertrofií není způsobena aldosteronem [Digoxinlike immunoreactivity in the serum of hyperthyroid rats with cardiac hypertrophy is not caused by aldosterone]. *Sb. Lek.* 82:305–308.

18. Schreiber, V., Štěpán, J., Kölbel, F., Přibyl., T., Jahodová, J., and Kubová, V. 1980. Failure of the aldosterone antagonist spironolactone to inhibit myocardial hypertrophy produced by experimental hyperthyroidism and accompanied by "apparent" digoxin immunoreactivity in the blood. *Physiol. Bohemoslov.* 29:577–579.

19. Sharma, V. K., and Banerjee, S. P. 1978. Specific ^{3}H-ouabain binding to rat heart and skeletal muscle: Effects of thyroidectomy. *Mol. Pharmacol.* 14:122–129.

20. Turto, H., and Lindy, S. 1973. Digitoxin treatment and experimental cardiac hypertrophy in the rat. *Cardiovasc. Res.* 7:482–487.

Force–Velocity–Length Relationship during Cardiac Hypertrophy
Time Course of Activation

Y. Lecarpentier, P. Gastineau, and P. Y. Hatt

I.N.S.E.R.M. U2
Hôpital Léon Bernard
94450 Limeil-Brévannes, France

J. L. Martin

E.N.S.T.A., Ecole Polytechnique
91120 Palaiseau, France

Abstract. Basic mechanical properties observed during cardiac hypertrophy were studied in left ventricular rat papillary muscles after exposure to chronic pressure and/or volume overloading. It is always possible, during such overloading conditions, to define the level of contractility in terms of a force–velocity–length (F–V–L) relationship regardless of time and initial length. Thus, during a determined period of the contraction phase and for a given total load, shortening velocity remained an univocal time-invariant function of shortening length, involving a time-independent maximum intensity of activation. The onset of this precise phase was reached relatively soon after stimulus. The time-independent F–V–L relation was observed both in controls and in hypertrophied heart muscles, whatever the degree and the type of induced hypertrophy, and even during the latest phases of congestive heart failure.

In the last 10 years, morphology, mechanics, and biochemistry have demonstrated many myocardial changes during the development of cardiac hypertrophy. Abnormalities in mechanical parameters such as shortening velocity or isometric tension have been found (2,25,26). But little is known about the tridimensional force–velocity–length (F–V–L) relationship and the time course of activation during chronic cardiac overloading. In normal heart muscle, instantaneous measurements of the four main variables, force, shortening velocity, shortening length, and time have led to a definition of the contractile state. First, a relationship was shown to exist between the shortening velocity and the shortening extent, regardless of initial length (22). Cardiac contractility was then defined as the time- and initial length-independent part of the F–V–L diagram (5). Any change in contractility obtained after various inotropic effects was found to be the result of a shift in the F–V–L surface (22). This relationship characterizes the mechanical performance of heart muscle and involves a maximum time course of active state when the muscle is operating on the F–V–L surface (24). Any change in maximum intensity of the activation processes is implicit in the shift of the force–velocity relationship brought about by inotropic effects (1,20,21).

Load-clamp techniques (5,7) have contributed to an understanding of further basic mechanical properties in normal heart muscle: during an afterloaded isotonic twitch (1) there is a precise stage during the contraction phase when the instantaneous shortening velocity is exclusively determined by the instantaneous extent of shortening, and (2) when an abrupt load clamp is applied at a given final total load, the instantaneous shortening velocity adapts almost immediately to the extent of shortening. These two properties depend neither on initial length nor on the moment when the load clamp is applied during this particular stage.

Our aim was to determine whether properties 1 and 2, observed in normal mammalian papillary muscle, were still persistent during cardiac hypertrophy and congestive heart failure. Quantitative parameters were deliberately excluded from this concise study.

We have found it was possible, using chronic overloading conditions, to define the level of contractility in terms of the time- and initial length-invariant relationship. We shall see that these basic mechanical properties did not disappear whatever the type and degree of chronic ventricular overloading and even in terminal stages of congestive heart failure, although quantitative modifications in overall mechanical behavior were found.

MATERIALS AND METHODS

This study was carried out on left ventricular papillary muscles from Wistar rats, whose hearts were subjected to different types of pressure and volume overloading, resulting in various degrees of cardiac hypertrophy. Heart weight, in many cases, attained two to three times that of normal rats; this is comparable to human cardiac hypertrophy. Some of the rats even suffered from congestive heart failure with dyspnea, pulmonary and subcutaneous edema, and hepatic congestion at the moment of sacrifice.

Five groups of Wistar rats were studied. Group 1 were controls ($N = 16$; heart weight: 0.85 ± 0.03 g). Group 2: aortic insufficiency (AI) was induced by a lesion of one sigmoid aortic valve with a catheter introduced into the right carotid artery ($N = 10$; heart weight: 1.91 ± 0.10 g). Group 3 had an aortocaval fistula (ACF): a communication between the abdominal aorta (between the left renal artery and aortic bifurcation) and inferior vena cava was induced as previously described (13) ($N = 12$; heart weight: 1.68 ± 0.08 g). Group 4: aortic stenosis (AS) was obtained with subtotal constriction of the abdominal aorta (16) ($N = 9$; heart weight: 1.25 ± 0.08 g). Group 5 had AS and AI: double pressure and volume overloading was successively induced in the same rat with a 15-day interval between the two operations ($N = 4$; heart weight: 2.26 ± 0.15 g).

Papillary muscles were quickly removed from the left ventricle and vertically suspended in a bathing solution containing (in mM): NaCl 118, KCl 4.7, $MgSO_4 \cdot 7H_2O$ 1.2, KH_2PO_4 1.1, $NaHCO_3$ 24, $CaCl_2 \cdot 6H_2O$ 2.5, and glucose 4.5. The preparations were electrically stimulated with rectangular pulses of 5 msec duration just above threshold by means of two platinum electrodes. Frequency of stimulation was 6 beats/min. The solution was bubbled with 95% O_2 and 5% CO_2 and maintained at pH 7.4 and 29°C. After a 1-hr stabilization period at L_{max}, the muscles recovered optimal mechanical performance. The force transducer system and the whole electronic device have been described elsewhere (6).

RESULTS

The experiments described in Figures 1, 2, and 3 show the mechanical behavior of different twitches at the same final total load. In the first experiment (Figure 1), preload was modified from one twitch to another by adapting the afterload in such a way that total load was the same for each

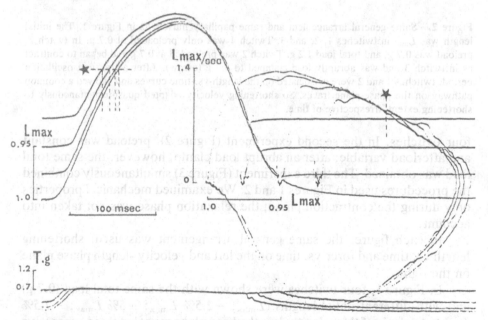

Figure 1. On the left: shortening length-vs.-time and force-vs.-time curves. On the right: superimposed velocity–length phase plane diagram. Four twitches have been shown with different initial lengths (L_{max}; -2.5% L_{max}; -5% L_{max}; -7.5% L_{max}) but with total load kept constant (0.7 g). Although the shortening length-vs.-time curves were dissociated, velocity–length phase planes presented a common pathway over a large part of the contraction phase. So shortening velocity as a function of length is independent of initial length and time during this particular stage of the contraction phase. The papillary muscle used in this experiment was removed from a left ventricle overloaded for 1 year by an aortocaval fistula; heart weight, 1.7 g; preload at L_{max}, 0.7 g.

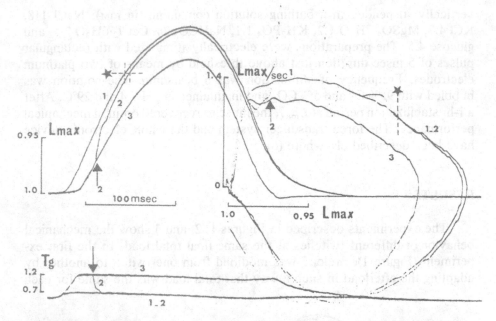

Figure 2.   Same general arrangement and same papillary muscle as in Figure 1. The initial length was L_{max} in twitches 1, 2, and 3. Twitch 1 was only preloaded at 0.7 g. In twitch 3, preload was 0.7 g, and total load 1.2 g. Twitch 2 was preloaded at 0.7 g and began to contract as in twitch 3 and was abruptly load clamped to 0.7 g (arrow). After a transient oscillation period, twitches 1 and 2 were dissociated on the length-vs.-time curves and showed a common pathway on the phase-plane traces. So shortening velocity adapted quasi-instantaneously to shortening extent, irrespective of time.

four twitches. In the second experiment (Figure 2), preload was constant and afterload variable; after an abrupt load clamp, however, the same total load was obtained. The third experiment (Figure 3) simultaneously combined the procedures used in Figures 1 and 2. We examined mechanical properties only during the contraction phase; the relaxation phase was not taken into account.

In each figure, the same general arrangement was used: shortening length vs. time and force vs. time on the left and velocity–length phase plane on the right.

In Figure 1, four twitches were shown with the same total load (0.7 g) and with different initial lengths (L_{max}; -2.5% L_{max}; -5% L_{max}; -7.5% L_{max}). Analysis of the velocity–length phase plane revealed three successive stages a, b, and c. Stage b corresponded to the common pathway of the traces on the velocity–length phase plane. During this particular stage of the contraction phase, instantaneous shortening velocity was entirely determined by instantaneous shortening length regardless of initial length. Moreover, a given extent of shortening occurred at different times when initial length was changed. Thus, during stage b, instantaneous velocity was independent of time and preload. This means that whenever a given degree

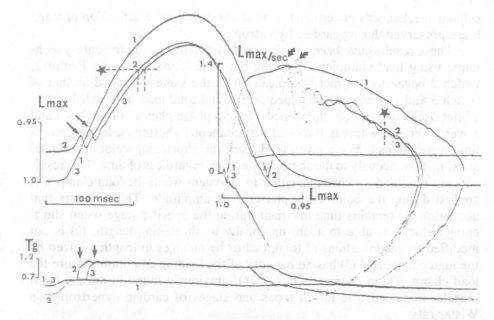

Figure 3. Same general arrangement and same papillary muscle as in Figure 1. The initial length was L_{max} in twitches 1 and 3 and $-2.5\%\ L_{max}$ in twitch 2. Twitches 2 and 3 were abruptly load clamped from 0.7 to 1.2 g at two different moments (arrows). After a brief oscillation period, velocity–length phase planes of twitches 2 and 3 coincided, although shortening length-vs.-time curves were dissociated. So shortening velocity is a time- and initial length-invariant function of shortening length.

of shortening occurs and for a constant total load, one and only one instantaneous shortening velocity will correspond to it. This univocal velocity–length function characterizes the level of contractility and implies a time-invariant course of active state during stage b.

Stage a in Figure 1 corresponded to the initial part of the twitches, from stimulus to the onset of stage b. After peak velocity, traces of the four phase planes remained dissociated because a given shortening extent was reached at different velocities. So, during stage a, a time-dependent and nonunivocal function linked instantaneous shortening velocity to shortening extent. This implies a time-variant intensity of active state until the onset of the common pathway on the phase plane. The end of stage a occurred when the activation processes leveled off. Stage c in Figure 1 constituted the third part of contraction when the velocity–length phase planes were dissociated again. Time and initial length influenced the relationship between shortening length and shortening velocity, as a given shortening velocity corresponded to several extents of shortening. This nonunivocal function suggests that intensity of active state varies during stage c.

In all hypertrophied hearts, a specific stage b, characterizing the time-independent activation, was found. This mechanical behavior was observed in both normal and chronically overloaded muscles. This implies that intracellular mechanisms governing the invariant time course activation of stage b are preserved during cardiac hypertrophy.

These results have been corroborated by means of complementary technique using load clamping (5) during the contraction phase. In Figure 2, twitch 2 began to contract isotonically with the same total load as that of twitch 3 and was abruptly clamped at the final total load of twitch 1. After a brief oscillation period, the velocity–length phase planes of twitches 1 and 2 were merged, whereas traces of instantaneous shortening length versus time were distinct. For a given total load, the shortening velocity adapted quasi-instantaneously to the shortening extent, regardless of time. This result was not modified by changing either the moment when the load clamp was applied during the contraction phase or its amplitude. This suggests that activation (1) remains time invariant during the specific stage when shortening velocity is able to adapt univocally to shortening length, (2) is not modified by modifications of total load or by changes in length induced by the load clamp, and (3) has no memory of the loading conditions before the load clamp. These characteristics (5,24), previously found in normal heart muscle, remained true for all types and stages of cardiac hypertrophy in Wistar rats.

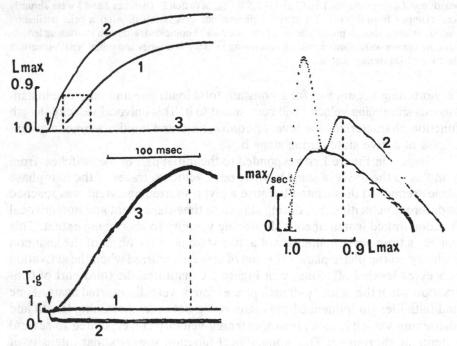

Figure 4.   Same general arrangement as in Figure 1. Only the contraction phase has been shown. The heart muscle used in this experiment was overloaded for 2 months by aortic insufficiency (heart weight 1.4 g and preload at L_{max} 0.8 g). Twitch 1 was only preloaded at 0.8 g. Twitch 2 was abruptly clamped to zero load just after stimulus. Maximum unloaded velocity occurred 25 msec after stimulus (17% of the time to peak tension).

Figure 3 combines the two experiments shown in Figures 1 and 2. Twitches 2 and 3, which began at two different initial lengths, were clamped at two different moments at the same final total load. After a brief oscillation period, traces of twitches 2 and 3 coincided on the velocity–length phase planes and were distinct on the length-vs.-time curves. Thus, for a given level of total load, shortening velocity was able to adapt univocally to shortening length. This quasi-instantaneous adaptation was time and initial length independent.

Another experimental procedure is shown in Figure 4. Twitch 1 was only preloaded, and twitch 3 contracted isometrically. Twitch 2 was abruptly clamped to zero load very soon after stimulus, and an adequate damping abbreviated the transient oscillation period. Maximum unloaded velocity was reached early in the contraction phase, about 25 msec after stimulus. Peaks of unloaded velocity and further courses of unloaded phase planes were found to be independent of initial length during cardiac hypertrophy. This result has previously been described in normal mammalian heart (5). The onset of the time-independent unloaded relationship began early at about 17% of the time to peak tension. Although the maximum value of unloaded velocity decreased during cardiac hypertrophy (19), the qualitative mechanical properties remained present. Values of V_{max} were (L_{max}/sec): Controls, 2.65 ± 0.12; AI, 2.61 ± 0.16; ACF, 1.98 ± 0.17; AS, 1.64 ± 0.11; AS + AI, 1.13 ± 0.14.

DISCUSSION

Stage b of the contraction phase characterizes the mechanical behavior of both normal and hypertrophied heart muscles. When total load is progressively incremented from preload until isometric tension, the whole range of stage b describes the specific time-invariant part of the tridimensional F–V–L surface which defines the level of contractility and the maximum activation of the muscle. This F–V–L relationship is globally lowered during chronic cardiac hypertrophy. Several abnormalities have been described during chronic pressure and volume overloading (10), both in membrane systems and in contractile apparatus. Activation appeared to be subject to quantitative changes; however, its time-invariant regulated part is maintained during stage b. A drop in the maximum level of constant activation may occur during cardiac hypertrophy as implied by the decreased maximum unloaded velocity (19).

Many authors have attempted to quantify the active state in striated muscle by mechanical measurements (17). The concept itself has been largely discussed (15) because the method used to measure it, the muscle length (27), and changes in length (3,12) may influence its intensity and time course. It has been found that shortening velocity in skeletal muscle increases very soon after stimulus and quickly attains a maximum value near V_{max} (14).

Moreover, the active state has been shown to develop relatively slowly in heart muscle (4,11,23). Measured with the quick-release technique, it is fully developed after 35% of time to peak tension (24). The duration of its maximum intensity (24) represents approximately 65% of the time to peak tension.

On the other hand, the time to maximum unloaded velocity, measured by zero-load clamp, occurs soon after the latent period at about 15–20% of time to peak tension (5). This suggests that activation may rapidly attain its maximum value after stimulus. In accordance with these results, we have found that maximum unloaded velocity was attained early during the contraction phase, at about 17 to 25% of time to peak tension (see Figure 4).

Instantaneous adaptation of velocity to length was not verified when load clamps were applied later, during the third part of the contraction phase, because of a decrease in activation. Further time course of contraction and relaxation appeared markedly modified, and the force–velocity–length relationship became load and time dependent. Load sensitivity obtained at the end of the contraction phase and during the relaxation phase is specific to mammalian heart muscle (8,9) and implies an efficient sarcoplasmic reticulum (18). This mechanical property is not found in frog ventricular muscle which has a sparse sarcoplasmic reticulum. However, we have always observed during cardiac hypertrophy the load and time sensitivity of the last part of the contraction phase. This suggests that, in chronic pressure- and volume-overloading conditions, intracellular membraneous systems may still regulate the onset, the duration, and the end of stage b according to the general loading conditions.

REFERENCES

1. Abbott, B. C., and Mommaerts, W. F. H. M. 1959. A study of inotropic mechanisms in the papillary muscle preparation. *J. Gen. Physiol.* 42:533–551.
2. Bing, O. H. L., Matsushita, S., Fanburg, B. L., and Levine, H. J. 1971. Mechanical properties of rat cardiac muscle during experimental hypertrophy. *Circ. Res.* 28:234–245.
3. Brady, A. J. 1965. Time and displacement dependence of cardiac contractility: Problems in defining the active state and force–velocity relations. *Fed. Proc.* 24:1410–1420.
4. Brady, A. J. 1966. Onset of contractility in cardiac muscle. *J. Physiol.* (*Lond.*) 184:560–580.
5. Brutsaert, D. L. 1974. The force–velocity–length–time interrelation of cardiac muscle. In: R. Porter, and D. W. Fitzsimons (eds.), *The Physiological Basis of Starling's Law of the Heart*, pp. 155–175. Elsevier, Excerpta Medica, North-Holland, Amsterdam.
6. Brutsaert, D. L., and Claes, V. A. 1974. Onset of mechanical activation of mammalian heart muscle in calcium- and strontium-containing solutions. *Circ. Res.* 35:345–357.
7. Brutsaert, D. L., Claes, V. A., and Sonnenblick, E. H. 1971. Velocity of shortening of unloaded heart muscle and the length–tension relation. *Circ. Res.* 29:63–75.
8. Brutsaert, D. L., De Clerck, N. M., Goethals, M. A., and Housmans, P. R. 1978. Relaxation of ventricular cardiac muscle. *J. Physiol.* (*Lond.*) 283:469–480.
9. Brutsaert, D. L., Housmans, P. R., and Goethals, M. A. 1980. Dual control of relaxation: Its role in the ventricular function in the mammalian heart. *Circ. Res.* 47:637–652.
10. Dhalla, N. S., Das, P. K., and Sharma, G. P. 1978. Subcellular basis of cardiac contractile failure. *J. Mol. Cell. Cardiol.* 10:363–385.

11. Edman, K. A. P., and Nilsson, E. 1968. Mechanical parameters of myocardial contraction studied at a constant length of the contractile element. *Acta Physiol. Scand.* 72:205–219.
12. Edman, K. A. P., and Nilsson, E. 1972. Relationships between force and velocity of shortening in rabbit papillary muscle. *Acta Physiol. Scand.* 85:488–500.
13. Hatt, P. Y., Rakusan, K., Gastineau, P., and Laplace, M. 1979. Morphometry and ultrastructure of heart hypertrophy induced by chronic volume overload (aorto–caval fistula in the rat). *J. Mol. Cell. Cardiol.* 11:989–998.
14. Hill, A. V. 1951. The transition from rest to full activity in muscle: The velocity of shortening. *Proc. R. Soc. Lond. [Biol.]* 138:329–338.
15. Jewell, B. R., and Wilkie, D. R. 1960. The mechanical properties of relaxing muscle. *J. Physiol. (Lond.)* 152:30–47.
16. Jouannot, P., and Hatt, P. Y. 1975. Rat myocardial mechanics during pressure-induced hypertrophy development and reversal. *Am. J. Physiol.* 229:355–364.
17. Julian, F. J., and Moss, R. L. 1976. The concept of active state in striated muscle. *Circ. Res.* 38:53–59.
18. Lecarpentier, Y. C., Chuck, L. H. S., Housmans, P. R., De Clerck, N. M., and Brutsaert, D. L. 1979. Nature of load dependence of relaxation in cardiac muscle. *Am. J. Physiol.* 237:H455–H460.
19. Lecarpentier, Y., Martin, J. L., Gastineau, P., and Hatt, P. Y. 1980. Mammalian heart mechanical properties during pressure and volume cardiac hypertrophy. *J. Mol. Cell. Cardiol.* 12(Suppl. 1):92.
20. Sonnenblick, E. H. 1962. Force–velocity relations in mammalian heart muscle. *Am. J. Physiol.* 202:931–939.
21. Sonnenblick, E. H. 1962. Implications of muscle mechanics in the heart. *Fed. Proc.* 21(Suppl.):975–990.
22. Sonnenblick, E. H. 1965. Instantaneous force–velocity–length determinants in the contraction of heart muscle. *Circ. Res.* 16:441–451.
23. Sonnenblick, E. H. 1967. Active state in heart muscle. Its delayed onset and modification by inotropic agents. *J. Gen. Physiol.* 50:661–676.
24. Sonnenblick, E. H., and Parmley, W. W. 1967. Active state in heart muscle: Force–velocity–length relations, and the variable onset and duration of maximum active state. In: D. I. Abramson (ed.), *Circulation in the Extremities*, pp. 65–83. Academic Press, London, New York.
25. Spann, J. F., Buccino, R. A., Sonnenblick, E. H., and Braunwald, E. 1967. Contractile state of cardiac muscle obtained from cats with experimentally produced ventricular hypertrophy and heart failure. *Circ. Res.* 21:341–354.
26. Spann, J. F., Covell, J. W., Eckberg, A. L., Sonnenblick, E. H., Ross, J., Jr., and Braunwald, E. 1972. Contractile performance of the hypertrophied and chronically failing cat ventricle. *Am. J. Physiol.* 223:1150–1157.
27. Taylor, S. R., and Rüdel, R. 1970. Striated muscle fibers: Inactivation of contraction induced by shortening. *Science* 167:882–884.

Hemodynamics, Regional Myocardial Blood Flow, and Sarcoplasmic Reticulum Calcium Uptake in Right Ventricular Hypertrophy and Failure

R. K. H. Wyse, K. C. Welham,* M. Jones,† E. D. Silove,‡ and M. R. de Leval§

Department of Paediatric Cardiology
Institute of Child Health
London WC1N 3EH, England

Abstract. Either right ventricular hypertrophy (RVH) or failure (RVF) was produced by pulmonary arterial banding in 47 piglets aged 3–6 weeks. When sufficient time was allowed to elapse after banding, RVH was present in 30 and had progressed to RVF in 17. These two groups were compared with 24 control, i.e., normal pigs (C). Animals with RVF differed from RVH and C animals by having reduced cardiac output and clinical signs of failure. Both RVH and RVF had significantly elevated right ventricular peak systolic pressures (RVS), weights (GMRV), and RV/LV systolic pressure ratios (these variables all increased >100% compared with C). The RV $(dP/dt)_{max}$ correlated with RVS in C ($r = 0.687$, $P < 0.001$), but this relationship was absent in RVH with higher RVS and GMRV. The RV $(dP/dt)_{max}$ correlated closely with RV blood flow/g per min in C ($r = 0.638$, $P < 0.01$) and in RVH ($r = 0.462$, $P < 0.02$). Calcium uptake by RV sarcoplasmic reticulum (SR) was diminished in RVH compared to C and further diminished in RVF (38%, $P < 0.001$). Calcium uptake by LV SR also fell in RVF, suggesting that SR calcium uptake is merely a passive reflection of myocardial function. Our results also suggest that hemodynamic and subcellular changes seen in RVF may be detected during the compensated stage of RVH.

The establishment of a reliable and reproducible method of creating right ventricular hypertrophy (RVH) or failure (RVF) in this laboratory (12) has allowed a detailed study of these pathological states. The present study combines observations of the hemodynamic response to this stimulus to hypertrophy with determinations of sarcoplasmic reticulum calcium uptake. It is pertinent to combine these studies because they both consider events occurring in the stressed and unstressed sides of the heart and provide insight

---

* Present address: Department of Molecular and Life Sciences, Dundee College of Technology, Dundee, Scotland.

† Present address: Surgery Branch, National Heart, Lung and Blood Institute, National Institutes of Health, Bethesda, Maryland 20205, USA.

‡ Present address: The Children's Hospital, Ladywood Middleway, Birmingham, England.

§ Present address: Thoracic Unit, The Hospital for Sick Children, London WC1N 3JH, England.

97

into mechanisms of myocardial response to hypertrophy. Some animals were allowed to develop RVF because it has long been suspected that an abnormality of excitation–contraction coupling occurs in heart failure and that this abnormality may be mediated by inappropriate movements of calcium within the sarcoplasmic reticulum. This possibility has previously been investigated (3,4,6,10,11) with conflicting results. It still remains uncertain whether impairment of sarcoplasmic reticulum function represents a specific abnormality that promotes the precipitation of heart failure. It is also unclear from the literature whether the function of the sarcoplasmic reticulum is depressed during the development of RVH and before the onset of failure. Evidence obtained in the present study favors the suggestion that calcium uptake by the sarcoplasmic reticulum is a passive reflection of the contractile state of the heart.

MATERIALS AND METHODS

Production of Right Ventricular Hypertrophy of Failure

Either compensated RVH or RVF was produced by banding the pulmonary artery in Welsh breed piglets at 3 to 6 weeks of age. They were anesthetized with a mixture of halothane, nitrous oxide, and oxygen; after intubation with a 4 mm diameter cuffed endotracheal tube, anesthesia was maintained by a mixture of 0.75–1.5% halothane, 50% nitrous oxide, and oxygen. Intermittent positive-pressure ventilation was provided by a Manley ventilator (Hutchinson Blease, Ltd.) using an inflation pressure of 30 cm water and tidal volume of 200 ml. The electrocardiogram (lead II) was displayed throughout the procedure. The left hemithorax was entered through the third intercostal space and the pericardium opened. After mobilizing the pulmonary artery, it was encircled with a piece of Teflon® or cotton tape, and the vessel constricted. Care was taken to ensure that reduction of vessel diameter was at a level insufficient to produce changes in the electrocardium. The pericardium and overlying tissues were closed, and the animal allowed to recover.

Hemodynamic Studies

These studies were performed on 24 normal pigs and the 47 survivors of pulmonary arterial banding between 7 and 12 weeks after their initial operation. These survivors were split into two groups. Both groups included animals with RVH; group 2 also contained 16 animals in which RVF had been allowed to develop. Right ventricular failure was diagnosed according to the criteria of Welham et al. (12). Additionally, the liver was weighed at the end of the experiment in order to calculate liver-to-body-weight ratios. Myocardial blood flow was measured in group 1 animals ($N = 23$) and controls ($N = 17$) using radioactive microspheres. Calcium uptake by right and left ventricular sarcoplasmic reticulum was measured in group 2 animals

(N = 24) and controls (N = 7). Hemodynamic studies were performed on both groups by first anesthetizing with a mixture of halothane, nitrous oxide, and oxygen as before and inserting a cuffed endotracheal tube. Blood gas levels and pH were frequently monitored and kept within normal limits (1) by regulation of gas flow to the respirator. The chest was opened by a median sternotomy, and intermittent positive–pressure ventilation was provided by a Manley ventilator using an inflation pressure of 30 cm water and tidal volume of 600–800 ml. Nylon catheters (4F, Portex, Ltd.) were passed into the right ventricle via an external jugular vein and retrogradely via a carotid artery into the left ventricle and aorta. Catheter-tip micromanometers (Millar Instruments Inc., Model Pc-471) were used to monitor both left and right ventricular pressures. Two differentiators, built in this laboratory and incorporating buffer amplifiers, were used to measure the first derivitive of both ventricular pressure signals. The phase lags of the differentiators were 2 msec (LV dP/dt) and 5 msec (RV dP/dt), respectively. Cardiac outputs were measured as described by Welham et al. (12).

Measurement of Myocardial Blood Flow

Carbonized microspheres (15 ± 5 μm diameter) impregnated with strontium-85 (10.32 mCi/g) (3M Company, Minnesota) and diluted with excess normal saline were subjected to vigorous agitation and injection into the left atrium of group 1 animals and their controls. Reference blood samples were obtained by allowing blood to emerge from an arterial catheter for the minute immediately following microsphere injection. At the end of the experiment, the heart was dissected into right and left ventricular and septal segments and weighed. The right ventricle was dissected according to a numbered map, and each section was weighed and counted for radioactivity (Wallac DECEM-GTL) along with reference blood samples included to allow the determination of myocardial blood flow by standard methods. For the purposes of the current study, right ventricular blood flow per gram of muscle represents the mean of approximately 44 right ventricular samples per animal.

Isolation of Sarcoplasmic Reticulum

Sections of approximately equal weight (about 10 g) were taken from each ventricle in group 2 animals and their controls after the hemodynamic studies had been completed. These sections were trimmed of fat, diced, and homogenized in a Waring blender for 1 min in 3 volumes of a solution containing 320 mM sucrose, 120 mM potassium chloride, and 100 mM L-histidine hydrochloride at pH 7.4. Care was taken throughout the preparative procedure to maintain the temperature of the samples at 0°–4°C. The homogenate was centrifuged at 600 g (Mistral 6L) for 15 min, and the resulting supernatant fluid strained through muslin. This supernatant was centrifuged at 8800 g for 20 min, then at 30,000 g for 15 min; the resulting pellets were discarded. The 30,000-g supernatant, when centrifuged at 100,000 g for 1 hr, deposited a straw-colored pellet enriched in sarcoplasmic reticulum which was gently resuspended in fresh cold homogenizing solution using a hand-operated Teflon® homogenizer.

Measurement of Calcium Uptake

Aliquots of resuspended sarcoplasmic reticulum were incubated at 30°C and pH 7.1 in the following medium: 150 mM potassium chloride; 50 mM L-histidine monohydrochloride; 5 mM magnesium chloride; 5 mM ATP, Na salt; 5 mM potassium oxalate; 62.5 μM calcium chloride; ^{45}calcium chloride as a marker (specific activity 0.02 Ci/μg calcium). The total volume was 2 ml. After preincubation for 1 min, calcium uptake was started by adding 0.2 ml of the protein suspension (final protein concentration in the reaction medium 100 μg/ml) to the reaction vessel. After 2 min, some of the reaction mixture was rapidly filtered through a Millipore® filter (0.45 μm diameter pore size). Radioactivity of equal volumes (0.05 ml) of filtrate and original reaction medium was measured in a scintillation counter (Phillips PW4510) using 10 ml of Bray's solution as a scintillant (2). Calcium uptake calculated on a protein basis was determined from the differences between these values. Protein determinations were performed using Lowry's method (7) with serial dilutions of bovine serum albumin as standard. Absorbance was measured at 720 nm on a Pye Unicam SP500 spectrophotometer using a tungsten light source with a red filter. Values for calcium uptake by the sarcoplasmic reticulum isolated from control animals were compared with those from animals with hypertrophying or failing hearts.

A 2-min incubation period was selected for the present study in order to measure rate rather than total calcium uptake, and under these experimental conditions, the activity was linear over the first 5 min. Preparations of sarcoplasmic reticulum are known to contain protein contamination from other subcellular fractions (4,5). Known inhibitors of mitochondrial calcium uptake, sodium azide and rotenone, were used to help monitor this. They reduced the rate of calcium uptake by less than 3% in all preparations, suggesting that mitochondrial contamination was low; furthermore, there was consistently low succinic dehydrogenase activity in all preparations of sarcoplasmic reticulum, and these values did not alter significantly in hypertrophy or failure.

All reagents used were of analytical grade.

RESULTS

Animals with compensated right ventricular hypertrophy and those with right ventricular failure were differentiated from controls by having elevated right-ventricular-to-total-ventricular weight ratios (C, 0.222 ± 0.013; RVH, 0.451 ± 0.018; RVF, 0.458 ± 0.022). They were also distinguished from one another on the basis of cardiac outputs and elevated right ventricular peak systolic and end-diastolic pressures. For a detailed hemodynamic report on these animals, see Welham et al. (12). There was no difference in the liver-to-body weight ratios between C animals and animals with RVH (C, 23.0; RVH, 23.0 g/kg).

Figure 1 shows the relationship between RV $(dP/dt)_{max}$ and RV peak systolic pressure in control animals and animals with RVH. Controls showed a close correlation ($r = 0.687$; $P < 0.001$) between RV $(dP/dt)_{max}$ and RV peak systolic pressure. However, this relationship was absent in RVH animals in which RV peak systolic pressures were significantly higher than normal (C, 21.5 ± 1.2 mm Hg; RVH, 54.5 ± 2.1 mm Hg; $P < 0.001$). Thus, RV $(dP/dt)_{max}$ did not increase in response to elevated RV peak systolic pressures in the animals with RVH and, indeed, tended to diminish at very high RV pressures.

Figure 2 shows the relationship on the unstressed left side of the heart between LV $(dP/dt)_{max}$ and peak aortic systolic pressure in controls and in animals with RVH. Both controls ($r = 0.612$; $P < 0.05$) and animals with RVH ($r = 0.763$; $P < 0.001$) showed a close and similar relationship between LV $(dP/dt)_{max}$ and peak aortic systolic pressure. The hypertrophied right ventricle did not appear to affect this relationship.

The reaction of the RV coronary vascular bed to increased demand is shown in Figure 3 which describes the relationship between RV $(dP/dt)_{max}$ and RV blood flow per gram of muscle per minute in control animals and

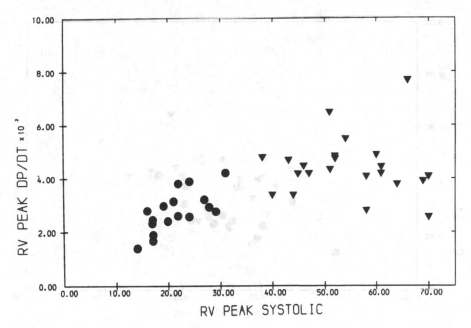

Figure 1.   The relationship between RV $(dP/dt)_{max}$ (mm Hg/sec) and RV peak systolic pressure (mm Hg) in normal, i.e., control animals (circles) and those with right ventricular hypertrophy (triangles).

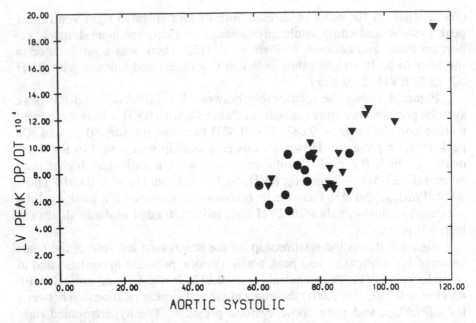

Figure 2. The relationship between LV $(dP/dt)_{max}$ (mm Hg/sec) and peak aortic pressure (mm Hg) in normal animals (circles) and those with right ventricular hypertrophy (triangles).

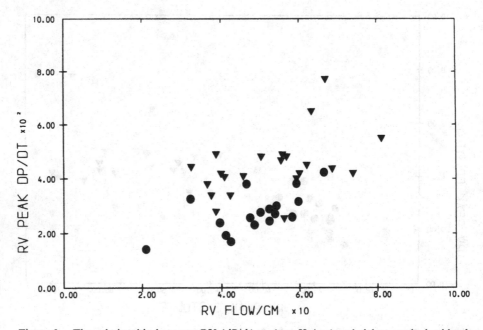

Figure 3. The relationship between RV $(dP/dt)_{max}$ (mm Hg/sec) and right ventricular blood flow per gram of muscle (expressed as ml/100 g per min) in normal animals (circles) and those with right ventricular hypertrophy (triangles).

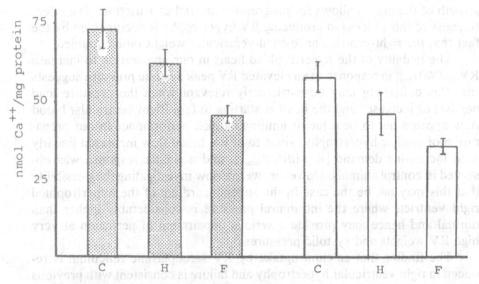

Figure 4. The effect of right ventricular hypertrophy and failure on calcium uptake by pig left (LV, shaded) and right (RV, unshaded) ventricular sarcoplasmic reticulum expressed as nmol Ca^{2+}/mg protein and measured as a linear rate over 2 min. Vertical bars are the standard errors of the means. C, normals; H, hypertrophied; F, failing.

in those with RVH. Both controls and animals with RVH showed similar increases in blood flow in response to increased RV $(dP/dt)_{max}$ (for controls, $r = 0.638$, $P < 0.01$; for RVH, $r = 0.462$, $P < 0.02$), which suggests that there was no impairment of blood flow in these hypertrophied right ventricles.

Values for calcium uptake by preparations of left and right ventricular sarcoplasmic reticulum from control animals, from those with RVH, and from those with RVF are shown in Figure 4. Calcium uptake by right ventricular sarcoplasmic reticulum was less than that from the left ventricle even in control animals (LV, 73.1 ± 6.6; RV, 57.4 ± 4.9 nmol Ca^{2+}/mg protein). Calcium uptake by right ventricular sarcoplasmic reticulum was reduced in RVH and RVF by mean values of 22% and 38% (35.4 ± 2.6 nmol Ca^{2+}/mg protein, $P < 0.001$), respectively (RVH vs. RVF, $P < 0.01$). Animals with RVH and RVF also had reduced mean values for left ventricular sarcoplasmic reticulum calcium uptake by 15% and 38% (45.6 ± 3.1 nmol Ca^{2+}/mg protein, $P < 0.001$), respectively.

DISCUSSION

Constriction of the pulmonary artery in swine causes an increased right ventricular work load. Our preparation has the advantage that the natural growth of the piglets allows for progressive arterial constriction. The effectiveness of this process in producing RV hypertrophy is documented by the fact that the right-ventricular-to-total-ventricular weight ratios doubled.

The inability of the hypertrophied heart in our preparation to increase RV $(dP/dt)_{max}$ in response to an elevated RV peak systolic pressure suggests that this deficiency may be particularly relevant when the pressure load persists or increases and the heart is starting to fail. Right ventricular blood flow appears not to be a factor limiting cardiac performance in our preparation of cardiac hypertrophy, since total RV blood flow increased linearly with increasing demand [RV $(dP/dt)_{max}$], and a similar response was observed in control animals. However, we are now investigating the possibility that this may not be the case in the subendocardium of the hypertrophied right ventricle where the intramural pressure is considerably higher than normal and hence may provide a serious impairment of perfusion at very high RV weights and systolic pressures.

The finding that calcium uptake by RV sarcoplasmic reticulum is reduced in right ventricular hypertrophy and failure is consistent with previous findings (8,11) by other workers. However, it is unlikely that this reduction represents a primary biochemical abnormality directly causing depression of contractile performance in these pathological states, since similar reductions of activity were found in sarcoplasmic reticulum isolated from the unstressed left ventricle.

Is the unstressed left side of the heart in RV hypertrophy or failure affected by events occurring on the side undergoing hemodynamic challenge? Our results show that there is a normal linear relationship of LV $(dP/dt)_{max}$ to aortic systolic pressure in both control animals and those with RVH. However, left ventricular sarcoplasmic reticulum did show a depression of function that was worse in RVF than in RVH even though the left ventricle was unstressed. Although such depression is known to occur in sarcoplasmic reticulum isolated from stressed ventricular muscle (11), the demonstration that it can also occur on the unstressed side of the heart suggests that the activity of the sarcoplasmic reticulum calcium pump reflects the overall contractile state of the heart rather than being a dominant factor in the control of contractility. Such a concept is consistent with the finding that physical training without associated hypertrophy was alone enough to increase calcium uptake by the sarcoplasmic reticulum (9). Certainly, the activity of this calcium pump is altered by rapid (8) and, in the present study, by chronic changes in work load. It may be that the effective stimulus in the hypertrophying heart is an intracellular calcium deficiency resulting from a decrease in the surface-to-volume ratio of the myocardial cells.

ACKNOWLEDGMENTS

The authors would like to thank Brian Reeson and Margaret L. Stevenson for their expert technical assistance and the British Heart Foundation for the provision of financial support for this project.

REFERENCES

1. Astrup, P., Jørgensen, K., Andersen, O. S., and Engel, K. 1960. The acid–base metabolism. A new approach. *Lancet* 1:1035–1039.
2. Bray, G. A. 1960. A simple efficient scintillator for counting aqueous solutions in a liquid scintillation counter. *Anal Biochem.* 1:279–284.
3. Harigaya, S., and Schwartz, A. 1969. Rate of calcium binding and uptake in normal animal and failing human cardiac muscle. Membrane vesicles (relaxing system) and mitochondria. *Circ. Res.* 25:781–794.
4. Ito, Y., Suko, J., and Chidsey, C. A. 1974. Intracellular calcium and myocardial contractility. V. Calcium uptake of sarcoplasmic reticulum fractions in hypertrophied and failing rabbit hearts. *J. Mol. Cell. Cardiol.* 6:237–247.
5. Katz, A. M., Repke, D. I., Upshaw, J. E., and Polascik, M. A. 1970. Characterisation of dog cardiac microsomes. Use of zonal centrifugation to fractionate fragmented sarcoplasmic reticulum, (Na^+ + K^+)-activated ATPase and mitochondrial fragments. *Biochim. Biophys. Acta* 205:473–490.
6. Lentz, R. W., Harrison, C. E., Jr., Dewey, J. D., Barnhorst, D. A., Danielson, G. K., and Pluth, J. R. 1978. Functional evaluation of cardiac sarcoplasmic reticulum and mitochondria in human pathologic states. *J. Mol. Cell. Cardiol.* 10:3–30.
7. Lowry, O. H., Rosebrough, N. J., Farr, A. L., and Randall, R. J. 1951. Protein measurement with folin phenol reagent. *J. Biol. Chem.* 193:265–275.
8. Nayler, W. G., McInnes, I., Chipperfield, D., Carson, V., and Kurtz, J. B. 1970. Ventricular function and the calcium-accumulating activity of the sarcoplasmic reticulum. *J. Mol. Cell. Cardiol.* 1:307–324.
9. Penpargkul, S., Repke, D. I., Katz, A. M., and Scheuer, J. 1977. Effect of physical training on calcium transport by rat cardiac sarcoplasmic reticulum. *Circ. Res.* 40:134–138.
10. Sordahl, L. A., McCollum, W. B., Wood, W. G., and Schwartz, A. 1973. Mitochondria and sarcoplasmic reticulum function in cardiac hypertrophy and failure. *Am. J. Physiol.* 224:497–502.
11. Suko, J., Vogel, J. H. K., and Chidsey, C. A. 1970. Intracellular calcium and myocardial contractility. III. Reduced calcium uptake and ATPase of the sarcoplasmic reticular fraction prepared from chronically failing hearts. *Circ. Res.* 27:235–247.
12. Welham, K. C., Silove, E. D., and Wyse, R. K. H. 1978. Experimental right ventricular hypertrophy and failure in swine. *Cardiovasc. Res.* 12:61–65.

Myocardial Energy Metabolism of Congestive and Hypertrophic Cardiomyopathy in Man

H. Abe

Department of Radiology,
Nihon University School of Medicine
Tokyo, 173 Japan

T. Yamada, K. Miyata, and A. Yoshida

Department of Internal Medicine
Josai Dental University
Saitama, Japan

Y. Yabe

Cardiovascular Diagnostic Laboratory Center
Toho University School of Medicine
Tokyo, Japan

Abstract. A key enzyme of glycolysis (pyruvate kinase) and main enzymes of the electron transport system (NADH cytochrome c reductase, succinic cytochrome c reductase, and cytochrome c oxidase) were measured in left ventricular biopsy specimens from six hypertrophic (HCM) and six congestive (CCM) cardiomyopathy. Pyruvate kinase was 104.0 and 45.0 mU/mg protein in HCM and CCM, respectively. NADH cytochrome c reductase, succinic cytochrome c reductase, and cytochrome c oxidase were 146.0, 9.9, and 775.0 mU/mg protein in HCM and 87.4, 5.2, and 502.0 mU/mg protein in CCM, respectively. From these data, it is evident that glycolysis and enzyme activities of the electron transport system are increased in HCM and decreased in CCM. Cardiac function reflects the state of these energy metabolism pathways in the myocardium. The changing energy metabolism in the right ventricle of the emphysema hamster seems to support this concept.

In recent years, different types of cardiomyopathy have become easily recognized by means of improved medical instrumentation such as cardiac catheterization, cineangiography, and echocardiography. However, the etiology of cardiomyopathy still remains unknown. The study of energy metoblism, which is closely related to energy production and oxygen utilization, plays an important role in the understanding of pathophysiology of the diseased heart muscle. In the present investigation, abnormalities of energy metabolism were examined in the left ventricular myocardium obtained from cardiomyopathy patients by a transcatheter endomyocardial biopsy technique. Furthermore, as an experimental model, energy metabolism in the right ventricle of the emphysema hamster was investigated in its hypertrophic and congestive stages resulting from cor pulmonale.

MATERIALS AND METHODS

Twelve patients with definite diagnoses of cardiomyopathy were entered in this study. There were six patients with hypertrophic cardiomyopathy (HCM) and six with congestive cardiomyopathy (CCM). In HCM, all patients were male, and the average age was 53 years, whereas in CCM, there were four males and two females, with an average age of 47 years.

Following right and left heart catheterization, coronary cinearteriography, and left ventriculography, myocardial specimens were obtained from the left ventricle by a transcatheter endomyocardial biopsy technique developed by the author.

Enzyme activities of the sonicated homogenate of the myocardial specimen were measured using the multiconvertible spectrophotometer. Pyruvate kinase, as a key enzyme of glycolysis, was measured by the method of Bücher. Main enzymes of the electron transport system, NADH cytochrome c reductase, succinic cytochrome c reductase, and cytochrome c oxidase, were measured by the method of King (2), Tisdale (5), and Wharton and Tzagoloff (6), respectively.

In addition to the clinical study, an experiment was designed to evaluate various stages of ventricular overload. In 40 cases of elastase-induced emphysemic hamsters, the same enzymes were measured in the right ventricles in the hypertrophic or congestive stage, 6 or 12 months after initiation of the experiment.

RESULTS

Hemodynamic data of patients with HCM and CCM are shown in Table 1. End-diastolic volume in CCM was significantly higher than that in HCM, whereas end-diastolic pressures were equally elevated in both groups. Wall thickness in HCM was increased to 15 mm, and that of CCM was 8 mm. Ejection fraction, mean V_{cf}, and dP/dt were markedly depressed in CCM.

Most histological sections of the HCM ventricle showed that myocardial cells were homogeneously hypertrophied and that the morphology of the mitochondria appeared normal. Although the myocardium of the CCM ventricle was still normal in appearance, the ultrastructure of the same biopsied specimen showed evidence of decreased glycogen granules and enlargement in the sarcoplasmic reticulum. However, the mitochondria remained intact, which may suggest that the energy production system in mitochondria still maintains its function.

Enzyme activities of the biopsied left ventricle are shown in Table 2. Activity of pyruvate kinase was 104.0 mU/mg protein per min in HCM,

Table 1.   Hemodynamic Data in Patients with HCM and CCM (Means ± S.D.)

	Age (yrs)	Cardiothoracic ratio (%)	Heart rate (beats/min)	Cardiac index (liter/min per m²)	LVP/EDP (mm Hg)	EDV (ml)	Ejection fraction (%)	Wall thickness (mm)	Mean V_{cf} (circ/sec)	dP/dt (mm Hg/sec)
HCM ($N = 6$)	53 ± 5	51 ± 6	61 ± 5	2.95 ± 0.53	108/15 ± 15/±7	135 ± 35	77 ± 7	15 ± 2	1.42 ± 0.29	1700 ± 352
CCM ($N = 6$)	47 ± 9	57 ± 2	54 ± 16	2.47 ± 0.27	107/15 ± 16/±10	249 ± 77	40 ± 12	8 ± 1	0.57 ± 0.20	1158 ± 136

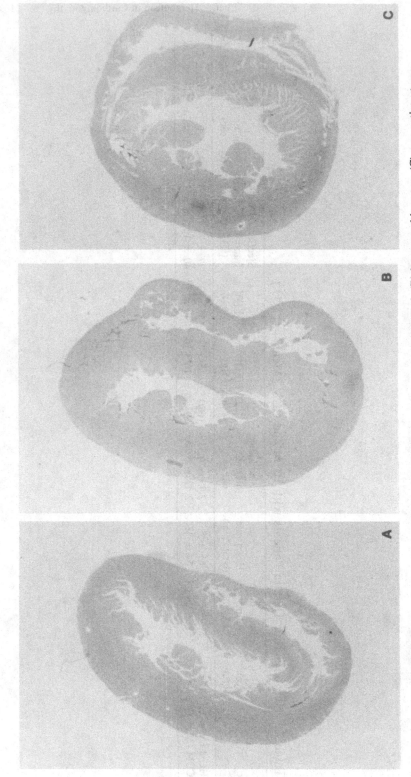

Figure 1. Gradual changes in the right ventricle of the emphysema hamster, (A) control, (B) hypertrophic stage, (C) congestive stage.

Table 2. Enzyme Activities in HCM and CCM[a]

	HCM	CCM
Pyruvate kinase	104.0	45.0
NADH cytochrome c reductase	146.0	87.4
Succinic cytochrome c reductase	9.9	5.2
Cytochrome c oxidase	775.0	502.0

[a] PH 7.4, 20°C, mean value of six patients in each group; values expressed in mU/mg protein per min.

whereas that of the CCM group was as low as 45.0 mU/mg protein per min. NADH cytochrome c reductase activity in HCM and CCM was 146.0 and 87.4 mU/mg protein per min, respectively.

On the other hand, succinic cytochrome c reductase in HCM was 9.9 and in CCM was 5.2 mU/mg protein per min. Cytochrome c oxidase was also higher in HCM than in CCM: activities of this enzyme were 775.0 and 502.0 mU/mg protein per min in HCM and CCM, respectively.

In the elastase-induced emphysema hamster, morphological changes in the right ventricles are apparent in its evolution from the hypertrophic to the congestive stage (Figure 1). Enzyme activities of pyruvate kinase,

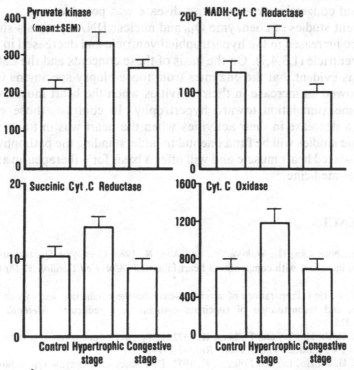

Figure 2. Enzyme activities in the right ventricle of the emphysema hamster (mU/mg protein per min).

NADH cytochrome c reductase, succinic cytochrome c reductase, and cytochrome c oxidase were measured in the right ventricles of the emphysema hamsters. It is evident that all four enzymes increased significantly in the compensatory hypertrophic stage and then decreased in the congestive stage, which is the end stage of right ventricular overload resulting from cor pulmonale (Figure 2).

DISCUSSION

Stress and overload to the ventricles would be expected to require a higher level of enzymes for contribution to the bioenergetic mechanisms supporting the biosynthesis of ATP. Under the hemodynamic conditions observed in HCM patients, it seems very likely that energy production would be supported by an increase in specific activities of enzymes of the mitochondrial electron transfer system. When the myocardium fails in CCM or in the late stage of ventricular overload, a deficiency of these enzymes in the ventricle involved will be observed. In animal experiments with elastase-induced emphysemic hamsters, gradual changes of the right ventricle from compensatory hypertrophy to the congestive stage were observed. Using this model, comparative study of the enzyme levels for normal, hypertrophied, and congestive types of heart disease was possible.

Recent studies of coenzyme Q_{10} and nuclear DNA synthesis show that they were increased in the hypertrophied ventricle and decreased in the thin dilated ventricle (1,3,4,7). On the basis of these concepts and the data in the table, it is evident that the enzymes from those biopsy specimens from the heart showed an increase in their activities when the heart muscles underwent some stimulation toward hypertrophy. In contrast, those enzymes showed a decrease in their activities when the heart was in failure. These enzymatic studies will be fundamental to understanding the pathophysiology of the diseased heart muscle and will offer a basis for a therapeutic approach in clinical medicine.

REFERENCES

1. Abe, H., Nagasaka, H., Wakiya, Y., and Abe, K. 1980. Coenzyme Q_{10} activity of myocardium in patient with compensated heart failure. *J. Mol. Cell Cardiol.* 12 (8) (Suppl. 1) 1.
2. King, T. E. 1967. Preparations of succinate–cytochrome c reductase and cytochrome b–c, particle, and reconstitution of succinate–cytochrome c reductase. *Methods Enzymol.* 10:216–225.
3. Littaru, G. P., Ho, L., and Folkers, K. 1972. Deficiency of coenzyme Q_{10} in human heart disease. Part I. *Int. J. Vitam. Nutr. Res.* 42:291–305.
4. Littaru, G. P., Ho, L., and Folkers, K. 1972. Deficiency of coenzyme Q_{10} in human heart disease. Part II. *Int. J. Vitam. Nutr. Res.* 42:413–434.

5. Tisdale, H. D. 1967. Preparation and properties of succinic–cytochrome *c* reductase (complex II–III). *Methods Enzymol.* 10:213–215.
6. Wharton, D. C., and Tzagoloff, A. 1967. Cytochrome oxidase from beef heart mitochondria. *Methods Enzymol.* 10:245–250.
7. Yabe, Y., and Abe, H. 1980. Changes in DNA synthesis in significantly hypertrophied human cardiac muscle. In: M. Tajuddin, P. K. Das, M. Tariq, and N. S. Dhalla (eds.), *Advances in Myocardiology*, Vol. 1, pp. 553–563. University Park Press, Baltimore.

Effects of Cardiac Work and Leucine on Protein Turnover

B. Chua, D. L. Siehl, E. O. Fuller,
and H. E. Morgan

Department of Physiology
The Milton S. Hershey Medical Center
The Pennsylvania State University
Hershey, Pennsylvania 17033, USA

Abstract. The purpose of these experiments was to assess effects of cardiac work and leucine in hearts supplied only glucose or substrate and hormone mixtures that simulated plasma. Rates of protein degradation greatly exceeded protein synthesis in Langendorff preparations supplied glucose. This severely negative nitrogen balance was brought closer to zero by provision of more complete substrate mixtures. Cardiac work further improved the nitrogen balance by stimulating protein synthesis in hearts supplied glucose (mixture 1), glucose–insulin–glucagon–lactate–β-hydroxybutyrate (mixture 2), or palmitate–β-hydroxybutyrate–glucose (mixture 3) and inhibiting protein degradation in hearts supplied glucose. Cardiac work did not affect the rates of either protein synthesis or degradation in hearts provided insulin–lactate–glucose (mixture 4). The increase in protein synthesis was associated with increased rates of peptide chain initiation. Addition of 1 mM leucine had an additional effect to restore nitrogen balance to zero or to achieve positive balance in working hearts supplied substrate and hormone mixture 2.

The role of ventricular pressure development in cardiac growth has received considerable attention over the past decade (8,9,12,19,20,23). Since the protein content of a heart is determined by the balance between the rates of protein synthesis and degradation, hypertrophy may arise from a change in either protein synthesis, degradation, or both. Studies carried out in intact animals indicated that rates of both protein synthesis and degradation increased in hypertrophying hearts, but the increase in synthesis was greater (12,23). The increase in the synthetic rate appeared to depend on increased RNA content. When the efficiency with which RNA was utilized was assessed during in vitro perfusion, the rate of protein synthesis, expressed as a function of RNA, was unchanged (9). On the other hand, in vitro cardiac work accelerated protein synthesis and facilitated peptide chain initiation in hearts supplied either glucose or palmitate as oxidizable substrate (7,8). In regard to protein degradation, Schreiber et al. found that acute pressure overload did not change the rate of release of amino acids from prelabeled protein (20).

Protein turnover is also regulated by a number of hormonal (5,15,18) and nonhormonal factors, such as availability of branched-chain amino acids (2–4,14,15). Leucine at 1 mM, but not isoleucine or valine, inhibited protein degradation and accelerated protein synthesis in hearts supplied glucose and normal plasma levels of other amino acids (2–4). Furthermore, an intraperitoneal injection of the three branched-chain amino acids or leucine alone resulted in the formation of polyribosomes in psoas muscle of starved rats that had been pretreated with glucose and insulin (1).

Recently, the method for perfusion of working rat heart has been modified to facilitate studies of protein turnover in hearts provided with substrate mixtures simulating plasma. In the present experiments, the effects of in vitro cardiac work on rates of protein synthesis and degradation and nitrogen balance were studied in perfused rat hearts supplied glucose or substrate mixtures simulating plasma concentrations of substrates after chow feeding (mixture 2), 2 days of fasting (mixture 3), or a large carbohydrate meal (mixture 4). In addition, the role of leucine in modifying protein turnover was assessed in both Langendorff preparations and working hearts supplied a substrate and hormone mixture (mixture 2).

MATERIALS AND METHODS

Perfusion of Hearts

Hearts were removed from heparinized male Sprague–Dawley rats (300 g) that had been fasted overnight and anesthetized with sodium pentobarbital (12.5 mg). Hearts were perfused as Langendorff and working preparations as described previously (13,16). A modified Krebs–Henseleit bicarbonate buffer, pH 7.4, was used in all experiments. In addition, one of the following substrate mixtures was added to the buffer: (1) glucose 15 mM, and bovine serum albumin 0.2%; (2) glucose 8 mM, insulin 100 μU/ml, glucagon 30 pg/ml, lactate 1 mM, DL-β-hydroxybutyrate 2 mM, and bovine serum albumin 0.2%; (3) palmitate 1.5 mM, DL-β-hydroxybutyrate 10 mM, glucose 8 mM, and bovine serum albumin 4%; or (4) lactate 2 mM, glucose 10 mM, insulin 400 μU/ml, and bovine serum albumin 0.2%. The lactate and β-hydroxybutyrate concentrations in the perfusate were maintained by constant infusion as detailed previously (13).

Analytical Procedures

The rates of protein synthesis were estimated as described earlier (11,13). Protein degradation was estimated from changes in perfusate phenylalanine content in the presence of 0.02 mM cycloheximide (3,13). When nitrogen balance was studied, the buffer contained 0.01 mM phenylalanine. This concentration of phenylalanine was sufficient to maintain a maximal rate of protein synthesis but was sufficiently low to allow for estimation of the phenylalanine that was released (11). Ribosomal subunits were analyzed as described previously (13). ATP and creatine phosphate were determined enzymatically (10). Aortic and atrial pressures were recorded on light-sensitive paper (Honeywell Visicorder, Model 1508C). Aortic flow was determined from the outflow from the compliance chamber; coronary flow was estimated by measuring fluid dripping from the heart. Significance of differences between means was established by Student's t-test.

RESULTS

The apparatus for the working heart (Figure 1) was greatly improved and simplified by the use of an oxygenator that was described by Hems et al. (6) for liver perfusion and used by Taegtmeyer et al. (22) for heart perfusion. The apparatus consisted of six major parts: cannula assembly, aortic compliance chamber, combined oxygenator and left atrial reservoir, heart chamber, buffer reservoir and filter, and peristaltic pump. The cannula assembly for mounting the aorta and left atrium and the aortic compliance chamber were detailed previously (13,16). The outflow from the compliance chamber was returned to the buffer reservoir via a length of Tygon® tubing with a hypodermic needle inserted into the distal end to offer outflow resistance. Use of a 20-gauge needle resulted in systolic and diastolic pressures of 145 and 75 mm Hg. The height of the overflow above the level of the heart provided a left atrial filling pressure of 9 mm Hg. Perfusate entered the top of the oxygenator and spread as a film over the entire surface of a series of glass bulbs. The lower end of the oxygenator terminated in the left atrial chamber and a side-arm to return excess buffer to the reservoir. A mixture of 95% O_2 plus 5% CO_2 entered the oxygenator via a side arm and was carried into the buffer reservoir through the overflow side arm. Oxygen tension of buffer leaving the oxygenator was approximately 620 mm Hg, whereas oxygen tension of the coronary effluent that was obtained from the pulmonary artery of working hearts averaged 210 mm Hg. Two salient features are worthy of mention. First, the circulating volume could be reduced to 35 ml in contrast to 65 ml in the earlier apparatus (16). This reduction in volume became important when rates of protein degradation were assessed by measuring phenylalanine concentrations in the perfusate. Second, in some experiments designed to simulate plasma conditions, albumin-containing buffer could be oxygenated without formation of foam.

Heart rate, aortic pressure, aortic and coronary flow, and levels of ATP and creatine phosphate were stable over 2 hr of perfusion with buffers that contained glucose or mixtures of glucose, lactate, and insulin or glucose, palmitate, and β-hydroxybutyrate (Figure 2). Regardless of the substrate mixture used, heart rate was approximately 300 beats per minute. The systolic and diastolic pressures stayed at 145 and 75 mm Hg. The aortic output and coronary flow were 45 and 25 ml per minute, respectively. These data indicated that the mechanical performance of the working heart preparation

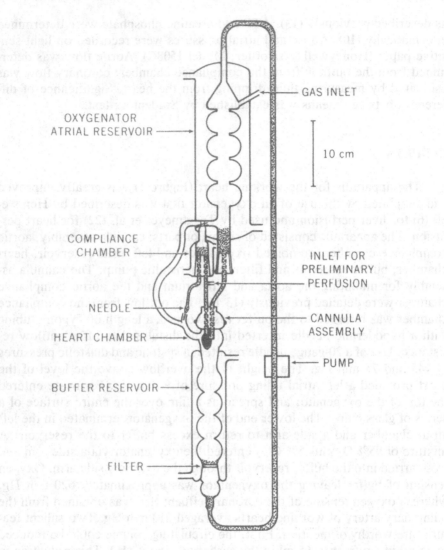

OXYGENATOR
ATRIAL RESERVOIR

GAS INLET

10 cm

COMPLIANCE
CHAMBER

INLET FOR
PRELIMINARY
PERFUSION

NEEDLE

CANNULA
ASSEMBLY

HEART CHAMBER

PUMP

BUFFER RESERVOIR

FILTER

Figure 1.   Modified apparatus for perfusion of working rat hearts. Reproduced from Morgan et al. (13) with the permission of the publisher of the *American Journal of Physiology*.

was similar to that found in vivo. ATP levels were maintained at 20 μmol per gram. The levels of creatine phosphate fell to 15 μmol per gram in hearts provided only glucose but were kept at 23 μmol per gram in hearts supplied more complete substrate mixtures.

In Langendorff preparations that were perfused with an aortic pressure of 60 mm Hg and supplied glucose as the oxidizable substrate (Table 1), nitrogen balance was severely negative, indicating that rates of protein degradation greatly exceeded synthesis. The extent of the negative balance, as indicated by net phenylalanine release, was reduced in working hearts. When a more physiological substrate mixture was supplied, net phenylalanine release was reduced approximately 60% in both Langendorff and working preparations. Cardiac work decreased phenylalanine release by 50%.

An improvement of overall nitrogen balance by work could involve a change in rates of either protein synthesis or degradation. The effects of cardiac work on protein turnover were further investigated by direct measurements of the rates of protein synthesis and degradation in Langendorff preparations and working hearts supplied glucose or the substrate mixture (Table 1). In hearts supplied glucose as substrate, cardiac work increased the rate of protein synthesis and decreased the rate of protein degradation. Provision of a more complete substrate mixture increased the rate of protein synthesis and decreased the rate of protein degradation in both Langendorff preparations and working hearts. Cardiac work stimulated protein synthesis

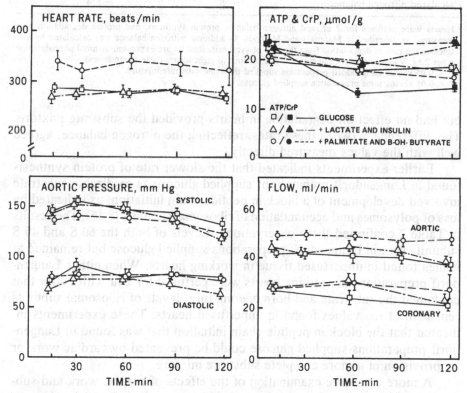

Figure 2. Stability of performance and energy levels in hearts with a 20-gauge needle in aortic outflow tract. Hearts were perfused for a period of 120 min, and the performance was monitored. Contents of ATP and Cr-P were measured at the end of perfusions of 60 and 120 min and expressed per gram dry weight. Substrate mixtures are denoted as follows: glucose 15 mM, bovine serum albumin 0.2% (□); lactate 2 mM, glucose 10 mM, insulin 400 μU/ml, and bovine serum albumin 4% (△); and palmitate 1.5 mM, DL-β-hydroxybutyrate 10 mM, glucose 8 mM, and bovine serum albumin 4% (○). Values are mean ± S.E. of 4–6 hearts. Reproduced from Morgan et al. (13) with the permission of the publisher of the *American Journal of Physiology*.

Table 1. Effect of Cardiac Work on Nitrogen Balance and Rates of
Protein Synthesis and Degradation[a]

	Condition of perfusion	
Parameter	Langendorff	Working
Glucose, 15 mM		
Measured nitrogen balance	−1900 ± 90(8)	−1172 ± 111(4)[b]
Synthesis	820 ± 38(4)	1117 ± 42(4)[b]
Degradation	2478 ± 80(8)	2213 ± 68(8)[b]
Calculated nitrogen balance	−1658	−1096
Glucose, 8 mM; insulin 100μU/ml; glucagon, 30 pg/ml; lactate, 1 mM; DL-β-OH-butyrate, 2 mM		
Measured nitrogen balance	−738 ± 64(7)[c]	−369 ± 74(4)[b,c]
Synthesis	1194 ± 29(4)[c]	1496 ± 43(4)[b,c]
Degradation	1776 ± 58(4)[c]	1670 ± 67(4)[c]
Calculated nitrogen balance	−582	−174

[a] Hearts were perfused for 2 hr, and nitrogen balance, protein synthesis, and protein degradation were measured as described in Materials and Methods. In addition, nitrogen balance was calculated by subtracting the rate of degradation from the rate of synthesis. Results are expressed as nmol phenylalanine/g per 2 hr. Values represent the mean ± S.E. of four to eight hearts (N in parentheses).
[b] $P < 0.05$ versus Langendorff preparation supplied the same substrate mixture.
[c] $P < 0.05$ versus same preparation supplied glucose.

but had no effect on degradation in hearts provided the substrate mixture. The difference between these rates, reflecting the nitrogen balance, agreed well with the values measured directly.

Earlier experiments indicated that the slower rate of protein synthesis found in Langendorff preparations supplied glucose as oxidizable substrate involved development of a block in peptide chain initiation, as indicated by loss of polysomes and accumulation of ribosomal subunits (8,15). The results in Table 2 confirmed these observations. Levels of both the 60 S and 40 S subunits rose in Langendorff preparations supplied glucose but remained at values found in unperfused tissue in working hearts. When either Langendorff preparations or working hearts were perfused for 2 hr with buffer that contained the substrate and hormone mixture, levels of ribosomal subunits remained at the values found in unperfused hearts. These experiments indicated that the block in peptide chain initiation that was found in Langendorff preparations supplied glucose could be prevented by cardiac work or by provision of a more complete substrate mixture.

A more extensive examination of the effects of cardiac work and substrate and hormone mixtures simulating concentrations found in vivo are summarized in Figure 3. The effects of cardiac work on nitrogen balance were largest in hearts supplied only glucose as substrate, denoted as mixture 1. This effect was caused by acceleration of protein synthesis and inhibition of protein degradation. Substrate mixture 2, which contained 8 mM glucose, 100 μU insulin/ml, 30 pg glucagon/ml, 1 mM lactate, and 1 mM L-β-hydroxybutyrate, reduced the magnitude of the negative nitrogen balance in Langendorff preparations by accelerating protein synthesis and restraining pro-

Table 2.   Effect of Cardiac Work on Distribution of
RNA in Ribosomal Subunits[a]

Conditions of perfusion	RNA content of ribosomal subunit peaks (μg RNA per mg RNA in heart homogenate)	
	60 S	40 S
Unperfused	65 ± 5(6)	41 ± 3(6)
	Glucose, 15 mM	
Langendorff	122 ± 7(8)[b]	82 ± 5(8)[b]
Working	77 ± 6(4)	49 ± 4(4)
	Glucose, 8 mM; insulin, 100 μU/ ml; glucagon, 30 pg/ml; lactate, 1 mM; DL-β-hydroxybutyrate, 2 mM	
Langendorff	59 ± 2(4)	35 ± 1(4)
Working	69 ± 4(4)	43 ± 4(4)

[a] Hearts were perfused for 120 min with the buffer which contained 15 mM glucose or the substrate and hormone mixture and normal plasma levels of amino acids. Values represent the mean ± S.E. The figures in parenthesis indicate the number of observations.
[b] $P < 0.05$ versus unperfused heart.

tein degradation. In hearts supplied this mixture, work increased synthesis further, had no effect on degradation, and brought the heart into nitrogen balance. Mixture 3 contained 1.5 mM palmitate, 5 mM L-β-hydroxybutyrate, and 8 mM glucose. As with mixture 2, nitrogen balance was less negative in Langendorff preparations because of faster synthesis and slower degradation. In hearts supplied mixture 3, cardiac work accelerated protein synthesis but had no effect on degradation. Nitrogen balance remained negative. Mixture 4 contained 2 mM lactate, 10 mM glucose, and 400 μU insulin/ml. As with the other substrate mixtures, protein synthesis was accelerated, and protein degradation was restrained. Nitrogen balance was achieved. Cardiac work had no further effect on any of these rates.

The results thus far indicated that working hearts supplied substrate mixtures simulating substrate and hormone concentrations found in plasma were essentially in nitrogen balance. It was of interest to examine the effects of other modulators such as leucine on the overall nitrogen balance and rates of protein synthesis and degradation under these simulated physiological conditions (Figure 4).

As shown previously (2–4), addition of 1 mM leucine accelerated protein synthesis and inhibited protein degradation in Langendorff preparations supplied glucose. In the presence of leucine, work inhibited proteolysis but had no effect on protein synthesis. In both preparations, leucine addition brought nitrogen balance closer to zero. When a substrate and hormone mixture was supplied, leucine did not have a significant effect on either synthesis or degradation, although there was a tendency to accelerate synthesis and inhibit degradation. When nitrogen balance was measured directly by net

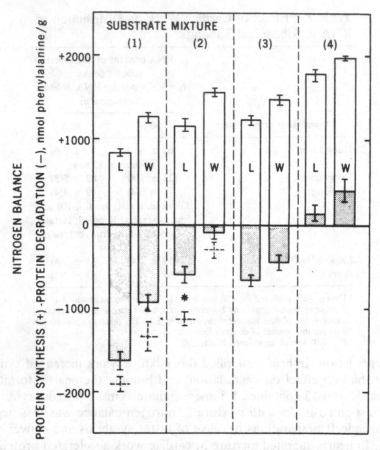

Figure 3.   Nitrogen balance in Langendorff preparations and working hearts perfused for 2 hr. Rates of protein synthesis are plotted above zero line. Rates of degradation are plotted downward from synthesis values. Nitrogen balance, as indicated by stippled area, was obtained by subtracting rate of degradation from rate of synthesis. Values of nitrogen balance determined directly are plotted as dashed lines. Substrate mixtures are: (1) glucose 15 mM; (2) glucose 8 mM, insulin 100 μU/ml, glucagon 30 pg/ml, lactate 1 mM, DL-β-hydroxybutyrate 2 mM; (3) palmitate 1.5 mM, DL-β-hydroxybutyrate 10 mM, glucose 8 mM; and (4) lactate 2 mM, glucose 10 mM, insulin 400 μU/ml. Outflow resistance in working hearts was offered by a 20-gauge needle. Asterisk indicates that nitrogen balance, as estimated by the two methods, was statistically different ($P < 0.05$). Reproduced from Morgan et al. (13) with the permission of the publisher of the *American Journal of Physiology*.

phenylalanine release, addition of 1 mM leucine converted the balance from slightly negative to positive in working hearts, indicating that the leucine had a small effect under simulated physiological conditions.

DISCUSSION

The present experiments indicate that a broad spectrum of both hormonal and nonhormonal factors accelerate protein synthesis and inhibit

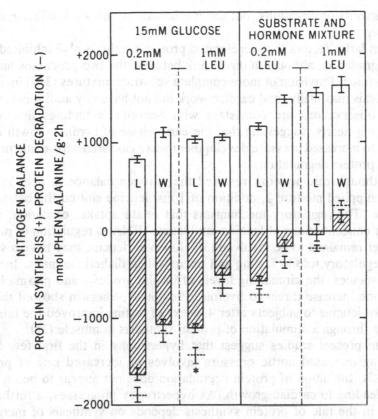

Figure 4.   Effect of 1 mM leucine on nitrogen balance in Langendorff preparations and working hearts perfused for 2 hr. Rates of protein synthesis and degradation are plotted as described in Figure 3. Nitrogen balance, as indicated by the shaded area, was obtained by substrating the rate of protein degradation from the rate of synthesis. Nitrogen balance as determined directly was plotted as dashed lines. Substrate mixtures are: (1) glucose 15 mM; (2) glucose 8 mM, insulin 100 μU/ml, glucagon 30 pg/ml, lactate 1 mM, DL-β-hydroxybutyrate 2 mM. Leucine was added to the perfusate as indicated. The asterisk indicated that nitrogen balance, as determined by the two methods, was statistically different ($P < 0.05$).

protein degradation in heart muscle. On the synthesis side, most of these factors act by accelerating the rate of peptide chain initiation more than the rate of elongation. Among the hormones, insulin, glucagon, and epinephrine were found to stimulate protein synthesis (5,18). A number of compounds, such as leucine (2–4), lactate (17), metabolites of fatty acids (17), and ketone bodies (3,17) also enhance the synthetic rates. Hence, provision of a substrate and hormone mixture would improve the nitrogen balance by stimulating protein synthesis. Protein synthesis proceeded below the maximal rate in hearts supplied mixtures 1–3. Imposition of cardiac work enhanced protein synthesis further. However, protein synthesis was maximally accelerated by insulin and lactate in the Langendorff preparation; consequently, cardiac work had no effect. These studies confirm and extend

Hjalmarson's observations, but the mechanism of the work effect remains unknown.

Similarly, factors that accelerated protein synthesis also inhibited protein degradation, although a direct link between the two processes has not been defined. Provision of more complete substrate mixtures (2–4) inhibited proteolysis maximally, and cardiac work did not have any additional effect. These observations are consistent with Schreiber's findings in isolated guinea pig hearts, suggesting that the early phase of cardiac growth in response to increased pressure development was associated with an unchanged rate of protein degradation.

Although cardiac work restored the nitrogen balance to near zero in hearts supplied mixture 2, addition of 1 mM leucine shifted the balance to positive. The regulatory mechanisms that relate uptake, oxidation, intracellular concentrations of leucine, and leucyl-tRNA to regulation of protein turnover remained to be resolved (3). However, leucine may have a significant regulatory role in fasting and uncontrolled diabetic animals. In these circumstances, the circulating levels of insulin are low, and plasma levels of leucine increase three- to fivefold. Previously, Sherwin showed that infusion of leucine to subjects after 4 weeks of fasting improved the nitrogen balance through a stimulation of protein synthesis in muscle (21).

The present studies suggest that hypertrophy in the first few hours following increased aortic pressure involves an increased rate of protein synthesis. Inhibition of protein degradation does not appear to be an early event leading to cardiac growth. As hypertrophy progresses, a further increase in the rate of protein synthesis depends on synthesis of increased numbers of ribosomes. Tissue content of rRNA rises during the rapid phase of cardiac growth following aortic banding and decreases during the cardiac atrophy that follows debanding or following hypophysectomy of normal rats (9). Factors that control synthesis, processing, and degradation of rRNA and synthesis and degradation of ribosomal proteins must be investigated to complete our understanding of the regulation of cardiac protein turnover.

ACKNOWLEDGMENTS

These studies were supported by National Institutes of Health Grants HL-18258, HL-20388, and HL-07223.

REFERENCES

1. Buse, M. G., Atwell, R., and Mancusi, V. 1979. *In vitro* effect of branched chain amino acids on the ribosomal cycle in muscles of fasted rats. *Horm. Metab. Res.* 11:289–292.
2. Chua, B., Siehl, D. L., Fuller, E. O., and Morgan, H. E. 1980. Branch chain amino acids and protein turnover in heart. In: *Fourth USA–USSR Symposium on Myocardial Metabolism*, pp. 305–324. U.S. Dept. of Health and Human Services (NIH Publication No. 80-2017), Bethesda.

3. Chua, B. L., Siehl, D. L., and Morgan, H. E. 1979. Effect of leucine and metabolites of branched-chain amino acids on protein turnover in heart. *J. Biol. Chem.* 254:8358–8362.
4. Chua, B., Siehl, D. L., and Morgan, H. E. 1980. A role for leucine in the regulation of protein turnover in working rat hearts. *Am. J. Physiol.* 239:E510–E514.
5. Chua, B., Watkins, C., Siehl, D. L., and Morgan, H. E. 1978. Effect of epinephrine and glucagon on protein turnover in perfused rat heart. *Fed. Proc.* 37:540.
6. Hems, R., Ross, B. D., Berry, M. N., and Krebs, H. A. 1966. Gluconeogenesis in the perfused rat liver. *Biochem. J.* 101:284–292.
7. Hjalmarson, Å. C., and Isaksson, O. 1972. *In vitro* work load and rat heart metabolism. I. Effect of protein synthesis. *Acta Physiol. Scand.* 86:126–144.
8. Hjalmarson, Å. C., and Isaksson, O. 1972. *In vitro* work load and rat heart metabolism. IV. Effect on ribosomal aggregation. *Acta Physiol. Scand.* 86:342–352.
9. Kao, R., Rannels, D. E., Whitman, V., and Morgan, H. E. 1978. Factors accounting for growth and atrophy of the heart. In: T. Kobayashi, Y. Ito, and G. Rona (eds.), *Recent Advances in Studies on Cardiac Structure and Metabolism.* Vol. 12: *Cardiac Adaptation,* pp. 105–113. University Park Press, Baltimore.
10. Lamprecht, W. I., and Trautschold, I. 1965. Determination with hexokinase and glucose-6-phosphate dehydrogenase. In: H. U. Bergmeyer (ed.), *Methods of Enzymatic Analysis,* pp. 543–551. Academic Press, New York.
11. McKee, E. E., Cheung, J. Y., Rannels, D. E., and Morgan, H. E. 1978. Measurement of the rate of protein synthesis and compartmentation of heart phenylalanine. *J. Biol. Chem.* 253:1030–1040.
12. Millward, D. J. 1980. Protein turnover in skeletal and cardiac muscle during normal growth and hypertrophy. In: K. Wildenthal (ed.), *Degradation Processes in Heart and Skeletal Muscle,* pp. 161–199. Elsevier/North Holland Biomedical Press, Amsterdam.
13. Morgan, H. E., Chua, B. H. L., Fuller, E. O., and Siehl, D. L. 1980. Regulation of protein synthesis and degradation during *in vitro* cardiac work. *Am. J. Physiol.* 238:E431–E442.
14. Morgan, H. E., Earl, D. C. N., Broadus, A., Wolpert, E. B., Giger, K. E., and Jefferson, L. S. 1971. Regulation of protein synthesis in heart muscle. I. Effect of amino acid levels on protein synthesis. *J. Biol. Chem.* 246:2152–2162.
15. Morgan, H. E., Jefferson, L. S., Wolpert, E. B., and Rannels, D. E. 1971. Regulation of protein synthesis in heart muscle. II. Effect of amino acid levels and insulin on ribosomal aggregation. *J. Biol. Chem.* 246:2163–2170.
16. Neely, J. R., Liebermeister, H., Battersby, E. J., and Morgan, H. E. 1967. Effect of pressure development on oxygen consumption by isolated rat heart. *Am. J. Physiol.* 212:804–814.
17. Rannels, D. E., Hjalmarson, Å. C., and Morgan, H. E. 1974. Effects of non-carbohydrate substrates on protein synthesis in muscle. *Am. J. Physiol.* 226:528–539.
18. Rannels, D. E., Kao, R., and Morgan, H. E. 1975. Effect of insulin on protein turnover in heart muscle. *J. Biol. Chem.* 250:1694–1701.
19. Schreiber, S. S., Briden, K., Oratz, M., and Rothschild, M. A. 1966. Protein synthesis in the overloaded heart. *Am. J. Physiol.* 211:314–318.
20. Schreiber, S. S., Oratz, M., Evans, C., Reff, F., Klein, I., and Rothschild, M. A. 1973. Cardiac protein degradation in acute overload *in vitro*. Reutilization of amino acids. *Am. J. Physiol.* 224:338–345.
21. Sherwin, R. S. 1978. Effect of starvation on the turnover and metabolic response to leucine. *J. Clin. Invest.* 61:1471–1481.
22. Taegtmeyer, H., Hems, R., and Krebs, H. A. 1980. Utilization of energy-providing substrates in the isolated working rat heart. *Biochem. J.* 186:701–711.
23. Zak, R., Martin, A. F., Reddy, M. K., and Rabinowitz, M. 1976. Control of protein balance in hypertrophied cardiac muscle. *Circ. Res.* 38(Suppl. 1):145–150.

The Rate of Cardiac Structural Protein Synthesis in Perfused Heart

Y. Ito

Sanraku Hospital
Tokyo 101, Japan

Y. Kira, K. Ebisawa, T. Koizumi, S. Matsumoto, and E. Ogata

The Fourth Department of Internal Medicine
Faculty of Medicine
The University of Tokyo
Tokyo, Japan

Abstract. Synthesis of cardiac structural protein was studied in perfused rabbit hearts using [^{3}H]lysine and perfluorochemical blood substitute. Relative synthesis rate was estimated in adult rabbit heart when both ventricles worked against zero pressure. The decreasing order was troponin complex, actinin complex, myosin, tropomyosin, and actin and was almost the same as that found in an in vivo study. The synthesis rates of myosin B in left and right ventricles were almost equal in hearts without left and right ventricular pressure load. In young rabbit heart with a right ventricular pressure load, an increase in the synthesis rate of right ventricular myosin B was observed along with the concomitant increase in that of left ventricle. As those increases were blocked by neither propranolol nor verapamil, it was suggested that these increases were not mediated by Ca^{2+} influx or β-adrenergic receptors.

Structural protein synthesis in normal and pressure-loaded hearts has been studied, and differences are recognized in synthesis rates of various structural protein fractions (6,13). Futhermore, in vivo study showed that the synthesis rate of myosin B is different between left and right ventricles (6).

This study was done to clarify more precisely the synthesis rates of cardiac structural protein fractions and the relationship between right and left ventricular myosin B synthesis in perfused rabbit hearts with or without a right ventricular pressure load.

MATERIALS AND METHOD

Heart Preparation

Young and adult female rabbits, about 1 kg, 4 to 6 weeks after weaning and about 3 kg, 5 months after weaning, respectively, were used in these experiments. Rabbits were anesthetized with ethyl ether and injected with heparin (300 U/kg) and curare (0.3 mg/kg) after intubation to maintain respiration with a respirator. The thorax was opened and the heart was resected after ligation of superior vena cava and inferior vena cava and then was soaked in cold saline to stop the heart beat. The aorta and pulmonary artery were cannulated with polyethylene cannulas, and the pulmonary veins were ligated. Perfusion was performed according to the modified Langendorff preparation. The coronary perfusion was performed from a reservoir via an aortic cannula at the constant pressure of 100 cm H_2O. The right ventricle was not subjected to any volume load other than coronary flow. Pulmonary pressure was maintained at zero in the control group and at 20 cm H_2O in the pressure-loaded group by elevation of the pulmonary cannula (Figure 1). The left ventricle was freed from load by a puncture through the left ventricular apical wall with an 18-gauge Teflon® tube in young rabbits and a 14 gauge Teflon® tube in adult rabbits.

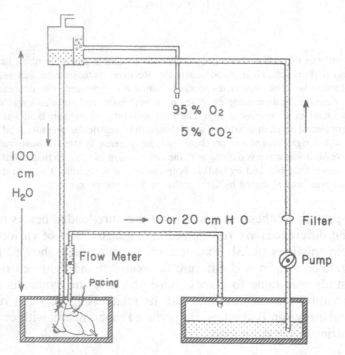

Figure 1. Perfusion apparatus for rabbit heart. Two hundred and fifty milliliters of Fluosol DA® 20% was used and recirculated 150 min as perfusate. Normal plasma levels of amino acids were added. Perfusion pressure was 100 cm H_2O. Left ventricular pressure was zero, and right ventricular pressure was zero in the control group and 20 cm H_2O in the pressure-loaded group. Heart rate is fixed at 250/min by atrial pacing, pH 7.4, 37°C. Constituents of Fluosol DA 20%: 14.0 w/v% perfluorodecalin, 6.0 w/v% perfluorotripropylamine, 3.0 w/v% hydroxystarch, 0.600 w/v% NaCl, 0.034 w/v% KCl, 0.020 w/v% $MgCl_2$, 0.028 w/v% $CaCl_2$, 0.210 w/v% $NaHCO_3$, 12.5 mM glucose, 2.7 w/v% pluronic F-68, 0.4 w/v% yolk phospholipid, and 0.8 w/v% glycerol.

Perfusions

Two hundred and fifty milliliters of Fluosol DA® (blood substitute, supplied by the Green Cross Corporation) with amino acids added in physiological concentrations was employed as perfusate to keep the oxygen supply more physiological (Figure 2); it was bubbled with gas mixture of 95% O_2 and 5% CO_2 to maintain the pH at 7.4. Constituents of Fluosol DA® are indicated in the legend to Figure 1. The perfusate was kept at 37°C, and heart and cannula were transferred to a temperature-controlled perfusion chamber. The heart rate was fixed at 250/min by atrial pacing after the spontaneous sinus rhythm became stable. Coronary flow rate was measured at the pulmonary artery by flow meter and expressed as the mean flow per minute during the perfusion.

Determination of Structural Protein Synthesis Rate

One hundred microcuries of l-[4,5-^{3}H]lysine was added to the perfusion system after the beginning of atrial pacing to a final concentration 0.4 μCi/ml. The turnover rate of cardiac structural proteins was estimated from the l-[^{3}H]lysine incorporation rate during the 150-min perfusion period. The perfusate was recirculated. Synthesis rate of myosin B was estimated in both right and left ventricle, and those of several structural protein fractions were estimated only in left ventricle.

Preparation of Structural Protein Fractions

Structural protein was extracted by the methods of Ebashi (2,3) and Sugita (11) with a slight modification as described previously (6). Actinin complex (10 S + α), tropomyosin, and troponin complex were prepared from myosin B as described below. Myosin B was dialyzed against 2 mM NaHCO$_3$ solution for about 48 hr and centrifuged at 68,000 × g for 90 min. The supernatant had specific amounts of solid ammonium sulfate added in order to obtain the actinin complex, tropomyosin, and troponin complex as follows. One hundred milliliters of the supernatant was mixed with 20 g of ammonium sulfate and centrifuged at 15,000 × g for 10 min. The resulting precipitate was collected, dialyzed against 2 mM NaHCO$_3$, and used as the complex of the actinin fraction. Troponin complex was precipitated by adding another 8 g of ammonium sulfate to 100 ml of its original volume after extraction of actinin complex by centrifugation at 15,000 × g for 10 min. Tropomyosin was precipitated by adding another 12 g of ammonium sulfate to 100 ml of its original volume after extraction of troponin complex by centrifugation at 15,000 × g for 10 min. They are all dialyzed against 2 mM NaHCO$_3$ solution before counting. The amino acid content of each structural protein fraction was analyzed by an amino acid analyser (JLC-8AH, Nihondenshi).

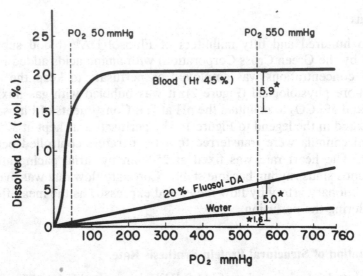

Figure 2. Oxygen dissociation curves of Fluosol DA®, whole blood, and water. The figure shows oxygen volume (vol %) that can be released from Fluosol DA, whole blood, and water when P_{O_2} drops from 550 to 50 mm Hg (from the Green Cross Corporation Technical Information Ser. No. 5).

Experiments on the Effects of Propranolol and Verapamil on Structural Protein Synthesis in Heart with Right Ventricular Pressure Load

Propranolol and verapamil were added to perfusate to final concentrations of 5.5×10^{-7} M and 1.2×10^{-6} M, respectively; then the heart was perfused at least for 30 min before the pulmonary artery pressure was elevated to 20 cm H_2O and [^{3}H]lysine was added to the perfusate.

RESULTS

Synthesis Rates of Cardiac Structural Proteins in Perfused Adult Rabbit Heart without Pressure Load

The average incorporation rates of [^{3}H]lysine into left and right ventricular myosin B of adult rabbits were $22,821 \pm 10,656$ cpm/mg myosin B and $21,454 \pm 9550$ cpm/mg myosin B, respectively. Each structural protein was extracted, and synthesis rates were calculated from the proteins [^{3}H]-lysine incorporation rates corrected for their lysine contents. The lysine contents of myosin heavy chain, light chain, actin, actinin complex, tropomyosin, and troponin complex per 10^5 g of each fraction were 89, 79, 67, 52, 85, and 122, respectively. Synthesis rates were described in relative terms with the rate of actin synthesis taken as 1.0 and compared with those of a previous in vivo study (6) (Table 1). The synthesis rate of actin was the lowest, and that of troponin complex the highest; the order of structural

Table 1.   Relative Synthesis Rates of Cardiac Structural Proteins
(Actin = 1.0)

	Actin	Tropomyosin	Heavy chain	Light chain	Actinin (10S ± α)	Troponin
Langendorff[a]	1.0	2.2	2.6	2.9	3.4	4.2 Native tropomyosin
In vivo	1.0	—	2.0	1.7	2.5	2.7

[a] [^{3}H]Lysine incorporation into actin is 23,169 ± 4638 cpm/mg lysine (mean ± S.E.M.).

protein synthesis rates was almost the same as that of the in vivo study except for minor differences in myosin heavy and light chain.

Effect of Right Ventricular Pressure Load on Myosin B Synthesis in Right and Left Ventricles

The myosin B synthesis rate was examined in perfused heart with or without a pressure load (20 cm H_2O) to the right ventricle. In young rabbit hearts, myosin B synthesis rates of right and left ventricles were both significantly increased by 260% in right and 50% in left ventricle in response to the right ventricle pressure load (Figure 3). On the other hand, adult rabbit hearts did not show any increase in myosin B synthesis with same pressure load to the right ventricle in contrast to young rabbits hearts (Figure 4).

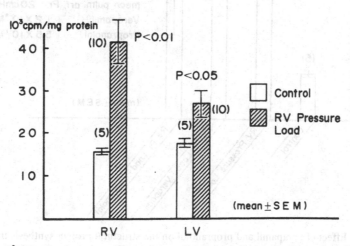

Figure 3.   [^{3}H]Lysine incorporation rate into right and left ventricular myosin B in young rabbit hearts with pressure load on right ventricle. Mean pulmonary pressure was 20 cm H_2O. In right and left ventricle the increase was 260% ($P < 0.01$) and 50% ($P < 0.05$), respectively. RV, right ventricle; LV, left ventricle.

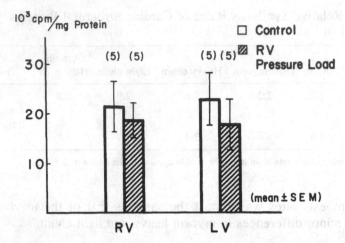

Figure 4. [³H]Lysine incorporation rate into right and left ventricular myosin B in perfused adult rabbit heart with pressure load on right ventricle. No increase was observed in contrast to the young rabbit heart, even with pressure load (20 cm H₂O) on right ventricle.

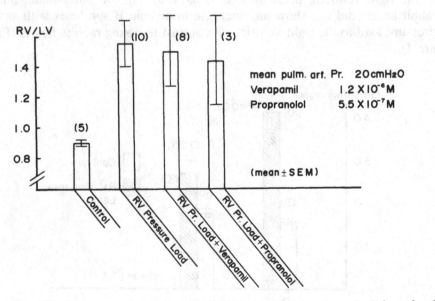

Figure 5. Effect of verapamil and propranolol on the structural protein synthesis in perfused young rabbit heart with pressure load on right ventricle. The ratios of right to left ventricular [³H]lysine incorporation rate of myosin B were determined. The two drugs did not show any effect on the ratios. The concentrations of verapamil and propranolol in perfusate were 1.2×10^{-6} M and 5.5×10^{-7} M, respectively.

Effect of Verapamil and Propranolol on Myosin B Synthesis in Young Rabbit Heart with Pressure Load on Right Ventricle

To examine the mechanism of increase in ventricular myosin B synthesis in young rabbit heart with right ventricular pressure load, effects of propranolol, an adrenergic β-receptor blocker, and verapamil, a Ca^{2+} antagonist, were studied. Neither verapamil nor propranolol could suppress the increase of myosin B synthesis in both ventricles, and the ratio of synthesis rates in right and left ventricle was not different from that in hearts without these agents (Figure 5).

DISCUSSION

There are few reports (6,13,14) on the turnover rates of various structural proteins of the heart. We have already shown (6) in adult rabbit that the turnover rate of actin is the lowest and that of native tropomyosin the highest in an in vivo study. In the present study, the turnover rates of various cardiac structural proteins were estimated in a perfused heart system. This system enabled us to examine more accurate and precise turnover rates of structural proteins because of high incorporation rates of [³H]lysine into structural proteins. The order of turnover rates in various structural proteins was almost the same as that found in the in vivo study previously reported (6) except for a minor difference in myosin heavy and light chain. This difference may be caused by the difference in experimental conditions, mainly, the difference in cardiac work in conditions in vivo and in vitro. The highest native tropomyosin turnover rate in the in vivo study was that of the troponin complex, and this finding was the same as that in skeletal muscle reported by Koizumi (7). Zak (13) reported the same order of half-lives of cardiac structural proteins in Sprague–Dawley rats in vivo as that found earlier in vivo in rabbit (6). The reason for the difference was not clear, but it may be a result of different species and experimental procedures.

Synthesis rates of myosin B in right and left ventricles were almost equal in the perfused heart of the present study when left and right ventricles contracted against zero pressure. With a right ventricular pressure load, right ventricular myosin B synthesis rate increased by 260% in young rabbit although not significantly in adult rabbit. These results suggested that young rabbit heart was more sensitive to pressure load and that heavier pressure load may be necessary for adult heart to induce the increased protein synthesis rate. Second, direct tension stress to the ventricular wall may be one of the main rate-limiting factors for the protein synthesis rate; this may explain why the structural protein synthesis rate of left ventricle was greater than that of right ventricle in our previous in vivo study (6).

The effect of right ventricular pressure load on left ventricular protein synthesis is still controversial. Zelis et al. (15) and Schreiber et al. (10)

showed coincidental increase in left ventricular protein synthesis in heart with right ventricular pressure load, whereas Everret et al. (4) recognized no increase. This difference may come from differences of species, animal age, and degree of right ventricular pressure load. Zelis et al. and Schreiber et al. suggested a mechanical factor for left ventricular myocardium as the inducer of increased left ventricular protein synthesis rate, since increased right ventricular tension would be expected to transmit to the left ventricle through the intra- and transventricular muscle bundle (12). Alternatively, humoral factors such as phosphorylation potential (9), creatine (5), prostaglandin (1), and norepinephrine (8) were also proposed as the stimulator of protein synthesis in heart. But in our study, propranolol, a β-adrenergic receptor blocker, and verapamil, a Ca^{2+} antagonist, could not inhibit the increase in structural protein synthesis of right and left ventricles. Furthermore, our perfusion system was devoid of systemic humoral as well as neurogenic factors. However, the existence of humoral factors derived from the pressure-loaded ventricle could not be ruled out.

In our preliminary coperfusion experiment in which two hearts with and without right ventricular pressure load were perfused with common recirculating perfusate, increased synthesis of myosin B was observed not only in the pressure-loaded heart but also in the heart without pressure load. This fact may suggest the possibility of some humoral factor, which would require further study. On the other hand, clinical experience indicates that hypertrophy of one ventricle resulting from any stress need not necessarily be associated with the clinically detectable hypertrophy of the other ventricle. The discrepancy between clinical and experimental findings is difficult to explain at present. There are several possibilities. First, moderate or marked cardiac hypertrophy could occur only when stress and a metabolic stimulating factor coexist and cooperate. Second, the normal unstressed heart may rapidly become insensitive to the metabolic stimulating factor unless stress coexists. Third, there may be an unknown feedback mechanism controlling the protein synthesis in the normal heart. Fourth, the protein degradation rate of normal unstressed heart may be faster than that of stressed heart. Further study is needed.

ACKNOWLEDGMENTS

We are thankful to Mrs. Kuroda for her technical assistance.

Original work presented in this chapter was supported by grants from the Ministry of Education, Japan, numbers 511101-71 and 577358-745.

REFERENCES

1. Chazov, E. I., Pomoinetsky, V. D., Geling, N. G., Orlova, T. R., Nekrasova, A. A., and Smirnov, V. N. 1979. Heart adaptation to acute pressure overload. An involvement of endogenous prostaglandins. *Circ. Res.* 45:205–211.

2. Ebashi, S. 1974. Regulatory mechanism of muscle contraction with special reference to Ca–troponin system. *Essays Biochem.* 1:1–36.
3. Ebashi, S., and Ebashi, F. 1964. A new protein component participating in the superprecipitation of myosin B. *J. Biochem.* (*Tokyo*) 55:604–613.
4. Everett, A. W., Taylor, R. R., and Sparrow, M. P. 1977. Protein synthesis during right ventricular hypertrophy after pulmonary artery stenosis in the dog. *Biochem. J.* 166:315–325.
5. Ingwall, J. S., Morales, M. F., Stockdale, F. E., and Wildenthal, K. 1975. Creatin: A possible stimulus for skeletal and cardiac muscle hypertrophy In: P. Roy and P. Harris (eds.), *Recent Advances in Studies on Cardiac Structure and Metabolism.* Vol. 8: *The Cardiac Sarcoplasm*, pp. 467–491. University Park Press, Baltimore.
6. Ito, Y., Ebisawa, K., Kira, Y., and Koizumi, T. 1980. Turnover rates and synthesis of cardiac structural proteins in normal and hypertrophied heart In: M. Tajuddin, P. K. Das, M. Tariq, and N. S. Dhalla (eds.), *Advances in Myocardiology*, Vol. 1, pp. 509–518. University Park Press, Baltimore.
7. Koizumi, T. 1974. Turnover rates of structural proteins of rabbit skeletal muscle. *J. Biochem.* (*Tokyo*) 76:431–439.
8. Laks, M. M. 1976. Norepinephrine—the myocardial hypertrophy hormone? *Am. Heart J.* 91:674.
9. Meerson, F. Z. 1975. Role of synthesis of nucleic acid and protein in adaptation to the external environment. *Physiol. Rev.* 55:79–123.
10. Schreiber, S. S., Rothschild, M. A., Evans, C., Reff, F., and Oratz, M. 1975. The effect of pressure or flow stress on right ventricular protein synthesis in the face of constant and restricted coronary perfusion. *J. Clin. Invest.* 55:1–11.
11. Sugita, H., Katagiri, T., Shimizu, T., and Toyokura, Y. 1973. Studies on the structural proteins in various neuromuscular diseases. In: B. A. Kakulas (ed.), *Basic Research in Myology* (International Congress Series, Volume 294), pp. 291–297. Excerpta Medica, Amsterdam.
12. Taylor, R. R., Covell, J. W., Sonnenblick, E. H., and Ross, J., Jr. 1967. Dependence of ventricular distensibility on filling of the opposite ventricle. *Am. J. Physiol.* 213:711–718.
13. Zak, R. 1977. Metabolism of myofibrillar proteins in the normal and hypertrophic heart. *Basic Res. Cardiol.* 72:235–240.
14. Zak, R., Martin, A. F., Dowell, R. T., and Rabinowitz, M. 1973. Turnover of myocardial components in cardiac hypertrophy. In: N. S. Dhalla (ed.), *Recent Advances in Studies on Cardiac Structure and Metabolism.* Vol. 3: *Myocardial Metabolism*, pp. 603–614. University Park Press, Baltimore.
15. Zelis, R., Wickman-Coffelt, J., Kamiyama, T., Peng, C. L., Salel, A. F., Amsterdam, F. A., and Mason, D. T. 1973. Acute right ventricular stress as a stimulus for left ventricular RNA and protein synthesis In: N. S. Dhalla (ed.), *Recent Advances in Studies on Cardiac Structure and Metabolism.* Vol. 3: *Myocardial Metabolism*, pp. 625–635. University Park Press, Baltimore.

DNA Synthesis and Mitotic Activity in Adult Atrial Cardiocytes in Culture

M. Cantin, M. Ballak, J. Beuzeron-Mangina, and C. Tautu

Laboratory of Pathobiology
Clinical Research Institute of Montreal
and
Department of Pathology
University of Montreal and Hôtel-Dieu of Montreal
Montreal, Quebec H2W 1R7, Canada

Abstract. Trypsin-dissociated adult rat atrial cardiocytes were exposed to [³H]thymidine for sequential 24-hr periods from day 3 to day 13 of culture. Following preparation for ultrastructural autoradiography, 1000 cells (at each daily interval) were examined with an electron microscope. Maximal incorporation occurred on day 5 when 63% of the cells were labeled. Small secondary peaks of incorporation occurred on days 8 and 11 following previous exposure to fresh serum. Mitotic activity never exceeded 0.5% of all cardiocytes examined. DNA synthesis and mitoses occurred only in immature cardiocytes characterized by subsarcolemmal filaments and Z-bands with or without specific granules; more mature cells were never labeled.

Modern investigative methods have revealed that, in mammals, the atrial myocardium is markedly different from its ventricular counterpart. The mammalian atrial cardiocyte is smaller, has a poorly developed T system, has a secretory-like apparatus made up of specific granules and a large Golgi complex (1), and, in contrast to adult ventricular cardiocytes, shows DNA synthesis and mitotic activity in certain circumstances (2). We now wish to report a technique of culture of adult rat atrial cardiocytes. These cells show intense DNA synthesis and moderate mitotic activity.

MATERIALS AND METHODS

Cardiocyte Culture

Each time a culture was started, the right and left atria were dissected from 40 hearts of 300- to 350-day-old Sprague–Dawley rats (Biobreeding Laboratories, Ottawa, Ontario, Canada). The tissues were placed separately in Eagle's minimal essential medium (MEM) [Grand Island Biological Company of Canada (GIBCO), Burlington, Ontario, Canada], washed twice in Hank's balanced salt solution (BSS) (GIBCO) without calcium and mag-

137

nesium, and dissociated at 37°C in 0.1% trypsin (DIFCO Laboratories, Detroit, Michigan, USA) in Ca^{2+}- and Mg^{2+}-free BSS buffered with HEPES at pH 7.4.

The complete dissociation procedure included seven steps, the first two steps each lasting 10 min, the third and fourth 15 min, and the fifth to seventh 20 min. After each step, the minced tissues were aspirated 20 times in a 10-ml pipette to disperse the cells, placed in a 15-ml centrifugation tube, and mixed with 5 ml of fetal calf serum (FCS) (GIBCO) to block enzyme activity. The cell suspensions were then centrifuged at 400 g for 5 min, and each pellet resuspended in 2 ml of complete medium (CM) made up of MEM buffered with HEPES at pH 7.4 and supplemented with 10% FCS, 1% glutamine, and 1% penicillin–streptomycin (GIBCO).

To obtain cultures enriched in cardiocytes, a modification of Kasten's original technique (3) of selective plating was used: the final cell suspension (made up of the last five dissociation steps) was mixed and placed in a gelatinized (2) 25-cm culture flask (Corning) at 37°C for three 1-hr periods followed by a 24-hr period to allow as many of the nonmyogenic cells as possible to attach to the gelatinized surface. The final supernatant was centrifuged at 400 g, resuspended in CM, counted in a hemocytometer, and cultured at an initial density of 2×10^6 to 3×10^6 cell in 6 ml of CM renewed after 4, 7, and 10 days. Cultures were incubated at 37°C with air as the gas phase in gelatinized 25-cm flasks (Corning).

Ultrastructural Autoradiography

Starting on the second day and for each successive day up to 12 days, the cells of one flask were exposed to 1.0 μCi/ml of medium of [methyl-^{3}H]-thymidine ([^{3}H]-TdR) (New England Nuclear, Boston, Mass.; specific activity 20.0 Ci/mmol) for the next 24 hr. Starting on the third day up to 13 days, the cells were rinsed with cacodylate buffer containing 2% sucrose and fixed in 2% glutaraldehyde (buffered with 0.1 M cacodylate HCl at pH 7.1) for 1 hr. They were then washed in cacodylate buffer to which 2% sucrose had been added. After the cells had been collected with a rubber policeman and centrifuged at 400 g for 15 min to obtain a pellet, they were postfixed for 1 hr in 2% osmium tetroxide (OsO_4) buffered with veronal acetate. The cells were then dehydrated in graded alcohols and embedded in Araldite. Semifine sections were stained with toluidine blue for orientation, and fine sections were cut with a diamond knife in an OMU 2 ultramicrotome. The fine sections were prepared for ultrastructural autoradiography according to the flat substrate technique as already described (4,5). Briefly, the fine sections were placed on collodion-coated slides, stained with uranyl acetate and lead citrate, and covered with a thin film of evaporated carbon. The slides were then dipped in dilute Ilford L_4 emulsion. The autoradiographs were exposed for 2 months. They were then developed, placed on copper grids, and examined with a Philips 300 electron microscope.

Index of DNA Synthesis

For each time interval (from the third to the 13th day) the autoradiographs were scanned consecutively until 1000 cells were examined: first for the presence of silver grains over their nucleus and then for the presence in these labeled cells of myofilaments with forming Z-bands and/or specific granules. Only cells with these characteristics were considered as cardiocytes having synthesized DNA (Figure 1).

RESULTS

Phase-Contrast Microscopy

The cultures were examined several times daily with an inverted phase-contrast microscope (Leitz). The cells did not start to attach before the end of the second day. They grew steadily and reached confluence on the eighth day of culture. Only occasional cells were found to beat at all time intervals. Once they reached confluence, they elongated and enlarged considerably to finally form a crisscross pattern of very large, branching cells. They have been maintained in culture for up to 40 days. There was no behavioral difference between the left and right atrium.

Ultrastructure

The entire spectrum of cell development from very immature to nearly mature cardiocytes was encountered in the cultures. The maturation of cells was asynchronous so that by the seventh day, cells with subsarcolemmal filaments accompanied by forming Z-bands and an abundant rough endo-

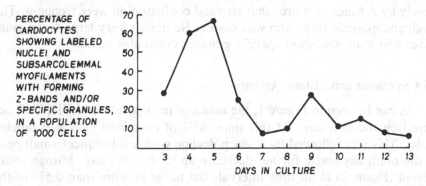

Figure 1. Ultrastructural radioautographic evaluation of the incorporation of tritiated thymidine by the adult rat atrial cardiocytes in culture. The trypsinized cells from either right or left atrium were plated in gelatinized flasks on day 0. The supernatant was plated anew on day 1. Cardiocytes did not start to attach before the end of day 2. Starting on day 2, and on each subsequent day, the cells were exposed to [³H]-TdR (1 μCi/ml) for 24 hr before harvesting. The media were renewed on days 4, 7, and 10. The cultures reached confluence on day 8.

plasmic reticulum with dilated cisternae were found side by side with more organized cells with adult-type myofilaments and Z-bands, a much less conspicuous rough endoplasmic reticulum, a large Golgi complex, and specific granules. By the 13th day, a majority of the cardiocytes were of the latter type. Here again, there was no difference between the left and right atrium.

Young Myocytes.   These cells possessed only scanty myofilaments, mostly just under the sarcolemma. Dense, amorphous collections of Z-band material were located either parallel to the sarcolemma and just under it or among the myofilaments and with their long axis perpendicular to the sarcolemma. The rough endoplasmic reticulum was very abundant at this stage. The Golgi complex was mostly paranuclear and composed of small vesicles sometimes containing progranules. Microtubules with or without thin ($\approx$75 Å) filaments were often present. Specific granules were scanty. The mitochondria were few in number, small, with normal contours. They possessed normal cristae. Prominent intramitochondrial granules were often noted. Lysosomes were rare, but autophagic vacuoles and residual bodies (C granules) were numerous in some cells. The nuclei were large with dispersed chromatin and often prominent nucleoli. Subsarcolemmal micropinocytotic vesicles were sometimes abundant. Transverse tubules were not present. Lateral sacs of the smooth endoplasmic reticulum were closely approximated to the sarcolemmal membrane. The sarcolemma appeared normal, but the cell coat (basement membrane) was often much thicker than that in mature cardiocytes. Desmosomes were present between many cells, but no intercalated disks were found.

More Mature Cardiocytes.   From the eighth day on, the cells started to elongate and enlarge markedly. Some reached a length corresponding to half the space delimited by two grid bars [the space between two grid bars (150 mesh) is 129 μm]. There was evident maturation of the cells as well: typical thick and thin filaments far from the sarcolemma and crossed transversely by Z-bands of more adult size and configuration were frequent. The rough endoplasmic reticulum was scarce. Numerous very large Golgi complexes and more abundant specific granules could also be seen.

DNA Synthesis and Mitotic Activity

As can be seen in Figure 1, the maximal incorporation of [³H]-TdR occurred on the fifth day. At this time, 63% of examined cells had labeled nuclei. This was followed by a sharp decline with a subsequent small peak on the ninth day and a further decrease up to the 13th day. Mitoses were present (Figure 2) at all time intervals but never in more than 0.5% of the cells examined. Binucleated cells sometimes with labeled nuclei were encountered from the fifth day on. Maturation seemed to impose stringent restrictions on DNA synthesis: no cell was labeled that contained myofilaments away from the subsarcolemmal area (Figures 3 and 4); the presence of mature Z-bands away from the subsarcolemmal area was likewise never

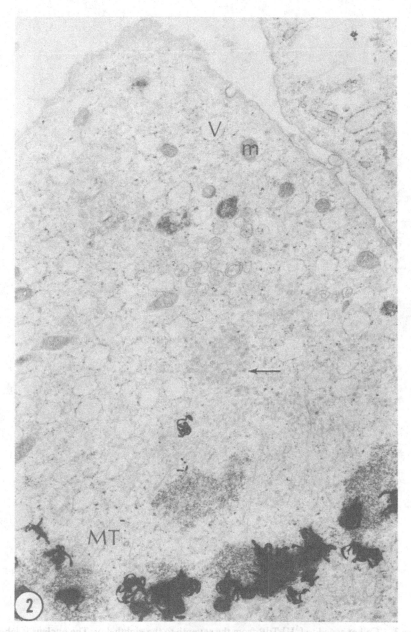

Figure 2.   Cell in metaphase from a culture exposed to [³H]-TdR from the fifth to the sixth day. Silver grains are present over dividing DNA among which microtubules (MT) from the mitotic spindle may be seen. The small Golgi vesicles contain progranules (arrow). Small mitochondria (m) and vesicles (V) of the rough endoplasmic reticulum are also present, (×21,600).

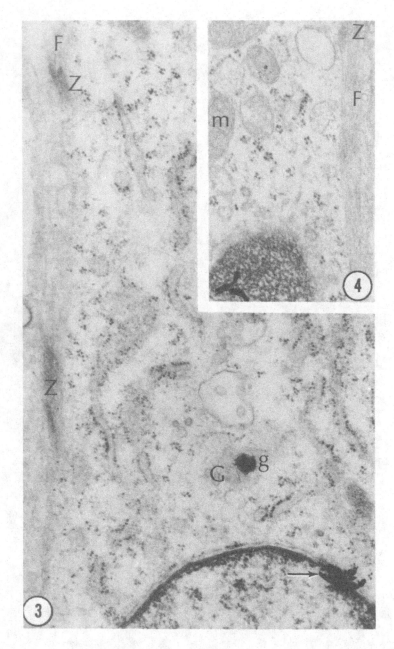

Figure 3.   Cell exposed to [³H]-TdR from the seventh to the eighth day. The nucleus is labeled (arrow). The cell contains subsarcolemmal filaments (F) with forming Z-bands (Z) parallel to the sarcolemma. The cytoplasms also contain numerous saccules of rough endoplasmic reticulum, small polyribosomes, and small Golgi vesicles (G). Specific granule (g) (×33,750).

Figure 4.   Cell exposed to [³H]-TdR from the eighth to the ninth day. The nucleus is labeled. Subsarcolemmal filaments (F) with densities (Z) corresponding to forming Z-bands are present. Mitochondria (m) and polyribosomes may also be seen (×35,100).

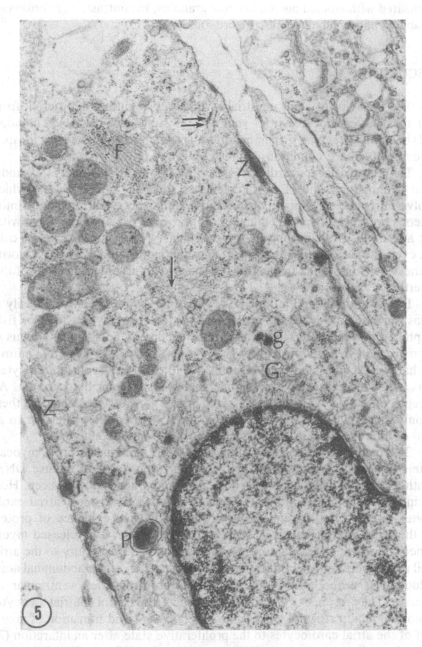

Figure 5.   Cell exposed to [³H]-TdR from the sixth to the seventh day. The nucleus is unlabeled. Typical mature myofilaments (F), both thick and thin, are present away from the sarcolemma and are decorated with numerous ribosomes. Subsarcolemmal Z-bands (Z) of more mature type than in previous micrographs may be seen. Specific granules (g) are near the Golgi complex (G). Phagolysosome (P). Mitochondria are more numerous and larger with dense granules. Microtubules (arrow) are abundant. Note the great decrease in rough endoplasmic reticulum (double arrow) (× 16,070).

associated with labeled nuclei. Specific granules, in contrast, were observed in labeled and unlabeled cells (Figure 5).

DISCUSSION

The behavior of adult rat atrial cardiocytes in culture is different from that of atrial cardiocytes from young (2- to 3-day-old) rats (1). The adult cells beat only irregularly, their maturation is much slower, and their lifespan in identical culture conditions is much longer.

That these cells are cardiocytes is evident from the presence of Z-bands, even if immature, and of subsarcolemmal "primary filaments" (6) which evolve into characteristic thick and thin myofilaments. The frequent simultaneous presence of specific granules in these cells differentiates them without any doubt from fibroblasts (myofibroblasts) and smooth muscle cells (7), even at the most immature stage. The later maturation of a large majority of these cells into bona fide cardiocytes is also an argument in favor of this assertion.

DNA synthesis and mitotic activity can be induced relatively easily in areas surrounding an injury in the adult ventricular myocardium of fish, amphibia, and reptiles. The cardiocytes immediately adjacent to a focus of necrosis seem to partially dedifferentiate prior to DNA synthesis and mitosis so that they acquire a striking resemblance to early embryonic cardiocytes. This is not the case, however, in mammalian ventricular myocardium. Although conflicting evidence exists, there is now general agreement that there is only sluggish DNA synthesis in the nuclei of myofibers adjacent to an area of infarction in rat and mice and very little mitotic activity.

The picture is completely different in adult mammalian atrial myocardium. Following an infarction of the rat left ventricle, an intense DNA-synthesizing activity is present in both atria, and mitoses may be seen. Here again, preceeding the outburst of reactive hyperplasia, most atrial cardiocytes undergo dedifferentiation with morphological evidence of protein synthesis. Z-disk breakdown occurs in prometaphase, and released myofilament bundles are pushed towards the periphery. Local injury to the atrial wall and hyperfunction of the heart after constriction of the abdominal aorta induces less pronounced cardiocyte proliferation than left ventricular infarction. The presence of a small (2–3%) proliferative pool of atrial myocytes in normal adult rat is not sufficient to explain the rapid transition of nearly half of the atrial cardiocytes to the proliferative state after an infarction (7). The same argument is also valid in the present experiment.

To the best of our knowledge, there are no previous reports of DNA-synthesizing adult mammalian cardiocytes in culture. Although adult rat ventricular cardiocytes can be cultured (8), they do not appear to show mitotic activity. It is possible that the dissociation technique presently used is partly responsible for initiation of DNA synthesis in atrial cells. The trypsinization of cells is known to damage myofilaments and, in young cardiocytes, is followed by an intense wave of protein synthesis and cell division (1).

Apart from their intrinsic biological interest, the present findings for the first time offer the opportunity to study in vitro the factors responsible for the block of DNA synthesis and mitotic activity characteristic of mature mammalian cardiocytes.

ACKNOWLEDGMENTS

This work was supported by a group grant from the Medical Research Council of Canada to the Multidisciplinary Research Group on Hypertension of the Clinical Research Institute of Montreal, by a grant from the Medical Research Council of Canada (grant MT-1973), and by the Quebec Heart Foundation.

REFERENCES

1. Cantin, M., Araujo-Nascimento, M. de F., Benchimol, S., and Désormeaux, Y. 1977. Metaplasia of smooth muscle cells into juxtaglomerular cells in the juxtaglomerular apparatus, arteries and arterioles of the ischemic (endocrine) kidney. An ultrastructural–cytochemical and radioautographic study. *Am. J. Pathol.* 87:581–602.
2. Cantin, M., Tautu, C., Ballak, M., Yunge, L., Benchimol, S., and Beuzeron, J. 1980. Ultrastructural cytochemistry of atrial muscle cells. IX. Reactivity of specific granules in cultured cardiocytes. *J. Mol. Cell. Cardiol.* 12:1033–1051.
3. Chamley-Campbell, J., Campbell, G. R., and Ross, R. 1979. The smooth muscle cell in culture. *Physiol. Rev.* 59:1–61.
4. Jacobson, S. L. 1977. Culture of spontaneously contracting myocardial cells from adult rat. *Cell Struct. Funct.* 2:1–9.
5. Kasten, F. H. 1973. Mammalian myocardial cells. In: P. F. Kruse, Jr. and M. K. Patterson, Jr. (eds.), *Tissue Culture Methods and Applications*, pp. 72–81. Academic Press, New York.
6. Legato, M. J. 1972. Ultrastructural characteristics of the rat ventricular cell grown in tissue culture, with special reference to sarcomerogenesis. *J. Mol. Cell. Cardiol.* 4:299–317.
7. Rumyantsev, P. P. 1977. Interrelations of the proliferation and differentiation processes during cardiac myogenesis and regeneration. *Int. Rev. Cytol.* 51:187–273.
8. Yunge, L., Benchimol, S., and Cantin, M. 1980. Ultrastructural cytochemistry of atrial muscle cells. VIII. Radioautographic study of synthesis and migration of proteins. *Cell Tissue Res.* 207:1–11.

DNA Synthesis in Atrial Myocytes of Rats with Aortic Stenosis

P. P. Rumyantsev

Institute of Cytology of the Academy of Sciences of the USSR
Leningrad 190121, USSR

Abstract. Indices of labeled myonuclei have been determined in hypertrophying hearts of adult Wistar rats by autoradiography after single-pulse or repeated [³H]thymidine administration. After single [³H]thymidine injections, only 1.36 ± 0.66 and $1.32 \pm 0.87\%$ labeled myonuclei were observed in the left and right atria, respectively. In the experiments with multiple [³H]thymidine administration, the first injection of this precursor was given on the seventh day after aortic constriction; thereafter, 30 or 42 injections of [³H]thymidine were given at 12-hr intervals up to the fourth postoperation week. Following 30 repeated [³H]thymidine injections, 29.75 ± 4.65 and $16.78 \pm 3.33\%$ labeled myonuclei were visible in left and right atrial muscle cells, respectively. The cumulative labeling index for left atrium myocytes clearly correlates ($r = 0.65$–0.73) with an increase in the weight of the heart. Increase in heart weight to more than 160% of controls corresponds to [³H]thymidine labeling of 38.06 ± 4.65 and $21.67 \pm 4.16\%$ in left and right atrial myocytes, respectively, whereas in hearts weighing less than 140% of controls, [³H]thymidine labels only $8.20 \pm 1.93\%$ in the left atrium and $3.94 \pm 1.57\%$ in the right one. In the ventricles, cumulative indices of myonuclear labeling do not exceed $0.217 \pm 0.11\%$ even in hearts weighing nearly 180% of controls. Cumulative frequencies of labeling for AV system myocytes are almost ten times higher (1.97 ± 0.38). These results, together with our data concerning mycocardial infarction (27–29,31), make it necessary to reconsider the role of cardiomyocyte hyperplasia in different experimental and pathological conditions, paying special attention to the proliferative behavior of the atrial muscle cells. DNA synthesis in atrial myocytes seems to be stimulated by heart hyperfunction.

It is generally believed that adult mammalian cardiomyocytes do not respond by reactivation of their DNA synthesis and mitoses to heart hyperfunction, infarction, or various kinds of injuries. This concept is based on evidence obtained as a rule from investigations of the ventricular myocytes of adult mammals (for literature see 13,19,26,28,29,38,39). The possibility of variations in the proliferative behavior of different types of cardiac myocytes comprising the mammalian heart has been neglected for almost a century. However, both the myocytes of the specialized impulse-conducting system of the heart and those of the atria are known to differ from their ventricular counterparts in their morphological, physiological, and biochemical properties. Moreover, they are known to be heterogeneous and each consists of several subpopulations of cells (see 5,6,10,17). It is interesting to note that Schiaffino and his co-workers (35) were recently able to show immunocytochemical differences among myofibrils of ventricular, atrial, and Purkinje muscle cells.

Some time ago we unexpectedly observed a relatively high number of DNA-synthesizing and mitotically dividing myonuclei in atria of rats with experimental left ventricular infarction. Although single [³H]thymidine injections made 5–7 days after infarction resulted in the labeling of only about 4% of the auricular myonuclei, when the administration of this precursor was repeated 33 to 34 times between the third and the 19th days after infarction, up to 50 to 60% of the myonuclei of both atria were tagged. The ventricular muscle cells displayed, in these experiments with multiple [³H]-thymidine injections, almost no DNA-synthesizing and mitotically dividing nuclei except for the myofibers surrounding necrotized muscles, where 0.11 ± 0.075 and 6.23 ± 1.48% myocytes were labeled, respectively, after single and 33 to 34-fold repeated [³H]thymidine injections (27–29).

It seems likely that compensatory atrial myocytes hyperplasia following ligation of the left coronary artery results from postinfarction hyperfunction rather than from other possible factors (chalone imbalance, release of diffusible growth-stimulating substances from the necrotic tissues, and so on). This assumption is compatible with the fact that extracardiac atrial myocytes, which surround the pulmonary veins in rats and other rodents, remain largely unlabeled following left ventricle infarction and multiple [³H]-thymidine labeling (29). These extracardiac myocytes, which are in all respects similar to typical atrial muscle cells (14), are indeed unlikely to be considerably overloaded after infarction.

In order to assess more directly the supposed role of heart hyperfunction in reactivation of atrial myocyte replication, we have performed experiments with multiple [³H]thymidine injections following coarctation of the abdominal aorta of rats. The highest frequencies (40–50%) of ³H-thymidine-labeled atrial myonuclei were observed, as a rule, in animals with a pronounced increase in heart weight (170–190% of controls). This is compatible with the hypothesis that hyperfunction triggers renewed DNA synthesis and mitosis of atrial myocytes.

MATERIAL AND METHODS

Constriction of the abdominal aorta was performed in adult female Wistar rats weighing 176.2 ± 1.5 g (first experimental series) or 149.3 ± 3.1 g (second experimental series) according to the method of Beznak (7) as modified by Kogan (15). Twenty-seven rats of the first experimental series as well as unoperated controls received, at 10 a.m., single [³H]thymidine injections (for postoperation stages, see Figures 1 and 2). Twenty-two rats from the second experimental series received multiple [³H]thymidine injections at 12-hr intervals (one at 10 a.m., and another at 10 p.m. each day) beginning from the seventh day postoperation. The total number of injections was 30 in 16 rats that were sacrificed on days 21–24 after operation and 42 in six rats sacrificed by day 28 (see Figure 2). [³H]Thymidine with

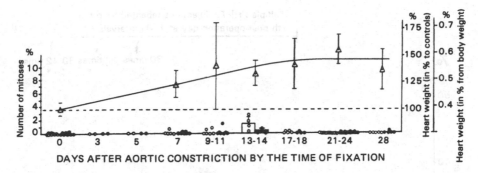

Figure 1.   Heart weight (triangles) and mitotic activity of the left (open circles) and right (filled circles) atrial myocytes after aortic constriction in rats. Vertical bars are 95% confidence limits for heart weight and S.E.M. for mitoses. Each circle represents the mitotic index for one animal.

a specific activity of 18 Ci/mmol (Soviet production) was used at the dose of 0.5 to 0.8 mCi/g body weight per injection. The intervals between repeated [3H]thymidine injections were chosen to correspond roughly to the duration of the adult rat atrial myocyte S phase, which lasts 11–13 hr (32). Therefore, multiple [3H]thymidine injections at this time interval were believed to provide for the labeling of nearly all the myocytes entering DNA synthesis at any time throughout the period of the continuous precursor administration. This approach was shown to be highly effective for the accumulation of 3H-thymidine-labeled myocytes in atria of rats with ligated left coronary arteries (28–31).

An additional smaller group included three rats that received five successive injections of [3H]thymidine beginning from the 12th postoperative day.

Hearts of all the animals were excised under ether anesthesia and weighed after careful removal of the blood from their cavities. Material was fixed in Carnoy fluid and embedded in paraffin. Sections 5μm thick were processed by a standard technique for autoradiography using type "M" liquid emulsion (Soviet production) and stained with hematoxylin–eosin. The frequencies of 3H-thymidine-labeled and of mitotically dividing myonuclei were determined by counting at least 1000 atrial myocytes. In some animals, similar counts were performed for myocytes and nonmuscle cells in the left ventricles and for cells of the atrioventricular conducting system of the heart.

RESULTS

Heart weight increased steadily after the operation, reaching nearly maximal mean values (140–150% of controls) on the third postoperative week (Figure 1). During the first week, there was some swelling of the left

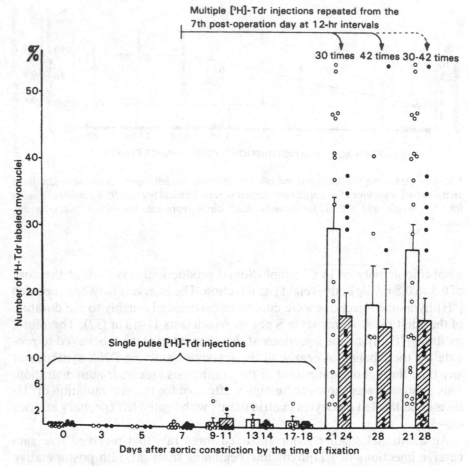

Figure 2.   The number of labeled myonuclei after single-pulse [³H]thymidine injections and after multiple administration of the precursor beginning from day 7 postoperation at different stages following aortic constriction in rats. Cumulative percentages for 30-fold and 42-fold repeated injections are shown separately and together (two graphs on the right). Open circles represent an individual labeling index for left atrium myocytes, and filled circles one for the right atrium myocytes. Vertical bars in corresponding graphs are S.E.M.

atrium myofibers which became slightly basophilic. No such changes were observed in the right atrium myocardia. Beginning with the seventh post-operative day and especially at the end of the second week, a variable number of ³H-thymidine-labeled and/or mitotically dividing myonuclei were observed in both atria of some of the operated animals (Figures 1,2). The morphology of the DNA-synthesizing and dividing myocytes (Figures 3,4) is identical in all respects to that of proliferating muscle cells previously observed in atria of rats with ligated left coronary arteries (27–30,32,33).

Replicating myocytes are distributed within both atria rather diffusely. There is no doubt about the location of labeled or dividing nuclei within muscle cells because of their predominant central position and because of the absence of a pronounced myocyte dedifferentiation. This was proved using electron microscopic autoradiography of the atrial cells proliferating following infarction (27–29).

During the second postoperative week, the individual indices of ^{3}H-thymidine-labeled and dividing atrial myonuclei fluctuated from a zero level up to 6 and 2.7%, respectively, their mean maximal values in the left atria being $1.36 \pm 0.66\%$ for the former and $1.44 \pm 0.50\%$ for the latter (Figures 1,2). In some animals, the sum of DNA-synthesizing and dividing atrial myonuclei attained 4–7%. By the middle of the third postoperative week, mitoses disappeared almost completely, but low frequencies (0.5–1.0%) of DNA-synthesizing myonuclei still occurred in both atria (Figures 1,2).

These data showed a delay of 3–5 postoperative days in the burst of atrial myocyte proliferation after aortic constriction as compared with left

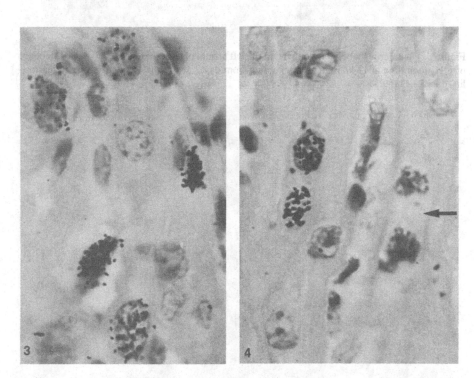

Figure 3.   Atrial myocyte proliferation by day 13 after aortic constriction in rats. Three left atrium myonuclei are labeled with [^{3}H]thymidine injected 2 hr before fixation. Haematoxylin–eosin, ×1150.

Figure 4.   Right atrial myocytes of the same animal as that represented in Figure 3; labeling of two adjacent myonuclei (presumably belonging to a binucleate cell) and an unlabeled myocyte telophase (arrow). Haematoxylin–eosin, ×1150.

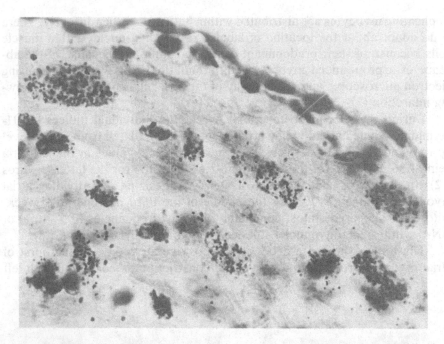

Figure 5.   Numerous labeled myonuclei in the left atrium of a rat that had received 30 injections of [³H]thymidine at 12-hr intervals beginning from day 7 after aortic constriction. Hematoxylin–eosin, ×1150.

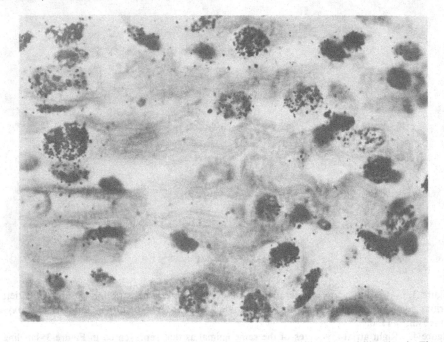

Figure 6.   Abundant labeled myonuclei in the right atrium of a rat treated like that in Figure 5. Hematoxyline–eosin, ×1150.

ventricular myocardial infarction; the response was, moreover, 2.5 times lower and more inconstant as compared with the rekindling of DNA synthesis and mitosis observed in atria following left ventricular myocardial infarction in rats (27–29). However, the total period of time during which some sluggish myonuclear replication occurs was quite long, lasting 1.5 weeks or more after a prereplicative period of 7–9 days. It was therefore possible that during that time additional small bursts of DNA synthesis and mitosis might occur in atria of the hyperfunctioning hearts. For this reason, multiple [3H]thymidine injections were performed in order to accumulate labeling of all of the replicating myonuclei.

In three rats that received five [3H]thymidine injections, 0.2, 2.1, and 5.8% of the myonuclei were labeled in the left atria, and 0.1, 0.7, and 5.5% in the right atria, respectively. It was supposed that five repeated precursor injections do not cover a sufficiently long period of time to provide for accumulation of numerous labeled myonuclei. This was proven in the main series of experiments with 30-fold repeated [3H]thymidine injections beginning from the seventh postoperative day (Figures 2,5,6). By days 21–24, the mean percentage of labeled myonuclei was found to attain 29.75 ± 4.65 and 16.78 ± 3.33% ($P < 0.05$) in the left and right atria, respectively. Forty-twofold repeated [3H]thymidine injections resulted in no additional increase in the myonuclear labeling frequency (Figure 2). Therefore, the results obtained with 30 and 42 successive [3H]thymidine injections were included in a common graph which gives practically the same values as in the subgroup with 30-fold precursor administration (Figure 2).

In the experiments with the multiple [3H]thymidine injections, there is a still more striking variation (from nearly 0.5–4% to 54%) of the individual indices of labeled myonuclei in both atria as compared with those observed

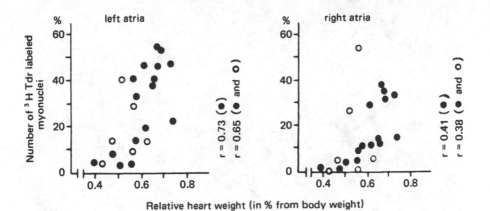

Figure 7.   Correlation between heart weight and percentage of labeled left and right atrium myocytes. Filled circles are individual labeling indices for rats that received 30 repeated [3H]-thymidine injections, and open circles those for rats that received 42 injections of this precursor at 12-hr intervals beginning from 7th postoperative day.

Table 1.   Cumulative Indices (%) of Labeled Myonuclei from Atria of
Rats with Different Degrees of Heart Hypertrophy[a]

Animal groups	Heart weight (% of controls)	Number of animals	Left atrium	Right atrium	Significance of difference between left and right atrium
1	Less than 140	6	8.20 ± 1.93	3.94 ± 1.57	$P > 0.1$
2	140–160	6	26.17 ± 6.54*	20.80 ± 8.18†	$P > 0.6$
3	160 and more	10	38.06 ± 4.65***	21.67 ± 4.16**	$P < 0.02$

[a] Data are expressed as mean ± S.E.M. The animals received 30–42 injections of [³H]thymidine at 12-hr intervals beginning on day 7 after aortic constriction. Symbols indicate the significance of the difference from group 1: †$P > 0.05$; *$P < 0.05$; **$P < 0.01$; ***$P < 0.001$.

using single precursor pulses. This fact led us to compare the extent of reactivation DNA synthesis with that of the increase in weight of the heart. The level of DNA synthesis reactivation in atrial myonuclei was found to depend on the degree of heart hypertrophy, the correlation coefficients (r) being 0.73 for the left atria but only 0.41 for the right one (Figure 7).

As seen from Table 1, the mean cumulative indices of ³H-thymidine-labeled atrial myonuclei in hearts weighing more than 160% of the controls

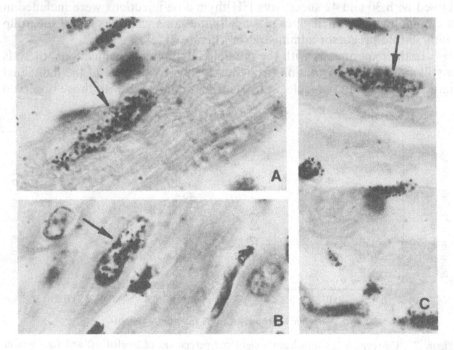

Figure 8.   Occasional labeled myonuclei (arrows) from the left ventricle. The rat received 30 injections of [³H]thymidine at 12-hr intervals beginning from day 7 after aortic constriction. Hematoxylin–eosin, ×1150.

reach 38.06 ± 4.65 and 21.67 ± 4.16% for left and right atrium myocytes, respectively ($P < 0.02$), whereas in hearts weighing less than 140% of the controls, these indices are 4.6–5.5 times lower ($P < 0.001$–0.01).

In contrast to atrial myocardia, only occasional labeled myonuclei (Figure 8) were found in ventricles irrespective of the postoperative stages and the number of [^{3}H]thymidine injections. The profound difference in the proliferative behavior of atrial and ventricular myocytes is clearly seen from the data of Table 2: the mean accumulated frequency of labeled myonuclei in the left ventricles is more than 200 times lower than that in the corresponding atria, the maximal individual cumulative index being only 0.616% (Table 2).

Detailed analysis of the proliferative behavior of the conducting system myocytes from hyperfunctioning hearts as well as that of nonmuscle cells was beyond the scope of this work. The cumulative index of labeled myonuclei in the AV node and the adjacent portions of the bundle of His determined for four animals that received 30–42 [^{3}H]thymidine injections and whose hearts weighed 154.6 ± 11.84% of controls was found to be 1.97 ± 0.38%. This value is indicative of an almost tenfold increase ($P < 0.01$) in cumulative frequency of DNA-synthesizing specialized myocytes compared to working ventricular muscle cells (cf. Table 2). These preliminary results concerning the myocytes of the conducting system will be completed in the near future.

The accumulated frequency of ^{3}H-thymidine-labeled nonmuscle cells from hypertrophied hearts was 275 times higher than that of working ventricular myocyte, only slightly exceeding the number of left atrium labeled myonuclei (Table 2). Hearts weighing 179.42 ± 3.86 and 122.94 ± 6.97%

Table 2. Cumulative Indices of Labeled Nuclei for Atrial and Left Ventricular Myocytes as Well as for Nonmuscle Cells of the Left Ventricle of Rat Hearts Displaying the Highest Degrees of Hypertrophy Observed in this Study[a]

| | | Cumulative indices of labeling (%) | | | |
| | | Myocytes | | | |
Animal no.	Heart weight (% of controls)	Left atrium	Right atrium	Left ventricle	Nonmuscle cells from left ventricle
1615	184.8	47.22	33.0	0.263	59.52
1618	180.7	40.47	12.32	0	65.43
1621	169.0	47.0	11.48	0.049	54.49
1631	172.6	54.28	35.13	0.156	57.12
1633	190.0	53.19	31.37	0.616	60.81
Mean ± S.E.M.	179.42 ± 3.86	48.43 ± 2.49	24.72 ± 5.27	0.217 ± 0.11	59.59 ± 1.76

[a] The animals received 30 repeated injections of [^{3}H]thymidine at 12-hr intervals beginning on day 7 after aortic constriction.

of controls contained practically the same percentages of labeled nonmuscle cells: $59.59 \pm 1.76\%$ in the former and $55.69 \pm 5.85\%$ in the latter.

DISCUSSION

The data obtained in this work confirm the previously established fact that atrial myocytes of adult rats resume DNA synthesis and mitosis much more readily than their ventricular counterparts. This increased capacity of atrial myocytes to proliferate is even more evident in rats with ligated left coronary arteries (27–30). Some characteristic traits of adult cardiomyocyte stimulated hyperplasia are compared in Table 3 in terms of the experimental conditions and the type of myocardial cells.

Ventricular working myocytes display a very limited accumulated frequency of labeling (up to 6% after multiple [^{3}H]thymidine injections) only within the narrow perinecrotic zone of postinfarction hearts (Table 3). Similar conditions of repeated [^{3}H]thymidine administration following aortic constriction result in the labeling of no more than 0.2% of left ventricle myocytes, which is nearly 30 times lower than the cumulative labeling index for the perinecrotic region (Tables 2,3). The number of [^{3}H]thymidine-tagged myonuclei in the ventricular myocardia located far from the infarcted region is also close to zero even in the experiments with multiple precursors injections (see Figure 23 of reference 28). It can be concluded from these data that hyperfunction is practically unable to trigger the transition of ventricular myocytes of the adult rat heart from the G_0 state into the mitotic cycle.

Numerous data reviewed by Pfitzer (24), Zak (38,39), Meerson (20), and Rumyantsev (28) as well as the results of several recent investigations (9,16,36) are in full accordance with the above statement. Exceptions include the reactivation of DNA synthesis in hyperfunctioning hearts of neonatal and very young animals (8,11,12,21,37) and the intriguing fact of the appearance of higher ploidy classes in the ventricular myocytes of hypertrophied human and primate hearts (2,3,24,25,34). The latter fact, however, has never been confirmed by autoradiography.

This work enables us to conclude that hyperfunction generates a stimulus (or stimuli) necessary for the step-by-step transition of numerous—up to 50% and even more—atrial myocytes from the nonproliferating G_0 state into the reactivated mitotic cycle. This kind of atrial myocyte stimulation seems to be similar if not identical after both ligation of the coronary artery and aorta banding but is more intense after extended infarctions (cf. 27,30). The latter result in considerable overloading of the atria, which are known to participate in the compensation of heart function (1,4,18). Therefore, the addition of numerous newly formed postmitotic atrial myocytes and/or their nuclei and genomes (if DNA synthesis is followed by acytokinetic mitoses or polyploidization) might be of great importance for compensating heart failure. Our counts of the total number of myonuclei are indicative of its

Table 3. Proliferative Behavior of Atrial, Ventricular, and Conductive System Myocytes of Rat Heart in Different Experimental Conditions[a]

Type of operation	Heart compartment	Duration of the prereplicative period (days postoperation)	Period of maximal proliferative activity (days postoperation)	Maximal number of a single-pulse ³H-thymidine-labeled myonuclei (Mean ± S.E.M.)	Maximal number of myocyte mitoses (Mean ± S.E.M.)	Cumulative indices of labeled myonuclei after 30–42 repeated [³H]thymidine injections (Mean ± S.E.M.)
Ligation of the coronary artery	Perinecrotic left ventricular myocardium	Unclear	Absent	0.114 ± 0.075	0.043 ± 0.034	6.23 ± 1.48
	Left ventricular myocardium far from infarcted region	Unclear	Absent	0.075 ± 0.032	0	0.21 ± 0.09
	Left atrium	4–5	5–9	3.63 ± 0.47	1.36 ± 0.22	62.44 ± 2.25
	Right atrium	5–6	6–9	2.16 ± 0.43	0.88 ± 0.33	52.30 ± 13.90
	AV node and bundle of His	?	?	0.195 ± 0.12	0.195 ± 0.12	3.73 ± 1.15
Constriction of the abdominal aorta	Left ventricle	?	Absent	—	—	0.217 ± 0.11
	Left atrium	7–9	9–17	1.36 ± 0.66	1.44 ± 0.50	29.75 ± 4.65
	Right atrium	7–9	9–17	1.32 ± 0.87	0.29 ± 0.15	16.78 ± 3.33
	AV node and bundle of His	?	?	—	—	1.97 ± 0.38
Local burning of auricle with heated needle	Perinecrotic myocardium of the left atrium	?	7–21	2.50 ± 1.10	1.40 ± 0.10	—
Linear crushing of the auricle	Perinecrotic myocardium of the left atrium	?	?	3.40 (only one animal studied)	2.15	—

[a] This table includes both the results of the present study and our data published elsewhere (27–32).

considerable increase at later stages after ligation of the coronary artery in rats (30). The exact nature of the hyperfunction-dependent stimulus that triggers the onset of atrial myocyte hyperplasia remains to be investigated with special attention to the molecular events preceding or accompanying DNA synthesis and mitosis (membrane changes, DNA polymerase and proteinase behavior, RNA and protein synthesis, and so on).

It would be quite wrong to conclude from the results of this work and those of our previous studies dealing with myocardial infarction that atrial myocytes possess very high proliferative capacity. Relatively high percentages of labeled atrial myocytes are achieved only because [^{3}H]thymidine is made available over a long period by frequently repeated injections. The number of proliferating myonuclei in the atria of the majority of rats with a ligated coronary artery or banded aorta at any given time does not in fact exceed 4–7% (Figures 1,2; Table 3). Atrial myocytes proliferate after coronary artery ligation almost twice as slowly as nonmuscle cells. This is evident from the data obtained by the method of labeled mitosis curves (30,32). Local injuries to the auricles result in rather sluggish myocyte proliferation (Table 3). Myocytes of hamster atria display no appreciable hyperplasia when pieces of auricles are transplanted into the anterior eye chamber (23). Atrial muscles, like all myocardia studied, are devoid of satellite-type dormant myoblasts which provide for regeneration of skeletal muscles (28,29). Therefore all of the necrotic areas in atria are generally filled by a scar tissue as a result of the overgrowth of rapidly proliferating nonmuscle cells.

The results discussed here call for further reconsideration of the role of cardiomyocyte hyperplasia versus hypertrophy in experimental and clinical pathology involving atrial overload. It would be interesting to compare the different properties of proliferating and nonproliferating fractions of atrial myocytes, taking into account the heterogeneity of these cells under normal conditions (6). It is not impossible that atrial myocyte reactivated hyperplasia could contribute in some way in the future to the prevention or recovery from atrial fibrillation.

The still rather incomplete data concerning the proliferative behavior of specialized myocytes of the conductive system of the heart suggest that these cells resume DNA synthesis after infarction or aorta banding nearly ten times more frequently than the bulk of the working ventricular myocytes located far from the necrotic areas (Table 3). Despite the low absolute values of the cumulative indices of DNA-synthesizing myocytes in this part of the myocardium (about 2–4% according to the data of Table 3), it cannot be excluded that the appearance of only a few newly formed specialized myocytes (or their nuclei and genomes) might contribute to the maintenance of failing heart function. Further investigations are necessary to clarify this promising but still very incomplete subject.

Numerous questions arise concerning the nature and significance of the profound differences in the proliferative behavior of various types of car-

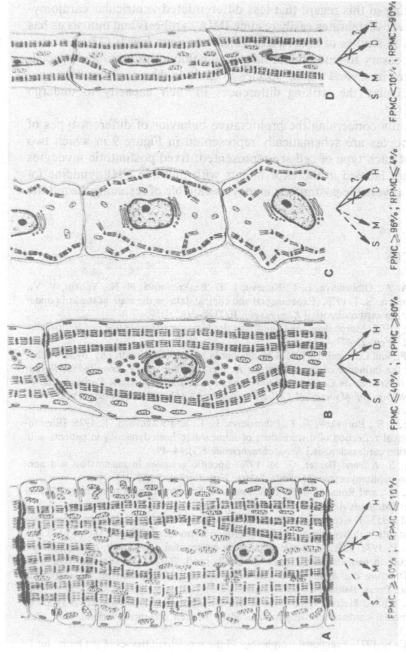

Figure 9. Schematic representation of the possible proliferative and nonproliferative responses of different cardiac myocytes to injury and/or overloading. Key: S, DNA synthesis; M, mitosis; D, complete dedifferentiation (free myoblast formation); H, hypertrophy; FPMC, fixed postmitotic (or static) cells; RPMC, reversible postmitotic cells. Solid arrows indicate very frequent events; dashed ones, extremely rare events; and crossed arrows, possible events, that do not occur. Assessment of the FPMC and RPMC percentages are estimated on the basis of the experiments with multiple [³H]thymidine injections (see text). (A) Rat ventricle, (B) rat atrium, (C) rat atrioventricular conductive system, (D) frog ventricle.

diomyocytes. The enhanced capacity of atrial myocytes for DNA synthesis and mitosis is probably related to the less differentiated state of these cells as compared to ventricular working myocytes (for literature see 28–30). It is worth noting in this regard that less differentiated ventricular cardiomyocytes of lower vertebrates easily resume DNA synthesis and mitosis as has been proved in studies of injured frog (28,29) or newt hearts (22).

It is necessary to study the proliferative behavior of atrial and specialized myocytes in several animal species to exclude the possibility that only rat hearts display the striking differences in their capacity to undergo hyperplasia.

Our results concerning the proliferative behavior of different types of cardiac myocytes are schematically represented in Figure 9 in which two categories of each type of cell are represented: fixed postmitotic myocytes which are not labeled in the experiments with multiple [^{3}H]thymidine injections and reversible postmitotic myocytes capable of resuming the mitotic cycle.

REFERENCES

1. Abinder, A. A., Olbinskaya, L. I., Kitaeva, I. T., Beskrovnova, N. N., Yankin, V. V., and Antonenko, N. I. 1976. [Experimental and clinical data on the state of the atria under post-infarction cardiosclerosis.] *Kardiologiia* 16(7):88–93.
2. Adler, C. P. 1972. Morphologische Grundlagen der Herzhypertrophie und des Herzwachstums. *Med. Welt.* 23:477–484.
3. Adler, C. P., and Costabel, U. 1975. Cell number in human heart in atrophy, hypertrophy, and under the influence of cytostatics. In: A. Fleckenstein and G. Rona (eds.), *Recent Advances in Studies on Cardiac Structure and Metabolism*. Volume 6: *Pathophysiology and Morphology of Myocardial Cell Alteration*, pp. 343–355. University Park Press, Baltimore.
4. Aslibekian, I. S., Borovkov, A. I., Olbinskaya, L. I., and Kitaeva, I. T. 1975. [Electrokymographical reflection of disturbances of intracardiac hemodynamics in patients with postinfarction cardiosclerosis.] *Krovoobrashchenie* 8(3):44–49.
5. Bencosme, S. A., and Berger, G. M. 1976. Specific granules in mammalian and non-mammalian cardiomyocytes. *Methods Achiev. Exp. Pathol.* 5:173–213.
6. Berger, G. M., and Rona, G. 1971. Functional and fine structural heterogeneity of atrial cardiocytes. *Methods Achiev. Exp. Pathol.* 5:540–590.
7. Beznak, M. 1953. The restoration of cardiac hypertrophy and blood pressure in hypophysectomized rats with large doses of LHP or growth hormone. *J. Physiol. (Lond.)* 120:23P.
8. Bishop, S. P. 1973. Effect of aortic stenosis on myocardial cell growth, hyperplasia and ultrastructure in neonatal dogs. In: N. S. Dhalla (ed.). *Recent Advances in Studies on Cardiac Structure and Metabolism.* Vol. 3: *Myocardial Metabolism*, pp. 637–656. University Park Press, Baltimore.
9. Bishop, S. P., and Melsen, L. R. 1976. Myocardial necrosis, fibrosis and DNA synthesis in experimental cardiac hypertrophy induced by sudden pressure overload. *Circ. Res.* 39:238–245.
10. Challice, C. E. 1971. Functional morphology of the specialized tissues of the heart. In: E. Bajusz (ed.), *Functional Morphology of the Heart*, pp. 121–172. Karger, Basel.
11. Dowell, R. T., and McManus, R. E. III 1978. Pressure-induced cardiac enlargement in neonatal and adult rats. Left ventricular functional characteristics and evidence of cardiac muscle cell proliferation in the neonate. *Circ. Res.* 42:303–310.

12. Hollenberg, M., Honbo, N., and Samorodin, A. J. 1976. Effects of hypoxia on cardiac growth in neonatal rats. *Am. J. Physiol.* 231:1445–1450.
13. Hudgson, P., and Field, E. J. 1973. Regeneration of muscle. In: G. H. Bourne (ed.), *The Structure and Function of Muscle.* Vol. 2, Pt. II, pp. 312–363. Academic Press, London, New York.
14. Klika, E., and Jarkovska, D. 1976. *The Myocardium of the Intrapulmonary Veins in Mammals.* Academia, Praha.
15. Kogan, A. Ch. 1961. [A new simple method of controlled constriction of the renal and other arteries in chronic experiment in small animals.] *Biull. Eksp. Biol. Med.* 51:112–114.
16. Kostirev, O. A., and Leontieva, T. A. 1973. [Autoradiographic study of the DNA synthesis in muscle and connective tissue heart cells injured by isopropilnoradrenalin.] *Biull. Eksp. Biol. Med.* 76:108–110.
17. Legato, M. J. 1973. Ultrastructure of the atrial, ventricular and Purkinje cells with special references to the genesis of arrhythmias. *Circulation* 47:178–189.
18. Makolkin, V. I., Shatichin, A. I., Abbakumov, S. A., and Leshkova, M. I. 1971. [Diagnostics of the atrial pathology using bloodless instrumental methods.] *Kardiologiia* 2(7):147–156.
19. McMinn, R. M. 1969. *Tissue Repair.* Academic Press, New York.
20. Meerson, F. Z. 1975. [*Heart Adaptation to the Overload and Heart Insufficiency.*] Nauka, Moscow.
21. Neffgen, G. F., and Korecky, B. 1972. Cellular hyperplasia and hypertrophy in cardiomegalies induced by anemia in young and adult rats. *Circ. Res.* 30:104–113.
22. Oberpriller, J. O., and Oberpriller, J. C. 1974. Response of the adult newt ventricle to injury. *J. Exp. Zool.* 187:249–253.
23. Oberpriller, J. O., and Oberpriller, J. C. 1977. Modified hamster atrial cardiac muscle cells isolated in the anterior chamber of the eye. *J. Mol. Cell. Cardiol.* 9:1013-1017.
24. Pfitzer, P. 1972. Die karyologischen Grundlagen der Hypertrophie. *Verh. Dtsch. Ges. Kreislaufforsch.* 38:22–34.
25. Pfitzer, P., and Schulte, H. D. 1972. The nuclear DNA content of myocardial cells of monkeys as a model for the polyploidization in the human heart. In: E. I. Goldsmith and J. Moor-Jankowski (eds.), *Medical Primatology 1972.* Proceedings of the Third Conference on Experimental Medicine and Surgery in Primates, Lyon 1972, Part I, pp. 379–389. Karger, Basel.
26. Polezhaev, L. V. 1972. *Organ Regeneration in Animals.* Charles C Thomas, Springfield, Illinois.
27. Rumyantsev, P. P. 1974. Ultrastructural reorganization, DNA synthesis and mitotic division of myocytes in atria of rats with left ventricle infarction. An electron microscopic and autoradiographic study. *Virchows Archiv.* [*Cell. Pathol.*] 15:357–378.
28. Rumyantsev, P. P. 1977. Interrelations of the proliferation and differentiation processes during cardiac myogenesis and regeneration. *Int. Rev. Cytol.* 51:187–273.
29. Rumyantsev, P. P. 1979. Some comparative aspects of myocardial regeneration. In: A. Mauro (ed.), *Muscle Regeneration,* pp. 335–355. Raven Press, New York.
30. Rumyantsev, P. P. 1981. New comparative aspects of myocardial regeneration with special reference to cardiomyocyte proliferative behavior. In: R. O. Becker (ed.), *Mechanisms of Growth Control,* pp. 311–342. Charles C Thomas, Springfield, Illinois.
31. Rumyantsev, P. P., and Kassem, A. M. 1976. Cumulative indices of DNA synthesizing myocytes in different compartments of the working myocardium and conductive system of the rat's heart muscle following extensive left ventricle infarction. *Virchows Archiv.* [*Cell. Pathol.*] 20:329–342.
32. Rumyantsev, P. P., and Mirakyan, V. O. 1968. [Increased activity of DNA synthesis and mitoses in rat atrial muscle cells under ventricular myocardial infarction and local injuries of auricles.] *Tsitologia* 10:1276–1287.
33. Rumyantsev, P. P., and Mirakyan, V. O. 1968. Reactive synthesis of DNA and mitotic division in atrial heart muscle cells following ventricle infarction. *Experientia* 24:1234–1235.
34. Sandritter, W., and Scomazzoni, G. 1964. Deoxyribonucleic acid content (Feulgen pho-

162   P. P. Rumyantsev

tometry) and dry weight (interference microscopy) of normal and hypertrophic heart muscle fibres. *Nature* 202:100–101.

35. Schiaffino, S., Cantini, M., Bormioli, S. P., and Sartore, S. 1979. Heterogeneity of cardiac muscle cells in vivo and in vitro. In: A. Mauro (ed.), *Muscle Regeneration*, pp. 357–361. Raven Press, New York.
36. Steinert, W., Pfitzer, P., Friedrich, G., and Stoepel, K. 1974. DNS-Synthese im Herzen von Ratten mit renalem Hochdruck bei Langzeitinfusion von ^{3}H-Thymidin. *Beitr. Pathol.* 153:165–177.
37. Wachtlová, M., Mareš, V., and Oštádal, B. 1977. DNA synthesis in the ventricular myocardium of young rats exposed to intermittent high altitude (IHA) hypoxia. An autoradiographic study. *Virchows Archiv.* [*Cell Pathol.*] 24:335–342.
38. Zak, R. 1973. Cell proliferation during cardiac growth. *Am. J. Cardiol.* 31:211–219.
39. Zak, R. 1974. Development and proliferative capacity of cardiac muscle cells. *Circ. Res.* 34–35(Suppl. 2):17–26.

DNA Synthetic Activity of Right and Left Ventricular Biopsy Specimens in Patients with Cardiomyopathy

Y. Yabe

Cardiovascular Diagnostic Laboratory Center
Toho University School of Medicine
Tokyo, Japan

H. Abe

Department of Radiology
Nihon University School of Medicine
Tokyo, 173 Japan

Y. Kashiwakura

Department of Cardiology
Urawa City Hospital
Urawa, Japan

Abstract. This investigation was designed to evaluate the difference in DNA activity between biopsy specimens obtained from right and left ventricles. Nucleic DNA in the myocardial cells of hypertrophied and congestive forms of cardiomyopathy was analyzed to investigate the relationship between cell function and clinical manifestations. Endomyocardial biopsy specimens were obtained simultaneously from right ventricular septal wall and left ventricular inferolateral wall by a transcatheter biotome. Measurement of DNA was based on the Feulgen reaction and dual wavelength cytophotometry. In this series, 12 patients with hypertrophic cardiomyopathy and four patients with congestive cardiomyopathy were studied. In the normal heart, the DNA value (arbitrary units) of the right ventricle was 138.6, whereas that of the left ventricle was 144.4. In the hypertrophic group, the mean DNA value in the right ventricle was 279.9, whereas that of the left ventricle was 317.5. In the congestive group, the DNA mean value in the right ventricle was 108.8, whereas that of left ventricle was 144.8. The linear relationship ($r = 0.67$) between right and left ventricular DNA values suggests that cellular function of one ventricle is affected by that of the other side. Higher DNA values of the left ventricle may indicate the difference in work load between the ventricles. The relationships among DNA values, LV wall thickness, LV mass, and parameters of contractility were statistically high.

Ideopathic cardiomyopathy is a distinct clinical entity of unknown etiology involving predominantly the heart muscle. However, clinical features and hemodynamic alterations are specific enough to justify a positive diagnosis. Myocardial biopsies have contributed greatly to proper diagnosis (2,3,6).

163

Almost all reports concerning biopsies of myocardial cells mainly used a morphological approach. It is also very important to analyze alterations at the cellular level by quantitative and qualitative histochemical evaluation. This report is concerned with biopsies of myocardial cells of patients who show cineangiographic features of idiopathic cardiomyopathy. Nuclear DNA in the myocardial cells of the hypertrophied and congestive forms of cardiomyopathy were analyzed to investigate the relationship between cell function and clinical manifestations. Moreover, we have tried to evaluate the difference in DNA activities between right and left ventricles.

MATERIALS AND METHODS

In this series, 12 patients with hypertrophic cardiomyopathy and four with congestive cardiomyopathy were studied (Table 1). Their ages ranged from 13 to 72 years. Twelve cases listed in the upper portion of Table 1 had hypertrophic cardiomyopathy (HCM), and the next four cases, numbered 13 through 16, displayed congestive cardiomyopathy (CCM). One case, numbered 17, without abnormal angiographic finding was also studied as a control.

All patients underwent selective left ventriculography and biventriculography to assess the wall thickness and the geometry of the left ventricle. Following these procedures, endomyocardial biopsy specimens were ob-

Table 1.   Clinical Features of 17 Cases

Pt. no.	Age	Sex	Cardiothoracic ratio	New York Heart Association	Left ventricular pressure (systolic/early diastolic/end diastolic)	CI	Ejection fraction	Wall thickness
1	13	F	44	III	110/2/7	6.6	0.82	9
2	50	M	46	II	112/5/10	2.6	0.62	12
3	60	M	47	I	150/0/15	4.6	0.58	14
4	54	M	54	I	142/2/11	3.1	0.50	14
5	72	M	52	II	142/11/17	2.4	0.81	16
6	15	M	38	I	130/4/17	3.2	0.86	9
7	45	F	50	I–II	135/2/18	3.1	0.87	17
8	49	M	46	I–II	163/10/14	3.2	0.84	19
9	30	M	47	I	117/5/14	4.8	0.80	14
10	61	F	65	II	147/8/19	3.1	0.64	19
11	50	M	50	I	125/0/15	3.80	0.76	14
12	45	M	49	I	112/0/20	4.68	0.74	16
13	42	M	56	III	119/9/28	2.0	0.35	6
14	57	M	57	II–III	128/11/20	2.6	0.32	5
15	46	M	55	III	224/25/49	2.3	0.30	6
16	52	M	56	II–III	100/7/22	2.7	0.34	6
17	40	M	38	I	126/0/10	3.5	0.60	9

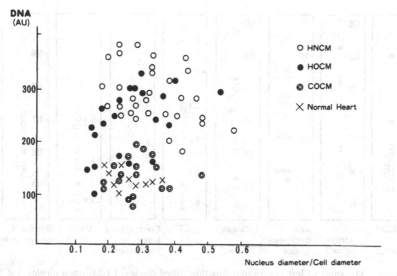

Figure 1.   Relationship between nuclear size and DNA values.

tained simultaneously from the right ventricular septal wall and the left ventricular inferolateral wall with the use of the transcatheter endomyocardial biotome. A report on this method has been presented by Abe and Kitamura (1).

The nucleic DNA volume was measured by Feulgen cytophotometry. Quantitative measurement of stained nucleic DNA was performed by the dual wavelength method using a computer-aided microspectrophotometer. As control, normal lymphocytes and normal adult myocardial cells from the heart without known heart disease were used, and theoretical diploid values were determined. The method of staining DNA and its measurement have been reported by Yabe and Kashiwakura (9) and Yabe and Abe (8).

RESULTS

Figure 1 demonstrates the relationship between DNA values in the right ventricle and the size of the nuclei. The size of a nucleus is divided by its cell diameter for normalization. In HCM cases, the nucleus–cell diameter ratio was 0.15 to 0.55, with a DNA content of 110–300. In hypertrophic, nonobstructive cardiomyopathy, this ratio was 0.2–0.55, with DNA content of 180–400. In CCM, this ratio was 0.18–0.49, with DNA content of 84–180. Normal heart muscle had a ratio of 0.19–0.35, with DNA content of 100–150 (Figure 1).

As clinical indices of left ventricular function, LVEDP, wall stress, LV wall thickness, LV mass, ejection fraction, contractility index, V_{max}, and stroke power index were measured. The LVEDP and diastolic wall stress showed high values in the CCM group. Left ventricular wall thickness and

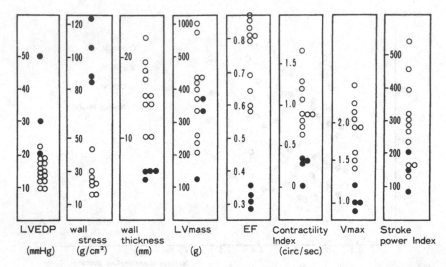

Figure 2.   Measures of left ventricular function: filled circles, CCM; open circles, HCM.

mass of all HCM cases were significantly greater than the normal values. The CCM cases, on the other hand, have smaller wall thickness and lower LV mass, distinctly different from the HCM group. With regard to ejection fraction, contractility index, V_{max}, and stroke power index, almost all in the HCM group either were normal or exceeded normal values (Figure 2). Comparison between ejection fraction V_{max}, and contractility index and DNA values in left ventricle yielded correlation coefficients (r) of 0.55, 0.60, and 0.78, respectively. These ejection phase indices increase with the amount of DNA in left ventricular myocardial cell nuclei (Figure 3).

Figure 4 demonstrates the difference in DNA kinetics between left and right ventricle in each case. In normal heart, the DNA value of the right ventricle was 138.6, whereas that of left ventricle was 144.4. In the hypertrophic group, the mean DNA value in the right ventricle was 279.9, and that of left ventricle was 317.5. However, in the HCM group, mean DNA values showed wide variation between 178 and 496. In CCM cases, the DNA mean values in the right ventricle was 108.8, and that of left ventricle was 144.4. DNA values of the CCM group were significantly low compared to control and distinctly different from those of the HCM group.

In all patients, the mean DNA value of the right ventricle was 231.3 ± 57.8, while that of left ventricle was 272.6 ± 62.9. The comparison of DNA values between right and left ventricle showed its predominance (+12%) in the left ventricular myocardial cells. The correlation between right and left ventricular DNA activities was $r = 0.67$.

DISCUSSION

Yabe and Abe showed in histogram form the DNA values of myocardial cell nuclei in patients with idiopathic cardiomyopathy (8). In the normal

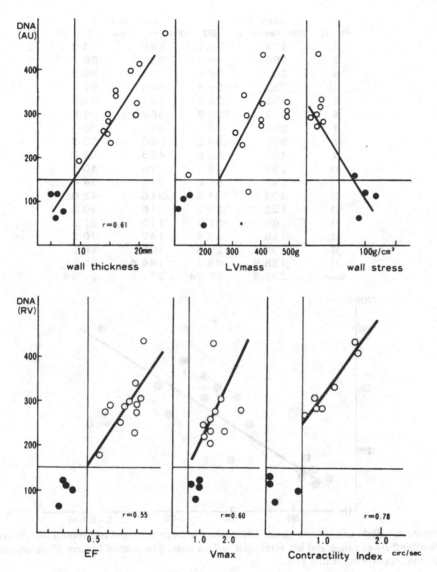

Figure 3.   Relationships between DNA values of left ventricles and various parameters of left ventricular function: filled circles, CCM; open circles, HCM.

heart, the mode and distribution of the nuclear DNA showed a diploid–tetraploid pattern, suggesting that nuclear DNA values of this cell population were almost constant. In the hypertrophic obstructive group, it showed a tetraploid–octaploid pattern. However, in the hypertrophic non-obstructibe group, there were two different kinetic expressions: tetraploid–octoploid and hexaploid–decaploid. Likewise, in the congestive group, two trypes of DNA pattern were noted and showed mainly hypodi-

Pt. No	Right Ventricle DNA mean value	SD	Left Ventricle DNA mean value	SD
1	178	79.0	299	73.0
2	256	48.0	332	88.0
3	287	76.0	326	96.0
4	237	59.4	449	97.5
5	196	73.2	141	40.3
6	343	123.7	362	104.8
7	298	78.5	316	100.1
8	290	86.0	280	100.0
9	436	52.6	496	55.0
10	237	39.9	278	40.5
11	295	54.0	315	34.4
12	306	34.0	316	48.0
13	153	34.3	216	50.0
14	69	31.7	110	21.5
15	116	40.4	147	70.5
16	97	27.5	106	18.5
17	138.6	43.3	144.4	32.5
mean	231.3	57.74	272.6	62.98

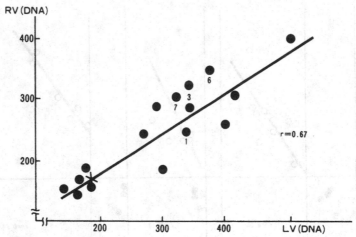

Figure 4.   Right and left ventricular DNA values in 16 patients and one control and the relationship between right and left ventricular DNA values. The control (patient 17) is indicated by the cross on the scatter plot.

ploidization. Therefore, DNA kinetics showed polyploidization in the HCM group compared to normal heart muscle cell nuclei. The multiplication of myocardial cell nuclei and significant increase of DNA values of each myocardial cell in patients with HCM results in hypertrophy of cell nuclei.

Sandritter and Scomazzoni (5) also reported that normal heart showed tetraploid and that cardiac hypertrophy showed octaploid or greater polyploidy (90% of the muscle cells). Therefore, we could differentiate DNA kinetics of hypertrophied cardiac muscle cell nuclei from the histogram of DNA values among the different types of cardiomyopathy. The ploidy grade of DNA indicates the stage of cardiomyopathy and the type of disease.

It is generally held that increased heart weight and hypertrophied myocardium result from an increase in the diameter of the muscle cells. We demonstrated a correlation between nucleic DNA values and size of nuclei. There was no significant difference in size of the nuclei among the different types of cardiomyopathy. However, in the HCM group, nuclear DNA content was almost in proportion to the increase in nuclear volume.

The contents of DNA showed wide variations with some correlation with the different types of disease. In particular, CCM cases were found in the lower range of DNA values, distinctly different from the HCM group.

Kunkel et al. also reported that cardiac muscle cells showed signs of hypertrophy of varying degree with enlargement of the nucleus and cell diameter in the hypertrophic and CCM groups (4). They reported finding normal mean cardiac muscle cell diameter in one patient with advanced CCM, although 31% showed a mild enlargement of the mean muscle fiber diameter. In analysis of left ventricular function in patients, the significant increase of LVEDP, LVEDV, and diastolic wall stress in CCM cases indicates that the disturbance of left ventricular diastolic performance may cause interstitial fibrosis.

In the entire HCM group, although significant increases of LV wall thickness and LV mass were noted, the ejection fraction, contractility index, V_{max}, and stroke power index either were within or exceeded normal values. These results suggest that myocardial contraction and myocardial function are not impaired in spite of significantly hypertrophied myocardium. Moreover, we have demonstrated that correlations between DNA values in left ventricle and LV wall thickness or parameters of left ventricular contractility were statistically significant.

Comparison of DNA values of right and left ventricles showed a predominance in the left ventricular myocardial cells, and the linear relationship ($r = 0.67$) between right and left ventricular DNA activity suggests that cellular function of one ventricle is affected by that of the other side. Higher DNA values of the left ventricular specimens than of those from the right ventricle may be associated with the difference in work loads of the ventricles.

We have reported that RNA in the nuclei showed changes completely parallel with those of DNA activities (7). In the nonobstructive hypertrophic group, the mean RNA value was 185.0, and in the hypertrophic obstructive group, 168.5. In the congestive group, it showed the lowest mean value, 81.0.

Myocardial energy metabolism in cardiomyopathy was investigated by Yamada et al. (10). Pyruvate kinase—a key enzyme of glycolysis and of the electron transport system (succinate cytochrome c reductase, NADM cytochrome c reductase, and cytochrome c oxidase)—was significantly increased in HCM compared to the congestive form. In CCM, pyruvate kinase activity was 45 mU/mg, which was less than that of HCM (104 mU/mg). Succinate cytochrome c reductase and NADH cytochrome c reductase and oxidase were 5.2, 87, and 397 mU/mg in CCM, whereas these enzymes were 9.9, 146, and 775 mU/mg in HCM, respectively.

These facts suggest that the increase of protein synthesis ability, especially in HCM, activates these enzymes of myocardial energy metabolism and does so in proportion to the activation of nucleic acid synthesis. Therefore, polyploidization in hypertrophied cardiac muscle cells plays an important role in maintaining cell function by accelerating RNA activity and contractile protein synthesis.

REFERENCES

1. Abe, H., and Kitamura, K. 1981. New trial of myocardial biopsy. *Jpn. Circ. J.* 45 (Suppl.) 22.
2. Brooksby, A. B., Jenkins, B. S., Coltart, D. J., and Webb-Peploe, M. M. 1974. Left ventricular endomyocardial biopsy. *Lancet* 2:1222–1225.
3. Konno, S., Sekiguchi, M., and Sakakibara, S. 1971. Catheter biopsy of the heart. *Radiol. Clin. North Am.* 9:491–510.
4. Kunkel, B., Lapp, H., Kober, G., and Kaltenbach, M. 1978. Light-microscopic evaluation of myocardial biopsies. In: M. Kaltenbach, F. Loogen, and E. G. Olsen (eds.), *Cardiomyopathy and Myocardial Biopsy*, pp. 62–70. Springer-Verlag, Berlin, Heidelberg, New York.
5. Sandritter, W., and Scomazzoni, G. 1964. DNA content (Feulgen photometry) and dry weight (interference microscopy) of normal and hypertrophic heart muscle fibres. *Nature* 202:100–115.
6. Shirey, E. K., Hawk, W. A., Mukerji, D., and Effler, D. B. 1972. Percutaneous myocardial biopsy of the left ventricle. Experience in 198 patients. *Circulation* 46:112–122.
7. Yabe, Y., and Abe, H. 1979. Changes in DNA and RNA synthesis of the cardiac muscle cell in patients with cardiomyopathy (myocardial biopsy). *J. Mol. Cell. Cardiol.* 77(Suppl. 7):68.
8. Yabe, Y., and Abe, H. 1980. Changes in DNA synthesis in significantly hypertrophied human cardiac muscle. In: M. Tajuddin, P. K. Das, M. Tariq, and N. S. Dhalla (eds.), *Advances in Myocardiology*, Vol. 1, pp. 553–563. University Park PRess, Baltimore.
9. Yabe, Y., and Kashiwakura, Y. 1978. Nucleic DNA and RNA in cardiac muscle cell of experimental myocardial infarction. In: T. Kobayashi, Y. Ito, and G. Rona (eds.), *Recent Advances in Studies on Cardiac Structure and Metabolism*. Vol. 12: *Cardiac Adaptation*, pp. 415–423. University Park Press, Baltimore.
10. Yamada, T., Abe, H., and Yabe, Y. 1980. Myocardial energy metabolism of congestive and hypertrophic cardiomyopathy in man. *J. Mol. Cell. Cardiol.* 12:181.

Comparative Changes in the ^{32}P Labeling of Adenine and Uracil Nucleotides in the Hypertrophying Rat Heart

A. Ray, J. Aussedat, J. Olivares, and A. Rossi

Laboratory of Animal Physiology, Scientific and Medical University of Grenoble
38041 Grenoble Cedex, France

Abstract. The turnover of cardiac adenine and uracil nucleotides was studied in the hypertrophying rat heart by means of the kinetics of incorporation of labeled phosphate into the α-phosphate groups of nucleotides. Cardiac hypertrophy was induced either by chronic isoproterenol treatment (5 mg·kg^{-1} body wt. daily, s.c.) or by abdominal aortic constriction. In both experimental models, although the labeling of α-P groups of adenine nucleotides was at first unmodified, the incorporation of [^{32}P]Phosphate into uracil nucleotides was accelerated early and the stimulation maintained for several days. The intramyocardial concentration of UTP and uracil nucleotides rose during the early phase of hypertrophy, while the ATP and adenine nucleotide pools were depleted. All of these alterations were more pronounced in isoproterenol-treated animals than in those with aortic stenosis. In this experimental model (isoproterenol treatment), the hypertrophy develops faster and is accompanied by a larger increase in cardiac RNA concentration. Thus, the increase in the rate of synthesis of uracil nucleotides may be interpreted as an adaptative change of nucleotide metabolism in response to an increased requirement of precursors for RNA synthesis. The possible limiting role of pyrimidine nucleotides in the hypertrophic process is discussed.

In response to a sustained work load, the cardiac muscle cell enlarges by increasing the rate of synthesis of its cellular components. In this process, an increase of RNA synthesis occurs very early (3). The myocardial free nucleotides, which provide energized precursors for the synthesis of RNA, probably play a key role in the early phase of cardiac hypertrophy. Alterations occurring in the adenine nucleotide pool have focused the attention of people working in this field (4,5,10,14,23,25–28) because of the role played by ATP in the energetic process. Less attention has been paid to the other nucleotides.

It is well know that the concentration of pyrimidine nucleotides is high in tissues in which active protein synthesis takes place. In contrast, the pool size of uracil nucleotides in the myocardium is about 20 times smaller than that of adenine nucleotides (12,17,19,21,22). Obviously, any alteration occurring in this pool may be of importance relative to the metabolism of RNA. Moreover, changes in the turnover rate of these nucleotides should take place among the early events of developing cardiac hypertrophy. Indeed, previous observations have revealed changes both in uracil nucleotide pool

171

size and rate of labeling (12), but no measurement of the rate of synthesis was made. The purpose of this work was to describe accurately the changes in pool size and rate of synthesis of uracil nucleotides in the early phase of cardiac hypertrophy. Two models of experimental cardiac hypertrophy were used in order to be able to detect these features. The rate of synthesis was measured by utilizing a method that was developed by our group (18,20). Parallel investigations on adenine nucleotides were performed to compare the time course alterations in the two pools.

MATERIAL AND METHODS

Animals and Experimental Procedure

Cardiac hypertrophy was induced in female Wistar rats (220 to 250 g) either by daily subcutaneous injection of isoproterenol (5 mg·kg^{-1} body weight) or by abdominal aortic stenosis with a hemostatic clip, a modification of the technique of Nair et al. (16). Sham operations were performed for comparison of results.

The hearts used for ATP and UTP level measurements were clamped by means of Wollenberger tongs (24) precooled in liquid nitrogen. The hearts used for nucleotide pools and specific activity measurements were rapidly excised; the ventricles were rinsed and wiped before chilling in liquid nitrogen.

The frozen ventricles were rapidly weighed. The wet weight was corrected to account for water content changes caused by edema or the clamping procedure.

The extent of cardiac hypertrophy was assessed by comparing the measured weight of the ventricles to the expected weight calculated from the regression line in terms of ventricle weight and body weight [heart weight (mg) = 1.86 body weight (g) + 183].

Biochemical Procedures

ATP and UTP Dosages.   Nucleotide extraction was performed by cold perchloric acid on frozen ventricles. ATP and UTP were determined by enzymatic methods (2,9,11).

RNA Dosage.   RNA was extracted from the acidinsoluble pellet using the technique of Munro and Fleck (15). The RNA concentration was determined by UV spectrophotometry.

Pool Size Determination.   The method has been described in detail in previous papers (18–20). In brief, the ventricles of five rats were pooled to obtain a sufficient quantity of purified uracil nucleotides. The nucleotides extracted from the tissue by cold perchloric acid were alkaline hydrolyzed into nucleoside monophosphates. AMP and UMP were separated by DOWEX 1 × 8 column chromatography, and the pool sizes were calculated from the UV absorbance of column chromatography eluates.

Labeling Procedures

[32P]Phosphate in the form of sodium salt in a saline solution (CEA, Saclay-F) was injected intravenously at the dose of 0.5 mCi·100 g^{-1} body weight.

Two kinetics were followed: ^{32}P incorporation after a constant labeling time (6 hr) at various stages of the hypertrophy or time course of labeling for a given stage of cardiac hypertrophy.

The specific activities of the α-phosphate groups were measured on AMP and UMP purified by paper chromatography.

The inorganic phosphate specific activity was measured in an aliquot of the initial perchloric acid extract freed of nucleotides by adsorption on activated charcoal. The phosphate content determination was achieved by the technique of Bartlett (1) or by the technique of Furchgott and De Gubareff (6) and the radioactivity was measured by Cerenkov counting.

Mathematical Analysis of Labeling Kinetics

Rates of incorporation of inorganic phosphate into the α-phosphate groups of the nucleotides were calculated from time course of labeling of inorganic phosphate and of α-phosphate groups of the nucleotides.

This model was based on the assumptions that intracellular nucleotide pools are not compartmented and that inorganic phosphate may be considered the proximate precursor of the α-phosphate groups of nucleotides (18). The validity of this method was discussed in previous papers (18,20), and the details of the calculation are given in a recent paper (17).

RESULTS

Changes in Heart Weight and RNA Concentrations

As shown in Figure 1, the time course of development of cardiac hypertrophy was different in the two experimental models. The myocardial weight rose rapidly and reached 143% of control value after five daily injections of isoproterenol. It increased more slowly and did not exceed 128% of that of sham operated rats 8 days after aortic constriction.

Within the same periods of time, RNA concentrations were, respectively, augmented to 139% and 133% of control value (2.04 ± 0.36 mg·g^{-1}, means ± S.E., $N = 18$).

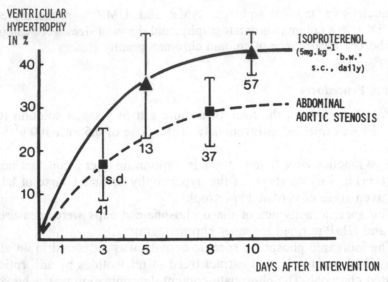

Figure 1.   Cardiac hypertrophy development induced by isoproterenol injections (▲) or aortic stenosis (■). Measured weights were compared with the expected weights calculated from the regression line in terms of ventricle weight and body weight (see methods). Results are means ± standard deviation. Number of experiments is indicated beneath each point.

Alterations of ATP and UTP Levels

It is well known that the myocardial ATP concentration falls soon after the initiation of isoproterenol treatment (4,10,23) or after pressure overload (5,26,27) and remains depressed for several days. Such a durable diminution is shown in Figure 2 for our two experimental models: from the sixth hour after the initiation of treatments, ATP level was reduced to about 75% of control value.

Changes in UTP level followed a different pattern. The first injection of isoproterenol induced a transient fall and subsequent increase in UTP. This augmentation was significant 6 hr after the first injection and remained present for the duration of the experiment. In the "aortic stenosis" model, the expansion of the UTP pool was delayed: maximal values were reached on the third day following aortic constriction and decreased significantly on the eighth day although still remaining above control value. In sham-operated animals, ATP and UTP levels did not differ from controls.

Rates of Synthesis of Adenine and Uracil Nucleotides

The purpose of the work was to estimate the most important modification in the rate of synthesis of adenine and uracil nucleotides that occurred during the development of cardiac hypertrophy.

We had first to define the single duration of ^{32}P exposure that could

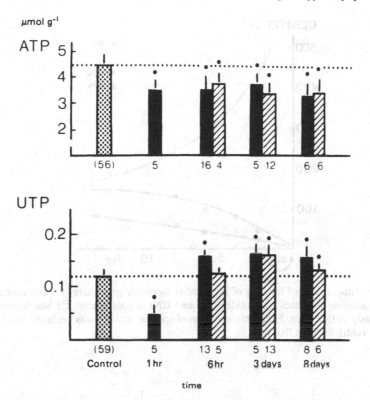

Figure 2. Changes in myocardial ATP and UTP concentrations following daily isoproterenol injections (■) or aortic stenosis (▨). Initiation of treatment at time zero. Results are means ± standard deviation. Number of experiments reported under each column. *Significant differences from controls (C); $P < 0.05$.

permit us to determine, by a rough investigation, the time periods in the two treatments when the variations in the rate of incorporation of radiophosphorus were the greatest. Based on previous work (18) and on analysis of the ^{32}P-incorporation time course into myocardial inorganic phosphate and nucleotide α-phosphate groups of controls (Figure 3), we chose a period for ^{32}P incorporation of 6 hr, which was long enough to permit the realization of an isotopic equilibrium between extracellular phosphate and the different intracellular precursors of nucleotide α phosphate groups.

The ratio of specific activity of α-phosphate groups relative to the specific activity of inorganic phosphate was taken as an index of the speed of labeling.

The comparative changes in the ^{32}P labeling of α-phosphate groups of myocardial adenine and uracil nucleotides, 6 hr after the injection of radiophosphorus, in the course of time of development of hypertrophy are illustrated in Figure 4. The labeling of adenine nucleotides was at first unmodified in the two experimental models. It then increased slowly, reaching

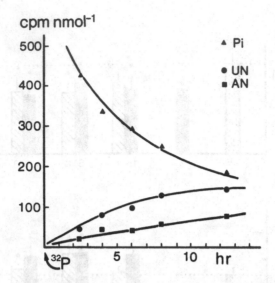

Figure 3.   Time course of labeling of myocardial inorganic phosphate (Pi) and α-phosphate groups of adenine and uracil nucleotides (AN and UN) in control rats; ^{32}P was administered intravenously at time zero. Each determination of specific activity was performed on batches of pooled ventricles from five rats.

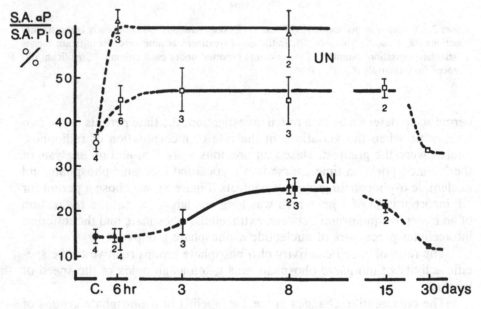

Figure 4.   Comparative changes in the ^{32}P labeling of α-P groups of myocardial adenine (▲, ■) and uracil (△, □) nucleotides in the course of development of hypertrophy in rats. Treatment: aortic stenosis (■, □); isoproterenol (daily s.c., 5 mg·kg^{-1}) (▲, △). Labeling: measurement of specific activities (S.A.) of α-phosphate groups of nucleotides (αP) and Pi over 6 hr after i.v. injection of ^{32}P. Results are means ± S.D. Number of batches indicated under each data point.

Table 1. Comparative Changes in Pool Sizes and
Synthesis Rates of Myocardial Adenine and Uracil
Nucleotides on the First Day of Isoproterenol Treatment
and 3 Days after Banding Aorta in Rats

	Pool sizes[a] (μmol · g^{-1})	Rates of synthesis[b] (nmol · g^{-1} · hr^{-1})
Controls		
Adenine nucleotides	5.58 ± 0.08 (23)	100
Uracil nucleotides	0.258 ± 0.009 (24)	16
Isoproterenol, day 1		
Adenine nucleotides	4.50 ± 0.23 (7)	90
Uracil nucleotides	0.448 ± 0.007 (6)	58
Aortic stenosis, day 3		
Adenine nucleotides	4.80 ± 0.17 (10)	150
Uracil nucleotides	0.388 ± 0.002 (10)	42

[a] Pool sizes: each measurement was made on five pooled rat hearts. Results are
means ± standard error; number of experiments in brackets.
[b] Rates of synthesis: each result was calculated from ^{32}P labeling kinetics data (five
groups of five pooled hearts each).

a maximal value several days after the initiation of treament, when the
hypertrophying process was almost over.

The incorporation of labeled inorganic phosphate into the α-phosphate
group of uracil nucleotides was stimulated quite early. It reached a maximal
value on the first day of isoproterenol treatment and the third day after the
placing of aortic constriction. For the same period of time, the ^{32}P labeling
of adenine and uracil nucleotides was not significantly different in sham-
operated animals than in controls. The complete study of the time course
of labeling of myocardial inorganic phosphate and α-phosphate groups of
adenine and uracil nucleotides at these times of the treatments permitted us
to determine maximal values of the rates of synthesis (Table 1).

Adenine nucleotide synthesis remained unchanged for the first day of
isoproterenol treatment and was multiplied by 1.5, the third day after aortic
stenosis. The alterations in uracil nucleotide synthesis were more pronounced. The first isoproterenol injection induced an increase of about 260%
in this parameter. The third day after banding the abdominal aorta, this rise
did not exceed 160%.

DISCUSSION

The decrease of myocardial level of ATP in several experimental models
of cardiac hypertrophy is a well-known fact (4,5,10,23). On the basis of such
observations, Meerson and Pomoinitsky (14) proposed that the breakdown
of cardiac ATP should be considered the trigger that gives rise to the stim-

ulation of protein synthesis leading to the development of cardiac hypertrophy. In our experiments, the intramyocardial concentration of ATP was indeed decreased during the early phase of developing cardiomegaly. However, in both experimental models, the cardiac ATP level remained depressed until the eighth day of the experiment when there was no continuous cardiac enlargement. In a recent paper, Zimmer et al. (28) reported that cardiac hypertrophy could develop even when ATP decline was prevented by feeding adenine nucleotide synthesis with exogenous precursor. Thus, the possible relationships between ATP breakdown and the protein synthesis in the myocardial cell are perhaps more complex, and further investigations on this question are needed.

The alterations occurring in the pyrimidine nucleotide pools in the course of developing hypertrophy have not been investigated. However, a possible role of these nucleotides in cardiac hypertrophy must be questioned because of their role as precursors of ribonucleic acids.

An expansion of the uracil nucleotide pool was detected after aortic constriction in rats (12), and previous investigations by our group revealed that the myocardial UTP level rose early after isoproterenol administration in rats (17,21,22). The results reported in the present paper demonstrate that the enlargement of UTP pool and of the sum of uracil nucleotides was also present in the hearts of rats with aortic stenosis. Moreover, this increase occurred at an early phase of cardiac hypertrophy and reached a maximal value within the first days after initiation of the hypertrophic process, so a possible correlation of these events with the process of hypertrophy may exist.

The cardiac hypertrophy development being a dynamic process means that knowledge of the changes in the pool sizes of nucleotides is not sufficient to assess the possible role of these compounds in cardiomegaly. Indeed, the turnover rates of nucleotides are a better index of the alterations accompanying cardiac hypertrophy. A study of the de novo synthesis of adenine nucleotides was achieved by Zimmer et al. (25–28). These experiments demonstrated that the rate of this synthesis was raised during the initial phase in almost every type of experimentally induced myocardial hypertrophy. However, this increase was low when compared to the size of the ATP pool, and normal ATP levels were not rapidly restored by this way. Concerning uracil nucleotides, qualitative observations of Matsushita and Fanburg (13) showed that the de novo synthesis of these nucleotides was probably very low in both normal and·hypertrophying rat heart. These authors observed that the only enzyme of the synthetic pathways of uracil nucleotides the activity of which was found to be significantly raised after aortic constriction was uridine kinase.

Since it is well established that the "salvage pathways" that utilize preformed bases and nucleosides to synthetize nucleotides may be more efficient than de novo synthesis in heart tissue (7), more complex information about the turnover of nucleotides must be drawn from experiments that estimate the total synthesis (de novo + salvage pathways).

A method suitable for this purpose was developed by our group and is discussed in previous papers (18,20). The total synthesis of nucleotides was estimated from the ^{32}P-labeling kinetics of the α-phosphate groups of nucleotides. The results demonstrate that a very fast and large increase of the synthesis of cardiac uracil nucleotides was induced by isoproterenol injections in rats (17,22). The present results show that a similar stimulation is present in hearts after aortic stenosis. In contrast, in both experimental models, the synthesis of adenine nucleotides was stimulated at a later stage and to a smaller extent.

Since the enlargement of the uracil nucleotide pool and the increase in the total synthesis of these nucleotides occur in both experimental models, such alterations must be considered to be features of cardiac hypertrophy. In order to roughly estimate the need for precursors created by the increase in RNA synthesis in the early phase of cardiac hypertrophy, a calculation from the known values of RNA concentration and from a presumed turnover rate of RNA is reported in Table 2.

These calculations show that the changes in the amount of pyrimidine nucleotides incorporated hourly into the RNA pool largely parallel the changes in the rate of synthesis or uracil nucleotides as measured by our method. Thus, it can be assumed that the synthesis of cardiac uracil nu-

Table 2. Comparison between Uracil Nucleotide Synthesis Rate and Putative Pyrimidine Nucleotide Requirement for Extra Synthesis and Turnover of RNA in the Early Stages of Hypertrophic Development[a]

	RNA content ($\mu g \cdot heart^{-1}$)	Incorporation of pyrimidine nucleotides into RNA ($nmol \cdot heart^{-1} \cdot hr^{-1}$)	Synthesis rate of uracil nucleotides ($nmol \cdot heart^{-1} \cdot hr^{-1}$)
Controls			
Heart weight (H.W.) = 650 mg	1,320	8	10
[RNA] = 2.04 mg $\cdot g^{-1}$			
Isoproterenol, 2 days			
H.W. × 1.18	1,870	33	44
[RNA] × 1.19			
Aortic stenosis, 3 days			
H.W. × 1.16	1,840	24	31
[RNA] × 1.19			

[a] All calculations were relative to a heart (ventricles) from a 250-g body weight rat. The increases of heart weight and RNA concentration during hypertrophy were taken into account. The amount of pyrimidine nucleotides (cytosine + uracil nucleotides) incorporated per hour into RNA were roughly calculated assuming that the time course increase in RNA concentration was linear and that the half-life of RNA was 5 days.

cleotides, which also feeds the cytidine nucleotide pool, plays a limiting role in the synthesis of RNA. The speed with which the synthesis of uracil nucleotides is raised in the initial phase of cardiac hypertrophy is a sign of the potential capacity of the myocardial cell to adapt its metabolism to physiopathological conditions.

In conclusion, it may be assumed that the synthesis of uracil nucleotides plays a limiting role in the synthesis of RNA in the heart. Additional experiments are now being undertaken in order to verify this hypothesis and to study a possible controlling role in the initiation of cardiac hypertrophy.

ACKNOWLEDGMENTS

This study was supported by grants from the Delegation Generale a la Recherche Scientifique et Technique (DGRST 77.7.1023 and 79.7.1001).

REFERENCES

1. Bartlett, G. R. 1959. Phosphorus assay in column chromatography. *J. Biol. Chem.* 234:466–468.
2. Buecher, T. 1947. Uber ein phosphatubertragendes Garungsferment. *Biochem. Biophys. Acta* 1:292–314.
3. Fanburg, B. L., Matsushita, S., and Raben M. S. 1973. Nucleic acid metabolism in cardiac hypertrophy. In: N. S. Dhalla (ed.), *Recent Advances in Studies on Cardiac Structure and Metabolism*. Vol. 3: *Myocardial Metabolism*, pp. 577–588. University Park Press, Baltimore.
4. Fleckenstein, A., Doring, H. G., and Leder, O. 1969. The significance of high-energy phosphate exhaustion in the etiology of isoproterenol-induced cardiac necrosis and its prevention by iproveratril, compound D 600 or prenylamine. In: M. Lamarche and R. Royer (eds.), *International Symposium on Drugs and Metabolism of Myocardium and Striated Muscle, Nancy, France,* pp. 11–12.
5. Fizel, A., and Fizelova, A. 1971. Cardiac hypertrophy and heart failure: Dynamics of change in high-energy phosphate compounds, glycogen and lactic acid. *J. Mol. Cell. Cardiol.* 2:187–192.
6. Furchgott, R. F., and De Gubareff, J. 1956. The determination of inorganic phosphate and creatine phosphate in tissue extract. *J. Biol. Chem.* 223:377–388.
7. Goldthwait, D. A. 1957. Mechanisms of synthesis of purine nucleotides in heart muscle extracts. *J. Clin. Invest.* 36:1572–1578.
8. Hattori, E., Yatsuki, K., Miyazaki, T., Sata, T., and Nakamura, M. 1969. Adenine nucleotides of myocardium from rats treated with isoproterenol and for Mg or K deficiency. *Jpn. Heart J.* 10:218–224.
9. Jaworek, D., Gruber, W., and Bergmeyer, H. U. 1974. Adenosine-5'-triphosphate. Determination with 3-phosphoglycerate kinase. *Methods Enzymat. Anal.* 4:2097–2101.
10. Kako, K. 1965. Biochemical changes in the rat myocardium induced by isoproterenol. *Can. J. Physiol. Pharmacol.* 43:541–549.
11. Keppler, D., Rudigier, J., and Decker, K. 1970. Enzymatic determination of uracil nucleotides in tissues. *Anal. Biochem.* 38:105–114.
12. Koide, T., and Rabinowitz, M. 1969. Biochemical correlates of cardiac hypertrophy. II: Increased rate of RNA synthesis in experimental cardiac hypertrophy in the rat. *Circ. Res.* 24:9–18.

13. Matsushita, S., and Fanburg, B. L. 1970. Pyrimidine nucleotide synthesis in the normal and hypertrophying heart. Relative importance of the de novo and salvage pathways. *Circ. Res.* 27:415–428.
14. Meerson, R. Z., and Pomoinitsky, V. D. 1972. The role of high-energy phosphate compounds in the development of cardiac hypertrophy. *J. Mol. Cell. Cardiol.* 4:571–598.
15. Munro, H. N., and Fleck, A. 1966. The determination of nucleic acids. *Methods Biochem. Anal.* 14:113–176.
16. Nair, G. K., Cutilletta, A. F., Zak, R., Koide, T., and Rabinowitz, M. 1968. Biochemical correlates of cardiac hypertrophy. I. Experimental model; changes in heart weight, RNA content, and nuclear RNA polymerase activity. *Circ. Res.* 23:451–462.
17. Olivares, J., Ray, A., Aussedat, J., Verdys, M., and Rossi, A. 1980. Increased myocardial pyrimidine nucleotide synthesis in isoproterenol-induced cardiac hypertrophy in rats. *Biochem. Biophys. Res. Commun.* 95:367–373.
18. Rossi, A. 1975. ^{32}P labelling of the nucleotides in α-position in the rabbit heart. *J. Mol. Cell. Cardiol.* 7:891–906.
19. Rossi, A. 1975. Incorporation of uridine by the perfused rabbit heart. *Life Sci.* 16:1121–1132.
20. Rossi, A., Mandel, P., and Dessaux, G. 1972. Cinetique de renouvellement du phosphate α des nucleotides libres dans le tissu myocardique de rat. *Arch. Int. Physiol. Biochem.* 80:59–77.
21. Rossi, A., Olivares, J., Aussedat, J., and Ray, A. 1979. Stimulation by isoproterenol of myocardial pyrimidine nucleotides synthesis in rats. *J. Mol. Cell. Cardiol.* 11:50.
22. Rossi, A., Olivares, J., Aussedat, J., and Ray, A. 1980. Increased uracil nucleotide metabolism during the induction of cardiac hypertrophy by β-stimulation in rats. *Basic Res. Cardiol.* 75:139–142.
23. Takenaka, F., and Higuchi, M. 1974. High-energy phosphate contents of subepicardium and subendocardium in the rat treated with isoproterenol and some other drugs. *J. Mol. Cell. Cardiol.* 6:123–135.
24. Wollenberger, A., Ristau, O., and Schoffa, G. 1960. Eine einfache Tecknik der extrem schnellen Abkuhlung grosserer Gewebstucke. *Pfluegers Arch.* 270:339–412.
25. Zimmer, H. G., and Gerlach, E. 1974. Effect of beta-adrenergic stimulation on myocardial adenine nucleotide metabolism. *Circ. Res.* 35:536–543.
26. Zimmer, H. G., and Gerlach, E. 1977. Studies on the regulation of the biosynthesis of myocardial adenine nucleotides. In: N. M. Muller, E. Kaiser, and J. E. Seegmiller (eds.), *Purine Metabolism in Man*, pp. 40–49. Plenum Press, New York.
27. Zimmer, H. G., Steinkopff, G., and Gerlach, E. 1972. Changes of protein synthesis in the hypertrophying rat heart. *Pfluegers Arch* 336:311–325.
28. Zimmer, H. G., Steinkopff, G., Ibel, H., and Koschine, H. 1980. Is the ATP decline a signal for stimulating protein synthesis in isoproterenol-induced cardiac hypertrophy? *J. Mol. Cell. Cardiol.* 12:421–426.

Increased Synthesis of the Phosphorylated Form of the Myosin Light Chains in Cardiac Hypertrophy in the Rat

B. Kwiatkowska-Patzer,* G. Prior, and R. Zak

Department of Medicine
University of Chicago
Chicago, Illinois 60637, USA

Abstract. The incorporation rate of [³H]leucine into cardiac myosin subunits was studied in rat hearts undergoing hypertrophy secondary to constriction of the ascending aorta. Cardiac myosin was prepared by a modified Shiverick's method on the second and fourth day after constriction. Myosin light chains were separated by urea and subjected to two-dimensional electrophoresis. Incorporation of [³H]leucine was determined in electrophoretically separated heavy and light chains by the method of Martin et al. (11). It was found that the incorporation rate of [³H]leucine into the phosphorylated form of the myosin light chain 2 is significantly increased in hypertrophic hearts as compared to sham animals.

In muscle, protein phosphorylation takes place both in the sarcoplasm and in the myofibrils. In 1972, Perrie et al. (17) discovered that the 18,000-dalton myosin light chain of rabbit skeletal muscle also undergoes phosphorylation. Phosphorylation of light chains in vitro has since been reported for myosin from skeletal (16), smooth (3,8,13), and cardiac muscle (12,20). Similar phosphorylation was described in myoblast myosin (21) and in nonmuscle myosin from platelets (1,2,10) and fibroblasts (15).

Much is known about protein kinase, the enzyme that catalyses the phosphorylation of myofibrillar proteins. This kinase may be activated by calcium (4,7,22,25) or by cyclic AMP (19). The myosin light chain kinase has been shown to be substrate specific (18). The enzyme dephosphorylating myosin has also been isolated from rabbit skeletal muscle (14).

The existence of the enzymes phosphorylating and dephosphorylating myosin light chains suggests a physiological role for these reactions. The efforts to find such a role were most successful for smooth muscle and nonmuscle myosin. Myosin phosphorylation has been found to increase ATPase activity in guinea pig vas deferens (6) and rat myoblasts (21). Phosphorylation of platelet myosin leads to an increase of actin-activated ATPase (1).

---

* Present address: Academy of Medicine, Warsaw, Poland.

Reddy and Wynborny (20) and Pemrick (16) recently reported an increase in actin-activated ATPase activity of phosphorylated myosin from skeletal and heart muscle. Moreover, it was suggested that myosin phosphorylation mediates calcium regulatory functions (6,9) and influences mechanochemical coupling (5).

The physiological role of myosin light chain phosphorylation in increasing the binding of cross bridges to actin filaments was also suggested (5).

MATERIALS AND METHODS

Sprague-Dawley female rats weighing 180–200 g were used for all experiments. Cardiac hypertrophy was induced by aortic constriction: tantalum clips were applied to the ascending aorta. Rats were sacrificed on the second and fourth days after aortic constriction. [³H]Leucine was injected into the tail vein 30 min before the sacrifice. Hearts were excised and homogenized in a Sorvall Omnimixer® at 14,000 rpm for 45 sec in Weber solution.

Myosin was extracted from muscle tissue with a high-ionic-strength solution. Purification was achieved by ammonium sulfate fractionation at 4°C in the presence of ATP and excess Mg^{2+} to dissociate actomyosin. The myosin fraction was then dissolved and dialyzed against a low-ionic-strength buffer to remove ammonium sulfate and reprecipitate the myosin. Heavy and light chains were separated using the Wikman-Coffelt method (26).

Myosin heavy chains were purified by phosphate disk electrophoresis. Myosin light chains were separated by our modification of two-dimensional electrophoresis (Figure 1). The first dimension was performed on a vertical polyacrylamide–urea slab gel (12% polyacrylamide, 8 M urea) using 20 mM

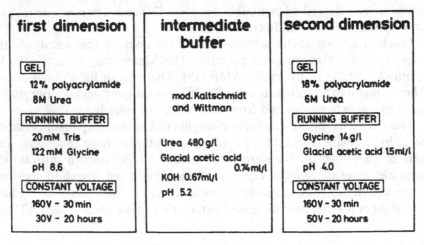

Figure 1.   Scheme of modified two-dimensional electrophoresis conditions.

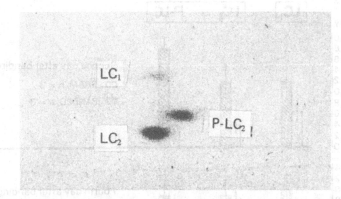

Figure 2.   Electrophoretic picture of myosin light chains after two-dimensional electrophoresis. LC$_1$, light chain 1; LC$_2$, light chain 2; P-LC$_2$, phosphorylated form of light chain 2.

Tris, 122 mM glycine running buffer, pH 8.6. Constant voltage (160 V) was used for 30 min, then 30 V for 20 hr. After the first dimension, the slab gel was placed into an intermediate buffer as modified by Kaltschmidt and Wittman (urea 480 g/liter, glacial acetic acid 0.74 ml/liter, KOH 0.67 ml/liter, pH 5.2).

A slice of the first-dimension gel was placed between two glass plates, and polyacrylamide gel with urea was poured over it. Gel for the second dimension contained 18% polyacrylamide and 6 M urea. The running buffer used for the second dimension contained glycine 14 g/liter, glacial acetic acid 1.5 ml/liter, pH 4.0. A voltage of 160 V for 30 min and 50 V for 20 hr was used (Figure 1). After electrophoresis, the proteins were visualized by staining with Coomassie brilliant blue R and destained electrophoretically. The light chains showed three spots for light chain 1, light chain 2, and the phosphorylated form of light chain 2, as indicated in Figure 2.

Subsequently, each spot was cut out and hydrolyzed in 6 N HCl at 110°C for 24 hr, and determination of specific radioactivity of [^{3}H]leucine was performed by the method of Martin et al. (11).

The presence of phosphate in the phosphorylated form of light chain 2 (P-LC-2) was proved in separate experiments by autoradiography following an injection of labeled ^{32}P-monosodium phosphate (48 hr prior to sacrifice of the animal). Cardiac myosin in these experiments was prepared in the presence of phosphatase inhibitors (iodoacetamide, sodium fluorate, and phosphate buffer) during homogenization.

Specific radioactivity of [^{3}H]leucine was measured in light and heavy chains and calculated as standard specific radioactivity for 100 g of rat body weight and for 100 μCi of injected [^{3}H]leucine.

Specific radioactivity of [^{3}H]leucine was also measured in heavy and light chains of cardiac myosin in sham-operated rats on the second and fourth day after the sham operation.

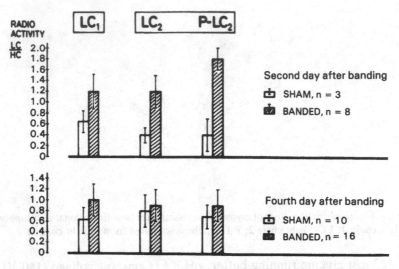

Figure 3.   Comparison of the turnover of myosin light chains on second and fourth days after aortic constriction. Results are expressed as a ratio of standard specific radioactivity (SSA) of light chain (LC) to standard specific radioactivity of heavy chain (SSA HC).

The results were expressed as a ratio of standard specific activity (SSA) of light chains (LC) to standard specific activity of heavy chains (SSA HC).

Materials used included L-[4,5-^{3}H]leucine (Amersham), [^{32}P]monosodium phosphate (New England Nuclear), acrylamide (Bio-Rad), bis-N,N-methylene-bis-acrylamide (Bio-Rad), and urea (Mallinkrodt).

RESULTS

As shown in Figure 3, we found that on the second day after aortic constriction the incorporation rate of [^{3}H]leucine into the phosphorylated form of myosin LC-2 was increased. The ratio of SSA P-LC-2 to SSA HC was 1.81 ± 0.20, whereas in sham-operated animals it amounted to 0.49 ± 0.13 ($P < 0.02$). In myosin LC-1, the leucine incorporation rate was also increased but much less: the ratio of SSA LC-1 to SSA HC was 1.2 ± 0.59 as compared to the control value of 0.64 ± 0.19. Similar results were obtained in LC-2: 1.02 ± 0.2 as compared to the control 0.38 ± 0.15.

On the fourth day after aortic constriction, the rate of [^{3}H]leucine incorporation, into all three light myosin subunits was only slightly increased.

DISCUSSION

These experiments strongly suggest that during the acute phase of cardiac hypertrophy the synthesis of the phosphorylated form of myosin LC-2 is significantly increased, much greater than that of other myosin subunits.

In our previous study, we showed that in hypertrophied heart during the period of rapid cardiac growth, the rate of [^{3}H]leucine incorporation into LC-2 separated in a phosphate electrophoretic system was significantly increased as compared to that from sham-operated animals (23, 27). In the present study, we managed to split LC-2 into the two subunits, and showed one of them to be a phosphorylated form of LC-2. By measuring the specific radioactivity of leucine, we found that the phosphorylated form of LC-2 is mainly responsible for the increase of leucine incorporation into LC-2.

REFERENCES

1. Adelstein, R. S., and Conti, M. A. 1975. Phosphorylation of platelet myosin increases actin-activated myosin ATP-ase activity. *Nature* 256:597–598.
2. Adelstein, R. S., Conti, M. A., and Anderson, W., Jr. 1973. Phosphorylation of human platelet myosin. *Proc. Natl. Acad. Sci. U.S.A.* 70:3115–3119.
3. Adelstein, R. S., Conti, M. A., and Hathaway, D. R. 1978. Phosphorylation of smooth muscle myosin light chain kinase by the catalytic subunit of adenosine 3'5'-monophosphate-dependent protein kinase. *J. Biol. Chem.* 253:8347–8350.
4. Aksoy, M. O., Williams, D., Sharkey, E. M., and Hathshorne, D. J. 1976. A relationhsip between Ca sensitivity and phosphorylation of gizzard actomyosin. *Biochem. Biophys. Res. Commun.* 69:35–41.
5. Barany, M., and Barany, K. 1980. Phosphorylation of the myofibrillar proteins. *Annu. Rev. Physiol.* 42:275–292.
6. Chacko, S., Conti, M. A., and Adelstein, R. S. 1977. Effect of phosphorylation of smooth muscle myosin on actin activation and Ca regulation. *Proc. Natl. Acad. Sci. U.S.A.* 74:129–133.
7. DiSalvo, J., Gruenstein, E., and Silver, P. 1978. Ca dependent phosphorylation of bovine aortic actomyosin. *Proc. Soc. Exp. Biol. Med.* 158:410–414.
8. Frearson, N., Focant, B. W. W., and Perry, S. V. 1976. Phosphorylation of a light chain component of myosin from smooth muscle. *FEBS Lett.* 63:27–32.
9. Hitara, M., Mikawa, T., Nonomura, Y., and Ebashi, S. 1977. Ca regulation in vascular smooth muscle. *J. Biochem. (Tokyo)* 82:1793–1796.
10. Lebowitz, E. A., and Cooke, R. 1978. Contractile properties of actomyosin from human blood platelets. *J. Biol. Chem.* 253:5443–5447.
11. Martin, A. F., Prior, G., and Zak, R. 1976. Determination of specific radioactivity of amino acids in proteins directly on polyacrylamide gels: An application to *l*-leucine. *Anal. Biochem.* 72:577–585.
12. McPherson, J., Fenner, C., Smith, A., Mason, D. T., and Wikman-Coffelt, J. 1974. Identification of in vivo phosphorylated myosin subunit. *FEBS Lett.* 47:149–154.
13. Mikawa, T., Nonmura, Y., and Ebashi, S. 1977. Does phosphorylation of myosin light chain have direct relation to regulation in smooth muscle? *J. Biochem. (Tokyo)* 82:1789–1796.
14. Morgan, M., Perry, S. V., and Ottawy, J. 1976. Myosin light chain phosphatase. *Biochem. J.* 157:687–697.
15. Muhlrad, A., and Oplatka A. 1977. Phosphorylation of fibroblast myosin. *FEBS Lett.* 77:37–40.
16. Pemrick, S. 1978. Phosphorylation of skeletal myosin enhances interaction with actin. *Circulation* 58(2):73.
17. Perrie, S. V., Smillie, L. B., and Perry, S. V. 1972. A phosphorylated light-chain component of myosin. *Biochem. J.* 128:105–106P.
18. Pires, E. M. V., and Perry, S. V. 1977. Purification and properties of myosin light chain kinase from fast skeletal muscle. *Biochem. J.* 167:137–146.

19. Reddy, Y. S., Pitts, B. J. R., and Schwartz, A. 1977. Cyclic AMP-dependent and independent protein kinase phosphorylation of canine cardiac myosin light chains. *J. Mol. Cell. Cardiol.* 9:501–513.
20. Reddy, Y. S., and Wyborny, L. E. 1978. Phosphorylation and ATPase activity of cardiac and skeletal myosins. *Physiologist* 21:97.
21. Scordilis, S. P., and Adelstein, R. S. 1977. Myoblast myosin phosphorylation is a prerequisite for actin-activation. *Nature* 268:558–560.
22. Sherry, J. M. P., Gorecka, A., Aksoy, M. O., Dabrowska, R., and Hartshorne, D. J. 1978. Roles of calcium and phosphorylation in the regulation of the activity of gizzard myosin. *Biochemistry* 17:4411–4418.
23. Sims, J. M., Patzer, B., Kumudavalli-Reddy, M., Martin, A. F., Rabinowitz, M., and Zak, R. 1978. The pathways of protein synthesis and degradation in normal heart and during development and regression of cardiac hypertrophy. In: T. Kobayashi, Y. Ito, and G. Rona (eds.), *Recent Advances in Studies on Cardiac Structure and Metabolism.* Vol. 12: *Cardiac Adaptation*, pp. 19–28. University Park Press, Baltimore.
24. Small, J. V., and Sobieszek, A. 1977. Ca-regulation of mammalian smooth muscle actomyosin via a kinase–phosphatase-dependent phosphorylation and dephosphorylation of the 20,000 Mr light chain of myosin. *Eur. J. Biochem.* 76:521–530.
25. Sobieszek, A. 1977. Ca-linked phosphorylation of light chain of vertebrate smooth-muscle myosin. *Eur. J. Biochem.* 73:477–483.
26. Wikman-Coffelt, J., Zelis, H., Fenner, C., and Mason, D. T., 1973. Studies on the synthesis and degradation of light and heavy chains of cardiac myosin. *J. Biol. Chem.* 248:5206–5207.
27. Zak, R. 1977. Metabolism of myofibrillar proteins in the normal and hypertrophic heart. *Basic Res. Cardiol.* 72:235–240.

Reconstitution of Heavy Chain and Light Chain 1 in Cardiac Subfragment-1 from Hyperthyroid and Euthyroid Rabbit Hearts

S. Ueda, K. Yamaoki, R. Nagai, and Y. Yazaki

Cardiovascular Research Unit
The Third Department of Internal Medicine
Faculty of Medicine
University of Tokyo
Tokyo 113, Japan

Abstract. It is now established that cardiac myosin from hyperthyroid rabbit hearts (TXM) exhibits high Ca^{2+} ATPase activity. The high Ca^{2+} ATPase activity of TXM was completely retained in cardiac myosin subfragment-1 (S-1) (1.33 ± 0.04 μmol Pi/mg per min; euthyroid, 0.51 ± 0.04). Cardiac S-1 from hyperthyroid and euthyroid rabbits (TXS-1 and NS-1) had the same pattern in SDS-polyacrylamide gel electrophoresis. The possible influence of heavy and light chains of TXM on increasing the ATPase activity was examined by reconstitution in the S-1 preparation. Crosswise reconstitution was performed using cardiac S-1 heavy chain (90,000 daltons) and light chain 1 (LC1) (27,000 daltons) from hyperthyroid and euthyroid hearts. Reconstitution was verified by using radiolabeled LC1. More than 95% of S-1 was recovered with full ATPase activity. When TXS-1 was reconstituted with LC1 from euthyroid hearts, the reconstituted molecule retained high ATPase activity. On the other hand, NS-1 reconstituted with LC1 from hyperthyroid hearts failed to increase the ATPase activity. The ATPase activity of S-1 was determined by the source of the heavy chain. These results suggest that the high Ca^{2+} ATPase activity of cardiac myosin and S-1 from hyperthyroid animals arises from the molecular alteration of the heavy chain induced by thyroxine administration.

It has been established that the administration of thyroid hormone elevates the ATPase activity of cardiac myosin (3,4,6,7,9,12). Several investigators have recently reported alterations in the myosin molecule (2,5), especially the heavy chain molecule, from hyperthyroid animal hearts. In this study, to clarify whether the heavy chain or light chain 1 determines the elevation of Ca^{2+} ATPase activity in hyperthyroid myosin, we have modified the reconstitution technique using solublized myosin subfragment-1 originally described by Wagner and Weeds (10) and applied it to subunits of this new cardiac myosin isozyme.

MATERIALS AND METHODS

Preparation of Cardiac Myosin, Subfragment-1, and Light Chain 1

Male albino rabbits (2.5 to 2.8 kg) were given daily injections of L-thyroxine (300 μg/kg) for 14 days. Rabbits were killed by a sharp blow, and the hearts were excised immediately. Cardiac myosin was purified according to our modified dilution technique, using DEAE-Sephadex A25 (12). Myosin subfragment-1 (S-1) was prepared by chymotryptic digestion of purified myosin, as described previously (10). Digestion was carried out for 10 min at 25°C in 0.12 M sodium chloride (pH 7.0). After centrifugation, the supernatant was applied to a Whatman DEAE-cellulose column. Cardiac light chain 1 (27,000 daltons) and light chain 2 (20,000 daltons) were dissociated from purified myosin with 5.0 M guanidine HCl (pH 8.0). After centrifugation, the supernatant was applied to a Whatman DEAE-cellulose column equilibrated with 50 mM potassium phosphate (pH 6.0). The early fractions of the single peak eluted with the ionic gradient (0.05 to 0.3 M potassium phosphate) were pooled as light chain 1.

Reconstitution of S-1

The subunits of S-1 (heavy chain, 90,000 daltons, and light chain 1, 27,000 daltons) were crosswisely reconstituted between euthyroid and hyperthyroid S-1. Tenfold (molar) purified light chain 1 (200 μM) was added to S-1 (20 μM) in a reaction mixture of 0.1 M imidazole HCl (pH 7.0) and 4.7 M ammonium chloride. After being stirred for 20 min at 4°C, the mixture was dialyzed against 50 mM imidazole HCl (pH 7.0) and 0.1 mM dithiothreitol. Reconstituted S-1 and free excess light chain 1 were separated on Sephadex S-200 equilibrated in the same buffer.

Determination of ATPase Activity of Myosin and S-1

The Ca^{2+} ATPase activity of myosin and S-1 was assayed in a medium containing 10 mM $CaCl_2$, 5 mM ATP, and 0.05 M Tris HCl (pH 7.5), and the K^+–EDTA ATPase activity of myosin and S-1 was assayed in a medium containing 0.6 M KCl, 1 mM EDTA, 5 mM ATP, and 0.05 M Tris HCl (pH 7.5), as described previously (12). The assays were run for 5 min at pH 7.5 and 25°C. The amount of Pi liberated was measured by the method of Fiske and SubbaRow (1). The Ca^{2+} ATPase activity of S-1 after thiol modification with N-ethylmaleimide was assayed in a medium containing 10 mM $CaCl_2$, 0.6 M KCl, 5 mM ATP, and 0.05 M Tris HCl (pH 7.5). Electrophoresis of myosin, S-1, and light chain 1 was performed with 7.5% SDS-polyacrylamide gels prepared according to Weber and Osborn (11). Protein was determined by the method of Lowry et al. (8).

RESULTS

SDS-polyacrylamide gel electrophoresis of cardiac S-1 showed three prominant bands. Comparison of the electrophoretic mobilities with proteins of known molecular weights gave values of 90,000, 75,000 and 25,000, re-

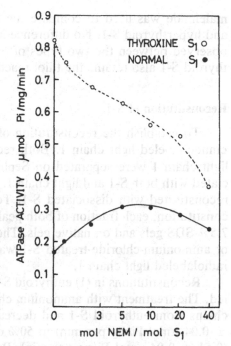

Figure 1. Effects of N-ethylmaleimide on ATPase activity of NS-1 (●) and TXS-1 (○). Subfragment-1 was incubated with N-ethylmaleimide in ratios indicated on the abscissa and described in the text. After removal of excess N-ethylmaleimide, ATPase activity was determined in the presence of 10 mM $CaCl_2$ and 0.6 M KCl.

spectively. The light chain 1 molecule was degraded by chymotryptic digestion, and light chain 2 completely disappeared. Light chain 1 separated from myosin was purified as a protein of 27,000 daltons. There was no difference between euthyroid and hyperthyroid myosin, S-1, or light chain 1, respectively, in SDS-polyacrylamide electrophoretic patterns.

ATPase Activities of Hyperthyroid S-1

The Ca^{2+} ATPase activity of hyperthyroid S-1 (1.33 ± 0.04 μmol Pi/ mg per min) was 2.2 times that of euthyroid S-1 (0.51 ± 0.04 μmol Pi/mg per min). The K^+–EDTA ATPase activity of S-1 did not differ between euthyroid and hyperthyroid hearts. The high level of Ca^{2+} ATPase activity of hyperthyroid myosin was completely retained in hyperthyroid S-1.

Titration with N-Ethylmaleimide

The Ca^{2+} ATPase of S-1 was assayed in high-molar potassium chloride as described in Materials and Methods (Figure 1). The Ca^{2+} ATPase activity of euthyroid S-1 was enhanced after thiol modification at a low concentration of N-ethylmaleimide and decreased above 9.0 mol N-ethylmaleimide per mol S-1. In contrast, the Ca^{2+} ATPase of hyperthyroid S-1 was no longer enhanced with thiol modification. To determine whether the lack of activation was caused by a difference in thiol modification rate, [^{14}C]-N-ethylmaleimide was used to compare the modification rate between euthyroid and hyperthyroid S-1. No difference in percent uptake of radioactivity was observed between the two types of S-1. These findings reveal that hyperthyroid S-1 also retains the thiol reaction specific for parent myosin.

Reconstitution of S-1

To establish the reconstitution of S-1, we used the $[^{14}C]$-N-ethylmaleimide-labeled light chain 1. Both reconstituted S-1 and free radiolabeled light chain 1 were separated on Sephadex S-200. Radioactivity was associated with both S-1 and light chain 1. About 6% of added light chain 1 was reconstituted with dissociated S-1. To further verify the formation of reconstitution, each fraction of both peaks was separately electrophoresed on 7.5% SDS gels and on native gels. These findings indicated that about 50% of ammonium-chloride-treated S-1 was certainly reconstituted with added radiolabeled light chain 1.

Reconstitutions in (1) euthyroid S-1 and (2) hyperthyroid S-1 were studied. The treatment with ammonium chloride dissociated about 50% of light chains from euthyroid S-1 and decreased the Ca^{2+} ATPase activity (0.26 $\pm$ 0.04 μmol Pi/mg per min) to 50% of the control value before treatment (0.51 $\pm$ 0.04 μmol Pi/mg per min). By addition of tenfold (molar) purified euthyroid light chain 1, the ATPase activity of ammonium-chloride-treated euthyroid S-1 was restored to 94% of the control value (0.48 $\pm$ 0.04 μmol Pi/mg per min). Addition of the same amount of hyperthyroid light chain 1 increased the Ca^{2+} ATPase activity of ammonium-chloride-treated euthyroid S-1 to a similar degree (0.47 $\pm$ 0.03 μmol Pi/mg per min). In the case of hyperthyroid S-1, the recovery of the Ca^{2+} ATPase activity (1.33 $\pm$ 0.05 μmol Pi/mg per min before treatment and 0.71 $\pm$ 0.04 μmol Pi/mg per min after treatment) was also obtained to a same extent after reconstitution with either euthyroid (1.26 $\pm$ 0.04 μmol Pi/mg per min) or hyperthyroid light chain 1 (1.25 $\pm$ 0.04 μmol Pi/mg per min). The reconstituted hyperthyroid S-1 showed higher ATPase activity than did the euthyroid S-1.

DISCUSSION

Hyperthyroid S-1 retains the increased Ca^{2+} ATPase activity, and specific thiol residues of the double-headed myosin molecule from hyperthyroid rabbit hearts. Since the light chain 2 molecule is removed by chymotryptic cleavage from S-1, it is not essential for the elevation of myosin Ca^{2+} ATPase activity. Crosswise reconstitution of the subunits between hyperthyroid and euthyroid S-1 has made it clear that the enzymatic alteration of hyperthyroid S-1 is mainly a result of the functional alteration of the heavy chain but not of light chain 1. Flink and his co-workers (2) have recently found that a structural alteration of the heavy chain molecule of cardiac myosin occurs in hyperthyroidism. Hoh and his co-workers (5) have also found that rat ventricular myosin consists of three myosin isozymes. These findings and our results reveal that the structural alterations of the heavy chains may be related to the elevation of Ca^{2+} ATPase activity in the hyperthyroid myosin. This suggests that thyroid hormone induces the synthesis of a new heavy chain consisting of a cardiac myosin isozyme in the rabbit.

REFERENCES

1. Fiske, C. H., and SubbaRow, Y. 1925. Colorimetric determination of phosphorus. *J. Biol. Chem.* 66:375–400.
2. Flink, I. L., Rader, J. H., and Morkin, E. 1979. Thyroid hormone stimulates synthesis of a cardiac myosin isozyme. Comparison of the two dimensional electrophoretic patterns of the cyanogen bromide peptides of cardiac myosin heavy chains from euthyroid and thyrotoxic rabbits. *J. Biol. Chem.* 245:3105–3110.
3. Goodkind, M. J., Dambach, G. E., Thyrum, P. T., and Luchi, R. J. 1974. Effects of thyroxine on ventricular myocardial contractility and ATPase activity in guinea pigs. *Am. J. Physiol.* 226:66–72.
4. Hjalmarson, A. C., Whitefield, C. H., and Mogan, H. E. 1970. Hormone control of heart function and myosin ATPase activity. *Biochim. Biophys. Res. Commun.* 41:1548–1589.
5. Hoh, J. F. Y., McGrath, P. A., and Hale, P. T. 1978. Electrophoretic analysis of multiple forms of rat cardiac myosin: Effects of hypophysectomy and thyroxine replacement. *J. Mol. Cell Cardiol.* 10:1053–1076.
6. Katagiri, T., Freedberg, A. S., and Morkin, E. 1974. Effects of N-ethylmaleimide on the ATPase activities of cardiac myosin from thyrotoxic rabbits. *Life Sci.* 16:1079–1087.
7. Kuczynski, S. F. 1973. *Quantitative and Qualitative Characterizations of Cardiac Actomyosin in Thyroxine-Induced Hypertrophy.* Ph. D. Thesis, New York Medical College, New York.
8. Lowry, O. M., Rosebrough, N. J., Farr, A. L., and Randall, R. J. 1951. Protein measurement with the Folin phenol reagent. *J. Biol. Chem.* 193:265–275.
9. Thyrum, P. T., Kritcher, E. M., and Luchi, R. J. 1970. Effect of L-thyroxine on the primary structure of cardiac myosin. *Biochim. Biophys. Acta* 197:335–336.
10. Wagner, P. D., and Weeds, A. 1977. Studies on the role of myosin alkali light chains. Recombination and hybridization of light chains and heavy chains in subfragment-1 preparations. *J. Mol. Biol.* 109:455–473.
11. Weber, K., and Osborn, M. 1969. The reliability of molecular weight determinations by dodecyl sulfate–polyacrylamide gel electrophoresis. *J. Biol. Chem.* 244:4406–4412.
12. Yazaki, Y., and Raben, M. S. 1975. Effect of the thyroid state on the enzymatic characteristics of cardiac myosin. A difference in behavior of rat and rabbit cardiac myosin. *Circ. Res.* 36:208–215.

Mechanisms of Degradation of Myofibrillar and Nonmyofibrillar Protein in Heart

J. M. Ord, J. R. Wakeland, J. S. Crie, and K. Wildenthal

Pauline and Adolph Weinberger Laboratory for Cardiopulmonary Research
Departments of Physiology and Internal Medicine
The University of Texas Health Science Center at Dallas,
Dallas, Texas 75235, USA

Abstract. The degradation of cardiac proteins is known to be altered by many physiological and pathological interventions, but the precise intracellular processes that regulate proteolysis and the relative roles of different proteolytic pathways in degrading different classes of protein remain poorly understood. Agents that interfere with lysosomal function produce major decreases in total protein breakdown; thus, lysosomes and lysosomal proteinases seem to be important in proteolysis. However, these same agents cause no change in the degradation of myofibrillar proteins, suggesting that this class of proteins is not dependent on lysosomal pathways for its turnover.

Although it is well known that cardiac protein degradation is susceptible to modification by many physiological and pathological interventions, the mechanisms by which this regulation occurs remain obscure. Also, it has not been clear if the pathways and regulation of degradation are the same for all proteins or, instead, if separate and distinct processes are involved in the breakdown of different types of proteins. Accordingly, the experiments described in this chapter were undertaken in an effort to provide information about the cellular mechanisms that might be involved in regulating cardiac proteolysis. In these early studies, emphasis was placed on analyzing the importance of lysosomal processes in degrading different classes of proteins, specifically, myofibrillar versus nonmyofibrillar proteins.

METHODS

Studies were made using fetal mouse hearts in organ culture (11). This preparation offers the advantage of long-term stability of metabolic function combined with precise control of experimental conditions. Cultured hearts of matched littermates were labeled with radioactive phenylalanine as described previously (14) and then maintained for 24 hr in control medium or medium supplemented with insulin (50 µg/ml), leupeptin (50 µg/ml), or chloroquine (0.1 mM) before being analyzed for rates of proteolysis. The rate of degradation of total protein was measured from the rate of release of radioactive phenylalanine from prelabeled TCA-precipitable protein (14). For experiments involving separate subclasses of protein, the "myofibrillar" pool was identified as those proteins that were located in the 1000 g precipitate following homogenization in a low-ionic-strength solution (16 mM NaH$_2$PO$_4$ plus 4 mM KH$_2$PO$_4$, pH 7.3) and were subsequently solubilized by rehomogenization in 0.6 M KCl plus 0.1% Triton X-100 (6); the rate of loss of labeled phenylalanine from this pool was used as an index of myofibrillar protein turnover. The proteins in this pool were further identified by SDS gel electrophoresis and found to be contaminated by ~15% with proteins that did not migrate with known myofibrillar proteins; the degree of contamination was the same in control and experimental hearts, however, suggesting that the behavior of the pool would be primarily a reflection of the turnover of mixed myofibrillar proteins. Differences were analyzed by Student's t-test for paired observations

RESULTS

The effect of insulin was similar on total protein and myofibrillar protein degradation (Table 1). Thus, insulin inhibited total proteolysis by 15% while reducing the breakdown of the myofibrillar protein pool by 14% in the same hearts ($P < 0.01$ for both).

In contrast, leupeptin had a much greater effect on the degradation of total protein than on that of the myofibrillar pool alone (Table 2). It reduced total proteolysis by 18% in these experiments ($P < 0.01$) but had no significant effect on the breakdown of myofibrillar proteins.

Like leupeptin, the lysosomotropic agent chloroquine produced different effects on the breakdown of myofibrillar protein than on that of the total protein pool (Table 3). Thus, interference with lysosomal function by chloroquine was accompanied by a 35% inhibition of total protein breakdown

Table 1.   Effect of Insulin on the Degradation of Total Protein and Myofibrillar Protein of Mouse Hearts in Organ Culture[a]

	Total protein (% degradation per day ± S.E.M.)	Myofibrillar protein (% degradation per day ± S.E.M.)
A. Control	42.9 ± 1.14	52.1 ± 2.35
B. Insulin	36.4 ± 1.31	45.1 ± 2.74
Difference (B − A)	−6.5 ± 1.11	−7.0 ± 1.83
% Difference (B − A)/A	−15%	−14%
P	<0.01	<0.01

[a] Values represent the average of matched hearts from 16 litters.

Table 2.   Effect of Leupeptin on the Degradation of Total Protein and Myofibrillar Protein of Mouse Hearts in Organ Culture[a]

	Total protein (% degradation per day ± S.E.M.)	Myofibrillar protein (% degradation per day ± S.E.M.)
A. Control	41.6 ± 0.91	52.1 ± 1.51
B. Leupeptin	34.4 ± 1.52	50.6 ± 1.45
Difference (B − A)	−7.2 ± 1.58	−1.5 ± 0.98
% Difference (B − A)/A	−18%	−3%
P	<0.01	>0.10

[a] Values represent the average of matched hearts from 16 litters.

($P < 0.01$), but there was no change in the degradation of the myofibrillar protein pool.

DISCUSSION

Chloroquine interferes with lysosomal proteolysis in many tissues including heart, apparently because it is concentrated within lysosomes and raises intralysosomal pH above the optimum of most lysosomal proteinases, and also because it directly inhibits lysosomal cathepsin B activity (10,15). Leupeptin deceases proteolytic capacity by inhibiting certain endogenous proteinases, especially those of the thiol class; along with some nonlysosomal proteinases, several important lysosomal enzymes (e.g., cathepsins B, H, and L) are inhibited by the agent (1). As in other tissues (2), inhibition of these enzymes in heart decreases the rate of total protein degradation (4,9,12).

Although the actions of chloroquine and leupeptin clearly include production of major defects in lysosomal proteolytic capacity, it remains possible that some of their effects might not be mediated via lysosomal processes. For example, chloroquine in large concentrations can also produce

Table 3.   Effect of Chloroquine on the Degradation of Total Protein and Myofibrillar Protein of Mouse Hearts in Organ Culture[a]

	Total protein (% degradation per day ± S.E.M.)	Myofibrillar protein (% degradation per day ± S.E.M.)
A. Control	43.7 ± 0.95	53.9 ± 1.52
B. Chloroquine	29.3 ± 1.24	54.6 ± 1.39
Difference (B − A)	−15.4 ± 0.97	+0.7 ± 1.43
% Difference (B − A)/A	−35%	+1%
P	<0.01	>0.10

[a] Values represent the average of matched hearts from 27 litters.

some nonspecific toxic effects on other organelles including mitochondria (8); leupeptin, although remarkable free of nonspecific toxicity (4), does inhibit some nonlysosomal proteinases that are thought to be of importance in heart. Thus, if chloroquine and leupeptin had been found to reduce myofibrillar protein degradation, one could not have concluded with absolute certainty that myofibrillar proteins are indeed broken down within lysosomes. On the other hand, the absence of any inhibitory effect of these agents on the rate of myofibrillar protein degradation implies strongly that the normal degradation of this molecule is accomplished via nonlysosomal mechanisms. These results also imply that none of the other proteinases that leupeptin is known to inhibit are of quantitative importance in degrading myofibrillar proteins.

It remains possible, of course, that after the initial steps of breakdown of myofibrillar proteins, their soluble subfragments could still be degraded within lysosomes. Nevertheless, it seems likely that the critical step in the degradation of the intact myofibrillar protein molecules themselves is not a lysosomal event.

To see if myofibrillar protein degradation is also immune to the action of other agents that are known to inhibit cardiac proteolysis, we tested the effect of insulin. Insulin inhibited the degradation of the myofibrillar pool to the same extent as that of total protein, thus indicating that the breakdown of this pool is indeed subject to physiological regulation. It has often been suggested that insulin's inhibition of proteolysis in heart and other tissues might be the result of its effect on lysosomes (5,7,13,14). In view of the differences observed in the present study between the inhibitory effects on myofibrillar protein degradation of insulin and of agents that are known to act primarily on lysosomes and lysosomal enzymes, it seems likely that insulin possesses important extralysosomal actions in addition to its putative lysosomal effects.

Finally, it should be noted that the isolation of the broad class of myofibrillar proteins by solubility characteristics serves as a rather crude screening procedure. It is therefore reassuring that in a separate set of experiments, in which a modified method of Hoh et al. (3) was used to separate intact myosin quantitatively and the rate of degradation of myosin was measured, results similar to those reported here for the total myofibrillar protein pool were obtained. Thus, in those experiments, interference with lysosomal proteolysis by chloroquine and leupeptin caused decreases of 25% or more in total protein degradation, but neither agent caused any reduction in the rate of degradation of myosin (16).

In summary, lysosomes are of importance in the normal degradation of cardiac protein. However, different types of cardiac proteins apparently are broken down through different mechanisms, and the degradation of myofibrillar proteins seems to be regulated solely by nonlysosomal mechanisms.

ACKNOWLEDGMENTS

This work was supported by the Moss Heart Fund and the National Institutes of Health (HL-14706 and HL-17669).

REFERENCES

1. Barrett, A. J. 1980. The many forms and functions of cellular proteinases. *Fed. Proc.* 39:9–14.
2. Dean, R. T. 1980. Regulation and mechanisms of degradation of endogenous proteins by mammalian cells: General considerations. In: K. Wildenthal (ed.), *Degradative Processes in Heart and Skeletal Muscle*, 3rd ed., pp. 3–30. North-Holland, Amsterdam.
3. Hoh, J. F. Y., McGrath, P. A., and Hale, P. T. 1978. Electrophoretic analysis of multiple forms of rat cardiac myosin: Effects of hypophysectomy and thyroxine replacement. *J. Mol. Cell. Cardiol.* 10:1053–1076.
4. Libby, P., Ingwall, J. S., and Goldberg, A. L. 1979. Reduction of protein degradation and atrophy in cultured fetal mouse hearts by leupeptin. *Am. J. Physiol.* 237:E35–E39.
5. Mortimore, G. E., and Ward, W. F. 1976. Behavior of the lysosomal system during organ perfusion. An inquiry into the mechanism of hepatic proteolysis. In: J. T. Dingle and R. T. Dean (eds.), *Lysosomes in Biology and Pathology*, Vol. 5, pp. 157–184. North-Holland, Amsterdam.
6. Ord, J. M. 1980. *The Effects of Various Hormones and Selective Inhibitors in the Turnover of Subclasses of Cardiac Protein.* Ph.D. Thesis, University of Texas Health Science Center at Dallas, Dallas.
7. Rannels, D. E., Kao, R., and Morgan, H. E. 1975. Effect of insulin on protein turnover in heart muscle. *J. Biol. Chem.* 250:1694–1701.
8. Ridout, R. M., Decker, R. S., and Wildenthal, K. 1978. Chloroquine-induced lysosomal abnormalities in cultured foetal mouse hearts. *J. Mol. Cell. Cardiol.* 10:175–183.
9. Ward, W. F., Chua, B. L., Li, J. B., Morgan, H. E., and Mortimore, G. E. 1979. Inhibition of basal and deprivation-induced proteolysis by leupeptin and pepstatin in perfused rat liver and heart. *Biochem. Biophys. Res. Commun.* 87:92–98.
10. Wibo, M., and Poole, B. 1974. Protein degradation in cultured cells. II. The uptake of chloroquine by rat fibroblasts and the inhibition of cellular protein degradation and cathepsin B_1. *J. Cell. Biol.* 63:430–440.
11. Wildenthal, K. 1971. Long-term maintenance of spontaneously beating mouse hearts in organ culture. *J. Appl. Physiol.* 30:153–157.
12. Wildenthal, K., and Crie, J. S. 1980. The role of lysosomes and lysosomal enzymes in cardiac protein turnover. *Fed. Proc.* 39:37–41.
13. Wildenthal, K., and Crie, J. S. 1980. Lysosomes and cardiac protein catabolism. In: K. Wildenthal (ed.) *Degradative Processes in Heart and Skeletal Muscle*, 3rd ed., pp. 113–129. North-Holland, Amsterdam.
14. Wildenthal, K., Griffin, E. E., and Ingwall, J. S. 1976. Hormonal control of cardiac protein and amino acid balance. *Circ. Res.* 38(Suppl. 1):138–144.
15. Wildenthal, K., Wakeland, J. R., Morton, P. C., and Griffin, E. E. 1978. Inhibition of protein degradation in mouse hearts by agents that cause lysosomal dysfunction. *Circ. Res.* 42:787–792.
16. Wildenthal, K., Wakeland, J. R., Ord, J. M., and Stull, J. T. 1980. Interference with lysosomal proteolysis fails to reduce cardiac myosin degradation. *Biochem. Biophys. Res. Commun.* 96:793–798.

Vasoactive Peptides and Regulation of Hemodynamics in Different Functional States of the Organism

A. M. Chernukh and O. A. Gomazkov

Institute of General Pathology and Pathological Physiology
Academy of Medical Sciences of the USSR
Moscow, USSR

Abstract. It is important to emphasize that the biochemical systems participating in humoral hemodynamic regulation may function at any level of the circulatory homeostasis: in the blood as a biological fluid constantly circulating along the vessels, at the microcirculatory bed where the exchange with tissues is realized, on the tonic activity of the resistive and capacitance vessels, defining the systemic blood pressure rate and organ redistribution, or, finally, on the main motive force of the blood, the heart. The interrelations of some molecular factors form the biochemical basis for the interaction of the main humoral systems. These factors are kallikrein for kinins and converting enzyme for the renin–angiotensin system, 9-ketoreductase and phospholipase for kinin and prostaglandin systems, and Hageman factors for coagulation, fibrinolysis, and kininogenesis systems. This main scheme includes "functional" connections, which are defined by a physiological interaction, and those between the central and peripheral nervous systems. We may, evidently, postulate an important biological regularity of a multifunctional participation of the same physiologically active factors in maintaining circulatory homeostasis. On the other hand, we have to emphasize the functional unity and joint correlating actions of different biochemical blood systems.

The development of an organism, its existence in a changeable environment, and its adaptation to physiological loads and pathological factors are defined by the coordinated activity of a variety of the regulatory mechanisms and regulated processes. The integrative and differentiating functional regulation at the level of the whole organism, organs, cell–tissue microsystems, and separate cell organelles is realized by a complicated combination of chemical factors formed in the process of evolution for specific roles in the organism's neurohumoral regulation. With the appearance and development of a pathological process, the activity of the complex system of neurohumoral regulation assumes specific features. In these cases, the disturbed and unregulated activity of physiological and biochemical systems may contribute to the progress of the disease.

To specify the basis of our work, we should like to define a "chemical regulator" as a substance that has quite specific biochemical and physiological peculiarities. In contrast to nonspecific chemical regulation by metabolites (e.g., oxygen and energetic metabolite transport, synthesis of nucleic acids and protein), which is directed, in principle, to all accessible organs and tissues, the physiological factors are addressed selectively. Neurotransmitters, vasoactive peptides, bioamines, prostaglandins (PG), and other factors are related to such substances. A main function of these substances is to transmit special information at the level of cells and the cell–tissue system; however, they are not involved directly in its response.

The presence of physiologically active substances (PAS) in organs, tissues, and individual cells is practically universal.

The following examples of PAS are of direct relevance to problems of interest to cardiologists: (1) molecular complexes circulating in the blood and able to be converted into an active form—kinins and angiotensins in blood plasma and serotonin and thromboxanes in platelets; (2) substances providing neural regulation of the heart and vessels and which are present in the terminals innervating practically all parts of the vascular bed; (3) general release of histamine—one of the more important regulators of vascular wall permeability—in tissues containing mast and some other cells; (4) localization of compounds able to synthetize PGs and cyclic nucleotides in membranes and intracellular organelles as well as myocardial and vascular cells. Thus, various regulatory mechanisms control practically all systems in the organism by means of PAS at all levels of integration.

It should be noted that the chemical origin of the regulatory substances may be quite different, from very simple organic compounds derived from the bioamine structure to complicated polymolecular substances such as peptides. Among the latter, "vasoactive polypeptides" are of greatest interest because of their importance in the regulation of different types of heart and vascular activity.

Our work has centered on two PAS groups: the kallikrein–kinin and renin–angiotensin blood systems. Being closely associated by biochemical factors and interrelating functionally, these two regulatory systems are of great importance for heart and vascular activity in various situations and in adaptation to changing environmental factors and in extreme situations. Finally, these systems play a major role in the pathogenesis of such diseases as myocardial infarction, hypertension, and shocks. We would like to underline the participation of these systems in the regulation of the blood circulation at different levels: blood as a biological system, microcirculation and function of the exchange vessels, vessel tonus, defining the features of regional blood flow, and, not least, in the function of the heart itself.

VASOACTIVE POLYPEPTIDES AND HEMOVASCULAR REGULATION

In 1949, Rocha e Silva et al. (20) found a PAS of an unknown nature. In dog blood taken immediately after the intravenous injection of trypsin or snake venom, there appeared a substance different from histamine and acetylcholine that possessed a hypotensive action and ability to slowly

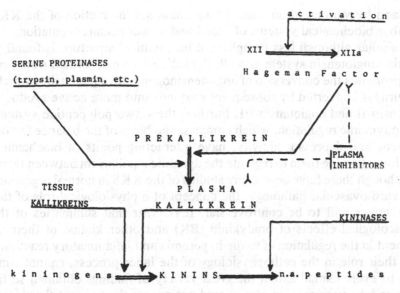

Figure 1.   Cascade structure of the kallikrein–kinin system. Solid arrows, activation; double arrows, conversion; dashed arrows, inhibition; n.a., nonactive.

shorten guinea pig intestine or rat uterus. This finding was supplemented by those of early publications by Frey, Kraut, and Werle (8,9) who found an enzyme with a hypotensive and diuretic action. These investigators identified polypeptide substances, which they called bradykinin and kallidin, and then determined their exceptionally high activity towards vascular smooth muscle and their ability to increase the tissue permeability.

Work in the 1950s and 1960s on bradykinin, kallikrein, and related components led to the creation of the concept of a total kallikrein–kinin system (KKS). A chain of biochemical reactions involving, sequentially, Hageman factor (or XII factor of blood coagulation), prekallikrein, kallikrein kininogen, and kinins led to kininogenesis in blood (Figure 1). The main system components are constantly present in blood plasma to be activated, when needed, in a specific zone of the vascular bed. The kininogenesis may also take place under the effect of tissue KK enzymes localized in kidneys, skin, and pancreatic and salivary glands in a granule form. Thus, one may speak about the existence of a whole system consisting of a chain of biochemically bound links.

Attention should be paid to the fact that an important feature in the organization of this system is the cascade principle of the interaction with the alternation of nonactive, activating and inhibiting components. Such a structure is of great biological significance, and it results in (1) the capacity for rapid formation of great quantities of the active substance, kinin; (2) multilateral regulation, activating and inhibiting the control at different stages and by various means; and (3) multicontact interaction of the KKS with other biochemical systems of blood and hemodynamic regulation.

A similar although less complicated biochemical structure is found in the renin–angiotensin system as well: the active enzyme, formed from pro-renin, promotes the conversion of angiotensinogen into angiotensin-I which, in its turn, is converted by subsequent enzymes into more active products, angiotensin-II and angiotensin-III. Further, these two polypeptide systems of hemodynamic regulation, which comprise the basis of the balance factors of pressor and depressor activity, have interacting points of biochemical regulation, allowing them to regulate the dynamic equilibrium between them.

Although there have been many studies of the KKS in normal organisms and in cardiovascular pathology, the concept of a physiological role of this system seems still to be controversial. It is clear that summaries of the pharmacological effects of bradykinin (BK) and other kinins, of their in-volvement in the regulation of tissue hyperemia and inflammatory reactions, and of their role in the pathophysiology of the labor process, cannot sum-marize to even a small extent the great variety of findings obtained so far in various laboratories. One also should not accept the concept that kinins have only a pathogenetic role as, for example, "shock mediators" or "pain mediators."

In our opinion, a typical error in many models is that only the properties of BK—a final product of a large and specialized biochemical system—are taken into account. Bradykinin was studied earliest from the pharmacolog-ical viewpoint when it was already present in the vascular bed. Hence, the very complicated and mobile relations of BK with the factors influencing its biosynthesis and decay, as well as the connections of KKS with other PASs of the organism, are left out of these accounts.

Several years ago, we formulated a concept of the physiological role of KK and BK as factors mediating the connection between vessel tonus and the rheological properties of blood circulating along a vessel (2,10). This hypothesis was based on numerous series of investigations in which KKS and related systems of the hemodynamic regulation were considered in different clinical conditions: during intensive physical exercise, in the dy-namics of adaptation of athletes to a chronic load, as well as in patients with different types of cardiovascular disturbances.

We proceeded from the fact that, because of its biochemical structure, KKS should be considered together with the systems of fibrinolysis and blood coagulation. Such a concept is formed from the following: (1) the presence of a common center in the initial activation of three systems, HF; (2) the existence of inhibitors common to the main enzymes of these three systems and HF, i.e., α-2-macroglobulin, CI-esterase inactivator, antith-rombin-III, and α-2-antiplasmin; (3) the leading role of KK in the regulation of HF biochemical activity and, hence, of all three systems.

The factors defining the vessel tonus or blood flow resistance may be divided into two groups: on one hand are the architectonic (geometric)

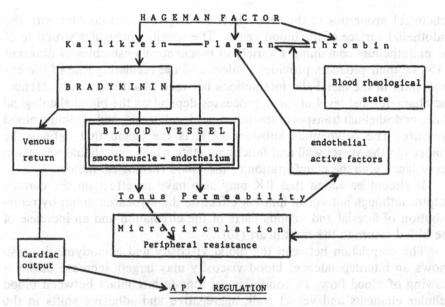

Figure 2. Conception of the physiological role of the blood kallikrein–kinin system in the regulation of hemovascular homeostasis, (AP) arterial pressure.

characteristics of the vessels, i.e., its diameter, extention, various ramifications, presence of the intimal wall changes; on the other hand are the rheological properties of the blood itself, a heterogenous, multicomponent biological system of a corpuscular nature. The blood viscosity is determined by the state of plasma and blood cells as well as their relative volume correlation. Such parameters as hematocrit, volume, erythrocyte form and rigidity, concentration of fibrinogen and other plasma proteins, tension and velocity shifts of blood layers, and aggregation of erythrocytes and platelets are the main factors determining the blood viscosity.

An important role belongs to the correlation between the factors of fibrinolysis and coagulation. In conditions of increased thrombogenesis, we bear in mind not only the limit in blood flow rate but also the degree of activation of the thrombin–plasmin systems which determine the fibrinogen concentration in blood and the state of the endothelial fibrin layer, playing a "lubricant" role and acting directly on the character of the bloodstream.

Here, the peculiarity of the KKS, because of its biochemical characteristics, lies in the fact that it is at an interface between the coagulation and fibrinolysis systems which determine to a large degree the blood rheological state (Figure 2). By its physiological characteristics, BK is a substance with pronounced vasomotor action. Thus, the KKS is responsible for the realization of the correlation between the factors regulating the blood state and the tonus and vessel permeability. In other words, a physiological role of BK is in conforming vessel tonus to blood rheological properties.

It would evidently be a great simplification to consider the physicobiochemical properties of the blood beyond its permanent contact with the endothelial surface of the blood vessel. The specific molecular structure of the endothelium containing a variety of biochemical ensembles of different PASs or their products provides evidence of the regulating role of the endothelium in the metabolic interactions between blood and tissue. Hence, the character and level of these processes depend on the blood rheological state, endothelium transport function, vessel wall tonus, and systemic blood pressure. The polypeptide substance BK is the ligand that defines the changes in the vessel wall and functional state of the endothelial vessels in accordance with the manifestation of the blood rheological factors.

It should be added that BK may also have an effect on the cardiac output, although not via an indirect effect on the myocardium but by redistribution of arterial and venous parts of the circulation and an increase of the blood return to the right heart (10).

The correlation between the blood viscosity and hemodynamics also shows an interdependence: blood viscosity may largely increase during a slowing of blood flow. In conditions of long-term contact between blood cellular elements and vessel wall, aggregative and adhesive shifts in the hemovascular system are more likely. The vasoactive kinins prevent or eliminate a disordering of the correlation between blood viscosity and flow in the circulatory system. In physiological conditions the compensatory mechanisms keep the blood flow normal even during a significant increase in the viscosity.

Up to recently, however, it was unclear how the interaction of several molecular components involved in the process of kininogenesis and blood coagulation is regulated. Is their combination at a moment of the activation—XII coagulation factor (HF)—random or strictly regular? In addition, what is the correlation between the blood flow velocity and biochemical reaction rates of the kininogenesis? In other words, how is local or generalized kinin action realized as a factor of the hemovascular regulation?

A rough estimate shows that the diameter of the lumen of the smallest capillary and the size of molecules participating in BK formation (HF, prekallikrein, kininogen, etc.), as well as the number of these molecules in blood, are so incommensurable that the "random" meeting of these molecules becomes practically impossible. According to the recent data on the molecular biochemistry of blood (5,6,15,16,18), these processes occur as follows: HF adsorbed by the negatively charged surface and undergoing an activating conformation change combines with the already existing macromolecular complexes containing prekallikrein, kininogen, and an inhibitor which is able to limit the enzymatic activity. Thus, the localization and high rate of the conjugate biochemical reactions are explained.

Recent investigations have also revealed a role of certain groups of phospholipids in blood cell membranes in the intiation of HF-contact activation. The membrane activation of erythrocytes, platelets, etc. leads to a

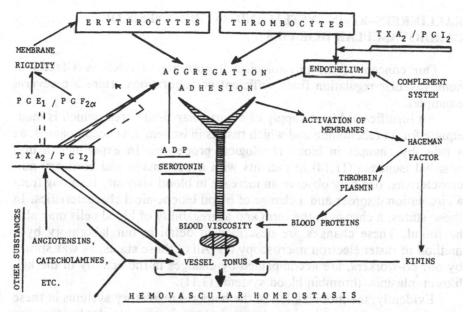

Figure 3.   Interaction among different groups of physiologically active substances in the regulation of vessel tonus and blood rheological properties.

change in conformation and increase in the adhesive and aggregative properties of these cells.

An important role in changing blood rheological properties belongs to both platelets and erythrocytes. In this case, as with the KKS and thrombin–plasmin systems, an active part of these processes requires other groups of PASs (Figure 3).

A number of factors lead to an increase in the aggregation or adhesion of blood cells. In all cases, a chain of biochemical processes promoting the release of serotonin, thromboxane, and ADP from the platelets into blood are triggered. These substances, on one hand, trigger an "aggregation avalanche" and, on the other hand, promote the endothelium synthesis of prostacyclin (PGI_2), possessing antiadhesive and antiaggregative properties. The balance of TXA and PGI_2 determines the equilibrium of the processes involved in platelet aggregation and disaggregation. In this connection, we think it reasonable to mention the work of Moncada et al. (17) showing the relationship between BK and PGI_2 release into the blood.

Thus, the scheme (Figure 3) demonstrating the KKS role in the regulation of vessel tonus in accordance with blood rheological properties may be supplemented with new data. We believe that such a regulation is realized by different biochemical systems of both plasma and cellular origin, and, hence, the unity of three components—blood plasma, corpuscular elements, and vessel wall—is provided.

KALLIKREIN–KININ SYSTEM AND PATHOGENESIS OF CARDIOVASCULAR DISEASES

Our concept of the physiological importance of KKS as a factor in hemovascular regulation finds sufficient corroborations. Here are several examples.

An insufficient blood supply of a particular tissue area, which is inadequate for its functioning and which results in ischemia, is accompanied, as a rule, by changes in blood rheological properties. In experimental myocardial ischemia (11,14) in patients with hypertension and coronary atherosclerosis, one may observe an increase in blood viscosity resulting from a circulation disorder and a change of blood biochemical characteristics. In these states, a change in the form and aggregability of blood cells may also be found. These changes are described in detail in our laboratory by a method of raster electron microscopy (1). All of these states, as was shown by our co-workers, are accompanied by changes in the activity of the kallikrein–plasmin–thrombin blood systems (3,11).

Evidently, the mobilization of the humoral regulatory systems in these situations must prevent increased thrombogenesis, provide clot lysis in sites distant from the injury, and promote the preservation of the normal blood flow.

Analyzing the changes in the activity of the KKS components, we divided several types of its reaction into different physiological or pathological states. These variations may characterize a stable state of the regulatory system, its activation under limited control, inhibition, or exhaustion. Such a formula is suitable for other systems of humoral regulation and may have, in our opinion, an essential significance for the evaluation of physiological and pathological shifts in the organism. We developed an original method for a simultaneous assay of the precursors and inhibitors of KK, plasmin, and thrombin in the blood by determining their argininesterase activity (12).

Figure 4a shows that patients with hypertension (stage IIA–IB) were given a hemodynamic test, that did not provoke changes in the indices of the Hageman factor system in the healthy persons. The patients responded to this effect by increased reactivity: intense output of PKK and prothrombin and an increase in the activity of the plasmin inhibitor.

Such great changes might also be observed in healthy persons in conditions of maximum physical exercise (Figure 4b)—work on a veloergometer to full capacity. And, as we saw, quite different reactions to such a maximum exercise may be observed in athletes who are used to undergoing a long adaptation to maximum physical influences. These tested subjects respond by a decrease in precursor level, i.e., loss of an increased level of these factors which they have acquired in the process of exercises.

These results represent interesting material for the evaluation of the theoretical aspects of the regulatory interaction of kallikrein–thrombin–

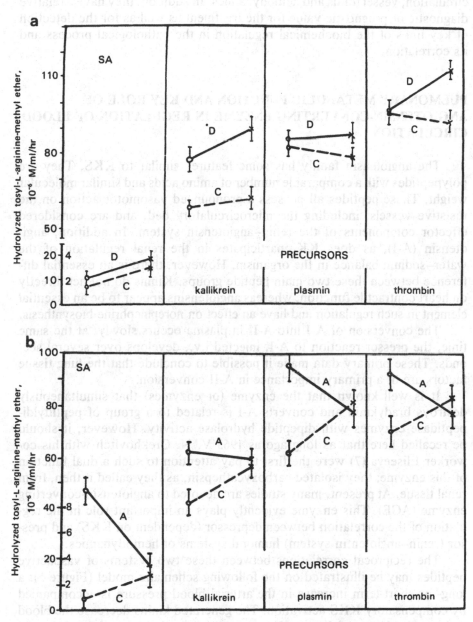

Figure 4. Changes in plasma content of kallikrein, plasmin, and thrombin precursors after physical exercise: a, walking in moderate rhythm for 30 min; b, veloergometer at full capacity. C, healthy untrained persons; A, athletes; D, patients with hypertension; SA, spontaneous activity.

plasmin—the main enzymatic factors providing a balance of blood micro-circulation, vessel tonus and hemodynamics. In addition, they have a relative diagnostic or prognostic value for the treatment as well as for the detection of key links of the biochemical regulation in the pathological process and its correlation.

PULMONARY METABOLIC FUNCTION AND KEY ROLE OF ANGIOTENSIN-CONVERTING ENZYME IN REGULATION OF BLOOD CIRCULATION

The angiotensin family has some features similar to KKS. They are polypeptides with a comparable number of amino acids and similar molecular weight. These peptides all possess a pronounced vasomotor action on the resistive vessels, including the microcirculatory bed, and are considered effector components of the renin–angiotensin system. In addition, angiotensin (A-I), as does KK, participates in the renal regulation of the water–sodium balance in the organism. However, there is an essential difference between these two main peptide groups. Kinins do not act directly on heart contractile function, whereas angiotensins appear to be an essential element in such regulation and have an effect on norepinephrine biosynthesis.

The conversion of A-I into A-II in plasma occurs slowly; at the same time, the pressor reaction to A-I, injected i.v., develops over several seconds. These primary data made it possible to conclude that the lung tissue factors are of a primary importance in A-II conversion.

It is well known that the enzyme (or enzymes) that simultaneously destroys bradykinin and converts A-I is related to a group of peptidyldipeptidase enzymes with dipeptide hydrolase activity. However, it should be recalled here that as long ago as 1963 V. N. Orekhovitch with his co-worker Eliseeva (7) were the first to pay attention to such a dual function of this enzyme: they isolated carboxycathepsin, as they called it then, from renal tissue. At present, many studies are devoted to angiotensin-converting enzyme (ACE). This enzyme evidently plays an important role in the regulation of the correlation between depressor (dependent on KKS) and pressor (renin–angiotentin system) humoral systems of hemodynamics.

The reciprocal correlations between these two systems of vasoactive peptides may be illustrated on the following schematic model (Figure 5): a long- or short-term increase in the arterial blood pressure is accompanied by compensatory KKS activation. The generated kinins decrease the blood pressure in the arterial part of the systemic circulation, and, at the same time, the products of kinin destruction inhibit the angiotensin-converting activity of peptidyldipeptidase. Hence, the greater the quantity of kinins generated in the blood, the greater is their physiological (hypotensive) and biochemical (inhibitory to ACE) action as related to the pressor factors which are connected with the angiotensin system. In turn, the kinin-induced

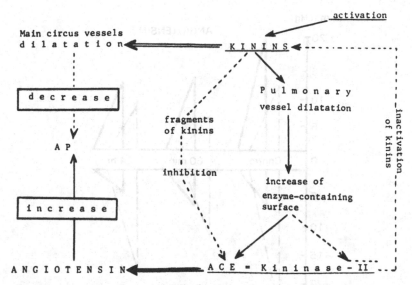

Figure 5.   Direct and "feedback" effects of bradykinin on the balance of blood pressor and depressor factors.

dilatation of vessels in the pulmonary circulation leads to an increase in the functioning area of the pulmonary microcirculatory bed, containing both the kininase and ACE activity. Such is probably the mechanism of a direct and "self-limiting" bradykinin action connected with its involvement in the regulation of a stable arterial blood pressure.

We have compared the pressor and depressor responses to A-I and BK in rats after intravenous and intraaortal injections in the dynamics of experimental myocardial infarction (Figure 6). A primary stage of acute myocardial ischemia produced by coronary arterial ligation was accompanied by a decrease in kininase activity and an increase in the angiotensin-converting activity. At late stages of experimental infarction, this correlation completely reverses (13). Hence, in defining the causes of the hemodynamic shifts in the norm and in pathology, it is necessary to take into account the so-called "double-edged" action of ACE as related to pressor or depressor polypeptides. In a study of the biochemical features of ACE, one must pay attention to the fact that the disturbances appearing in the organism under the influence of the pathological process may be a cause not only of a change in the general "total" ACE activity but of the transformation of its substrate specificity to a preferential effect on kinins or on A-I.

The findings of recent years have revealed new points of contiguity between the KK and renin–angiotensin polypeptide systems. The activation of plasma prorenin—the precursor of the active enzyme—appeared to be dependent on the Hageman factor (19,21). The significance of this discovery lies in the fact that it determines the second important line of interaction between pressor and depressor polypeptide systems of the organism. How-

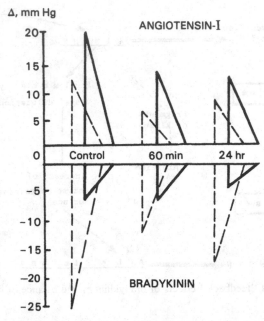

Figure 6.   Pressor and depressor responses to standard dosages of angiotensin-I and bradykinin in the dynamics of experimental myocardial infarction. Route of administration: solid line, intravenous; dashed line, intraaortic.

ever, it should be noted that the interaction of these biochemical systems controlling the vessel tonus is inseparable from the functions of coagulation and fibrinolysis connected with Hageman factor as well. Thus, blood flow regulation is provided via the interaction of different hemovascular homeostatic factors.

With regard to the key role of ACE, we bear in mind, first of all, the enzyme (or enzyme family with a similar substrate specificity) localized in the endothelium of the pulmonary circulation vessels. Hence, an important pathophysiological aspect of this problem is in the study on the peculiarities of a pulmonary metabolic function dependent on the pulmonary hemodynamics level, the quantity of "functioning" pulmonary microvessels and other factors. The metabolism of the other group of vasoactive substances, PGs, which are very important for hemodynamic regulation and heart work, is also connected with the lungs. In the case of PG inactivation, the function of the pulmonary microvessels is very significant. One can compare doses inducing standard hypotensive responses while injecting the drugs into the right or left auricle ("before" or "after" lungs). The arterial–venous difference of the effective doses is fivefold for BK and 22-fold for PGE_1. The polypeptide substance P, which possesses a greater molar vasomotor activity, is not subject to pulmonary biotransformation (4).

It should be emphasized that similarly to kinins and some other vasoactive substances, PGs themselves largely affect the pulmonary vessel resistance. At the same time, PGE_1, PGE_2, and $TXAB_2$ are released in large quantities from the lungs into the arterial blood flow. The activation of PG synthesis and their elimination takes place in alveolar hypoxia, pulmonary vascular embolia, and anaphylactic reactions as well as under the action of other PAS (kinins, serotonin, histamine) transported to the lungs with venous blood. Hence, among the humoral regulators, there occurs a peculiar "passing of the baton": before being destroyed in lungs, kinins induce the synthesis and release of the other depressor substance, PG.

Certainly, systemic blood pressure regulation and changes of this regulation under physical load as well as in hypertension, shock, etc. are also connected with the activity of renal humoral factors and, in particular, with the important controlling function of renal KKS, prostaglandin, and renin–angiotensin systems. Nevertheless, the new viewpoint—to value the genesis of hemodynamic disorders and to apply new forms of therapy "via lungs"—seems us to be a very interesting perspective.

Finally, reverting to the first part of this chapter which describes the factors of hemorheological regulation, we would like to note that in the pulmonary endothelium a higher specific protease and fibrinolytic activity as well as activity of thromboplastin and other coagulative factors are concentrated. Thus, taking into account the metabolism of prostaglandins, kinins, serotonin, and other substances influencing the biophysical properties and interaction of the formed blood elements, it becomes clear that the lungs are to be regarded as an important generalized regulator of hemovascular homeostasis.

REFERENCES

1. Chernukh, A. M., Alexeyev, O. V., and Ionov, B. V. 1981. [Interaction of erythrocytes in aggregation according to raster electron microscopy.] *Biull. Eksp. Biol. Med.* 2:226–228.
2. Chernukh, A. M., and Gomazkov, O. A. 1976. [On regularity and pathogenetic role of kallikrein–kinin system of organism.] *Patol. Fisiol. Eksp. Ther.* 1:5–16.
3. Chernukh, A. M., Gomazkov, O. A., Komissarova, N. V., and Lantsberg, L. 1981. [Changes in indices of Hageman factor system in human adaptation to intensive physical exercise.] *Patol. Fisiol. Eksp. Ther.* 5:25–28.
4. Chernukh, A. M., Oehme, P., and Gomazkov, O. A. 1980. [Hemodynamic characteristics of the polypeptide substance P in comparison with bradykinin and prostaglandin E_1.] *Biull. Eksp. Biol. Med.* 9:259–260.
5. Derkx, F. H., Bouma, B. N., and Schalekamp, M. 1979. An intrinsic factor XII–prekallikrein-dependent pathways activates the human plasma renin–angiotensin system. *Nature* 280:315–316.
6. Donaldson, V. H., Kleniewski, J., Saito, H., and Sayed, J. K. 1977. Prekallikrein deficiency and Fitzgerald trait clotting defect. Evidence that high molecular weight kininogen and prekallikrein exist as a complex in normal human plasma. *J. Clin. Invest.* 60:571–584.
7. Eliseeva, T. E., and Orekhovitch, V. N. 1963. [Isolation and study of specificity of carboxycathepsin.] *Dokl. Akad. Nauk. SSSR* 153:954–956.
8. Frey, E. K., and Kraut, H. 1928. Ein neues Kreislaufhormon und seine Wirkung. *Arch. Exp. Pathol. Pharmacol.* 133:1–56.

9. Frey, E. K., Kraut, H., and Werle, E. 1950. *Kallikrein (Padutin)*. Enke, Stuttgart.
10. Gomazkov, O. A. 1973. [Vasoactive kinins in physiology and pathology of cardiovascular system.] *Kardiologiia* 7:130–144.
11. Gomazkov, O. A. 1974. Das Kallikrein–Klinin-System bei Myokardischemie und Herzinfarct—Experimentelle Untersuchungen. *Med. Welt* 25:804–807.
12. Gomazkov, O. A., and Komissarova, N. V. 1976. [Method of simultaneous determination of precursors of kallikrein, plasmin, thrombin and their inhibitors in human blood plasma.] *Biull. Eksp. Biol. Med.* 5:632–634.
13. Gomazkov, O. A., Shimkovitch, M. V., and Chernukh, A. M. 1977. [Interrelation between kininase and angiotensin-converting activity under normal condition and in experimentally induced myocardial infarction.] *Kardiologiia* 17:103–108.
14. Gordon, R. J. 1974. Potential significance of plasma viscosity and hematocrit variations in myocardial ischemia. *Am. Heart J.* 87:175–182.
15. Griffin, J. 1978. Role of surface in surface-dependent activation of Hageman factor (blood coagulation factor XII). *Proc. Natl. Acad. Sci. U.S.A.* 75:1998–2002.
16. Meier, H. L., Pierce, J. V., Colman, R. W., and Kaplan, A. P. 1977. Activation and function of human Hageman factor. The role of high molecular weight kininogen and prekallikrein. *J. Clin. Invest.* 60:18–31.
17. Moncada, S., Mullane, K. M., and Vane, J. R. 1979. Prostacycline release by bradykinin in vivo. *Br. J. Pharmacol.* 66:96P–97P.
18. Movat, H. Z. 1978. The kinin system: Its relation to blood coagulation, fibrinolysis and formed elements of the blood. *Rev. Physiol. Biochem. Pharmacol.* 84:143–202.
19. Osmond, D. H., Lo, E. K., Loh, A. Y., Zingg, E. A., and Hedlin, A. H. 1978. Kallikrein and plasmin as activators of inactive renin. *Lancet* 2:1375.
20. Rocha e Silva, M., Beraldo, W., and Rosenfeld, G. 1949. Bradykinin, a hypotensive and smooth muscle stimulating factor releasing from plasma globulin by snake venom and by trypsin. *Am. J. Physiol.* 156:261–273.
21. Sealey, J. E., Altas, S. A., and Laragh, J. 1978. Linking the kallikrein and kinin system via activation of inactive renin. New data and hypothesis. *Am. J. Med.* 65:994–1000.

Pathogenesis of Immune-Mediated Carditis in Monkeys

I. S. Anand, N. K. Ganguly, A. K. Khanna, R. N. Chakravarti, and P. L. Wahi

Departments of Cardiology, Parasitology, and Experimental Medicine
Postgraduate Institute of Medical Education and Research
Chandigarh 160012, India

Abstract. An experimental model of carditis has been produced in the rhesus monkey by giving 12 weekly injections of streptococcal membrane antigen. Carditis was produced in as short a period as 14 weeks. There was evidence of myocarditis, endocarditis, and, in two animals, myocardial granuloma formation. No valvular lesions were seen. Measurement of immune responses showed that heart cross-reactive antibodies started appearing in the circulation after the second injection. By the sixth injection, there was evidence of complement consumption and appearance of circulating immune complexes. Antibody-dependent cell cytotoxicity started operating after the second injection, and by the sixth injection, peripheral lymphocytes had acquired hypersensitivity to membrane antigen. It is concluded that some of these immunologic responses might have played a role in the genesis of carditis.

Even though streptococcal sore throat is firmly implicated in the etiology of rheumatic heart disease, the pathogenesis of rheumatic carditis remains largely speculative (25). A large number of experimental models have been produced, using group A β-hemolytic streptotoccus or its products, in different experimental animals such as mice, rabbits, monkeys, baboons, and chimpanzees. As such, a variety of lesions have been seen, including focal inflammatory cell aggregates with areas of myocardial cell degeneration, nodular skin lesions, joint swelling, myocardial fibrinoid degeneration of collagen with granuloma formation, and even valvulitis (2,17,18,27,33). However, none of these models has shown a classical picture of pancarditis with Aschoff's nodules. Moreover, the mechanisms underlying these diverse experimental lesions have not been fully worked out.

The discovery by Kaplan and Meyserian of an antigenic cross reactivity between streptococci and heart muscle (13) led to the suggestion that an autoimmune mechanism may be involved in the genesis of rheumatic carditis. This hypothesis, and especially the role of humoral immunity in the pathogenesis of rheumatic carditis, was strengthened by the discovery of circulating antiheart-reacting antibodies in patients with rheumatic fever and the deposition of γ-globulin and complement in the myocardium of patients of rheumatic heart disease (10,12). The antigenic cross reactivity was later ascertained to be between the streptococcal protoplast membrane and car-

215

diac sarcolemma (30,32). This hypothesis is, however, far from satisfactory, as antiheart antibodies are found in a number of other conditions and not always in patients with rheumatic heart disease (9). Moreover, the granulomatous reaction of the Aschoff's nodule cannot be explained through antigen–antibody reaction (26,28). Furthermore, deposition of γ-globulin and complement has never been seen in Aschoff's nodules (11).

Recently, cellular hypersensitivity to group A streptococcal membrane antigen has been demonstrated in patients with rheumatic fever and rheumatic heart disease (22,24). It therefore appears that both humoral and cell-mediated immune responses play a role in the pathogenesis of rheumatic carditis.

In a preliminary study carried out at this institute, it was observed that repeated injections in rhesus monkeys of killed group A streptococcal L-forms (which are bags of streptococcal membranes) resulted in the production of granulomatous myocardial lesions (15). The present study was, therefore, undertaken to investigate the effects of repeated injections of purified streptococcal membrane antigen to rhesus monkeys in an attempt to produce a model of rheumatic or immune carditis. The ensuing humoral and cell-mediated immune parameters were also monitored to identify the possible immune mechanisms involved in the injury. Rhesus monkeys were chosen because they suffer natural group A streptococcal infection (16) and because their immune apparatus is similar to that of humans (5,6).

MATERIAL AND METHODS

The study was carried out on ten adult rhesus monkeys 4–5 kg in weight. They were tuberculin negative and were free of streptococcal infection. They were divided into three groups. The first group of four animals was kept on normal diet, whereas the second group of four monkeys was subjected to dietary protein calorie malnutrition for 8 weeks prior to the start of the experiment. This was done by giving them a diet containing half the protein and calories of that given to normals. Another two monkeys were kept as controls. All eight monkeys of groups I and II were then given 12 subcutaneous injections of 25 μg of purified streptococcal membrane antigen. Streptococcal membrane antigen was prepared by the method of Zabriskie and Freimer (32) as modified by Van de Rijn et al. (30). The rhamnose content of the membrane antigen was less than 0.1% of the streptococcal cell wall, and it was free of RNA, DNA, and muramyl peptides. The group A streptococcal strain used was M type I obtained from Colindale Laboratory, U.K.

The cross reactivity of the membrane antigen was tested against a saline-extracted antigen of monkey heart prepared according to the method of Chaturvedi et al. (1), and the antiserum was raised in rabbits against the heart antigen. A line of identity was seen between the streptococcal membrane and heart antigen. Membrane antigen injections were given at 1-week intervals for 12 weeks, the first two injections being combined with Freund's complete adjuvant. The two control monkeys were given two injections of Freund's complete adjuvant only. Thirty milliliters of blood in 15 units of preservative-free heparin and 10 ml of clotted blood were collected on four occasions, before the start of injections, after the second and sixth injections, and then 2 weeks after the 12th injection at sacrifice. The serum and plasma were stored in small aliquots at $-70°C$. The animals were sacrificed 2 weeks after the 12th injection, and the heart and kidney were examined histologically. The following parameters were measured in the plasma/serum, and on the peripheral lymphocytes.

HUMORAL PARAMETERS

Antistreptolysin O (ASO) and anti-DNAase B (ADNase B) were estimated according to the method of Rotta (23) and expressed as international units/ml. Antiheart-reacting antibody was estimated by an indirect hemagglutination (IHA) method using 60% ammonium sulfate precipitate of a saline-extracted heart antigen. The antimembrane antibody was titrated according to the method described by Grant (8). The cross adsorption of the above two antibodies was carried out using 700 μg of 60% ammonium sulfate precipitate of saline-extracted heart antigen in 10 ml of activated Sepharose 4B (Pharmacia Fine Chemicals, Ltd.).

Monkey C'3 was estimated according to Ganguly (5). Circulating immune complexes were estimated by C1q-binding radioimmunoassay (29).

Cellular Parameters

Lymphocytes. T and B cells were estimated according to the conventional rosetting method (15). Active or early T cells were estimated according to the method described by Quan and Burton (20). T_μ and T_γ cells were estimated according to Pichler and Krupp (19). Transformation of lymphocytes was studied using 50 μg of purified streptococcal membrane, 25 μg of concanavalin A (Con A), and 15 μg of phytohemagglutinin (PHA) (Burroughs Wellcome) per 3-ml culture of 2×10^6 lymphocytes. Antibody-dependent cell cytotoxicity (ADCC) was estimated by ^{51}Cr release of chicken RBC (3).

Macrophages. Macrophage maturation was estimated in 0.1-ml microcultures, in triplicate, on RPMI 1640 tissue culture medium with 20% fetal calf serum (21). Phagocytosis using Fc receptor sheep red blood cells and *Staphylococcus aureus* was carried out according to Furth et al. (4) and was expressed as percentage phagocytosis. Specific cytotoxicity was assayed on 60% of heart antigen coated on sheep RBC tagged with ^{51}Cr. It was expressed as percentage ^{51}Cr release.

Histopathology. The heart and kidney were examined histologically.

218   I. S. Anand et al.

RESULTS

Diet with restricted protein and calories caused a reduction in the body weight by an average of 32% in group I monkeys. There was loss of subcutaneous fat and a considerable loss of fur from most parts of the body. The animals became very sluggish in their physical activity, and their serum albumin fell from 4.3 g to 3.9 g/100 ml.

Figure 1 shows the ASO, ADNase B, antiheart-reacting antibody, and antimembrane antibody in normal and malnourished monkeys before and after the second, sixth, and 12th injections. There was a slight increase in the titers of ASO and ADNase B in normal monkeys from the second to sixth weeks. The rise in these titers in the malnourished monkeys was much more ($P < 0.05$) but followed the same pattern. Antiheart-reacting antibody

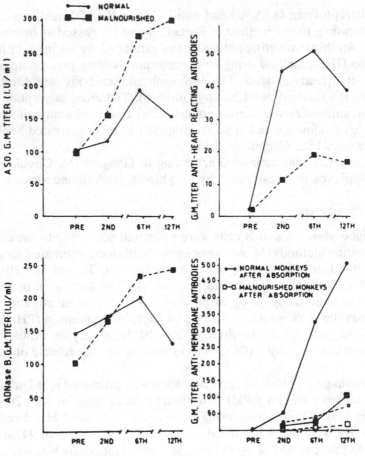

Figure 1.   Geometric mean titers of ASO, ADNase B, antiheart, and antimembrane antibodies in normal and malnourished monkeys before and after the second, sixth, and 12th injection of membrane antigen. Note the drop in the titers of antimembrane antibody on absorption with heart antigen.

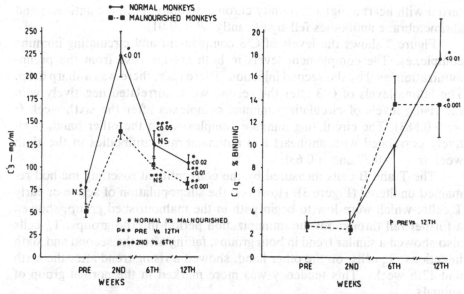

Figure 2.   Levels of C'3 and C1q binding before and after injection with membrane antigen. Dashed line in each column represents the mean preimmunization value for the normal monkeys, and the solid lines represent ±2 S.D.

showed a prompt increase by the second injection in both groups of monkeys, although the quantum of response was significantly lower in malnourished animals. The antimembrane antibodies, on the other hand, showed a marked increase only after the sixth week and kept rising thereafter. Once again, the response was lower in the malnourished group. After absorption of the

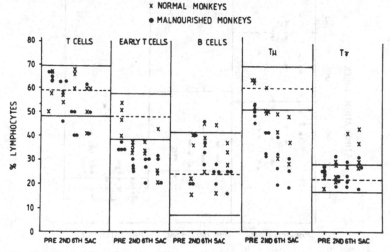

Figure 3.   B cells and T cells and their subpopulations before and after membrane antigen injections. Dashed and solid lines represent mean ± 2 S.D., respectively, of the normal preimmunized monkeys.

serum with heart antigen in affinity chromatography, both the antiheart and antimembrane antibodies fell significantly ($P < 0.01$).

Figure 2 shows the levels of C′3 complement and circulating immune complexes. The complement levels in both groups rose from the preimmunization level by the second injection. Thereafter, there was a sharp drop. The falling levels of C′3 after the second week correlated negatively with the rising levels of circulating immune complexes after the sixth week ($r = -0.883$). The circulating immune complexes, on the other hand, positively correlated with antiheart and antimembrane antibodies in the sixth week ($r = +0.77$ and $+0.63$).

The T and B cells measured by the conventional rosetting method remained unaltered (Figure 3). However, the subpopulation of active or early T cells, which were low to begin with in the malnourished group, showed a further fall throughout the immunization period in both groups. T_μ cells also showed a similar trend in both groups, falling after the second and sixth injections. T_γ cells, on the other hand, showed a rising trend after the sixth and 12th weeks. This tendency was more marked in the normal group of animals.

Figure 4 shows the lymphocytic blast transformation to PHA, Con A, and membrane antigen. The lymphocyte transformation by PHA was com-

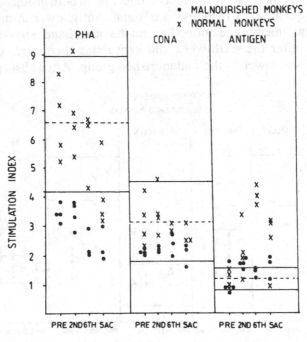

Figure 4.   Lymphocyte blast transformation to PHA, Con A, and membrane antigen in normal and malnourished monkeys before and after membrane injections. Dashed and solid lines represent the mean ± 2 S.D., respectively, of the preimmunized normal monkeys.

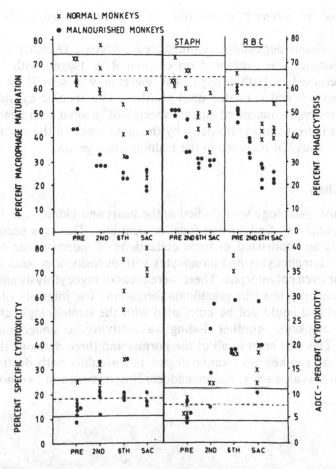

Figure 5. Macrophage maturation, cytotoxicity for *Staphylococcus aureus* and sheep RBC's, specific cytotoxicity, and ADCC in normal and malnourished monkeys before and after membrane injection. Dashed and solid lines in each panel represent the mean ± 2 S.D., respectively, of the preimmunized normal monkeys.

promised in both groups, although much more so in the malnourished group. Although the trend was visible after the second injection, maximal depression to PHA was seen at sacrifice. The response to Con A was preserved in both groups. When streptococcal membrane antigen was used as a mitogen, there was a stimulation of lymphocyte transformation, and this was visible after the second injection. The sensitization was most marked in the normal group of animals.

The maturation of macrophages from monocytes was depressed in the malnourished group in the preimmunization period, and it showed further depression by the second injection. In the normal group, the maturation function was affected by the sixth week (Figure 5). Very similar kinetics was seen for the phagocytosis function of the macrophage, both towards

Staphylococcus aureus and towards the Fc receptor-coated sheep RBCs (Figure 5).

The antibody-dependent cell-mediated cytotoxic (ADCC) reaction of the lymphocytes was measured on chicken RBC tagged with ^{51}Cr. The ADCC increased in both groups. The increase was significant after the second injection and persisted until sacrifice. The specific cytotoxicity of these macrophages measured against sheep RBC coated with heart antigen showed an increase in cytotoxicity by the sixth week in the normal group with only a marginal increase in the malnourished group.

Histopathology

The histopathology was studied in the heart and kidneys. In the heart, the most consistent finding was focal myocarditis. This was seen in all of the animals and consisted of focal collections of mononuclear cells, predominantly lymphocytes and monocytes with occasional plasma cells, histiocytes, or even polymorphs. There were areas of myocytolysis and in some places a tendency towards granuloma formation. The intensity of myocarditis varied and could not be correlated with the immunologic changes in individual monkeys. Another finding was perivascular collection of lymphocytes. This was seen in all of the normal and three malnourished monkeys. In one monkey an intense degree of vasculitis with destruction of vessel wall was also seen. Active endocarditis was seen in two normal and

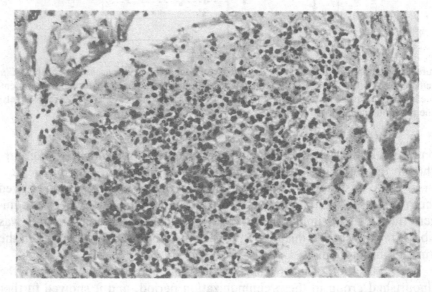

Figure 6.   Section of heart of monkey subjected to protein calorie malnutrition and given streptococcal membrane antigen. A granuloma in the myocardium is seen formed of degenerated muscle fibers with collection of lymphomononuclear cells, plasma cells, and a few giant cells. Hematoxylin and eosin, ×200.

two malnourished monkeys. Pericarditis was present in only one normal monkey. The most interesting lesion was a typical granulomatous myocarditis (Figure 6) seen in one malnourished and one normal monkey. It is possible that given more time focal areas of myocarditis might have developed into granulomas. There was no valvulitis or nodular lesion on the valves, nor was there any evidence of fibrin deposition.

The kidneys of all monkeys showed glomerular hypercellularity resulting from mesangial cell hyperplasia.

DISCUSSION

The major immunologic effect of malnutrition was a subdued antibody response in the malnourished monkeys. The complement levels remained unchanged. Most of the lymphocyte subpopulation remained within normal limits except for a depression of active or early T cells, which are short lived, and freshly developed lymphocytes. However, the lymphocytic response to PHA stimulation was compromised in the malnourished monkeys, although the response to Con A remained preserved. The maturation and the phagocytic function of the macrophages were depressed in the malnourished group. Their specific cytotoxicity against the heart antigen remained normal. Depression of immune response is known to occur with malnutrition. However, the effect of malnutrition on such varied immunologic parameters has as yet not been reported.

The rise in ASO and ADNase B seen especially in malnourished animals during the course of sensitization with streptococcal membrane antigen (which is free of streptococcal extracellular products) is hard to explain. Although throat cultures of these monkeys done at 1-week intervals were negative, mild subclinical infection with streptococci cannot be ruled out. This is especially so because these monkeys easily get infected with this organism in captivity (16). Furthermore, as the macrophage and some lymphocyte functions were affected in the malnourished monkeys, they might have become prone to infection. Nevertheless, the number of cells and their quantum of functions were such that hypersensitivity reactions could take place in both groups.

The appearance of cross-reacting antibodies in the monkeys was seen from 2 weeks onwards, and a sharp drop in the titers of antimembrane antibodies was noted on adsorption by heart antigen. The appearance of similar cross-reacting antiheart antibodies in patients with rheumatic heart disease, as seen by decreased fluorescence after absorption with streptococcal antigen, has been reported by Kaplan et al. (12). We used a different method to demonstrate the same effect in these monkeys. In addition, as two antibodies were monitored separately, their dynamics could also be studied. Whereas antiheart-reacting antibodies reached a plateau from the sixth week onwards, antimembrane antibodies continued to rise until sacrifice, probably because of continuous sensitization. This shows that a part of antimembrane antibody is very distinctive and is different from antiheart-reacting antibody.

The high levels of antiheart antibodies after the second week makes the myocardium vulnerable to attachment by these antibodies, thereby initiating myocardial injury by complement activation. The timing of the drop in the levels of C'3 correlates well with the rising levels of circulating antibodies as well as with the appearance of significant amounts of circulating immune complexes. Deposition of immune complex has been shown to occur in biopsy material from patients with rheumatic heart disease (12). We did not carry out immunofluorescence studies on our material, but our previous observations show the presence of complement and γ-globulin deposits in the myocardium of monkeys injected with a crude membrane antigen in the form of killed L-form streptococci (15). It is, therefore, likely that antibody- and complement-mediated injury is initiated by the second week. However, at about the same time, i.e., the second week, the antibody-dependent cell-mediated cytotoxicity also starts operating, and killer-cell-mediated injury of myocardial cells coated with antibody is also likely.

The number of T and B cells remained unaltered throughout the experiment. In acute rheumatic fever, the number of T cells is depressed but recovers following treatment (24). It is likely that the depression in T cells is caused by the preceding streptococcal infection through its toxic extracellular products. Such an infection was not given to these monkeys.

The helper cell population was affected during immunization as is reflected by lowered active or early T cell and T_μ cells. Some of the T-cell functions were also compromised, e.g., the response to PHA. It is not clear why only some of these T-cell populations and functions were depressed. A selective action of streptococcal membrane antigen in preferentially suppressing these subpopulations of T cells cannot be ruled out.

The increase in the population of cytotoxic T cells (T_γ) as well as the hypersensitivity state brought about through membrane sensitization of T cells was documented in these experiments. A similar sensitization of T cell to membrane antigen has also been shown to occur in patients with rheumatic heart disease (22,24). Furthermore, Yang and his colleagues have demonstrated that T cells sensitized to membrane antigen are cytotoxic to cultured myocardial cells in vitro (31). It follows, therefore, that additional myocardial injury in our monkeys through these mechanisms is possible. Moreover, the hypersensitivity phenomenon may well be the mechanism of formation of an Aschoff's nodule, since no immune complexes have been demonstrated in these nodules, and, at best, they can be categorized as hypersensitivity reactions (14).

We believe that the myocardial lesions seen in this study were immunologically mediated. This is because vasculitis and perivascular cuffing with lymphocytes, focal myocarditis with mononuclear infiltration, and granuloma formation with giant cells were the dominant lesions. Our data do not allow us to pinpoint the exact role that humoral or cell-mediated immune responses might have played or the time at which they had their effect.

Although our model is by no means an animal counterpart of human rheumatic carditis, there are a number of similarities: myocardial lesions are fairly similar, but valvulitis was not seen. This is not surprising in view of the fact that membrane antigen used in this study has no cross reactivity with valve tissue. The use of group A polysaccharide antigen, which has antigenic cross reactivity with the glycoproteins of heart valve (7), could have yielded different results. More work needs to be done, perhaps by using multiple cross-reactive antigens over a long period of time with more frequent blood sampling to see if a model more akin to the human counterpart can be produced.

REFERENCES

1. Chaturvedi, U. C., Davies, J. W., and Flewett, T. H. 1973. Separation and characterization of cardiac antigen proteins. *Clin. Exp. Immunol.* 15:613–622.
2. Cromartic, W. J., and Craddock, J. G. 1966. Rheumatic-like cardiac lesions in mice. *Science* 154:285–287.
3. Eckhardt, R., Kloos, P., Dierich, M. P., Meyer, Z., and Buschenfelde, K. H. 1977. K-lymphocytes (killer cells) in Crohn's disease and acute virus B-hepatitis. *Gut.* 18:1010–1016.
4. Furth, R., Van Zwet, T. L., and Leijh, P. C. J. 1978. *In vitro* determination of phagocytosis and intracellular killing by polymorphonuclear and monophagocytes. In: D. M. Weir (ed.), *Handbook of Experimental Immunology,* pp. 31.1–32.19. Blackwell Scientific, Oxford.
5. Ganguly, N. K., Chugh, K. S., Pal, Y., and Sapru, R. P. 1977. Comparative values of C'3 in normal rhesus monkeys. *Indian J. Med. Res.* 66:570–575.
6. Ganguly, N. K., Sapru, R. P., and Mohan, C. 1977. Comparative evaluation of anti-hyaluronidase, antistreptolysin O and streptozyme tests in acute rheumatic activity. *Indian J. Med. Res.* 66:802–808.
7. Goldstein, I., Halpern, B., and Robert L. 1967. Immunological relationship between streptococcus A polysaccharide and the structural glycoproteins of the heart valves. *Nature* 213:44–47.
8. Grant, J. 1978. Immunological methods in bacteriology. In: D. M. Weir (ed.), *Handbook of Experimental Immunology,* pp. 39.1–39.15. Blackwell Scientific, Oxford.
9. Hess, E. V., Fink, C. V., Taranta, A., and Ziff, M. 1964. Heart muscle antibodies in rheumatic fever and other diseases. *J. Clin. Invest.* 43:886–893.
10. Kaplan, M. H. 1965. Autoantibodies to heart and rheumatic fever, the induction of autoimmunity to heart by streptococcal antigen cross reactive with heart. *Ann. N.Y. Acad. Sci.* 124:904–915.
11. Kaplan, M. H. 1965. Induction of acute autoimmunity to heart in rheumatic fever by streptococcal antigen(s). Cross reaction with heart. *Fed. Proc.* 24:109–112.
12. Kaplan, M. H., Bolande, R., and Rakita, L. 1964. Presence of bound immunoglobulins and complement in the myocardium in acute rheumatic fever. *N. Engl. J. Med.* 271:637–645.
13. Kaplan, M. H., and Meyserian, M. 1962. An immunological cross reaction between group A streptococcal cells and human heart tissue. *Lancet* 1:706–710.
14. Kaplan, M. H., and Suce, K. H. 1964. Immunological relation of streptococcal and tissue antigens III. *J. Exp. Med.* 119:651–666.
15. Mohan, C. 1979. *Pathogenecity of Group A Beta Haemolytic Streptococcus and Its L-Forms in Rhesus Monkeys.* Ph.D. Thesis, Postgraduate Institute of Medical Education and Research, Chandigarh, India.

16. Mohan, C., Ganguly, N. K., Chakravarti, R. N., and Chitkara, N. L. 1977. Prevalence of haemolytic streptococcal infection in rhesus monkeys. *J. Hyg. Epidemiol. Microbiol. Immunol. (Praha)* 21:203–208.

17. Murphy, G. E., and Swift, H. F. 1950. The induction of rheumatic like cardiac lesions in rabbits by repeated focal infection with group A streptococci. Comparison with the cardiac lesions of serum disease. *J. Exp. Med.* 91:485–498.

18. Ohanion, S. H., and Schwab, J. H. 1967. Persistence of group A streptococcal cell walls related to chronic inflammation of rabbit dermal connective tissue. *J. Exp. Med.* 125:1137–1148.

19. Pichler, W. J., and Krupp, M. 1977. Receptors of IgM coated erythrocytes on chronic lymphocytic leukemia cells. *J. Immunol.* 118:1010–1015.

20. Quan, P. C., and Burtin, P. 1978. E-rosette forming cells at 29°C: An assay for the immune status of cancer patients. *J. Cancer* 38:606–611.

21. Qurrie, G. A., and Hedley, D. W. 1977. Monocyte and macrophage in malignant melanoma. Peripheral blood macrophage precursors. *Br. J. Cancer* 36:1–6.

22. Read, S. R., Fischetti, V. A., Utermohlen, V., Falk, R. E., and Zabriskie, J. B. 1974. Cellular reactivity studies to streptococcal antigens. Migration inhibition studies in patients with streptococcal infections and rheumatic fever. *J. Clin. Invest.* 54:439–450.

23. Rotta, J., and Tawil, G. S. 1976. *Manual of Reference Procedures in Streptococcal Bacteriology and Serology.* WHO Technical Report, World Health Organization, Geneva.

24. Sapru, R. P., Ganguly, N. K., Sharma, S., Chandnani, R. E., and Gupta, A. K. 1977. Cellular reactions to group A beta haemolytic streptococcal membrane antigen and its relation to complement levels in patients with rheumatic heart disease. *Br. Med. J.* 2:422–424.

25. Stollerman, G. H. 1975. *Rheumatic Fever and Streptococcal Infection.* Grune & Stratton, New York.

26. Taranta, A. 1972. Rheumatic fever: Clinical aspects, In: J. L. Hollander and D. J. McCarty, (eds.), *Arthritis and Allied Conditions,* pp. 764–820. Lea & Febiger, Philadelphia.

27. Taranta, A., Cuppari, G., and Quagliata, F. 1969. Dissociation of hemolytic and lymphocyte transforming activities of streptolysin preparation. *J. Exp. Med.* 129:605–622.

28. Thomas, E. 1952. *Rheumatic Fever: A Symposium.* University of Minnesota Press, Minneapolis.

29. Varier Jones, J., and Cumming, R. N. 1977. Test for circulating immune complexes. In: R. A. Thompson (ed.), *Techniques of Clinical Immunology,* pp. 136–156. Blackwell Scientific, Oxford.

30. Van de Rijn, I., Zabriskie, J. B., and McCarty, M. 1977. Group A streptococcal antigens cross reactivity with myocardium purification of HRA and isolation and characterization of streptococcal antigen. *J. Exp. Med.* 146:579–599.

31. Yang, L. C., Soprey, P. R., Wittner, M. K., and Fox, E. N. 1977. Streptococcal induced cell mediated immune destruction of cardiac myofibres *in vitro. J. Exp. Med.* 146:344–360.

32. Zabriskie, J. B., and Freimer, E. H. 1966. An immunological relationship between the group A streptococcus and mammalian muscle. *J. Exp. Med.* 124:661–678.

33. Zimmerman, R. A., Krushan, D. H., Wilson, E., and Douglas, J. D. 1970. Human streptococcal disease syndrome compared with observations in chimpanzees, III. Immunologic responses to induced pharyngitis and the effect of treatment. *J. Infect. Dis.* 122:280–289.

Immunologic Studies in Infective Endocarditis

P. L. Wahi, K. K. Talwar, N. K. Ganguly, A. K. Khanna, P. S. Bidwai, and I. S. Anand

Departments of Cardiology and Parasitology
Postgraduate Institute of Medical Education and Research
Chandigarh 160012, India

Abstract. Some immunologic changes in patients with infective endocarditis were measured during therapy with antibiotics. T cells and C3 levels were low in 29 and 59% of the subjects, respectively. The circulating immune complexes were high and showed a negative correlation with serum C3 levels. Teichoic acid antibodies with titer of above 5 were generally seen only in cases of bacteremia in which endothelial damage had taken place. The antibody was specific for gram-positive organisms because it was negative in gram-negative bacteremia. The antibody showed a fall during treatment and hence could be used to monitor efficacy of antibiotic therapy.

Infective endocarditis is known to be associated with various immunologic alterations: hypergammaglobulinemia (13), positive rheumatoid factor (18), reduced complement level (19), high circulating immune complexes (3,9), and cryoglobulins (10). The course of these alteration during the treatment of infective endocarditis is not well worked out. This study was planned to investigate the humoral and cell-mediated immune responses during the course of treatment of infective endocarditis. In addition, blood samples were screened for the presence of antibodies to teichoic acid antigen of both staphylococcal and streptococcal cell wall with the purpose of improving the diagnostic indices of infective endocarditis.

MATERIALS AND METHODS

Twenty-seven cases of infective endocarditis proved on the basis of clinical criteria and positive culture and/or autopsy data formed the subject of this study. There were 20 male and seven female patients. Ages ranged from 12 to 40 years. The history of onset of illness prior to admission ranged from 2 weeks to 4 months.

The following immunologic parameters were studied: the serum complement (C'3 fraction) and circulating immune complexes (CIC). These parameters were studied in the first, second, third, and sixth week of the therapy period. The C'3 was estimated by the single radial immunodiffusion technique (14). The circulating immune complexes were estimated by the

227

methods of konglutinins binding (20), C1q binding assay (5), and complement consumption technique according to method described by Lachman and Thompson (12).

The cell-mediated immunity was studied from the lymphocytes of the peripheral blood of patients with infective endocarditis in the first and sixth weeks of therapy. The proportions of T-cell and B-cell rosettes were counted according to the technique previously reported from this laboratory (7). The [^{3}H]thymidine uptake of lymphocytes was studied in response to stimulation with phytohemagglutinins (PHA) and teichoic acid antigen prepared according to the modified method described by Sapru et al. (17). Teichoic acid antigen was prepared from *Streptococcus viridans* and *Staphylococcus pyogenes* cell wall (6), purified by a modified method of Moskowitz (16), and finally purified by thin-layer chromatography. The indirect hemagglutination technique was used for estimation of antibodies.

RESULTS

There was no significant difference in the mean levels of T (51.9 ± 12.4) and B (29.7 ± 6.5) lymphocytes from those of controls (T, 62 ± 8.6; B, 29 ± 7.5). The early T-cell population (41.4 ± 12.9) showed a significantly elevated mean value ($P < 0.001$) compared to the mean of the control (17 ± 6.3). The level dropped subsequently after the sixth week of therapy (Table 1), although the mean value (25.4 ± 4.7) was still higher than that of the control population. The T-cell population was low in 29% of cases during the first week, and even on the sixth week of therapy, low values were seen in 35% of cases. The early T-cell population, was high in 70.6% of cases at the first week.

The [^{3}H]thymidine uptake by lymphocytes in response to PHA was same as in the normal control. In contrast, uptake of [^{3}H]thymidine after exposure to teichoic acid antigen was considerably increased ($P < 0.01$) as compared to the control group (Table 2).

The C3 mean levels were significantly low in patients with infective

Table 1. T Cell Subpopulations and B Cells in Cases of Infective Endocarditis

	Infective endocarditis		Control
	First week	Sixth week	
T cell	51.9 ± 12.4	48.25 ± 11.8	62.0 ± 8.6
Early T cell	41.4 ± 12.9[a]	25.4 ± 4.7[a]	17.0 ± 6.3
B cell	29.7 ± 6.5	28.5 ± 7.8	29.0 ± 7.5

[a] $P < 0.001$.

Table 2.   Mean Stimulation Index ($\pm$ S.D.) of [^{3}H]Thymidine Uptake by Lymphocytes on Stimulation with PHA and Teichoic Acid Antigen in Patients with Infective Endocarditis

	Infective endocarditis	Control	Significance
PHA stimulation index	3.93 $\pm$ 2.70	3.1 $\pm$ 0.73	N.S.
Teichoic acid antigen stimulation	2.78 $\pm$ 1.06	1.2 $\pm$ 0.44	$P = 0.001$

endocarditis in the first and second weeks ($P < 0.001$). The mean value showed a rising trend from the first week to the sixth week following start of therapy. It was low in 59% of subjects in the first week of therapy and was still low in 40% of subjects in the sixth week of therapy; 2% of the subjects in the first week and 20% in the sixth week demonstrated high levels.

The circulating immune complexes (CIC) were high in 54% of cases when estimated with the C1q binding method. Using the other techniques of complement consumption and KG binding, the high levels of CIC were detected in 70% of cases. The mean value of CIC in the first, second, third, and sixth weeks was significantly higher than that in the control group (Table 3). In 73% of the patients, the CIC value demonstrated a fall towards the normal range from the first week to the sixth week of therapy (Table 3).

There was a significant negative correlation of C3 with the level of circulating immune complexes up to the third week of antibiotic therapy (Table 4). The correlation between the two was not significant in the sixth week of therapy period.

Antiteichoic acid antibodies were positive in 56% of the cases. The geometric mean of the positive titer was 10.29 $\pm$ 12.18 in patients with infective endocarditis and was significantly higher than the geometric mean in 11 subjects with bacteremia but without endocarditis (1.58 $\pm$ 1.76). The geometric mean in subjects with infective endocarditis with positive titer was 88.64 $\pm$ 4.18, and in those with positive culture was 128 $\pm$ 3. Five out of nine subjects showed a fourfold rise in the second week of therapy,

Table 3.   Mean Binding (%) of Circulating Immune Complexes in Cases of Infective Endocarditis[a]

	Infective endocarditis				Control
	First week	Second week	Third week	Sixth week	
C$_1$q	9.61 $\pm$ 8.82	8.9 $\pm$ 8.58	5.78 $\pm$ 6.96	7.63 $\pm$ 8.98	1.9 $\pm$ 0.86
CIC	23.94 $\pm$ 19.34	22.59 $\pm$ 19.36	16.07 $\pm$ 11.85	18.7 $\pm$ 15.86	8.0 $\pm$ 3.5
KG binding	10.6 $\pm$ 8.69	13.53 $\pm$ 11.48	8.06 $\pm$ 8.33	7.15 $\pm$ 6.48	2.4 $\pm$ 0.96

[a] $P < 0.001$ in all weeks for all parameters compared to controls.

Table 4.   Correlation Coefficient (r) of C3 with
CIC, C1q, and KG Binding during Different
Weeks of Infective Endocarditis[a]

	C1q	CIC	KG binding
Week 1	−0.672**	−0.218	−0.587*
Week 2	−0.753**	−0.206	−0.766**
Week 3	−0.580*	−0.683*	−0.689*
Week 6	−0.510	−0.412	−0.405

[a] Significance of correlation with C3: *$P < 0.01$; **$P < 0.001$.

whereas a similar number showed a fall in the second week of therapy.
Teichoic acid antibodies in all normal controls were negative (Table 5).

DISCUSSION

Although various immunologic mechanisms are known to be involved
in the pathogenesis of various manifestations of infective endocarditis, the
course of these alterations during illness and after therapy is not well worked
out (3,9,10,13,18,19). This study highlights certain aspects of various immunologic changes in patients with infective endocarditis and their fate
during the course of therapy with antibiotics.

T cells were low in 29% of the subjects. Following therapy with antibiotic for 6 weeks, about 35% of the cases still demonstrated low T cells.
The depressed immune state seems to persist until late in this disease. The
presence of a high percentage of early T cells indicates an enhanced response
of freshly primed cells from the thymus in response to infection which
ultimately drops down to normal a value as the process of infection subsides.
Increased [³H]thymidine uptake following stimulation with teichoic acid
antigen revealed acquisition of sensatization to teichoic acid antigen which

Table 5.   Geometric Mean Titer of Antiteichoic Acid Antibodies in
Infective Endocarditis, Bacteremia without Endocarditis, and Superficial
Abscess without Endocarditis[a]

	Infective endocarditis		Bacteremia without endocarditis ($N = 11$)	Superficial abscess without endocarditis ($N = 14$)
Control ($N = 25$)	Positive antibodies alone ($N = 13$)	Positive antibodies and culture ($N = 5$)		
10.29 ± 1.3*	88.6 ± 4.2**	128 ± 3**	1.58 ± 1.76	1.1 ± 0.38

[a] Significance of correlation: *$P < 0.001$ compared to other groups; **$P < 0.001$ compared to bacteremia
without endocarditis and superficial abscess group.

is a component of the cell wall of the gram-positive organisms, and the mechanism might be related to the damage to the heart valve when the microorganisms are lodged there.

C3 levels were low in 59% of subjects with infective endocarditis and high in 2% of the subjects, as compared to the value obtained in the control group. Increased C3 values have been described by Arnold et al. (1) in infective endocarditis cases. The values in a large number of cases in the present study might be low because most of the cases in the present series had reported between 2 and 4 weeks after the onset of illness. Low values of C3 have been described in cases of infective endocarditis by Mohammed et al. (15) and Gutman et al. (8). The C3 level demonstrated a rise towards the normal range during the course of therapy of infective endocarditis. The circulating immune complexes were high and demonstrated a negative correlation with serum C3 levels. This indicates that a complement-mediated injury may have occurred during the course of infective endocarditis. The CIC also demonstrated a fall toward the normal range in about 73% of the subjects. The direct evidence of immune complex deposition including C3 has been described by Keslin et al. (11) and Boulton-Jones et al. (2).

Cole (4) has postulated a diagnostic tetrad for diagnosis of infective endocarditis and included estimation of immune complexes in it; he also attributed petecheal rashes, Osler nodes, Roth's spots, Janeway's lesions, hematuria, retinal hemorrhages, vasculitis, splinter hemorrhages, and arthralgia to immune complex formation during the course of the disease. The data on circulating immune complexes CIC in cases of infective endocarditis is meager. Mohammed et al. (15) demonstrated CIC in three out of five cases of endocarditis. In the present study, although raised levels of CIC were seen in all cases of endocarditis, binding greater than 10% was seen only in 18% of cases.

REFERENCES

1. Arnold, S. B., Valone, J. A., Askenas, P. L., Kashgarian, M., and Freedman, L. R. 1975. Diffuse glomerulonephritis in rabbits with *Streptococcus viridans* endocarditis. *Lab. Invest.* 32:681.
2. Boulton-Jones, J. M., Sissons, J. G. P., Evans, D. J., and Peters, D. K. 1974. Renal lesions of subacute infective endocarditis. *Br. Med. J.* 2:11–14.
3. Cabne, J., Godeau, P., Hereman, G., Acar, J., Digeon, M. and Francois, J. 1979. Fate of circulating immune complexes in infective endocarditis. *Am. J. Med.* 66:277–282.
4. Cole, P. 1975. The engima of infective endocarditis. *Hosp. Update* 1:128–138.
5. Creighton, W. D., Lambert, P. H., and Miescher, P. A. 1973. Detection of antibodies and soluble antigen–antibody complexes by precipitation with polyethylene glycol. *J. Immunol.* 111:1219–1227.
6. Elliott, S. D., McCarty, M., and Sancefield, R. C. 1977. Teichoic acids of group D streptococci with special reference to strains from pig meningitis. *J. Exp. Med.* 145:490.
7. Ganguly, N. K., Mohan, C., Sapru, R. P., and Kumar, M. 1977. T and B cell populations in the peripheral blood of rhesus monkeys. *Int. Arch. Allergy Appl. Immunol.* 53:290.

8. Gutman, R. A., Striker, G. E., Gilliland, B. C., and Cutler, R. E. 1972. The immune complex glomerulonephritis of bacterial endocarditis. *Medicine (Baltimore)* 51:1–25.
9. Hereman, G., Godean, P., Cabane, J., et al. 1975. Etude immunologique des endocarditis infectieuses subaigiues par recherche de complexes immune circulants. *Nouv. Presse Med.* 4:2311.
10. Hurwitz, D., Quismorio, F. P., and Friou, G. 1975. Cryoglobulinemia in patients with infective endocarditis. *Clin. Exp. Immunol.* 19:131.
11. Keslin, M. H., Messner, R. P., and Williams, R. C., Jr. 1973. Glomerulonephritis with subacute bacterial endocarditis. *Arch. Intern. Med.* 132:578–581.
12. Lachman, P. J., and Thompson, R. A. 1970. Reactive lysis: The complement mediated lysis of unsensitized cell 11. The characterisation of activated factor as C 56 and the participation of C8 and C9. *J. Exp. Med.* 4:643.
13. Laxdal, T., Messner, R. P., Williams, R. C., Jr., and Quie, P. G. 1968. Opsonic agglutinating and complement fixing antibodies in patients with subacute bacterial endocarditis. *J. Lab. Clin. Med.* 71:638.
14. Mancini, G., Carbonara, A. O., and Heremans, J. F. 1965. Immunochemical quantitation of antigens by single radial immunodiffusion. *Int. J. Immunochem.* 2:235–254.
15. Mohammed, I., Thompson, B., and Holborow, E. J. 1977. Radiobioassay for immune complexes using macrophages. *Ann. Rheum. Dis.* 36(Suppl. 1):49.
16. Moskowitz, M. 1966. Separation and properties of red cell sensitizing substances from streptococci. *J. Bacteriol.* 91(6):2200–2204.
17. Sapru, R. P., Ganguly, N. K., Sharma, S., Chandnani, R. E., and Gupta, A. K. 1977. Cellular reaction to group A beta haemolytic streptococcal membrane antigen and its relation to complement levels in patients with rheumatic heart disease. *Br. Med. J.* 2:422–424.
18. William, R. R., Jr., and Kunkel, H. 1962. Rheumatoid factor complement and conglutinin abberrations in patients with subacute bacterial endocarditis. *J. Clin. Invest.* 41:666.
19. Williams, R. C., Jr. 1958. Serum complement in connection with tissue disorders. *J. Lab. Clin. Med.* 52:273.
20. Zubler, R. H., Lange, G., Lambert, P. H., and Miescher, P. A. 1976. Detection of immunecomplexes in unheated sera by a modified 125 C1q binding test. Effect of heating on the binding of C1q by immune complexes and application of test to systemic lupus erythematosus. *J. Immunol.* 116:232–235.

Adaptation of the Organism during Long-Lasting Survival with a Total Artificial Heart

J[aromír] Vašků, P. Hanzelka, J. Černý,
J[an] Vašků, E. Urbánek, M. Dostál, P. Guba,
V. Pavlíček, Z. Gregor, V. Krčma, H. Janečková,
O. Šotolová, T. Sládek, B. Hartmannová,
E. Šotáková, P. Wendsche, L. Krček, P. Urbánek,
and M. Gregorová

Institute of Pathological Physiology
Faculty of Medicine
IInd Surgical Clinic
University of J. E. Purkinje
and
Research Center for Heart Support and Total Heart Substitution
Regional Institute of National Health
Brno, Czechoslovakia

Abstract. The present chapter is a report of the current status of our testing of total artificial heart (TAH) implants in over 50 calves. Our 50th TAH experiment was performed with the calf Hasan; the experiment lasted 150 days. The TAH used in this experiment was TNS-BRNO-II, made of polymethylmethacrylate with polyurethane diaphragm and valves. Basic physiological functions normalized very soon after surgery. Blood flow through the device gradually increased from 7.5 to 11.5–12.5 liter/min at the end of the experiment. Central venous pressure (CVP) increased to 2.0–2.5 kPa in later months; atrial pressures were automatically maintained at the same level, ca. 1 kPa on both sides during the whole experiment. Anticoagulant therapy kept the prothrombin time two- to threefold above normal. The experiment was terminated by a sudden impairment of the blood coagulation mechanism, marked GI bleeding, and acute cerebral anemic anoxia. Autopsy revealed no thrombi at the artificial valves; there was thick pseudo-neointima in the outer portion of the diaphragm; inlet orifices were clean, without traces of pannus on either side. There were no signs of infection of organs detectable by the autopsy, but bacteriological examination revealed *Klebsiella* infection. Another experiment with the TAH, no. 51, was started immediately after experiment no. 50 was terminated. The calf, named Dalibor, recovered very quickly from surgery and anesthesia; about 3 weeks after surgery, basic physiological functions were stabilized , and during the subsequent course there were no problems in postoperative care. The calf was anticoagulated with warfarin (Coumadin®) until the 102nd day when slight GI bleeding occurred, and the administration of warfarin was inter-rupted. Only antiaggregation therapy with dipyridamole (Curantyl®) and aspirin was used from that time. Dalibor survived for 142 days in full health and died of accidental causes. During the calf's survival period, its CVP oscillated between 3 and 2.8 kPa, and blood flow through the TAH averaged 13 liter/min. The technical equipment used in both these experiments functioned without the slightest disturbance. In both experiments, the internal milieu of the calves showed absolute adaptation and normalization of all basic parameters, especially in the second calf, Dalibor. A third calf, no. 52, Samson, of this group survived 104 days; the cause of death was diaphragm leakage in the right-hand pump. The longest survival to date was achieved in calf no. 53, Florian, which survived 155 days; the cause of death was microthrombembolization in the CNS. The last calf of this group, no. 54, Waldemar, survived 31 days; the experiment was terminated because of a thrombembolism into the superior mesenteric artery. The mean survival of our five calves that lived longer than 1 month was 116 days. During their survival time, the basic physiological functions of all of these animals were fully normalized; the calves gained weight, and their condition was very good. These facts have documented excellent adaptation of these animals to the TAH. The control and driving unit used in our experiments with the TAH is an apparatus produced in our institute and designated Chirasist TN 3.

Work on total artificial heart research was started by our research group in December, 1974. Our previous results have been published elsewhere (11,13,14). Published results from some leading centers have shown the possibility of maintaining a calf with the total artificial heart (TAH) in good condition for several months (1,5,6). Although in our first three groups of experiments the survival time of our calves did not exceed 2 weeks, in the present, fourth group we have been able to attain survival time of over 100 days in four calves. Our basic aim is to elaborate standard methods for preoperative preparation of animals, for implantation surgery, and for the postoperative regimen, which would be organized according to the basic needs of the calf's physiology.

The TAH was developed in our research centre in two directions. At first, we used hybrid devices made of polymethylmethacrylate with polyurethane valves and diaphragm. These devices, designated TNS-BRNO-I and TNS-BRNO-II, were used in our second and third groups of experimental animals, whereas TAH experiments in our first experimental group were performed with the Soviet TAH, KEDR. In two long-surviving calves, no. 50, Hasan, and no. 51, Dalibor, of our fourth group, as well as in calves no. 53 and 54, a polymethylmethacrylate device, TNS-BRNO-II, was used. An artificial heart made totally of polyurethane, designated TNS-BRNO-III, was implanted in the remaining calf of the fourth group, calf no. 52, Samson.

MATERIALS AND METHODS

The devices used in our experiments have been described elsewhere (2,3). Summarizing the essential technical data, the polymethylmethacrylate (PMM) total artificial heart TNS-BRNO-II consists of two ventricles, each consisting of a blood and a pneumatic (or gas) chamber (Figure 1). Between these chambers is situated a polyurethane diaphragm which is firmly fixed to the edge groove of the PMM ventricle. Every ventricle has inlet and outlet mouth pieces, with a polyurethane flap inlet and a polyurethane roof outlet valve. The tangential connection of the mouthpieces with the bottom of the ventricle ensures optimal streaming of blood inside the ventricle. Thus, the occurrence of dead angles is prevented, where the blood can stagnate and thus initiate thrombus formation. To the mouthpieces, the polyurethane quick connectors with polyester cuffs and vascular prostheses are fixed, the cuffs being sewn to the remnants of the biological atria. The maximum beat volume of this artificial heart is 100 ml. This type of TAH has been used in the long-surviving calves nos. 50 and 51.

Further development of our TAH led to the TNS-BRNO-III (Figure 2). This device does not differ in its basic construction parameters from the previous one but is totally made of polyurethane. The left ventricle of this TAH has a greater volume, 120 ml, whereas the right one is only 100 ml. This is very important from the point of view of more physiological regulation of TAH activity. This device was first implanted into calf no. 52, Samson.

Both types, TNS-BRNO-II and TNS-BRNO-III, can be implanted by the method of Olsen in which the biological outlet valves are preserved; the TAH is therefore equipped only with with artificial inlet valves (7).

These artificial hearts are driven by the pneumatic principle, using continuous electropneumatic transducers. The driving and control unit in this experiment, Chirasist TN-3, was of our own construction and consisted of control component RJ-TN3/01 and driving component PJ-TN3/01.

The calves used in the experiments of the 4th group were hybrids with essential components of the Holstein strain (no. 50, Hassan, no. 51, Dalibor, no. 53, Florian, and no. 54, Waldemar); one calf was a pure Danish red strain (no. 52, Samson). The detailed preoperative preparation is described elsewhere (12).

After anesthesia had been started, the chest was opened through a right lateral thoracotomy, with the fifth rib removed, and after heparinization, cardiopulmonary bypass was induced. The biological ventricle with the great arteries was cut off above the level of the arterial valves and proximal to the atrioventricular valve ring. Grafts were attached to each of the two ventricles and anastomosed by continuous sutures to both atria, aorta, and pulmonary artery. The atrial and aortic quick connectors were fixed to the mouthpieces of the ventricle, and the air was removed through the venting port. Left heart pumping was started to maintain the left atrial pressure slightly above atmospheric pressure. The connection of the right pump was carried out in the same manner, and the total pumping of both artificial ventricles was started. The duration of surgery varied between 3 and 3.40 hr; that of cardiopulmonary bypass was about 90–100 min. The following hemodynamic parameters were continuously followed: cardiac output by computation of the heart rate and the right pump stroke volume, right and left atrial diastolic pressures from the measurement of air pressure directly on both sides of the artificial heart, and further left and right driving pressures; CVP was measured by the direct method.

From the laboratory parameters, blood gases and acid–base balance were continuously followed using the Astrup analyzer. Further, WBC, RBC,

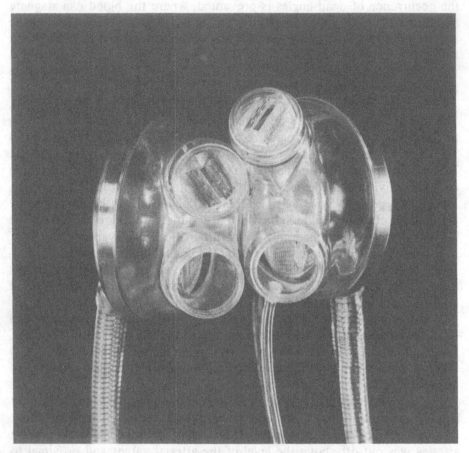

Figure 1.   Czechoslovak total artificial heart (TAH) TNS-BRNO-II made of polymethylmethacrylate. Left and right ventricles with inflow and outflow mouthpieces are shown. In the
outflow ones the polyurethane roof valves are clearly visible. Pneumatic driving tubes reinforced
with wire are connected to the pneumatic chambers.

platelets, Quick PT, PTT, factor VII, blood recalcification time (BRT), and
fibrinogen values were regularly estimated. Total and free Hb and Hct were
measured. Total serum proteins and protein fractions were estimated; blood
electrolytes, enzymes (SGOT, SGPT, LDH, and alkaline phosphatase),
blood glucose, lactate, creatinine, BUN, and total and direct bilirubin were
regularly estimated as well.

Biochemical components of urine, protein, bile components, and blood
were regularly estimated, and urine sediment was also examined regularly.

Regular laboratory estimation of these indicators has supplied a very
precise picture of all basic physiological functions important for the adaptation of the organism to the TAH.

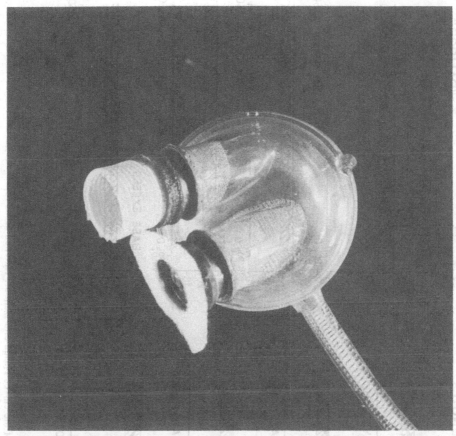

Figure 2. Left ventricle of the Czechoslovak TAH TNS-BRNO-III. The mouthpieces have quick connectors. The connectors are firmly fixed to the mouthpieces, and their polyester parts are prepared for suturing to the left atrium (circular cuff) and aorta (Lavsan aortic graft).

RESULTS

The Course of Experiment No. 50, Hasan

The calf recovered from the surgery and anesthesia within 8 hr. In the 42nd hour, the chest draining tube was removed, and anticoagulation therapy with warfarin (Coumadin®, aspirin, and Curantyl® (dipyridamol) was started, maintaining the prothrombin time on two to three times above normal for the whole experiment's duration. At the beginning of the third postoperative week, definite normalization of all basic physiological functions was reached. Until the 95th day, there were no serious problems in the postoperative regime.

The internal milieu, indicated by blood gases and acid–base balance, was completely within normal limits during the whole experiment. From the

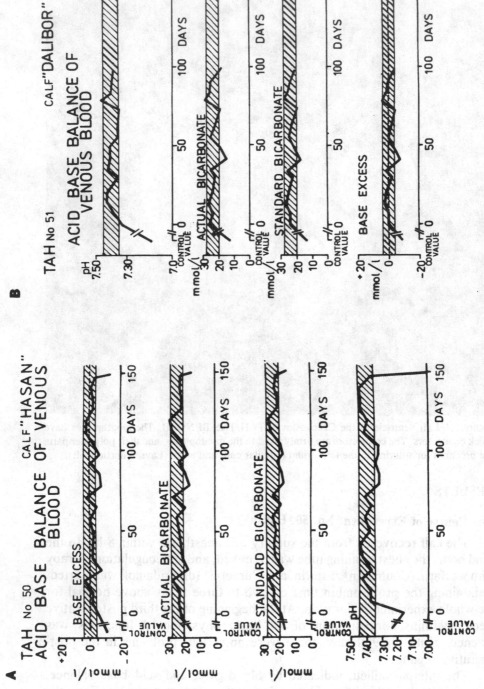

Figure 3.   Record of acid–base balance of the calves Hasan and Dalibor. Hatched areas represent normal ranges.

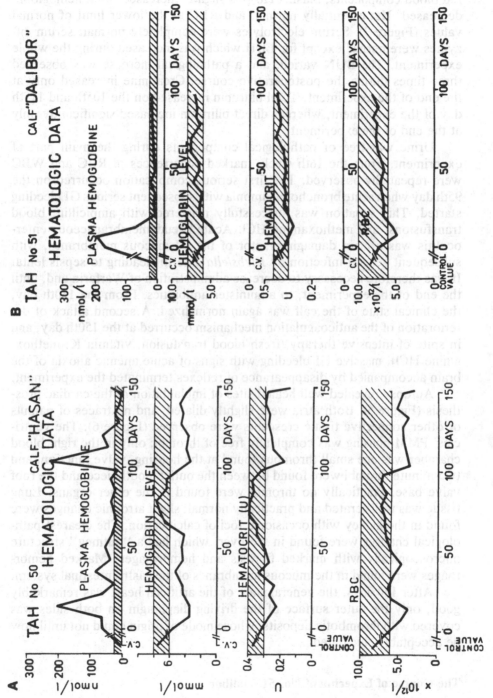

Figure 4.   Some hematologic data on the calves Hasan and Dalibor.

red blood components, plasma Hb was slightly increased, total hemoglobin decreased, Hct essentially normal, and RBC at the lower limit of normal values (Figure 3). Serum electrolytes were completely normal; serum enzymes were normal except for LDH which was increased during the whole experiment. The BUN varied, and a pathological increase was observed three times during the postoperative course. Creatinine increased only at the end of the experiment. Total bilirubin increased on the 105th and 115th day of the experiment, whereas direct bilirubin increased significantly only at the end of the experiment.

Urine was free of pathological components during the main part of experiment. From the 16th week, marked occurrences of RBC and WBC were repeatedly observed. The first serious complication occurred on the 95th day when acute bronchopneumonia with subsequent serious GI bleeding started. This situation was successfully mastered with ampicillin, blood transfusions, and methoxamine HCl. Acute pseudomembranaceous enterocolitis was a main damaging factor of the GI mucous membranes, with subsequent general infection by *Klebsiella* enteritis leading to sepsis lenta. It was therefore necessary to decrease administration of Warfarin and, until the end of the experiment, to administer antibiotics. From the 130th day, the clinical state of the calf was again normalized. A second attack of deterioration of the anticoagulation mechanism occurred at the 150th day, and in spite of intensive therapy (fresh blood transfusion, vitamin K, methoxamine HCl), massive GI bleeding with signs of acute anemic anoxia of the brain accompanied by disappearance of reflexes terminated the experiment.

Autopsy revealed well healed sites of implantation of the cardiac prosthesis (Figure 5). Both atria were slightly dilated, and no traces of pannus or other connective tissue crescents were observed (Figure 6). The ventricles' PMM housing was completely free of thrombi; only in the right blood chamber was one small thrombus found at the housing–valve junction, and two minute thrombi were found between the outlet mouthpiece and the roof valve base. Practically no thrombi were found in the other organs. Lung tissue was well aerated and practically normal; slight atrophic changes were found in the kidney with occasional foci of calcification. The clearest pathological changes were found in the liver, which had a "nutmeg" structure microscopically with marked fibrosis and hemorrhages. Marked hemorrhages were found in the mucous membranes of the gastrointestinal system.

After 150 days, the general state of the artificial heart was remarkably good; only the outer surface of the driving diaphragm on both sides was covered with thrombotic deposits, whose mode of origin could not until now be acceptably elucidated.

The Course of Experiment No. 51, Dalibor

In this calf, the same TNS-BRNO-II was used; the surgical procedure, preoperative care, and postoperative management of the calf did not differ

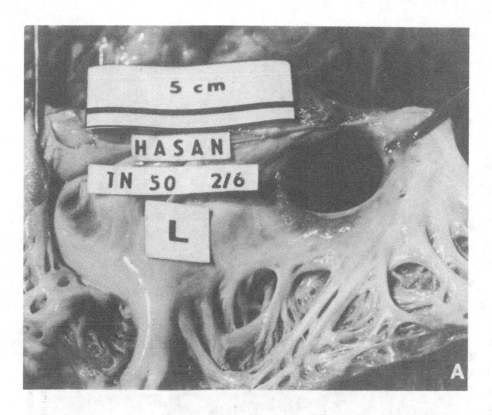

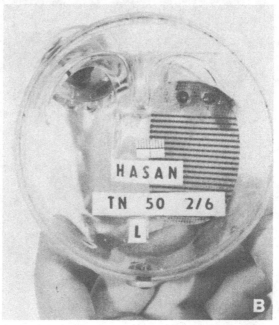

Figure 5.   Calf no. 50, Hasan. (A) Completely healed suture of the polyester cuff of the quick connector to the biological left atrium. No trace of pannus or other connective tissue crescents are visible in the atrial wall. Atrial trabeculae are slightly hypertrophied. (B) Inside of the blood chamber of the left artificial ventricle without the slightest trace of thrombi. The flap inflow valve, after 150 days of pumping, is preserved without any disturbance.

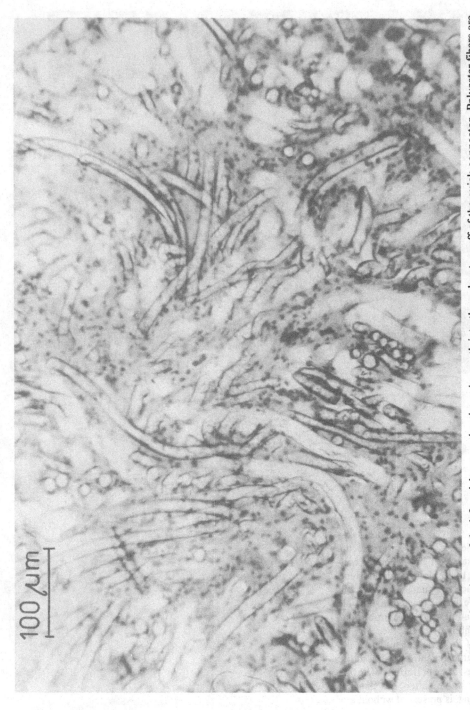

Figure 6.   Histological picture of the left atrial connective tissue ingrowth into the polyester cuff of the quick connector. Polyester fibers are encompassed by connective tissue cells and firmly fixed by collagen fibers. Hematoxylin and eosin stain. Calf no. 50, Hasan.

from that given the calf Hasan (Figure 7). The only difference was that the left ventricle was fixed to the chest wall. After implantation, it became obvious that the calf's chest was too narrow for the TAH dimensions, and compressive effects appeared in the right inflow tract. After fixation, the compressive phenomenon disappeared. The calf was anticoagulated slightly less then Hasan, maintaining a quick PT of 20–30%; from the 102nd day, because of slight GI hemorrhage, the administration of warfarin was completely interrupted. Until it died of accidental causes on day 142, the calf was in excellent physiological condition; all laboratory tests (as for Hasan) showed a fast and complete normalization of physiological and metabolic functions, and from the initial 73 kg at the time of surgery, the calf grew to more than 160 kg. The pumping frequency was about 130/min, and the flow rate about 13 liter/min; the vitality of the animal was remarkable. From the laboratory findings, only high serum LDH, elevated urine potassium, and low urine phosphorus excretion were remarkable. All other parameters were within normal limits.

The Course of Experiment No. 52, Samson

This calf had implanted the total polyurethane heart, TNS-BRNO-III. Its recovery from the surgery was remarkably good. The only complication until the 21st day of survival was diarrhea of medium intensity lasting several days. The calf was very reactive and sensitive, and its laboratory parameters were completely normal by the end of the second week. The calf died on day 104 as a result of leakage in the diaphragm of the right pump.

Driving and control regimens in calves 50 and 51 were practically the same, maintaining the left atrial pressures on both sides at the constant level of about 1 kPa using the automatic diastolic regulator.

The relative systolic time on the left side is variable; every systole has its optimal duration according to the blood volume filling the ventricle during the previous diastole. The duration of right systolic time is derived manually according to the function of the indication chamber.

The calf No. 52 had a somewhat different driving and control system. The peak systolic pressure was generally, in all experiments, 30–40 kPa on the left side and 10–20 kPa on the right side. In calves 50 and 51, CVP was gradually increased over the time of survival: in Hasan it was about 2.5 kPa at the experiment's termination; in Dalibor CVP oscillated between 2.8 and 3 kPa. We presume that the changes in the liver might have been caused by these CVP pressure elevations.

The Course of Experiments 53, Florian, and 54, Waldemar

Experiment no. 53 achieved the longest survival we have attained to date with the TAH: the calf, Florian, lived 155 days; the cause of death was microthrombembolism in the central nervous system.

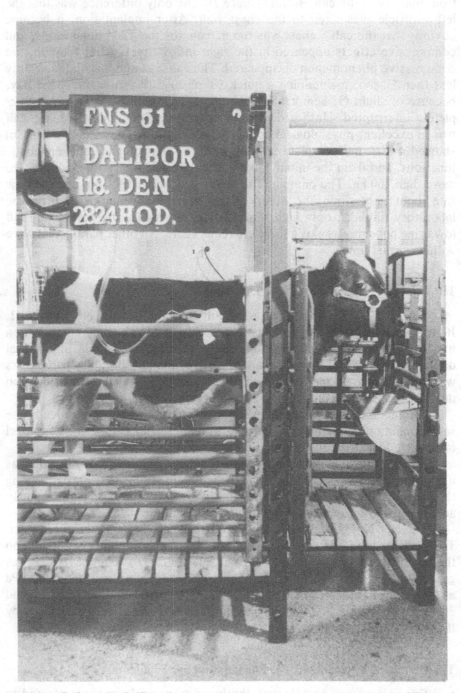

Figure 7.   Calf no. 51, Dalibor, in its special cage 118 days after implantation of the total artificial heart.

Calf no. 54, Waldemar, survived 31 days. This experiment was terminated because of a thrombembolism in the superior mesenteric artery.

DISCUSSION

These experiments are important contributions to our experience with long-term surviving calves with the TAH. Generally, we could confirm a number of problems that were pointed out in other places where this research is performed (4,8–10).

On the other hand, some observations, made by some authors, e.g., pannus formation in the atrium, could not be observed in our calf surviving 150 days. Also in the first 121 days of survival of a second calf, clinical signs of pannus (brisket edema, low output, high atrial pressures) could not be seen. Finally the autopsy revealed the medium size pannus formation in the left inflow port.

We started practical work on TAH in 1975, and until now we have performed 54 full experiments with TAH. We hope that we have contributed to the delineation of some basic laws that must be respected if the calf is to survive for a long time. Our two long-living calves (no. 50 and no. 51) were the only two cases in the world's research on TAH in which the polymethylmethacrylate device could achieve such long survival without the slightest generation of thrombi within the device (as was confirmed at autopsy). Further, we can point out an extremely dangerous combination of experimental accidents, i.e., infection with subsequent hemorrhage. Thrombi in the blood ventricles were found in the calf no. 54 and marked diaphragm mineralization on both sides, complicated with the secondary thrombotic deposits was observed in the calf no. 53.

We have also verified our system of individual driving and control of each ventricle using the diastolic regulator and have shown the variable systolic time on the left side to be a useful approach to the physiology of TAH regulation. We could further confirm the high stability and durability of our technical equipment, both the pump device and the driving and control unit. We will proceed further towards more precise physiological elaboration of TAH function, which would maintain as far as possible all basic vital functions of an animal in a completely normal equilibrium for the longest possible time of survival. In these experiments we have gained a great deal of new information which will be very useful in our further research on TAH.

REFERENCES

1. Fukumasu, H., Iwaya, F., Olsen, D. B., Lawson, J. H., and Kolff, W. J. 1979. Surgical implantation of the Jarvik-5 total artificial heart in a calf. *Trans. Am. Soc. Artif. Intern. Organs* 25:232–238.

2. Hanzelka, P., Krčma, V., Svoboda, P., Trbušek, V., Urbánek, P., Vašků, J[an], Vašků, J[aromír], Urbánek, E., and Dostál, M. 1980, BRNO-I, an implantable diaphragm-type artificial heart: Technical aspects of design. *Artif. Organs* 4:65–67.
3. Hanzelka, P., Vašků, J[an], Urbánek, P., Vašků, J[aromír], and Urbánek, E. 1979. Determination of cardiac output of the artificial heart from the drive air flow. *Artif. Organs* 3:277–278.
4. Hennig, E., Grosse-Siestrup, C., Krautzberger, W., Kless, H., and Bücherl, E. S. 1978. The relationship of cardiac output and venous pressure in long surviving calves with total artificial heart. *Trans. Am. Soc. Artif. Intern. Organs,* 24:616–623.
5. Lawson, J. H., Fukumasu, H., Olsen, D. B., Jarvik, R. K., Kessler, T. R., Coleman, D., Pons, A. B., Blaylock, R., and Kolff, W. J. 1979. Six month survival of a calf with an artificial heart. *J. Thorac. Cadiovasc. Surg.* 78:150–156.
6. Lawson, J., Olsen, D. B., Kolff, W. J., Liu, W. S., Hershgold, E. J., and van Kampen, K. 1976. A three month survival of a calf with an artificial heart. *J. Lab. Clin. Med.* 87:848–858.
7. Olsen, D. B., and Kolff, W. J. 1982. The total artificial heart. In: D. Liotta, and C. Cabrol (eds.), *Cardiac Surgery Today*, Maloine Editeur, Paris (in preparation).
8. Shaffer, L. J., Donachy, J. H., Rosenberg, G., Phillips, W. M., Landis, D. L., Prophet, G. A., Olsen, E., Arrowood, J. A., and Pierce, W. S. 1979. Total artificial heart implantation in calves with pump of an angled port design. *Trans. Am. Soc. Artif. Intern. Organs* 25:254–259.
9. Tsushima, N., Kasai, S., Koshino, I., Jacobs, G., Morinaga, N., Washizu, T., Kiraly, R., and Nosé, Y. 1977. 145 days survival of calf with total artificial heart (TAH). *Trans. Am. Soc. Artif. Intern. Organs* 23:526–534.
10. Vašků, J[aromír]. 1980. [Pathophysiological aspects of the present research state of the mechanical assisted circulation and of the total heart replacement.] *Bratisl. Lek. Listy* 73:649–661.
11. Vašků, J[aromír], Černý, J., Hanzelka, P., Dostál, M., Guba, P., Urbánek, E., Sládek, T., Urbánek, P., Šotolová, O., Krček, L., Vašků, J[an]. 1978. First experience with short and long term survival with the Czechoslovak TAH—TNS-BRNO-I. *ESAO Proc.* 5:99–103.
12. Vašků, J[aromír], Černý, J., Hanzelka, P., Vašků, J[an], Urbánek, E., Dostál, M., Urbánek, P., Guba, P., Pavlíček, V., Krček, L., Sládek, T., Hartmannová, B., Filkuka, J., Janečková, H., Šotolová, O., Šotáková, E., Doležel, S., Krčma, V., Cídl, K., and Bednařík, B. 1981. 150-Day survival of a calf with a polymethylmethacrylate total artificial heart: TNS-BRNO-II. *Artif. Organs* 5:388–400.
13. Vašků, J[aromír], Doležel, S., Černý, J., Dostál, M., Urbánek, E., Hanzelka, P., Vašků, J[an], Guba, P., Hartmannová, B., and Sládek, T. 1979. Changes in the monoaminergic innervation of the biological atrial remnants after implantation of TAH (Total Artificial Heart). *ESAO Proc.* 6:9–13.
14. Vašků, J., Urbánek, E., Černý, J., Urbánek, P., Dostál, M., Hanzelka, P., Dařena, F., and Sládek, T. 1977. Our first experiences with the total heart replacement by artificial heart. *ESAO Proc.* 4:380–408.

A Possible Mechanism of Adriamycin Cardiotoxicity

Inhibition of NADP-Linked Isocitrate Dehydrogenase

T. Minaga, M. Yasumi, K. Nakamura, I. Kimura,
A. Kizu, and H. Ijichi

Second Department of Medicine
Kyoto Prefectural University of Medicine
Kyoto 602, Japan

Abstract. In heart muscle, NADP-linked isocitrate dehydrogenase activity is particularly high when compared with that of the other representative NADPH-generating enzyme, glucose-6-phosphate dehydrogenase. Approximately 80% of cardiac NADP-linked isocitrate dehydrogenase activity originates in the mitochondria. Adriamycin inhibited the activity of both mitochondrial and cytoplasmic NADP-linked isocitrate dehydrogenase dose dependently but had no effect on glucose-6-phosphate dehydrogenase. The inhibition was kinetically distinguished as noncompetitive. Preincubation of crude cardiac enzyme preparations with adriamycin enhanced the inhibition time dependently for 45 min. However, there was no evidence to suggest that the metabolites of adriamycin produced in this system were active as inhibitors. Adriamycin-binding protein was fractionated by affinity chromatography, but NADP-linked isocitrate dehydrogenase activity was not detected in this fraction.

Adriamycin, an anthraquinone antitumor antibiotic derived from *Streptomyces peucetius var. caesius,* has been shown to be very effective against leukemia and many solid tumors (6,7,11). However, the clinical applications of this antibiotic have been limited by unfavorable side effects (8). Several hypotheses have been proposed to explain the mechanism of cardiotoxicity induced by adriamycin (15,23,26), but the precise mechanisms still remain unknown. It was reported recently that adriamycin cardiotoxicity was reduced by prior treatment with vitamin E. Myer suggested that lipid peroxidation was inhibited by vitamin E (21), and Folker demonstrated the increase in endogenous coenzyme Q_{10} by vitamin E (12). The relationship between vitamin E deficiency and muscular dystrophy is well known (14). Vitamin E deficiency induces a decrease of NADP-linked isocitrate dehydrogenase (ICDH) activity and a decrease of NADPH concentrations in the muscle (4,10). These findings prompted us to study the possible relationship of the depression of NADPH-generating systems to adriamycin cardiotoxicity.

In this chapter, we have demonstrated the effect of adriamycin on the two cardiac NADPH-generating enzymes, and we suggest that the inhibitory action against NADP-linked ICDH may be involved in the mechanism of cardiotoxicity of adriamycin.

MATERIALS AND METHODS

Materials

Male Wistar rats weighing about 200 g were used. Adriamycin and [^{3}H]-adriamycin were donated by Kyowa Hakko Co. (Tokyo). Thin-layer chromatography plates of silica gel 60 (layer thickness 0.25 mm) were obtained from E. Merck. Isobutyric acid, n-butyl alcohol, formic acid, ethyl formate, dioxane, and NH$_4$OH were of analytical grade. Cyanogen bromide, acetonitrile, DL-isocitrate-Na$_3$, glucose-6-phosphate, NAD, NADP, ADP, proteinase, and triethanolamine hydrochloride were purchased from Sigma Chemal Co. Sepharose 4B was obtained from Pharmacia Fine Chemicals, Sweden. A Shimadzu double-beam spectrophotometer (UV-210) was used for the enzyme assay.

Assay for Enzyme Activity

NAD- and NADP-linked ICDH activities were assayed according to the methods of Bert et al. (5) and Alp et al. (1), respectively. Glucose-6-phosphate dehydrogenase (G6PDH) was assayed as described by Gloch et al. (13).

Thin-Layer Chromatography

Adriamycin metabolites were investigated by TLC according to the method of Negishi and Takahira (22). Three different solvent systems were used: (1) isobutyric acid:NH$_4$OH:water (66:1:33), (2) n-butyl alcohol:dioxane:water (2:2:1), and (3) the upper layer of the mixture benzyl alcohol:formic acid:ethyl formate:water (4:1:4:5). Adriamycin and its metabolites were distinguished by the radioactivities from 1-cm cut sections of TLC plates.

Protein Determination

Protein was determined by the method of Lowry et al. (18).

Affinity Chromatography

Sepharose 4B was activated as described by March et al. (20), and then adriamycin was coupled to it. Tris HCl buffer, 10 mM (pH 7.4), and 0.2 M glycine buffer (pH 2.1) with 2 M NaCl were used for equilibration and elution, respectively.

Tissue Preparations

Rats were killed by decapitation. The hearts were dissected immediately and minced on ice-cold Petri dishes.

Twenty-percent homogenates were prepared by loose glass–teflon homogenization using 0.25 M sucrose. Mitochondrial fractions were then prepared according to the method of Hatefi et al. (16). Final mitochondrial pellets were suspended in 10 mM triethanolamine buffer (pH 7.4) and sonicated for 1 min at an amplitude of 6 μm. The sonicated fluids were used for the assay of both NAD-linked and mitochondrial NADP-linked ICDH activity.

Twenty-percent homogenates were prepared by Polytron at 4°C using 10 mM triethanolamine buffer (pH 7.5). These were sonicated under the same conditions as dscribed above and were used for the detection of total (mitochondrial plus cytoplasmic) NADP-linked ICDH activity.

Ten-percent homogenates were prepared by Polytron at 4°C using 0.25 M sucrose. These were centrifuged at 20,000 g, and the supernatants were used for G6PDH assay.

RESULTS

As shown in Table 1, heart muscle is a particularly rich source of NADP-linked ICDH when compared with liver, kidney, and skeletal muscle. Another NADPH-generating enzyme, G6PDH, showed little activity in these organs including heart muscle.

Cytoplasmic NADP-linked ICDH activity was estimated by subtraction of mitochondrial NADP-linked ICDH activity from the total (mitochondrial plus cytoplasmic) ICDH activity. The ratio of mitochondrial to cytoplasmic NADP-linked ICDH activity was 4:1 by protein basis. Adriamycin inhibited approximately equally both mitochondrial and cytoplasmic NADP-linked ICDH. Figure 1 shows that the total NADP-linked ICDH of rat heart was inhibited by adriamycin dose dependently. However, cardiac NAD-linked ICDH and G6PDH were not inhibited by adriamycin.

The inhibition of NADP-linked ICDH by adriamycin has been kineti-

Table 1. Comparison of the Activity of NADPH-Generating Enzymes in Several Organs (nmol/min per mg protein ± S.D.)

	NADP-linked ICDH	G6PDH
Liver	225.0 ± 52.0	21.0 ± 8.4
Kidney	360.0 ± 50.0	17.1 ± 2.4
Heart	1179.0 ± 29.0	5.6 ± 0.6
Skeletal muscle	76.0 ± 25.0	2.2 ± 1.1

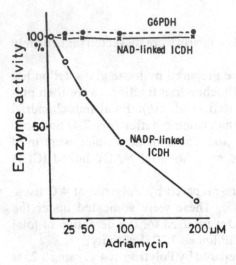

Figure 1. Dose-dependent inhibition by adriamycin of glucose-6-phosphate dehydrogenase and NAD- and NADP-linked isocitrate dehydrogenase.

cally distinguished as noncompetitive inhibition (26). The K_m value of cardiac NADP-linked ICDH is 66 μM for isocitrate and 30 μM for NADP, respectively.

Figure 2 shows that the inhibition of NADP-linked ICDH by adriamycin is enhanced by the incubation of adriamycin with the cardiac enzyme preparations before the assay of enzyme activity. In order to resolve the reasons for this, the following possibilities were considered.

The first possibility is that adriamycin metabolites formed during preincubation may be active inhibitors of ICDH. The same reaction mixtures as used in ICDH assay, containing the cardiac enzyme preparation preincubated for 30 min, were deproteinized, and the supernatants were developed by thin-layer chromatography using the three different solvent systems de-

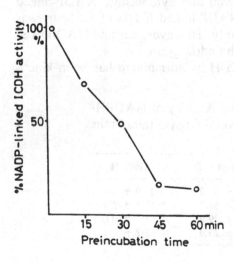

Figure 2. The enhancement of the inhibition by adriamycin of NADP-linked isocitrate dehydrogenase by increasing preincubation time with heart homogenate prepared as described in text.

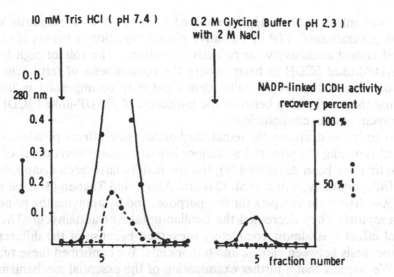

Figure 3.   Affinity chromatography of adriamycin.

scribed in Materials and Methods. However, metabolites were not detected in these systems.

The second possibility is that NADPH formed during the assay of this enzyme activity may react with adriamycin and produce the reduced metabolites (2). In order to exclude this, exogenous NADPH was added to the reaction mixtures, and the time course of NADPH concentrations was followed. As the optical density originating from NADPH was not decreased during the reaction time of the enzyme assay, this interference is unlikely, and these results suggest that adriamycin metabolites were not responsible for the inhibition of NADP-linked ICDH activity.

The third possbility is that NADP-linked ICDH may be inactivated during incubation by an interaction between adriamycin and the enzyme protein. Adriamycin-binding protein (19) from cardiac tissue preparations was isolated by affinity chromatography as shown in Figure 3, but NADP-linked ICDH activity was not found in the eluted binding protein, which had an affinity for adriamycin. Therefore, the adriamycin-binding proteins were also considered to be unrelated to the mechanism of enhancement of the inhibition by preincubation.

DISCUSSION

NADP-linked ICDH is present in both mitochondria and cytoplasm (5), whereas NAD-linked ICDH and G6PDH are located only in mitochondria (1) and cytoplasm (13), respectively. Cardiac NAD-linked ICDH and G6PDH were not inhibited by adriamycin as shown in Figure 1. However, NADP-linked ICDH, which had very high activity in heart muscle as shown in the table, was inhibited. NADH, the reduced form of NAD, is primarily used for the generation of ATP by oxidative phosphorylation, whereas NADPH is used almost exclusively for reductive reactions. The role of high levels of NADP-linked ICDH in heart, where the biosynthesis of fatty acid and steroid is less active, is not fully known but may be important in understanding the relationship between the inhibition of NADP-linked ICDH by adriamycin and its cardiotoxicity.

In order to decrease the lethal cardiotoxic side effects of adriamycin without reducing the powerful antitumor activity, newer derivatives of this antibiotic have been developed (9), but the results have been disappointing (17). Independently, Trout et al. (24) and Atassi and Tagnon (3) have used a DNA–adriamycin complex for this purpose, and by applying the principle of pinocytosis, they decreased the cardiac uptake of adriamycin. The cytocidal effect was almost completely preserved because of the differences in pinocytosis between cardiac and tumor cells. We confirmed these results (25). We suggest that a further examination of the essential mechanisms of cardiotoxicity and the reduction of cardiac uptake of adriamycin will lead to the reduction in cardiotoxicity.

ACKNOWLEDGMENTS

We wish to thank Academic Press, New York, for their kind permission to use figures from *Biochemical and Biophysical Research Communications* (26). We also thank Dr. W. G. Wilson, Medical Director, Japan Wellcome Co., for his help with the English manuscript.

REFERENCES

1. Alp, P. R., Newsholme, E. A., and Zammit, V. A. 1976. Activities of citrate synthase and NAD-linked and NADP-linked isocitrate dehydrogenase in muscle from vertebrates and invertebrates. *Biochem. J.* 154:689–700.
2. Asbell, M. A., Schwartzbach, E., Bullock, F. J., and Yesair, D. W., 1972. Daunomycin and adriamycin metabolism via reductive glycosidic cleavage. *J. Pharmacol. Ther.* 182:63–69.
3. Atassi, G., and Tagnon, H. J. 1974. Comparison of adriamycin with the DNA-adriamycin complex in chemotherapy of L 1210 leukemia. *Europ. J. Cancer.* 10:399–403.
4. Barry, T. A., and Rosenkrantz, H. 1962. The level of isocitric acid dehydrogenase in tissues of vitamin E-deficient rabbits. *J. Nutr.* 76:447–452.
5. Bert, E., and Bergmeyer, H. U. 1974. Isocitrate dehydrogenase. In: H. U. Bergmeyer, (ed.), *Methods of Enzymatic Analysis*, Vol. 2, pp. 624–627. Academic Press, New York.
6. Blum, R. H., and Carter, S. K. 1974. Adriamycin, a new anticancer drug with significant clinical activity. *Ann. Intern. Med.* 80:249–259.
7. Bonadonna, G., Monfardini, S., De Lena, M., and Rossai-Bellani, F. 1969. Clinical evaluation of adriamycin, a new antitumor antibiotic. *Br. Med. J.* 3:503–506.
8. Bristow, M. R., Thompson, P. D., Martin, R. P., Marson, J. W., Billingham, M. E., and Harrison, D. C. 1978. Early anthracycline cardiotoxicity. *Am. J. Med.* 65:823–832.
9. Crooke, S. T., Duvernay, V. H., Galvan, L., and Prestayko, A. W., 1978. Structure–activity relationships of anthracyclines relative to effects on macromolecular syntheses. *Mol. Pharmacol.* 14:290–298.

10. Dhalla, N. S., Fedelesova, M., and Toffler, I. 1971. Biochemical alterations in skeletal muscle of vitamin E deficient rats. *Can. J. Biochem.* 49:1202–1208.

11. Di Marco, A., Gaetani, M., and Scarpinate, B. 1969. Adriamycin (NSC-123,127): A new antibiotic with antitumor activity. *Cancer Chemother. Rep. [Part 1]* 53:33–37.

12. Edwin, E. E., Diplock, A. T., Bunyan, J., and Green, J. 1961. Studies on vitamin E. *Biochem. J.* 79:91–104.

13. Gloch, G. H., and Mc Lean, P. 1953. Further studies on the properties and assay of glucose-6-phosphate dehydrogenase and 6 phosphogluconate dehydrogenase of rat liver. *Biochem. J.* 55:400–408.

14. Gortner, R. A., Jr., and Milano, A. F. 1963. Effect of tocopherol depletion on muscle nucleic acid and creatine levels in the frog. *Am. J. Physiol.* 204:168–170.

15. Gosolvez, M., Van Rossam, G. D. V., and Blanco, M. F., 1979. Inhibition of sodium–potassium activated adenosine 5′ triphosphate and ion transport by adriamycin. *Cancer Res.* 39:257–261.

16. Hatefi, Y., Jurtshuk, P., and Haavik, A. G. 1961. Studies on the electron transport system. XXXII. Respiratory control in beef heart mitochondria. *Arch. Biochem. Biophys.* 94:148–155.

17. Kajiwara, H., Shimamoto, F., and Nakagami, K. 1980. Aclacinomycin cardiomyopathy. In: *Abstracts, 3rd Congress of Cardiac Metabolism, Kyoto, Japan,* p. 20.

18. Lowry, O. H., Rosenbrough, N. J., Farr, A. L., and Randall, R. J. 1951. Protein measurement with the folin phenol reagent. *J. Biol. Chem.* 193:265–275.

19. Lucacchini, A., Martini, C., Segnini, D., and Ronca, G. 1979. Evidence of soluble proteins binding adriamycin by affinity chromatography. *Experientia.* 35:1148–1149.

20. March, S. C., Parikh, I., and Cuatrecasas, P. 1974. A simple method for cyanogen bromide activation of agarose for affinity chromatography. *Anal. Biochem.* 60:149–152.

21. Myer, C. E., McGuire, W. P., Liss, R. H., Ifrim, I., Grotzinger, K., and Young, R. C. 1977. Adriamycin: The role of lipid peroxidation in cardiac toxicity and tumor response. *Science* 197:165–167.

22. Negishi, T., and Takahira, H. 1973. [The absorption, excretion, distribution and metabolism of adriamycin.] *Kiso To Rinsho* 7:425–431.

23. Olson, H. M., and Capen, C. C. 1977. Subacute cardiotoxicity of adriamycin in the rat. *Lab. Invest.* 37:386–394.

24. Trout, A., Campeneere, D. D., and De Duve, C. 1972. Chemotherapy through lysosomes with a DNA–daunomycin complex. *Nature [New Biol.]* 239:110–112.

25. Yasumi, M., Minaga, T., Nakamura, K., Kimura, I., Maeda, M., Yoneda, S., Kizu, A., and Ijichi, H. 1980. The studies on cardiotoxicity by adriamycin. In: *Abstracts, 3rd Congress of Cardiac Metabolism, Kyoto, Japan,* p. 19.

26. Yasumi, M., Minaga, T., Nakamura, K., Kizu, A., and Ijichi, H. 1980. Inhibition of cardiac NADP-linked isocitrate dehydrogenase by adriamycin. *Biochem. Biophys. Res. Commun.* 93:631–636.

Effects of Propranolol and Hydrocortisone Pretreatment on Radiation-Induced Myocardial Injury in Rats

M. R. Tajuddin, S. K. Johri, M. Tariq, and V. Ram

Faculty of Medicine
Aligarh Muslim University
Aligarh, India

Abstract. Earlier studies in our laboratory (23) showed evidence of dose-related acute injury to the myocardium after exposure of rats to ionizing radiation. Biochemical, histological, and electrocardiographic parameters were studied. In further continuation of this study, the effects of intervention by pretreatment with propranolol (10 mg/kg body weight) and hydrocortisone (10 mg/kg body weight) have been studied. The above drugs were administered to male albino rats weighing 150 to 200 g 30 min before exposure to 6000-rad single-dose γ radiation over the precordial area. The parameters observed were cardiac glycogen, serum enzymes, lactate, pyruvate, blood sugar, adrenal ascorbic acid, and histology of the myocardium. The beneficial effects of this procedure are discussed.

Radiation-induced myocardial injury has been reported (3,20) in patients undergoing radiotherapy for intrathoracic malignancies and carcinoma of the breast. Animal experiments have confirmed that structural, functional, and biochemical changes observed are proportional to the intensity of γ radiation (21). Reduction or reversal of the known injury pattern was the basis for assessment of the protective value of the drugs used in this study. This may be a useful and simple therapeutic preventative procedure in clinical radiotherapy.

MATERIAL AND METHOD

Male albino rats weighing 150 to 200 g were divided into four groups. Group I were normal controls. Group II were anesthetized with sodium pentobarbital, and the precordial region was exposed to a single dose of 6000 rads of γ radiation. Groups III and IV were anesthetized and given propranolol (10 mg/kg body weight) and hydrocortisone (10 mg/kg body weight), respectively, 30 min prior to exposing the precordial region to a single dose of 6000 rads of γ radiation. Anesthesia and drugs were administered intraperitoneally. The animals in groups III and IV were maintained on propranolol and hydrocortisone, respectively, for 72 hr, using the same dosage every 8 hr. They were then sacrificed, and blood, heart, and adrenal

255

glands were collected for biochemical and histological examination. Biochemical parameters studied were cardiac glycogen (12), adrenal ascorbic acid (16), blood sugar, (1), serum lactate and pyruvate (6,9), serum cholesterol (7,8,26), SGOT (15,25), and SLDH (24). For histology, light microscopy was done using eosin and hematoxylin stains. Previous studies (22) showed that an 8000-rad single-dose exposure produces irreversible necrotic changes 72 hr after exposure. In the present study, a single-dose exposure of 6000 rads was found suitable for production of acute and consistent reproducible injury 72 hr after exposure.

RESULTS

Histological changes (Figure 1) were studied in the myocardium of controls and of animals pretreated with propranolol and hydrocortisone. The changes observed in animals exposed to a 6000-rad single dose were cloudy swelling of myocytes, inflammatory response, and pericapillary mononuclear cell infiltration. There was significant reduction in inflammatory response in the hydrocortisone-pretreated group but no effect on the cloudy swelling of myocytes. Dilatation of capillaries was observed in the group treated with propranolol. The results of biochemical changes in the various groups are given in Table 1. The EKG changes in lead II were nonspecific in all groups, consisting of ST and T changes with tachycardia.

DISCUSSION

Propranolol acts by β-adrenergic blockade, reducing the harmful catecholamine effects (14) on hypoxic myocardium. Myocardial hypoxia resulting from radiation exposure (20) is accompanied by stress-induced catecholamine release. The resulting harmful effects mediated by β receptors are oxygen wastage, rapid depletion of carbohydrate energy stores, and release of cardiotoxic free fatty acid subsequent to lypolysis (2,14). Propranolol also acts as an antistress factor through higher centers, reducing anxiety which is a potent stimulus for catecholamine release.

Inflammatory edema, perivascular infiltration, and cell swelling are recognized features of acute radiation-induced myocardial injury (11,20). Hydrocortisone reduces inflammatory response by decreasing capillary permeability and reducing congestion. Cellular edema is reduced by the lysosomal stabilizing action of hydrocortisone (5). Lysosomal membrane instability in hypoxic states causes release of proteolytic lysosomal enzymes and cell swelling (5). These glucocorticoid properties are greater in dexamethasone and methyl prednisolone, but hydrocortisone possesses less antiinsulin activity. Adequate insulin levels act beneficially in hypoxic states (4) by facilitating glucose uptake by the cell and preserving carbohydrate energy stores by increasing phosphorylase activity. Insulin also reduces cAMP-mediated lipolysis, preventing release of cardiotoxic free fatty acid (2,14,21).

The histological changes observed in this study were caused by acute radiation injury as early as 72 hr following exposure of rat precordium to a single dose of 6000 rads of γ rays. There was edema of the myocardial fibers and pericapillary mononuclear cell infiltration, causing luminal narrowing and affecting intramyocardial pressure and perfusion. As suggested by Ellinger, two types of injury are probably involved: direct dose-related structural damage, which is not reversible, and indirect cell injury secondary to obliterative vascular changes, which can be prevented by pharmacological intervention. Hydrocortisone pretreatment produces a significant reduction in the inflammatory response but had no effect on the cloudy swelling of myocytes. This may either be because of ineffective lysosomal membrane stabilization in the dose range used or because of some other mechanism which is not lysosome mediated. It may be caused by the damaging effect of highly reactive free hydroxyl and hydrogen ions formed by ionization of cell water. Dilatation of the capillaries was observed in the propranolol-pretreated group, suggesting improvement in microcirculation, probably mediated by inhibition of the vasoconstrictive action of catecholamines. Propranolol also acts on the higher centers, reducing anxiety-induced stress, a property absent in cardioselective β blockers.

Cardiac glycogen levels were significantly depleted ($P < 0.01$) in the animals exposed to a 6000-rad single dose. There was a significant reduction in glycogen depletion ($P < 0.01$) or possibly conservation of glycogen stores in animals treated with propranolol compared to the untreated group. Hydrocortisone showed no glycogen-conserving effect. Glycogen is the main source of energy in the hypoxic myocardium (17,19).

Glycogenolysis is accelerated by stress-induced catecholamine release (18). Low levels of myocardial glycogen and impaired myocardial performance (23) are, therefore, the result of stress-induced catecholamine release and myocardial hypoxia. Propranolol block the catecholamine effect mediated via β receptors with simultaneous reduction in myocardial oxygen demand. Both actions result in conservation of glycogen stores, which is beneficial for myocardial function.

Adrenal ascorbic acid level were significantly depleted in animals after a 6000-rad single-dose exposure ($P < 0.01$), indicating significant stress. Animals treated with propranolol had a significantly reduced ($P < 0.01$) degree of depletion, indicating reduction of stress. The antistress action of propranolol might be mediated via higher centers which balance parasympathetic and sympathetic activity. Blood sugar levels showed a significant rise in group II compared with controls ($P < 0.01$). This is explained by stress-induced hyperglycemia (2,10) as a result of exposure to radiation. Catecholamine release in stress accelerates glycogenolysis by activation of phosphorylase (17). Adrenal glucocorticoids released in stress conditions also have a hyperglycemic effect. Propranolol-treated animals showed a

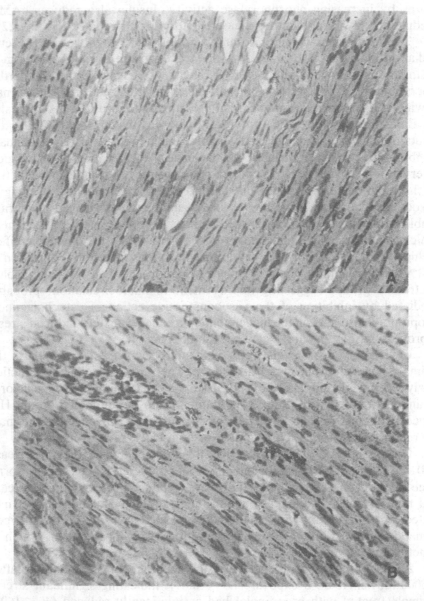

Figure 1. (A) Normal rat myocardium (group I). (B) Rat myocardium (group II) showing perivascular mononuclear cell infiltration and swelling of myocardial fibers. (C) Rat myocardium

significant reduction in the hyperglycemic response, possibly because of a reduction in glycogenolysis by the antistress action of propranolol.

Hydrocortisone showed no significant effect on hyperglycemia. This may be because of insufficient dosage with inadequate glucocorticoid activity coupled with adrenal suppression as a result of hydrocortisone administration. Serum cholesterol levels were significantly ($P < 0.01$) raised in

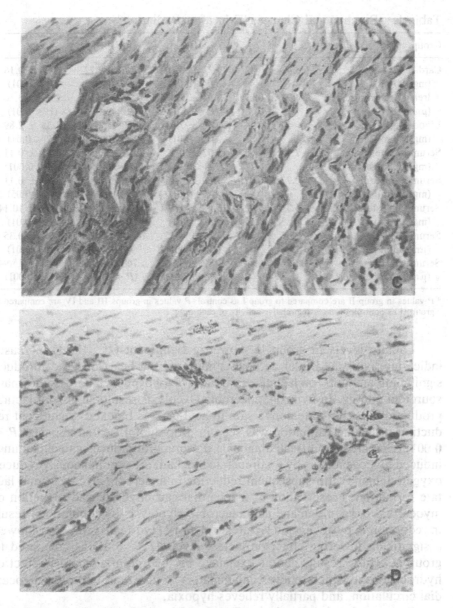

(group III) showing minimal perivascular infiltration; the myocardium otherwise appears normal. (D) Rat myocardium (group IV) showing perivascular mononuclear cell infiltration and edema of myocardial fibers. All are stained with hematoxylin and eosin, ×280.

group II. There is a direct correlation between stress and serum cholesterol levels (10,11). In the animals treated with propranolol, the rise in serum cholesterol was significantly ($P < 0.01$) less than that in group II, indicating an antistress activity of propranolol. Hydrocortisone-treated animals showed no significant change in serum cholesterol compared to group II.

Table 1.   Biochemical Changes 72 hr after Radiation[a]

Group	I	II	III	IV
Cardiac glycogen (mg/100 ml)	3.43 ± 0.12	1.23 ± 0.10 ($P < 0.01$)	1.56 ± 0.22 ($P > 0.05$)	2.14 ± 0.16 ($P < 0.01$)
Adrenal ascorbic acid (μg/mg)	4.74 ± 0.07	0.94 ± 0.07 ($P < 0.01$)	1.25 ± 0.14 ($P > 0.05$)	2.35 ± 0.10 ($P < 0.01$)
Blood sugar (mg/100 ml)	54 ± 0.14	151.50 ± 7.33 ($P < 0.01$)	89.50 ± 37.59 ($P > 0.05$)	53.33 ± 2.89 ($P < 0.01$)
Serum lactate (mg/100 ml)	7.76 ± 0.03	15.52 ± 0.12 ($P < 0.01$)	12.93 ± 0.57 ($P < 0.05$)	8.12 ± 0.11 ($P < 0.001$)
Serum pyruvate (mg/100 ml)	0.72 ± 0.01	1.60 ± 0.10 ($P < 0.01$)	1.76 ± 0.14 ($P > 0.05$)	1.30 ± 0.11 ($P > 0.05$)
Serum cholesterol (mg/100 ml)	145.33 ± 0.02	215.00 ± 17.61 ($P < 0.01$)	200.33 ± 8.26 ($P > 0.05$)	168.33 ± 10.14 ($P < 0.01$)
Serum GOT (μmol/min per liter)	9.37 ± 0.02	27.43 ± 0.35 ($P < 0.001$)	14.74 ± 0.37 ($P < 0.01$)	24.11 ± 0.35 ($P < 0.01$)
Serum LDH (μmol/min per liter)	324 ± 6.69	812 ± 8.91 ($P < 0.001$)	748 ± 20.08 ($P < 0.05$)	342 ± 15.94 ($P < 0.001$)

[a] P values in group II are compared to group I as control. P values in groups III and IV are compared to group II as control for assessing relative activity of each drug.

Lactate levels in group II showed a significant ($P < 0.01$) increase, indicating hypoxia. Under aerobic conditions, the heart does not produce significant amounts of lactate, as oxidative phosphorylation is the main source of energy. In hypoxia, anaerobic glycolysis results in greater lactate production, as pyruvate conversion to acyl-CoA is blocked. Significant reduction in lactate formation was seen in propranolol-treated animals ($P < 0.001$) compared to untreated animals. Propranolol reduces catecholamine-induced glycogenolysis by β-adrenergic blockade. It simultaneously reduces oxygen demand with subsequent reduction in anaerobic glycolysis and lactate formation. Preservation of myocardial carbohydrate and reduction of myocardial oxygen demand and anaerobic glycolysis by propranolol result in reduction in pyruvate and lactate formation. Hydrocortisone also showed a significant lowering effect on lactate levels ($P < 0.01$) as compared to group II. These results can be explained by the antiinflammatory effect of hydrocortisone which relieves inflammatory congestion, improves myocardial circulation, and partially relieves hypoxia.

Pyruvate levels were insignificantly ($P > 0.05$) raised in group II as compared to controls. There was no significant alteration in the pyruvate levels in group III and IV as compared to group II. The high lactate levels observed in group II indicate a rapid conversion of pyruvate to lactate, thus explaining the insignificant alterations in pyruvate levels.

Significant elevation of serum enzymes SGOT ($P < 0.01$) and SLDH ($P < 0.01$) was observed in group II compared to control, suggesting myocardial damage. Elevation of SLDH in group II was significantly reduced by propranolol ($P < 0.001$) and hydrocortisone ($P < 0.05$). The SGOT values were lower in propranolol- ($P < 0.01$) and hydrocortisone-treated ($P < 0.01$) groups compared to group II. This again is suggestive of protection from myocardial damage by propranolol and hydrocortisone.

The present study suggests that stress and myocardial hypoxia are the two major factors involved in radiation damage to the myocardium and that these can be considerably modified by pharmacological intervention with drugs. Propranolol beneficially alters the metabolism in the irradiated hypoxic myocardium by preserving glycogen stores, by reducing the stress; factor by acting on higher levels, controlling catecholamine release (13) and their damaging effect on the myocardium, and by relieving hypoxia by reducing catecholamine-induced vasoconstriction, resulting in improved microcirculation. Hydrocortisone reduces the damage caused by inflammatory edema and congestion, improves the microcirculation, and partially relieves hypoxia. It is difficult to assess any repair potential to the myocardium by pharmacological intervention in short-term experiments. The possible benefits of using these drugs prophylactically may be considered in patients undergoing long-term radiotherapy for thoracic malignancies in close proximity to the precordium.

REFERENCES

1. Asatoor, A. M., and King, E. J. 1954. Simplified colorimetric blood sugar method. *Biochem. J.* 56:44.
2. Bing, R. J. 1965. Cardiac metabolism. *Physiol. Rev.* 45:171–225.
3. Burch, G. E., Sohal, R. S., Sun, S. C., Miller, G. C., and Colcolough, H. L. 1968. Effects of radiation on the human heart. *Arch. Int. Medicine* 21:P230.
4. Calva, E., Mujica, A., Bisteni, A., and Sodi-Pallares, D. 1965. Oxidative phosphorylation in cardiac infarct. Effect of glucose–KCl–insulin solution. *Am. J. Physiol.* 209:371–375.
5. Dluhy, R. G., Lauler, D. P., and Thorn, W. T. 1973. Symposium on steroid therapy—pharmacology and chemistry of adrenal glucocorticoids. *Med. Clin. North Am.* 57(5):1155–1165.
6. Friedeman, T. E., and Greaser, J. B. 1935. The determination of lactic acid. *J. Biol. Chem.* 100:291–308.
7. Groover, M. E., Jeringan, J. A., and Martin, C. D. 1960. Variation in serum lipid concentration and clinical coronary disease. *Am. J. Med. Sci.* 237:133–139.
8. Hamarsten, J. F., Charles, W., Cathey, R., Remond, F., and Wolf, S. 1957. Serum cholesterol, diet, and stress in patients with coronary artery disease. *J. Clin. Invest.* 36:897.
9. Havel, R. J., Carlson, L. A., Ekelund, L. G., and Holmgren, A. 1964. Studies on the relation between mobilization of free fatty acids and energy metabolism in man—Effects of norepinephrine and nicotinic acid. *Metabolism* 13:1402.
10. Kinney, J. M., Long, C. L., and Duke, J. H. 1970. Carbohydrate and nitrogen metabolism after injury. *Ciba Found. Symp* 105–126.
11. Leaf, A. 1973. Cell swelling, a factor in ischaemic tissue injury. *Circulation* 48:455–458.
12. Montgomery, R. 1957. Determination of glycogen. *Arch. Biochem. Biophys.* 67:378–386.
13. Opie, L. 1980. Cardiac metabolism, catecholamines, calcium, cyclic AMP, and substrates. In: M. Tadjuddin, P. K. Das, M. Tariq, and N. S. Dhalla (eds.), *Advances in Myocardiology*, Vol. 1, pp. 3–20. University Park Press, Baltimore.
14. Rabb, W. 1944. Cardiotoxic substances in the blood and heart muscle in uraemia. *J. Lab. Clin. Med.* 29:715.

15. Reitman, S., and Frankel, S. 1957. A colorimetric method for the determination of serum glutamic oxaloacetic and glutamic pyruvic transaminases. *Am. J. Clin. Pathol.* 28:56–70.
16. Roe, J. H., and Kuether, C. A. 1943. The determination of ascorbic acid in whole blood and urine through the 2,4-dinitrophenylhydrazine derivative of dehydroascorbic acid. *J. Biol. Chem.* 147:399–407.
17. Scheuer, J. 1967. Myocardial metabolism in cardiac hypoxia. *Am. J. Cardiol.* 19:385–392.
18. Scheuer, J. 1972. Pathogenic significance of disproportion between myocardial oxygen supply and consumption. *Myocardiology* 1:721.
19. Smithen, C., Christodoulon, J., and Brachfield, N. 1974. Protective role of increased myocardial glycogen stores induced by propranolol. In: *7th Annual Meeting of the International Study Group for Research in Cardiac Metabolism, Quebec, June 18–21.*
20. Stewart, J. R., and Fajardo, L. F. 1971. Radiation induced disease: Clinical and experimental aspects. *Radiol. Clin. North Am.* 9:511.
21. Stewart, J. R., Fajardo, L. F., Cohen, K. E., and Page, V. 1968. Experimental radiation induced heart disease in rabbits. *Radiology* 91:814–817.
22. Stoner, H. B. 1958. Studies on the mechanism of shock. The quantitative aspects of glycogen metabolism after limb ischemia in the rat. *Br. J. Exp. Pathol.* 39:635–651.
23. Tajuddin, M. R., Kumar, S., Tariq, M., Tyagi, S. P., and Gupta, R. 1980. Effect of radiation on myocardial metabolism and structure. In: M. Tajuddin, P. K. Das, M. Tariq, and N. S. Dhalla (eds.), *Advances in Myocardiology.* Vol. 2, pp. 244–238. University Park Press, Baltimore.
24. Tajuddin, M., Tariq, M., Bilgrami, N. L., and Kumar, S. 1980. Biochemical and pathological changes in the heart following bile duct ligation. In: M. Tajuddin, P. K. Das, M. Tariq, and N. S. Dhalla (eds.), *Advances in Myocardiology.* Vol. 2, pp. 209–212. University Park Press, Baltimore.
25. Wroblesskl, F., and La Due, S. 1956. Serum glumatic pyruvic transaminase in cardiac and hepatic disease. *Proc. Soc. Exp. Biol. Med.* 91:569–571.
26. Zlatkis, A., Zab, B., and Boyle, J. A. 1953. A new method for the direct determination of serum cholesterol. *J. Clin. Med.* 41:486.

Inhibition of Vitamin D₃-Induced Vascular Calcification by Carbocromen

E. Schraven, D. Trottnow, and R. E. Nitz

Department of Medical Biological Research
Cassella AG, Frankfurt/Main, Federal Republic of Germany

Abstract. High doses of vitamin D_3 induce myocardial lesions, necrotic alterations, and calcification of the vascular smooth muscle, (Mönckeberg arteriosclerosis) (6). These effects are accompanied by an increased calcium influx into the wall of the aorta and mesenterial vessels (1). Prophylactic application of $MgCl_2$ nearly prevents this calcium overload, whereas KCl or calcium antagonists are less active. In our studies, the uptake of calcium-45 4 days after a single dose of vitamin D_3 (90,000 IU/200 g) was increased in rat heart and aorta by a factor of 3 to 7, and up to 30-fold in mesenterial vessels. Application of carbocromen (10 mg/kg b.i.d.) for 4 days decreases the vitamin D_3-induced radiocalcium uptake by 44 (aorta) to 67% (mesenterial vein), $MgCl_2$ (15 mmol/kg b.i.d.) by 46 (mesenterial vein) to 92% (mesenterial artery), and verapamil (5 mg/kg b.i.d.) by 15 (aorta) to 44% (mesenterial vein).

The pharmacology of vitamin D is closely related to calcium metabolism. In human beings, overdosage of vitamin D leads to kidney damage and Ca deposits in the tissue. In animal experiments, very high doses of vitamin D_3 induce myocardial lesions and the so-called Mönckeberg arteriosclerosis which is characterized by necrotic alterations and calcification of the vascular smooth muscle (6). These effects are accompanied by an increased calcium influx into the wall of the aorta and mesenterial vessels (1).

In 1969, Neville and Holdsworth (4) first suggested a possible involvement of cAMP in the vitamin D-mediated calcium absorptive mechanism. Since the cardioprotective agent carbocromen (chromonar) is also an inhibitor of phosphodiesterase, we studied the effect of this drug on vitamin D_3-potentiated Ca^{2+} uptake into the heart and vascular smooth muscle.

METHODS

The experiments were started by a single injection of 90,000 IU vitamin D_3 hydrosol/200 g body weight. Male Sprague–Dawley rats with a body weight of 200–220 g were used. The animals were kept on a standard diet and had free access to food and water. Drugs were given twice daily by a stomach tube during the first 3 days. On the fourth day, the animals received the last application of drug. Immediately after this, 20 μCi/kg $^{45}CaCl_2$ dissolved in Locke solution was injected intraperitoneally. Control animals were treated in the same manner with saline. Six hours after the application

263

Table 1.   Effect of Vitamin D_3 (90,000 IU/200 g) on the Incorporation Rate of ^{45}Ca in Rats[a]

	Control	Vitamin D_3
Right ventricle	0.64 ± 0.03 (38)	2.57 ± 0.28 (114)
Rest of the heart	0.57 ± 0.04 (38)	3.76 ± 0.46 (114)
Aorta	1.67 ± 0.05 (38)	7.38 ± 0.82 (114)
Inferior mesenteric artery	21.2 ± 2.5 (31)	31.1 ± 2.2 (108)
Mesenteric vein	8.99 ± 1.49 (38)	7.69 ± 0.75 (114)
Tibia	161.8 ± 9.3 (20)	52.4 ± 1.5 (53)
Skull	72.5 ± 3.7 (20)	31.4 ± 0.9 (53)

[a] Data are expressed in dpm(organ)/dpm(plasma) ± S.E.M.; number of animals in parentheses.

of $CaCl_2$ the animals were anesthetized with ether, blood was withdrawn from the right ventricle by puncture, and heart, vessels, and bones were dissected as quickly as possible. The cleaned material was weighed and dissolved in Lumasolve®. After addition of a toluol–ethanol scintillation cocktail, the radioactivity was measured with a Tricarbscintillation counter, and the uptake rate was calculated as dpm/g of tissue divided by dpm/ml plasma.

RESULTS

Table 1 shows the incorporation of calcium-45 in control and vitamin D-treated rats. In control animals, the uptake is lowest (0.64) in the heart

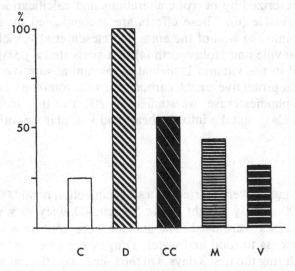

Figure 1.   Uptake of Calcium-45. Effect of carbocromen (10 mg/kg, N = 18) (CC), $MgCl_2$ (15 mmol/kg, N = 5) (M), and verapamil (5 mg/kg, N = 10) (V) on the vitamin D_3-induced (D) calcium overload in rat right ventricle. The effect of vitamin D_3 is defined as 100%; C is control.

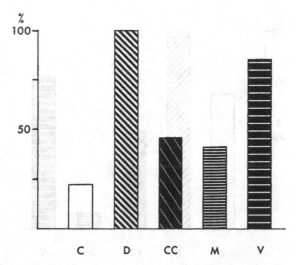

Figure 2.   Effect of carbocromen, MgCl₂, and verapamil on the vitamin D₃-induced calcium overload in aorta. Concentrations and abbreviations are as in Figure 1.

and highest (about 160) in the tibia. In the mesenteric artery, the radioactivity is more than 20 times higher than that in blood. Vitamin D increases the calcium uptake in heart and aorta four- to six-fold compared to control values. There was no effect in the mesenteric vein and a marked decrease in tibia and skull. Compared to the plasma radioactivity, there was a 30-fold increase of calcium-45 in the mesenteric artery under the influence of vitamin D.

In the right ventricle (Figure 1), carbocromen, MgCl₂, and verapamil produced similar responses. The effect of vitamin D was markedly reduced but not completely abolished. Verapamil was most effective, with a decrease of about 80%, whereas carbocromen reduced the vitamin D effect by 60%; MgCl₂ in a concentration of 15 mmol/kg caused a reduction of nearly 70%.

In the aorta (Figure 2), carbocromen and MgCl₂ produced the same effect as they had in the right ventricle. Both substances prevented the vitamin D-induced calcium overload by 57 and 75% respectively. It should be noted that verapamil, in contrast, decreased the vitamin D effect in this organ to only a small extent (19%). In the mesenteric vessels, the vitamin D effect itself was less pronounced than in heart and aorta. Whereas in the artery (Figure 3), vitamin D increased the uptake significantly but less than in the heart; in the vein (Figure 4) it had no effect.

In the mesenteric artery, MgCl₂ reduced the calcium uptake rate dramatically, and in the presence of carbocromen, the incorporation of calcium was also less than in control animals. Also, in these vessels, verapamil was less active than carbocromen and MgCl₂. It decreased the uptake, but this effect was statistically not significant.

In the mesenteric vein, carbocromen was most effective and reduced

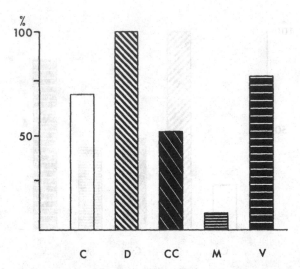

Figure 3.   Effect of carbocromen, $MgCl_2$, and verapamil on the vitamin D_3-induced calcium overload in mesenteric artery. Concentrations and abbreviations are as in Figure 1.

the uptake rate by 67%. $MgCl_2$ and especially verapamil were less active but showed the same tendency.

DISCUSSION

In the present study, it was shown that high doses of vitamin D remarkably increased the uptake of calcium into heart, aorta, and mesenteric

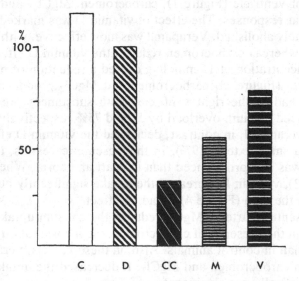

Figure 4.   Effect of carbocromen, $MgCl_2$, and verapamil on the vitamin D_3-induced calcium overload in mesenteric vein. Concentrations and abbreviations are as in Figure 1.

arteries. This effect could be at least partially antagonized by Ca^{2+} antagonists such as verapamil, by $MgCl_2$, and by carbocromen, a cardiotherapeutic agent. All of these substances were equipotent in heart muscle, but in vessel walls, the Ca^{2+} antagonist verapamil was much less effective than $MgCl_2$ and carbocromen.

These findings are consistent with those of other groups, mainly those of Fleckenstein (1,2), who also demonstrated that Ca^{2+} antagonists such as verapamil and $MgCl_2$ can antagonize the vitamin D effect. These authors claimed from their findings a protective effect of $MgCl_2$ and Ca^{2+} antagonists against deleterious Ca^{2+} overload induced by vitamin D. The same protective effect could be demonstrated for the cardiotherapeutic agent carbocromen. This drug hemodynamically has no Ca^{2+}-antagonistic potency but shows a number of other cardioprotective activities.

Scholtholt et al. (5) pointed out that carbocromen inhibits cardiotoxic side effects of digitalis glycosides, and Kipŝidze and Kikawa (3) demonstrated a marked reduction of the remaining scars after experimental infarction in dogs following oral treatment with carbocromen. Whether the protective effect of carbocromen, especially against overdosage of vitamin D, is related to its phosphodiesterase inhibition or to other metabolic effects of the drug remains to be clarified by further studies.

REFERENCES

1. Frey, M., Siegel, H., Janke, J., and Fleckenstein, A. 1976. Prevention of vitamin D₃-induced vascular calcification in rats by prophylactic treatment with $MgCl_2$. *Pfluegers Arch.* 365:R6.
2. Janke, J., Hein, B., Pachinger, O., Leder, O., and Fleckenstein, A. 1972. Hemmung arteriosklerotischer Gefäßprozesse durch prophylaktische Behandlung mit $MgCl_2$, KCl und organischen Ca^{++}-Antagonisten (Quantitative Studien mit Ca^{45} bei Ratten). In: E. Betz (ed.), *Vascular Smooth Muscle*, pp. 71–72. Springer-Verlag, Berlin.
3. Kipŝidze, N. N., and Kikawa, G. M. 1971. Die Wirksamkeit von Carochromen bei der oralen Behandlung und Prophylaxe des experimentellen Herzinfarktes. *Arzneim. Forsch. (Drug Research)* 21:1623–1628.
4. Neville, E., and Holdsworth, E. S. 1969. A "second messenger" for vitamin D. *FEBS Lett.* 2:313–316.
5. Scholtholt, J., Fiedler, V., Göbel, H., Nitz, R.-E., and Pötzsch, E. 1976. Wirkungen von Carbocromen auf toxische Digitaliseffekte. *Arzneim. Forsch. (Drug Research)* 26:876–881.
6. Selye, H. 1958. Prophylactic treatment of an experimental arteriosclerosis with magnesium and potassium salts. *Am. Heart J.* 55:805–809.

CARDIAC HYPOXIA, ISCHEMIA, AND INFARCTION

Mitochondrial Function in Normal and Hypoxic States of the Myocardium

J. R. Williamson and T. L. Rich*

Department of Biochemistry and Biophysics
University of Pennsylvania School of Medicine
Philadelphia, Pennsylvania 19104, USA

Abstract. The relationships among isometric tension development, the oxidation–reduction states of pyridine nucleotides and cytochrome c, and the oxygenation state of myoglobin have been assessed using the arterially perfused rabbit interventricular septum under different conditions of contraction rate, perfusate $[Ca^{2+}]$ and pH, catecholamine stress, and hypoxia. Hypoxia was produced either by decreasing oxygen availability with maintained flow (high-flow hypoxia) or by decreasing the flow rate (ischemia). Under normoxic conditions, increased work caused a fall of the cytosolic adenine nucleotide phosphorylation potential, $\Delta G_{(ATP)c}$, an oxidation of the pyridine nucleotides, and a reduction of cytochrome c; the opposite occurred with decreased work. Thus, the redox potential span from NADH to cytochrome c, ΔE_h, varied with the energy demand such that ΔE_h and $\Delta G_{(ATP)c}$ changed in the same direction. Under hypoxic conditions, all respiratory components became more reduced, and myoglobin was partially deoxygenated. The percentage change of developed tension under hypoxic conditions was approximately proportional to the percentage change of oxidized cytochrome c. When high-flow hypoxia and ischemia were compared at the same rates of oxygen delivery, the developed tension at any level of cytochrome c reduction was always lower with ischemia than with high-flow hypoxia. This difference was attributed to the low intracellular pH of ischemic tissue. Myoglobin deoxygenation was linearly related to cytochrome c reduction under all conditions of hypoxia, indicating steep oxygen gradients. The results support the concept of heterogeneous oxygenation of the tissue with mixed populations of aerobic and anaerobic mitochondria in the hypoxic state. In the full aerobic state, the control of mitochondrial respiration in situ appears similar to that of isolated mitochondria.

It is well recognized that aerobic metabolism is essential for the support of physiological levels of cardiac work and also for the eventual survival of the myocardium. Cardiac respiration is linearly related to cardiac work, and under fully aerobic conditions, complex relationships regulate the rate of ATP production to meet the tissue requirements for ATP utilization. In the intact heart, oxygen delivery is determined by blood flow through the coronary circulation. Autoregulation of the coronary flow occurs in response to chemical signals generated by the state of tissue oxygenation, but hypoxia develops when vasodilation has reached its limit, when the arterial perfusion

---

* Present address: Cardiovascular Research Laboratory, Department of Physiology, UCLA Medical Center, Los Angeles, California 90024, USA.

271

pressure falls, or with physical obstruction of an artery (2). Studies with isolated perfused rat hearts have shown that when oxygen supply is inadequate to meet the energy requirements for a given work load, coronary perfusion becomes heterogeneous, with relatively large unperfused anoxic zones appearing throughout the myocardium, although the surrounding tissue remains adequately oxygenated (26,28,29). Under these conditions, the heart as a whole may be considered hypoxic, and its work performance is suboptimal compared with the fully aerobic tissue.

Mitochondrial oxidative phosphorylation is the source of most of the ATP utilized for cardiac contraction. Energy for oxidative phosphorylation is derived from electron transport. According to the chemiosmotic theory of oxidative phosphorylation, the electron transport carriers are spatially arranged in the mitochondrial inner membrane such that protons are generated on the cytosolic C-side of the membrane and electrons on the matrix M-side (18). The net effect is an electrogenic efflux of protons and production of an electrical potential (negative inside) and pH gradient (alkaline inside) across the membrane. A large part of the free energy change associated with electron transport is thus conserved in the proton electrochemical gradient ($\Delta\bar{\mu}H^+$). This proton electrochemical gradient is thought to serve as a transducing mechanism which couples electron transport to ATP synthesis. ATP synthesized in the mitochondria is transported across the mitochondrial membrane for utilization by cytosolic energy-consuming reactions by an electrogenic exchange of external ADP^{3-} with internal ATP^{4-} via a specific carrier in the membrane. The driving force for this reaction is the membrane potential which favors entry of ADP^{3-} over ATP^{4-} and causes the extramitochondrial ATP/ADP ratio to be greater than that in the mitochondrial matrix (13). In well-coupled mitochondria, which have a low nonspecific permeability to protons, redox-linked electrogenic proton efflux is balanced by entry of electrogenic protons to drive the ATP synthetase and the adenine nucleotide translocator. Under these conditions, the rate of respiration is proportional to the difference between the thermodynamic driving force of the redox span across the three coupling sites and the thermodynamic back pressure exerted by the extramitochondrial phosphorylation potential (24,34,39).

There are relatively few studies concerned with mitochondrial function in the intact heart, and it has been questioned whether oxidation–reduction changes of mitochondria in situ behave similarly to those of isolated mitochondria when electron transport flux changes (11,12). Measurement of the oxidation–reduction state of the components of the electron transport chain provides one of the few selective, nondestructive techniques whereby mitochondrial function in the intact tissue can be investigated (4). In the present study, we have used the arterially perfused interventricular septum to study the relationship between tension development and the redox state of respiratory components under conditions of varied work load and oxygen supply.

METHODS

Studies were made with the arterially perfused interventricular septum from male albino rabbits (2–3 kg) as previously described (14,21). The perfusion medium contained 120 mM NaCl, 4.5 mM KCl, 1.2 mM MgSO$_4$, 1.2 mM KH$_2$PO$_4$, 28 mM NaHCO$_3$, 1.5 mM CaCl$_2$, 5 mM glucose, and 10^{-2} units/ml of insulin and was filtered through 8.0-μm porocity Millipore® filters prior to use. Perfusion fluid at 28°C was pumped through the cannulated septal artery at the rate of 6 ml/g per min unless otherwise indicated. The perfused septum was mounted vertically, and 5-mm light guides were positioned horizontally on both sides of the relatively flat muscle surfaces. A time-shared dual-wavelength spectrophotometer fitted with eight interference filters, allowing four separate dual-wavelength pairs to be monitored simultaneously, was used for light-transmission measurements (3). Light from a tungsten iodide source was alternately passed through appropriate filters located in a rotating disk. The transmitted light was conducted by a fiber-optic light guide to a photomultiplier and, after demodulation and amplification, was recorded on a multichannel recorder with a 5-sec time constant. The following wavelength pairs were used for optical measurements: 605–620 nm for cytochrome aa_3, 550–540 nm for cytochrome c, 560–577 nm for cytochrome b, and 620–587 nm for myoglobin. Changes of pyridine nucleotide fluorescence from the septum surface were monitored separately using a DC fluorometer constructed by the Johnson Research Foundation Workshop (3,8). Excitation light (366 nm) from a water-cooled 100-watt mercury arc lamp passed through optical fibers in a light guide positioned adjacent to the tissue surface, while fluorescent light (420–510 nm selected by secondary filters) and 366-nm reflected light passed through different fibers in the same fiber-optic light guide to two photomultipliers. Fluorescence changes were corrected for the small reflectance changes by subtraction of the respective signals (10).

RESULTS AND DISCUSSION

Effect of Tension Development on Mitochondrial Redox State

Figure 1 shows the responses of the pyridine nucleotide fluorescence and the corresponding absorbance changes attributed to cytochrome c, myoglobin, and cytochrome oxidase to a 4-min anoxic interval. Each of the parameters changed simultaneously and returned essentially to their original values on reoxygenation of the tissue. Isometric tension fell gradually by about 50% during the anoxic perfusion.

The redox potentials (E'_h) of the different respiratory chain components were calculated from the Nernst equation:

$$E'_h = E'_m + 2.3\, RT/nF \log \text{(oxidized/reduced)}$$

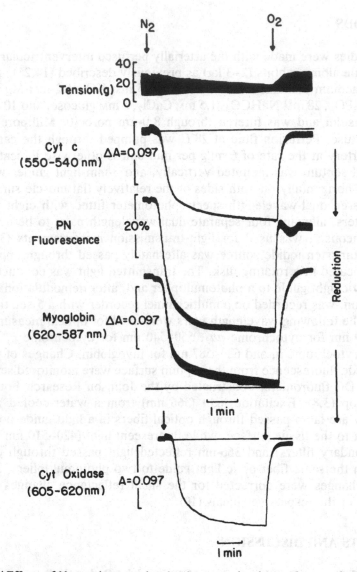

Figure 1. Effects of N_2 anoxia on tension development, absorbance changes of cytochrome c, cytochrome oxidase, and myoglobin, and fluorescence changes of pyridine nucleotides in perfused rabbit septum. The substrate was 1 mM pyruvate, and the contraction rate was 42 beats/min.

where E'_m is the condition-dependent midpoint potential. The ratio of oxidized to reduced component was determined for different metabolic states by separately measuring the absorbance change between the fully oxidized and fully reduced state. Figure 2 shows that oxidation of cytochrome c and cytochrome oxidase was achieved by addition of amobarbital (Amytal®), whereas reduction was achieved by the subsequent addition of cyanide. Changes of myoglobin absorbance were relatively small, indicating that artifacts introduced by the overlapping spectra of the different components were not a serious problem with the wavelength pairs chosen. Amobarbital caused a partial reduction of the pyridine nucleotides, with full reduction being obtained after addition of cyanide. Full oxidation of the pyridine nucleotides was achieved by titration with the uncoupling agent FCCP (data not shown). On the basis of these calibrations, it is estimated that for the perfused rabbit septum under aerobic conditions with pyruvate as substrate, cytochrome b is 60% oxidized, cytochrome c is 70% oxidized, and cytochrome oxidase is 80% oxidized (23).

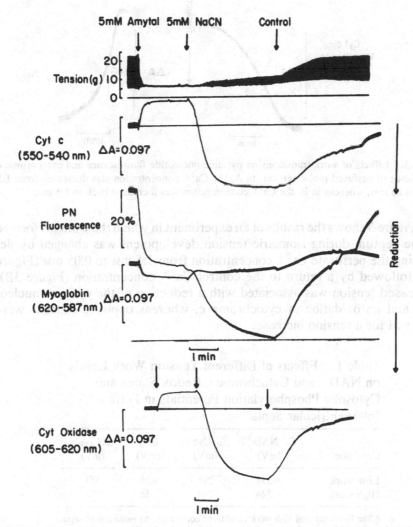

Figure 2.   Effects of amobarbital and cyanide on tension development, absorbance changes of cytochrome c, cytochrome oxidase, and myoglobin, and fluorescence changes of pyridine nucleotides in perfused rabbit septum. The substrate was 1 mM pyruvate, and the contraction rate was 42 beats/min.

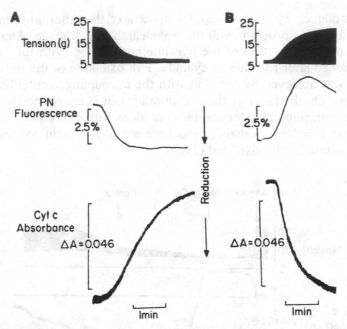

Figure 3.   Effects of work transitions on pyridine nucleotide fluorescence and cytochrome c absorbance in perfused rabbit septum. In A, the Ca^{2+} concentration was decreased from 1.5 mM to 0.05 mM, whereas in B, the Ca^{2+} concentration was increased back to 1.5 mM.

Figure 3 shows the results of an experiment in which the work performed by the septum during isometric tension development was changed by decreasing the perfusate Ca^{2+} concentration from 1.5 mM to 0.05 mM (Figure 3A), followed by a return to the control Ca^{2+} concentration (Figure 3B). Decreased tension was associated with a reduction of the pyridine nucleotides and an oxidation of cytochrome c, whereas opposite changes were observed for a tension increase.

Table 1.   Effects of Different Tension Work Levels on NAD^+ and Cytochrome c Redox States and Cytosolic Phosphorylation Potentials in Perfused Interventricular Septa[a]

Condition	E_h (NAD^+) (mV)	E_h (Cyt c) (mV)	ΔE_h (mV)	$\Delta G_{(ATP)c}$ (mV)
Low work	−331	295	626	553
High work	−326	232	558	538

[a] The low-work and high-work conditions correspond to perfusion of septa with 0.05 mM and 1.5 mM Ca^{2+}, respectively. E_h (NAD^+) was calculated using a midpoint potential value at 28°C and pH 7.4 of −337 mV. E_h (cyt. c) was calculated using a midpoint potential of 235 mV (5). $\Delta G_{(ATP)c}$ was calculated as previously described (28). Values are means for four separate experiments.

In Table 1, the redox potential span from NADH to cytochrome c (ΔE_h) for the conditions of low and high Ca^{2+} are compared with the cytosolic phosphorylation potential $\Delta G_{(ATP)c}$. The latter parameter was calculated as previously described (28). Increased work (tension development) was associated with the expected fall of the cytosolic phosphorylation potential. However, ΔE_h also decreased with an increase of work, indicating that a near-equilibrium relationship was maintained between the redox state of the respiratory chain carriers and the state of phosphorylation of the adenine nucleotides (7). Similar effects were observed when the isometric tension work was increased by altering the heart rate from 30 to 120 beats/min (22). The fact that the system is in near equilibrium, however, does not imply that regulation does not exist (c.f. ref. 7 and further discussion below).

The relationship between tension development and changes in the redox state of the pyridine nucleotides and cytochrome c is further illustrated in Figure 4. Tension was decreased by changing the pH of the perfusion fluid from 7.4 to 6.7. This was associated with a reduction of pyridine nucleotides and an oxidation of cytochrome c (c.f. Figure 3A). When the contraction rate was increased from 60 to 90 beats/min for 1 min at pH 6.7, developed tension increased, and there was an associated oxidation of pyridine nucleotides and reduction of cytochrome c. Since developed tension must be coupled with an increased rate of ATP utilization and oxygen consumption,

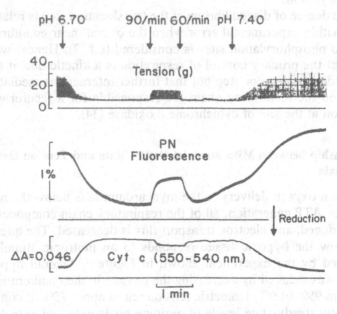

Figure 4.   Effects of acidosis on tension development, pyridine nucleotide fluorescence, and cytochrome c absorbance in perfused rabbit septum. The initial contraction rate was 60 beats/min, which was changed to 90 beats/min for 1 min during the interval shown in the figure. Acidosis was produced by increasing the percent CO_2 of the equilibrating gas mixture.

it is apparent that a reduction of cytochrome c occurs when electron transport flux increases. Other data show that the direction of the redox changes of cytochrome a and cytochrome oxidase was the same as that of cytochrome c (22).

The greatest loss of free energy in the respiratory chain is at the step of cytochrome c oxidase, and it has been proposed that mitochondrial respiratory control resides entirely at the terminal oxidation step (7,38). In support of this contention are the findings that the reactions of the respiratory chain between NADH and cytochrome c are in near equilibrium with the extramitochondrial phosphorylation potential and that flux through cytochrome c oxidase at high oxygen tensions is dependent both on the level of reduced cytochrome c and on the phosphorylation potential (38). The mechanism of energy coupling and flux regulation at the third phosphorylation site is not well understood (6,32,33). However, effects exerted by the extramitochondrial phosphorylation potential through the proton electrochemical gradient on ΔE_h in causing a reduction of cytochrome c, a, and aa_3 are clearly of importance in causing increased flux through the terminal irreversible step of the electron transport chain. Other studies (1,15,16) have concluded that during active mitochondrial respiration the intramitochondrial and extramitochondrial ATP/ADP ratios are not in thermodynamic equilibrium and that adenine nucleotide translocation across the mitochondrial membrane is rate limiting in the overall reaction of oxidative phosphorylation.

The degree of disequilibrium at the translocation step is relatively small and is within experimental error when the overall near equilibrium for the first two phosphorylation sites is considered (c.f. 7). Hence, we favor the view that the primary control of respiration is a kinetic one at the adenine nucleotide translocator step but that further interactions mediated through $\Delta\bar{\mu}H^+$ on the respiratory chain are responsible for a feedforward kinetic regulation at the site of cytochrome c oxidase (34).

Relationship between Mitochondrial Redox State and Tension Development in Hypoxia

When oxygen delivery to the myocardium falls below the needs of the tissue for ATP generation, all of the respiratory chain components become more reduced, and electron transport flux is decreased. The question arises as to how the hypoxic tissue responds to an inotropic stimulus. This is illustrated by the experiment shown in Figure 5. Overall hypoxia in the septum was induced by decreasing the oxygen in the equilibrating gas mixture from 95% to 9%. Isometric tension fell to about 75% of control values, while new steady-state levels of pyridine nucleotide and cytochrome c reductions and myoglobin oxygenation were rapidly achieved. Cytochrome c reduction increased to 30% of its anoxic value, pyridine nucleotide reduction to 80% of the anoxic value, and myoglobin became 25% deoxygen-

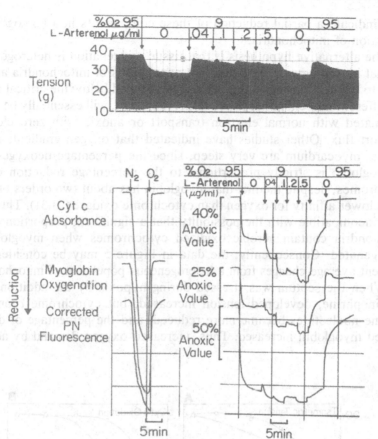

Figure 5. Effects of L-norepinephrine (arterenol) addition during hypoxic perfusion of rabbit septum on tension development, absorbance changes of myoglobin and cytochrome c, and fluorescence changes of pyridine nucleotides. Hypoxia was induced by decreasing the O_2 content of the perfusion fluid from 95% to 9% saturation.

ated. These are average changes for the total population of cells in the volume of tissue under observation.

The data can be interpreted from two points of view. In the first, the tissue oxygenation can be considered uniform, with all the mitochondria responding to the same oxygen tension. Cytochrome oxidase in vitro has a high affinity for oxygen, and the respiratory rate of suspension of cells or mitochondria is independent of oxygen tension above a few μM (17,20,30). When the oxygen tension falls below this critical value, the electron transport chain is oxygen limited, and the degree of reduction of the mitochondrial electron transport components becomes linearly dependent on the oxygen concentration (20,30,36). Consequently, partial reduction of the pyridine nucleotides and cytochrome c shown in Figure 5 during the hypoxic state could indicate a partial reduction of these components in a homogeneous population of mitochondria.

The alternative hypothesis is that tissue oxygenation is heterogeneous and that in the hypoxic state different populations of mitochondria are exposed to oxygen tensions either well above or well below the critical value. The different mitochondrial populations, therefore, will essentially be either oxygenated with normal electron transport or anoxic with zero electron transport flux. Other studies have indicated that oxygen gradients in the hypoxic myocardium are very steep, since the percentage deoxygenation of myoglobin is strictly proportional to the percentage reduction of the cytochromes, despite the fact that myoglobin has about two orders of magnitude lower affinity for oxygen than cytochrome oxidase (23,31). This finding is incompatible with the possibility that a significant proportion of the mitochondria contain aerobic oxidized cytochromes when myoglobin is deoxygenated. Consequently, the data in Figure 5 may be considered to represent average changes from a heterogeneous population of mitochondria.

When the septum was stressed during hypoxia by the addition of L-norepinephrine, developed tension increased, but cytochrome c and the pyridine nucleotides became more reduced, and the percentage of deoxygenated myoglobin increased. Thus, increased oxygen demand by aerobic

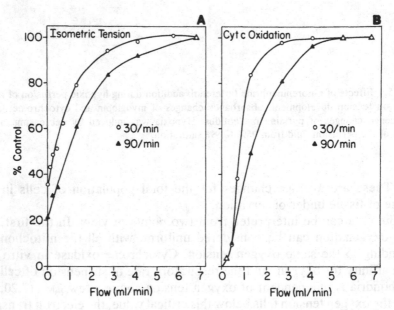

Figure 6.   Effects of varying perfusion flow rate on (A), isometric tension development and (B), cytochrome c redox state in perfused rabbit septum. The perfusion fluid was saturated with 95% O_2 and 5% CO_2, and the contraction rate was either 30 or 90 beats/min. Values shown are plotted as a percentage of the respective controls at the maximum flow rate of 7 ml/min. The septum was allowed to equilibrate for 4 min after each change of flow rate.

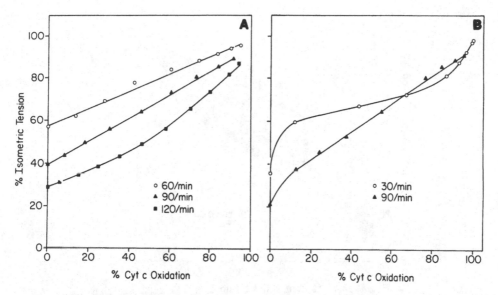

Figure 7.   Effect of contraction rate on the relationship between (A), tension development and (B), cytochrome c redox state in perfused rabbit septum. In A, hypoxia was induced by decreasing the percent O_2 of the gas mixture in equilibrium with the perfusion fluid while maintaining the flow rate of 7.1 ml/g wet wt. per min. In B, ischemia was induced by decreasing the flow rate as in Figure 8.

areas of the tissue was accompanied by a greater proportion of the tissue becoming anoxic.

Figure 6 shows the effect of stepwise decreases of flow rate on developed tension and percent cytochrome c oxidation in perfused septa paced at either 30 or 90 beats/min. When the flow rate fell below a critical value, tension development and percent cytochrome c oxidation both decreased. At the higher contraction rate, these changes both occurred at a higher critical flow rate, consistent with the higher control rate of respiration.

Similar relationships were observed when hypoxia was induced by decreasing the oxygen tension of the perfusion fluid while maintaining the flow rate constant. Figure 7 shows a comparison of the relationships obtained between percent change of isometric tension and percent change of cytochrome c oxidation with high-flow hypoxia (Figure 7A) and ischemia (Figure 7B) at different contraction rates. Except for the lower contraction rate with ischemia, essentially a linear relationship was obtained between the isometric tension and cytochrome c oxidation. For any given degree of hypoxia, e.g., when cytochrome c is 50% oxidized, the tension decreased with an increase of the contraction rate. Thus, at any given work load, the severity of hypoxia as determined by the cytochrome c redox state was approximately linearly related to cardiac function.

The comparative relationships between tension development and cytochrome c oxidation in high-flow hypoxia and ischemia for a rate of con-

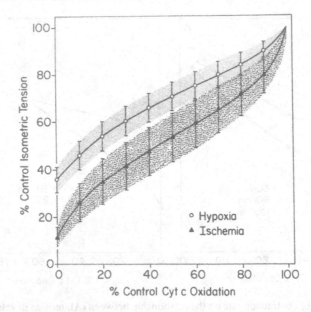

Figure 8.   Comparison of the relationship between tension development and cytochrome c redox state under conditions of high-flow hypoxia and ischemia in perfused rabbit septum. Relative levels of tension development and cytochrome c oxidation were calculated for the same rates of O_2 delivery during high-flow hypoxia or ischemia. Values shown are means ± standard error of the mean for seven muscles in each group.

traction of 90 beats/min are shown in Figure 8. Titrations with high-flow hypoxia and ischemia were made with the same calculated oxygen delivery rate for the two situations. It is evident that the quantitative relationship between tension development and cytochrome c oxidation is different with high-flow hypoxia and ischemia. Basically, for any given degree of reduction of cytochrome c, the tension is lower with ischemia than when the same

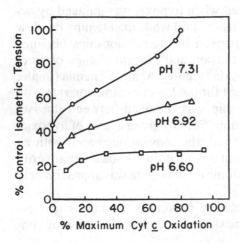

Figure 9.   Effects of pH on the relationship between tension development and cytochrome c redox state in perfused rabbit septum. The contraction rate was 90 beats/min, and the pH was decreased from the control value of 7.31 by increasing the percent of CO_2 in the gas mixture in equilibrium with the perfusion fluid.

degree of hypoxia is induced by deceasing the oxygen tension but leaving the flow rate unchanged. These data suggest that some factor other than oxygen delivery is inhibiting tension development during ischemia.

It is well known from a number of studies with isolated perfused hearts (9,19,25,27) that the intracellular pH falls to lower values during ischemia than when acid end products of metabolism such as lactate and CO_2 are removed by a relatively high flow rate of the perfusion medium. Furthermore, it is well know that respiratory acidosis causes a fall cardiac contractility (27,35). Figure 9 shows the relationship between tension development and cytochrome c oxidation with septa perfused at pH 6.6., 6.9, and 7.3 for conditions of high-flow hypoxia. At any given level of cytochrome c reduction, the tension development was inhibited by increased H^+ ion concentration. It is thus apparent that with increasing severity of ischemic hypoxia, as denoted by a decreased percent oxidation of cytochrome c, there is an accompanying fall of intracellular pH with its associated negative inotropic effect.

The present finding that the percent reduction of cytochrome c is approximately linearly dependent on the developed tension of the perfused septum over almost the entire range of cytochrome c reduction supports the suggestion that the cytochrome c redox state under conditions of varying hypoxia is titrating the number of anoxic cells or mitochondria in the tissue. This argument is reinforced by the fact that under all conditions of hypoxia, cytochrome c reduction was strictly proportional to myoglobin deoxygenation (23). In a recent study, Wilson et al. (36,37) observed a slowly increased reduction of cytochrome c when the oxygen tension was lowered to a critical value, which was compensated by a fall of the cytosolic adenine nucleotide phosphorylation potential. These authors claim that in intact cells reduction of cytochrome c is dependent on oxygen tension at all levels from air saturation and below.

An examination of the data presented by Wilson et al. (36) suggests, however, that considerably more experiments are required to establish this conclusion. First, no assessment of possible cellular oxygen heterogeneity caused, for instance, by inadequate stirring was made. Similar experiments with isolated heart cells in which the endogenous myoglobin oxygenation state was monitored simultaneously with the cytochrome redox state (23) showed that this was a problem with the cell concentrations reported by Wilson et al. (36). Second, the time response of the oxygen electrode was not compared with the time response of the cytochrome c measurements. Third, only total cellular ATP and ADP contents were measured rather than the cytosolic values. Because of the large difference between the cytosolic and mitochondrial ATP/ADP ratios, misleading conclusions can be reached when the total cell ATP/ADP ratio is assumed equal to the cytosolic ATP/ADP ratio (see 39). We conclude, therefore, that the apparent oxygen dependence of cytochrome c reduction observed by Wilson and co-workers at oxygen tensions above the critical value required for impairment of electron transport flux is caused by unrecognized oxygen gradients in the cell suspensions.

Data presented in this report support the concepts of steep tissue oxygen gradients and a defined critical tissue oxygen tension below which localized areas of anoxia occur identified by complete reduction of NAD^+ and cytochromes (23,26,29). Accordingly, hypoxia is visualized as a state of heterogeneous tissue oxygenation, or heteroxia. In contrast to other reports (11,12), it may also be concluded that the same principles govern the regulation of mitochondrial oxidative phosphorylation in situ as obtained in suspensions of isolated mitochondria.

REFERENCES

1. Akerboom, T. M. M., Bookelman, H., and Tager, J. M. 1977. Control of ATP transport across the mitochondrial membrane of isolated rat liver cells. *FEBS Lett.* 74:50–54.
2. Berne, R. M., and Rubio, R. 1979. Coronary circulation. In: R. M. Berne, N. Sperelakis, and S. R. Geiger (eds.), *Handbook of Physiology: The Cardiovascular System*, Vol. 1, pp. 873–952. American Physiological Society, Bethesda.
3. Chance, B., Legallais, V., Sorge, J., and Graham, N. 1975. A versatile time-sharing multichannel spectrophotometer, reflectometer and fluorometer. *Anal. Biochem.* 66:498–514.
4. Dutton, P. L., Leigh, J. S., and Scarpa, A. 1978. *Frontiers of Biological Energetics*, Vol. II, pp. 1341–1554. Academic Press, New York.
5. Dutton, P. L., Wilson, D. F., and Lee, C. P. 1970. Oxidation reduction potentials of cytochromes in mitochondria. *Biochemistry* 9:5077–5082.
6. Erecinska, M., and Wilson, D. F. 1978. Cytochrome c oxidase: A synopsis. *Arch. Biochem. Biophys.* 188:1–14.
7. Erecinska, M., Wilson, D. F., and Nishiki, K. 1978. Homeostatic regulation of cellular energy metabolism: Experimental characterization *in vivo* and fit to a model. *Am. J. Physiol.* 234:C82–C89.
8. Franke, H., Barlow, C. H., and Chance, B. 1976. Oxygen delivery in perfused rat kidney: NADH fluorescence and renal functional state. *Am. J. Physiol.* 231:1082–1089.
9. Garlick, P. B., Radda, G. K., and Seeley, P. J. 1979. Studies of acidosis in the ischemic heart by phosphorus nuclear magnetic resonance. *Biochem. J.* 184:547–554.
10. Harbig, K., Chance, B., Kovách, A. G. B., and Reivich, M. 1976. *In vivo* measurement of pyridine nucleotide fluorescence from cat brain cortex. *J. Appl. Physiol.* 41:480–488.
11. Hempel, F. G., Jöbsis, F. F., La Manna, J. C., Rosenthal, M. R., and Saltzman, H. A. 1977. Oxidation of ceregral cytochrome aa_3 by oxygen plus carbon dioxide at hyperbaric pressure. *J. Appl. Physiol.* 43:872–877.
12. Jöbsis, F. F. 1977. What is a molecular oxygen sensor? What is a transduction process? *Adv. Exp. Med. Biol.* 78:3–18.
13. Klingenberg, M., and Rottenberg, H. 1977. Relationship between the gradient of the ATP/ADP ratio and the membrane potential across the mitochondrial membrane. *Eur. J. Biochem.* 73:125–130.
14. Langer, G. A., and Brady, A. F. 1968. The effects of temperature upon contraction and ionic exchange in rabbit ventricular myocardium: Relation to control of active state. *J. Gen. Physiol.* 52:682–713.
15. Lemasters, J. J., and Sowers, A. E. 1979. Phosphate dependence and atractyloside inhibition of mitochondrial oxidative phosphorylation. *J. Biol. Chem.* 254:1248–1251.
16. Letko, G., and Küster, U. 1979. Competition between extramitochondrial and intramitochondrial ATP-consuming processes. *Acta Biol. Med. Germ.* 38:1379–1385.
17. Longmuir, I. S. 1957. Respiration rate of rat liver cells at low oxygen concentrations. *Biochem. J.* 65:378–382.

18. Mitchell, P. 1976. Vectorial chemistry and the molecular mechanics of chemiosmotic coupling: Power transmission by proticity. *Biochem. Soc. Trans.* 4:399–430.
19. Neely, J. R., Whitmer, J. T., and Rovetto, M. J. 1975. Effect of coronary blood flow on glycolytic flux and intracellular pH in isolated rat hearts. *Circ. Res.* 37:733–741.
20. Oshino, N., Sugano, T., Oshino, R., and Chance, B. 1974. Mitochondrial function under hypoxic conditions: The steady states of cytochrome $a + aa_3$ and their relation to mitochondrial energy states. *Biochim. Biophys. Acta* 368:298–310.
21. Rich, T. L., and Brady, A. J. 1974. Potassium contracture and utilization of high energy-phosphates in rabbit hearts. *Am. J. Physiol.* 226:105–113.
22. Rich, T. L., and Williamson, J. R. 1978. Correlation of isometric tension and redox state in perfused rabbit interventricular septum. In: P. L. Dutton, J. S. Leigh, and A. Scarpa (eds.), *Frontiers of Biological Energetics*, Vol. 2, pp. 1523–1532. Academic Press, New York.
23. Rich, T. L., and Williamson, J. R. 1982. Assessment of oxygen gradients in cells and perfused interventricular septum by optical techniques. *Am. J. Physiol.* (submitted).
24. Rottenberg, H. 1979. Non-equilibrium thermodynamics of energy conversion in bioenergetics. *Biochim. Biophys. Acta* 549:225–253.
25. Salhany, J. M., Peiper, G. M., Wu, S., Todd, G. L., Clayton, F. C., and Eliot, R. S. 1979. ^{31}P nuclear magnetic resonance measurements of cardiac pH in perfused guinea pig hearts. *J. Mol. Cell. Cardiol.* 11:601–610.
26. Steenbergen, C., Deleeuw, G., Barlow, C., Chance, B., and Williamson, J. R. 1977. Heterogeneity of the hypoxic state in perfused rat heart. *Circ. Res.* 41:606–615.
27. Steenbergen, C., Deleeuw, G., Rich, T., and Williamson, J. R. 1977. Effects of acidosis and ischemia on contractility and intracellular pH of rat heart. *Circ. Res.* 41:849–858.
28. Steenbergen, C., Deleeuw, G., and Williamson, J. R. 1978. Analysis of control of glycolysis in ischemic hearts having heterogeneous zones of anoxia. *J. Mol. Cell. Cardiol.* 10:617–639.
29. Steenbergen, C., and Williamson, J. R. 1980. Heterogeneous coronary perfusion during myocardial hypoxia. In: M. Tajuddin, B. Bhatia, H. H. Siddiqui, and G. Rona (eds.), *Advances in Myocardiology*, Vol. 2, pp. 271–284. University Park Press, Baltimore.
30. Sugano, T., Oshino, N., and Chance, B. 1974. Mitochondrial functions under hypoxic conditions: The steady states of cytochrome *c* reduction and of energy metabolism. *Biochim. Biophys. Acta* 347:340–358.
31. Tamura, M., Oshino, N., Chance, B., and Silver, I. A. 1978. Optical measurements of intracellular oxygen concentration of rat hearts *in vitro*. *Arch. Biochem. Biophys.* 191:8–22.
32. Wikström, M., and Krab, K. 1979. Proton pumping cytochrome *c* oxidase. *Biochim. Biophys. Acta* 549:177–222.
33. Wikström, M. F., and Saari, H. T. 1975. Conformational change in cytochrome aa_3 and ATP synthetase of the mitochondrial membrane and their role in mitochondrial energy transduction. *Mol. Cell. Biochem.* 11:17–33.
34. Williamson, J. R. 1979. Mitochondrial function in the heart. *Annu. Rev. Physiol.* 41:485–506.
35. Williamson, J. R., Safer, B., Rich, T., Schaffer, S., and Kobayashi, K. 1975. Effects of acidosis on myocardial contractility and metabolism. *Acta Med. Scand.* [*Suppl.*] 587:95–111.
36. Wilson, D. F., Erecinska, M., Drown, C., and Silver, I. A. 1979. The oxygen dependence of cellular energy metabolism. *Arch. Biochem. Biophys.* 195:485–493.
37. Wilson, D. F., Owen, C. S., and Erencinska, M. 1979. Quantitative dependence of mitochondrial oxidative phosphorylation on oxygen concentration: A mathematical model. *Arch. Biochem. Biophys.* 195:494–504.
38. Wilson, D. F., Owen, C. S., and Holian, A. 1977. Control of mitochondrial respiration: A quantitative evaluation of the roles of cytochrome *c* and oxygen. *Arch. Biochem. Biophys.* 182:749–762.
39. Van der Meer, R., Akerboom, T. P. M., Groen, A. K., and Tager, J. M. 1978. Relationship between oxygen uptake of perfused rat liver cells and the cytosolic phosphorylation state calculated from indicator metabolites and a redetermined equilibrium constant. *Eur. J. Biochem.* 84:421–428.

Cardiac Synthesis and Degradation of Pyridine Nucleotides and the Level of Energy-Rich Phosphates Influenced by Various Precursors

M. Siess, U. Delabar, and H. J. Seifart

Department of Pharmacology
Faculty of Medicine
University of Tübingen
D-7400 Tübingen, Federal Republic of Germany

Abstract. This chapter is concerned with the question of whether under normoxic and anoxic conditions the myocardial concentrations of pyridine nucleotides (NAD, NADP), adenine nucleotides (AN), and creatine phosphate (CP) can be influenced by addition of various precursors of these compounds to the perfusion solution in order to improve anoxic survival of cardiac cells. After i.p. injection of 10 mmol nicotinamide/kg guinea pig, a NAD level increased by 40–58% can be observed for a period of 12–24 hr, but there is no change in the AN and CP concentrations. In isolated atria of guinea pigs under normoxic conditions, the atrial concentration of NAD increases threefold over a 24-hr period if 10–20 mM nicotinamide is added to the Krebs–Henseleit solution with 15 mM glucose. Analysis of metabolites after incubation with 20 mM [^{14}C]nicotinamide showed that this increase resulted from new synthesis of NAD by activation of the nicotinamidase that deamidates nicotinamide to nicotinic acid via the Preiss–Handler pathway. Simultaneously, the high concentration of nicotinamide inhibits the degradation of NAD by the glycohydrolase. However, a high concentration of nicotinamide also impairs the new synthesis of AN from adenine and ribose in the salvage pathway. The anoxic degradation of NAD could be protected, compared with controls, by this high nicotinamide concentration. After aerobic incubation with 10 μM [^{14}C]nicotinamide, no deamidation to nicotinic acid could be observed, and a small but significant incorporation into NAD by the Dietrich pathway could be measured. This pathway is obviously located in the mitochondria. No increased NAD concentration could be observed, and in anoxia there was no protective effect. With 10 μM [^{14}C]nicotinic acid, a twofold higher synthesis of [^{14}C]-NAD could be observed than is seen with 10 μM [^{14}C]nicotinamide. Here, the Preiss–Handler pathway was operating for NAD synthesis. The glycohydrolase was not inhibited as observed with 20 mM nicotinamide. The total NAD level increased by 42%. The degradation of [^{14}C]-NAD to [^{14}C]-nicotinamide (N_{am}) could be observed in atria as well after its penetration in the nutritive solution. [^{14}C]Nicotinamide was also used for new synthesis of mitochondrial NAD via the Dietrich pathway. Therefore, we assume that the physiological precursor for cardiac NAD synthesis is nicotinic acid. Higher concentrations of nicotinic acid (50 μM) together with adenine and ribose significantly enhanced the total NAD level under aerobic conditions by 77%, ATP by 37%, and AN by 24% during a 24-hr period. Adenine (100 μM) and ribose (500 μM) increased the ATP and AN level in the same range under these conditions. Low concentrations of nicotinamide and nicotinic acid have little effect on the change of anoxic NAD concentration which is shifted to NADH or degraded. The anoxic loss of AN can be protected effectively only if the PRPP pool and the ATP pool have not been decreased to a great degree in the myocardial cell. Standstill before anoxic conditions are started or strongly reduced cardiac work (30 beats/min) in the anoxia test reported can save ATP by 70% through unrestricted anaerobic glycolysis during a 2-hr anoxic period, as compared with the aerobic values. In contrast, in spontaneously beating atria with a high frequency of 200 beats/min when anoxia was started, after 2 hr of anoxia the ATP level decreased strongly to 23%. The addition of adenine (100 μM) and ribose (500 μM) during anoxia produced only a weak but significant protective effect, whereas with higher anoxic ATP values in the anoxia test, the ATP and AN concentrations could be protected with concentrations of ribose (15 mM) and adenine (0.1 mM) comparable to the aerobic values. No protection of CP could be obtained by addition of CP(5–10 mM) or precursors during the 2-hr anoxic period. Therefore, strongly reduced contractile work or cardiac arrest before anoxic conditions are started, as most energy protective effect, may be beneficial for anoxic myocardial survival combined with addition of AN and NAD precursors to myocardial perfusion solutions during cardioplegia.

Cardiac energy metabolism is based on the biological oxidation of free fatty acids, glucose, and lactate as the main substrates for ATP production in the different steps of energy coupling in the respiratory chain localized in the mitochondria; NAD is a regulating link at the entrance to this chain (31).

NAD serves as a coenzyme of the various dehydrogenases located in mitochondria or in the cytosol, its most important role being that of a hydrogen acceptor in the fatty acid oxidation spiral and in aerobic glycolysis (17).

Under anoxic conditions, anaerobic glycolysis producing lactate serves as the only source of energy for the survival of the cardiac muscle cell. It has been shown by many scientists (17) that cytosolic NAD is the most important limiting factor in anaerobic glycolysis, and as long as lactate can leave the cell and NADH is oxidized to NAD, we can observe, as a reverse Pasteur effect, a 6- to 20-fold increased anaerobic glucose consumption with a considerably increased anaerobic ATP production rate (9,17,28). This can prolong the anaerobic survival of the heart in standstill. We have also observed under special conditions a long-lasting strongly reduced anoxic contractile activity in an anoxia test, as reported elsewhere (29).

Under aerobic conditions the concentrations of pyridine nucleotides, adenine nucleotides (AN), and creatine phosphate (CP) are in equilibrium with the mechanical work of contraction and the energy production. The energy supply by oxidation of substrates is regulated by the ATP/ADP quotient in the mitochondria as well as the ratio of NADH to NAD, which is correlated with the lactate/pyruvate quotient. However, under extreme metabolic situations such as anoxia, ischemia, or a pharmacologically induced disproportion between an increased cardiac work and the oxygen supply, an enhanced degradation of these important compounds is observed if they can not be sufficiently rapidly synthesized during energy deficiency. Metabolites of pyridine nucleotides, AN, and CP as well as various enzymes are leaking out through the cell membrane with detrimental effects for cardiac cell survival, as has been reported by G. Rona, M. Boutet, and I. Hüttner (this volume). It therefore seems reasonable to study possible ways of avoiding the leakage of these most important compounds for energy metabolism during energy deficiency.

The first possibility to be mentioned is the adaption of cardiac work to

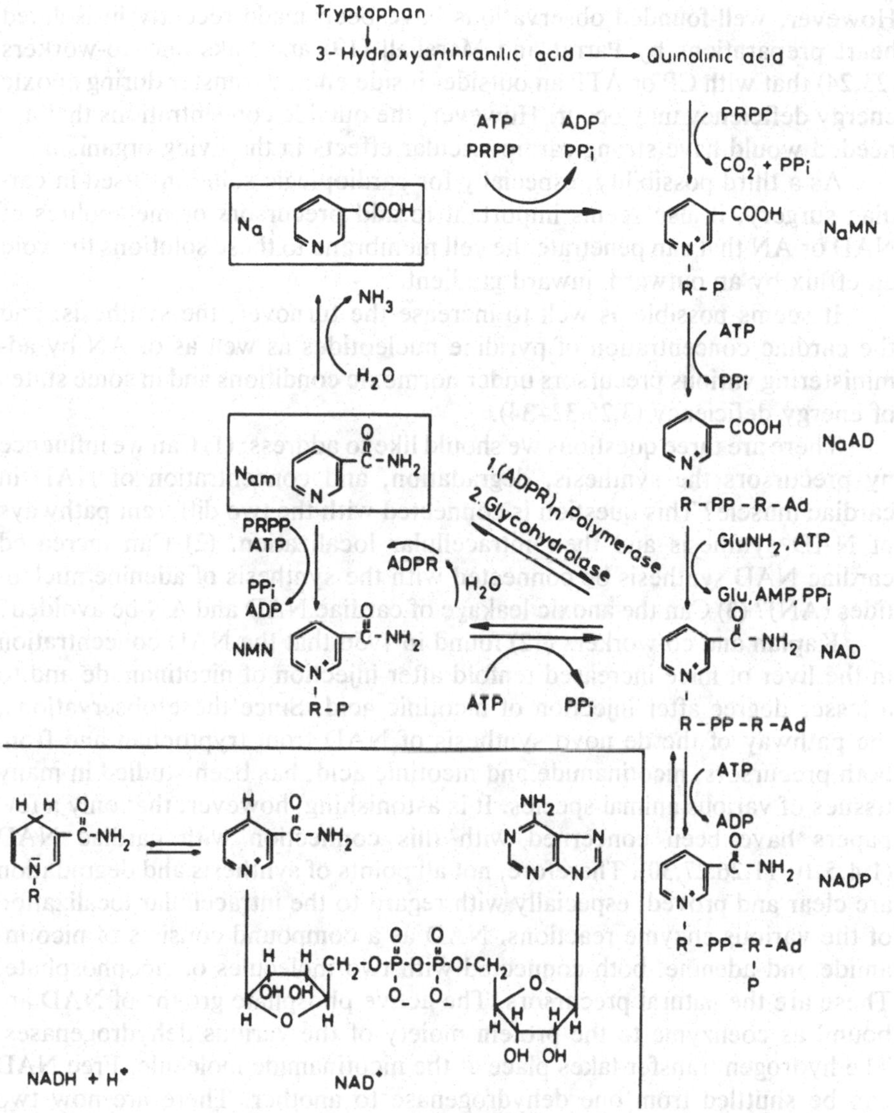

Tryptophan
↓
3-Hydroxyanthranilic acid ⟶ Quinolinic acid

ATP   ADP
PRPP   PPi

PRPP

CO_2 + PPi

N_a —COOH

N_aMN —COOH
R-P

ATP
PPi

N_aAD —COOH
R-PP-R-Ad

NH_3
H_2O

N_{am} C-NH₂

1.(ADPR)n Polymerase
2. Glycohydrolase

GluNH₂, ATP
Glu, AMP, PPi

PRPP
ATP
PPi
ADP

ADPR H_2O

NMN C-NH₂
R-P

ATP   PPi

NAD C-NH₂
R-PP-R-Ad

ATP
ADP

NADP C-NH₂
R-PP-R-Ad
P

NADH + H⁺   NAD⁺

CH₂-O-P-O-P-O-CH₂

Figure 1. Pathways of NAD synthesis and degradation. The abbreviations used are: N_{am}, nicotinamide; N_a, nicotinic acid; NMN, nicotinamide mononucleotide; NAD, nicotinamide adenine dinucleotide; NADP, nicotinamide adenine dinucleotide phosphate; N_aMN, nicotinic acid mononucleotide; N_aAD, nicotinic acid adenine dinucleotide (deamido-NAD); PRPP, 5-phosphoribosyl-1-pyrophosphate; ATP, adenosine triphosphate; PPi, pyrophosphate; Glu, glutaminic acid; GluNH₂, glutamine; ADPR, adenosine diphosphate ribose.

a reduced energy supply. This can be done with drugs by pharmacological intervention in the electromechanical or energy-coupling processes as well as by a decrease of the contractile work, especially the heart rate (18).

Since ATP, CP, and NAD cannot penetrate the cell membrane (6), it seems to be difficult to transfer energy from outside into the cardiac cells.

However, well-founded observations have been made recently in isolated heart preparations by Parrat and Marshall (19) and Saks and co-workers (23,24) that with CP or ATP an outside–inside energy transfer during anoxic energy deficiency may occur. However, the outside concentrations that are needed would have strong cardiovascular effects in the living organism.

As a third possibility, especially for cardioplegic solutions used in cardiac surgery, it also seems important to add precursors or metabolites of NAD or AN that can penetrate the cell membrane to these solutions to avoid an efflux by an outward–inward gradient.

It seems possible as well to increase the turnover, the synthesis, and the cardiac concentration of pyridine nucleotides as well as of AN by administering various precursors under normoxic conditions and in some states of energy deficiency (3,25,32–34).

There are three questions we should like to address: (1) Can we influence by precursors the synthesis, degradation, and concentration of NAD in cardiac muscle? This question is connected with the two different pathways of NAD synthesis and their intracellular localization. (2) Can increased cardiac NAD synthesis be connected with the synthesis of adenine nucleotides (AN)? (3) Can the anoxic leakage of cardiac NAD and AN be avoided?

Kaplan and co-workers (12) found in 1956 that the NAD concentration in the liver of mice increased tenfold after injection of nicotinamide and to a lesser degree after injection of nicotinic acid. Since these observations, the pathway of the de novo synthesis of NAD from tryptophan and from both precursors, nicotinamide and nicotinic acid, has been studied in many tissues of various animal species. It is astonishing, however, that only a few papers have been concerned with this connection with cardiac NAD (1,4,5,10,11,26,27,30). Therefore, not all points of synthesis and degradation are clear and proved, especially with regard to the intracellular localization of the various enzyme reactions. NAD as a compound consists of nicotinamide and adenine, both connected with two molecules of ribophosphate. These are the natural precursors. The active phosphate groups of NAD are bound as coenzyme to the protein moiety of the various dehydrogenases. The hydrogen transfer takes place at the nicotinamide molecule. Free NAD can be shuttled from one dehydrogenase to another. There are now two generally accepted pathways from the precursors nicotinamide and nicotinic acid (Figure 1).

THE PREISS–HANDLER PATHWAY

In the first step, deamidation of nicotinamide to nicotinic acid takes place by the nicotinamidase. Nicotinic acid is now converted to N_aMN, and in the next step, by transfer of adenosine phosphate, N_aAD is produced. In a special reaction, the nicotinic acid moiety is amidated to NAD (21,22). NAD can be converted to NADP. The NADP concentration in the heart is, however, low related to NAD. Therefore, it is understandable that the pentose phosphate shunt which is dependent on NADP plays no important role in the heart under normal conditions. By the glycohydrolase NAD is hydrolyzed to nicotinamide and ADPR which can be degraded to PRPP or polymerized to macromolecules (ADPR)$_n$ (7,13).

DIETRICH PATHWAY

The second, so-called Dietrich pathway starts with the connection of nicotinamide with ribophosphate to form NMN and, in the next step, NAD (4,5). As one can see, the Preiss–Handler pathway needs, from nicotinic acid to NAD, 3 ATP, and the Dietrich pathway 2 ATP. Important for both pathways is the 5-phosphoribosyl-1-pyrophosphate (PRPP) pool.

WHICH PATHWAY IS OPERATING IN THE HEART?

We shall see that this depends on the precursor and its concentration. An open question until now has been whether the two different pathways can be correlated with the compartmentation of NAD in the cytosol and in the mitochondrial membrane which is impermeable for the NAD molecule. Since NAD is located at the inner part of this membrane, it would be difficult to understand how NAD is transferred from cytosol to this area (6). There have been interesting studies in the heart by Severin and co-workers from 1966 to 1974 carried out to localize the enzymes of the different steps of NAD synthesis and degradation (26,27).

A general view about the localization of the various enzymes of the Preiss–Handler pathway and the Dietrich pathway as well as the degradation of NAD, according to the findings of Severin et al. (26,27) in the heart of rabbits and that Grunicke et al. (8) in the liver of rats, is shown in Table 1. It is interesting that both authors could find no synthesis of N_aMN, N_aAD, or NAD with nicotinic acid in mitochondria. NAD synthesis in the Preiss–Handler pathway is localized in cytosol and nucleus. The conversion of NAD to NADP takes place in the cytosol. The steps of the Dietrich pathway have been localized by both authors in the mitochondria. There is only one difference: the conversion of NMN to NAD in cardiac muscle could be found by Severin et al. (27) only in the nucleus but not in ultrasonic particles of mitochondria or intact mitochondria, whereas Grunicke et al. (8) could observe in intact mitochondria of liver cells, but not in ultrasonic particles, synthesis from NMN to NAD. Since Severin, however, also localized the enzyme NAD pyrophosphatase which degrades NAD to NMN in the mitochondria, it seems to us likely that NMN can be converted to NAD in cardiac muscle mitochondria as well as in the nucleus. This would explain a separate pathway of synthesis in the mitochondria as well as the

Table 1. Localization of the Various Enzymes of the Preiss–Handler Pathway and Dietrich Pathway as Well as the Degradation of NAD

Enzyme systems and enzyme code numbers (E.C.)	Cytosol	Mitochondria	Nucleus	Sarcoplasmic reticulum, microsomes
Preiss–Handler pathway				
$N_a \rightarrow N_aMN$: nicotinate phosphoribosyltransferase (2.4.2.11)	+	0(8,26,27)		++(26,27)
$N_aMN \rightarrow N_aAD$: nicotinate mononucleotide adenylyltransferase (2.7.7.18)		0(8,26,27)	++	++(26,27)
$N_aAD \rightarrow NAD$: NAD-synthetase (6.3.5.1)		0(8,26,27)	++	++(20)
Phosphorylation				
$NAD \rightarrow NADP$; NAD-kinase (2.7.1.23)	++(26,27)			
Degradation				
$NAD \rightarrow NMN$: NAD-pyrophosphatase (3.6.1.22)		+(26,27)	+(26,27)	
NAD ⎱ N_{am}: NAD(NADP)-glycohydrolase (3.2.2.5)	++(26,27)	+(26,27)		
$NADP$ ⎰				
$N_{am} \rightarrow N_a$: nicotinamidase (3.5.1.19)				
Dietrich				
D-R-5P $\rightarrow$ PRPP: ribosephosphate-pyrophosphokinase (2.7.6.1)	++(26,27)	++(8,26,27)[a]		
$N_{am} \rightarrow$ NMN: NMN-pyrophosphorylase (2.4.2.12)		++(8,26,27)		
NMN $\rightarrow$ NAD: NMN-adenylyltransferase (2.7.7.1)		++(8)[b]	++(26,27)	

[a] Outer mitochondrial membrane.
[b] Inner mitochondrial membrane.

degradation to NMN in this compartment. The NMN can be resynthesized here or can move into the cytosol and nucleus where it can be resynthesized to NAD.

Degradation of NAD to nicotinamide as well as to NMN and the deamidation reaction from nicotinamide to nicotinic acid are located for the most part in the sarcoplasmic reticulum (SR). In the following chapter, we shall discuss the possibilities of increasing the cardiac NAD level under aerobic conditions by administering the precursors nicotinamide and nicotinic acid in high pharmacologically active concentrations (in millimolar range) as well as in low physiological external levels (in micromolar range). The incorporation and degradation and the pathways used at different concentrations are also illustrated. We studied further the influence of precursors on AN synthesis together with nicotinamide and nicotinic acid on NAD and AN levels under normoxic conditions. Under anoxic conditions, the leakage of NAD and AN was studied as well as the basic conditions that help to avoid breakdown and efflux of these important compounds for anoxic survival and aerobic resuscitation of cardiac muscle.

MATERIALS AND METHODS

Isolated spontaneously beating or resting atria of guinea pigs as well as electrically driven left atria were prepared and incubated in Krebs–Henseleit solution (Na$^+$, 142.2; K$^+$, 5.9; Ca^{2+}, 2.5; Mg^{2+}, 1.2; Cl$^-$, 128; HPO$_4^{2-}$, 1.1; SO$_4^{2-}$, 1.2; HCO$_3^-$, 24 mM; including 15 mM glucose) and gassed with 95% O$_2$, 5% CO$_2$ or in anoxia with 95% N$_2$, 5% CO$_2$ at a temperature of 30°C or 35°C as reported previously (29). Pyridine and adenine nucleotides as well as CP have been determined in atrial tissue and related to 100 mg wet weight (w.w.) or to 1 mg protein measured with the method of Lowry et al. (14). The wet weight of 100 mg atrial tissue corresponds to 8.94 mg protein. The various metabolites of NAD synthesis and degradation are determined after incubation with [^{14}C]nicotinamide or [^{14}C]nicotinic acid in atrial tissue and in the nutrition solution by combined paper, thin-layer, and column chromatography. The methods and some of the results are published elsewhere in detail (2,3).

RESULTS AND DISCUSSION

The Cardiac NAD Level after Injection of Nicotinamide into Living Guinea Pigs

Severin and Tseitlin (26) found an increased NAD level (+175%) in the hearts of rabbits after injection of nicotinamide (500 mg/kg ~ 4 mmol/kg) which reached the maximum between 24 and 36 hr, a long time period. These authors also observed with this treatment an increase of the NAD

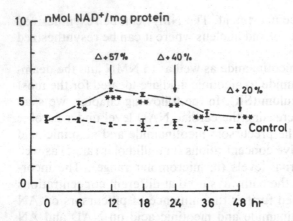

 nMol NAD⁺/mg protein graph values: Δ+57%, Δ+40%, Δ+20%, Control; x-axis 0 6 12 18 24 36 48 hr

Figure 2. NAD level in isolated atria of guinea pigs at different time intervals after i.p. injection of 10 mM nicotinamide/kg at 8:00 a.m. The atria were incubated for 30 min in Krebs–Henseleit solution plus 15 mM glucose and 10 mM nicotinamide at 35°C and then freeze-clamped in liquid nitrogen. $N = 4$; bars show S.E.M.; *$P < 0.05$; **$P < 0.01$; ***$P < 0.001$.

level lowered by an epinephrine myocarditis back to normal values. This was accompanied by an increased ATP and total AN level in both groups.

We have observed this in a similar way after i.p. injection of 10 mmol nicotinamide/kg in guinea pig atria (Figure 2). We observed an increased NAD level up to +58% after 12 hr and to +40% after 24 hr. This was not connected with an increased concentration of ATP, AN, and CP in our findings.

The Cardiac NAD Level in Isolated Atria

Incubation with High Pharmacologically Active Concentrations of Nicotinamide and Nicotinic Acid. Aerobic incubation with 20 mM nicotinamide leads to a positive inotropic effect in contrast to nicotinic acid which decreases contractile activity in this concentration. We can observe with nicotinamide during a 16- to 24-hr incubation a threefold increase in the enzymatically determined total NAD with ¹⁴C labeling of around 50% after 24 hr. Since there are no AN precursors in the external nutrition solution, the endogenous AN pool was alone responsible for the adenine moiety of the

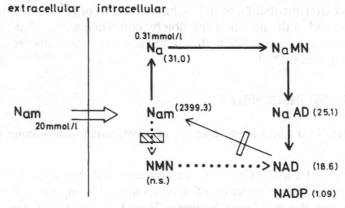

Figure 3. Incubation with 20 mM [¹⁴C]nicotinamide (specific activity: 0.5 μCi/μmol) at 30°C. The ¹⁴C-labeled nucleotides and metabolites were calculated in nmol/100 mg w.w. per 24 hr (mean in parentheses); $N = 5$; n.s., no significant radioactivity.

new synthesized [^{14}C]-NAD in the amount of 15% of the total AN. It is astonishing that without the precursor nicotinamide in the Krebs–Henseleit solution the NAD level remained unchanged during the 24-hr incubation time. This implies that without precursor the endogenous turnover of NAD might be very slow. Otherwise, we would expect a loss by diffusion of metabolites (3).

The increase of the NAD level by nicotinamide is concentration dependent in the range between 1 and 20 mM with two different kinetics (3). We assume that the first steep slope in the range between 1 and 5 mM can be connected with the activation of the nicotinamidase, and the second slope between 5 and 20 mM with the inhibition of the glycohydrolase.

Washout experiments changing from 20 mM labeled [^{14}C]nicotinamide after 8 hr to 20 mM cold nicotinamide let us calculate that the increased level of NAD can be explained by new synthesis as well as by inhibited degradation in the ratio of 2 : 1. Washout experiments with a nicotinamide-free incubation medium showed a decline of total NAD to normal values over 8 hr. Only in the first hour of washout the specific activity declined from 0.32 to 0.25, which then remained constant until, after 8 hr normal NAD values were reached (3).

According to our analysis of the radioactivity in the different metabolites, we came to the following conclusions. Nicotinamide, in contrast to nicotinic acid, penetrates the cell membrane completely in proportion to the external concentration. Since the Michaelis constant of the nicotinamidase in the SR is, according to our findings, high and in the 5 mM range, nicotinamidase converts nicotinamide to nicotinic acid with a significant atrial concentration of 0.31 mM (Figure 3).

We can find in the N_aAD spot after 24 hr of incubation the very high concentration of 25.1 nmol/100 mg w.w., which exceeds the radioactivity of NAD with 18.6 nmol/100 mg w.w. by the factor 1.35. The incorporation in NADP with 1.09 nmol/100 mg w.w. is very small, but we have to keep in mind that the NADP concentration in relation to NAD in the heart is very small. We found no activity in NMN. Since it is well known that high concentrations of nicotinamide inhibit the glycohydrolase reaction, we can assume that a stagnation in the last steps of the Preiss–Handler pathway will occur. The Dietrich pathway seems, in our observations, not to operate, perhaps because of inhibition of the NMN phosphorylase by the high concentration of nicotinamide (5).

However, we have to consider that the specific radioactivity of 20 mM nicotinamide in these experiments was not very high, and a very small degree of labeling in NMN cannot be completely excluded.

From these observations in isolated atria, we can conclude that the observed increase of the NAD level in cardiac tissue as well as in other organs after a high dosage of nicotinamide results from the same mechanism: increased new synthesis via the Preiss–Handler pathway and decreased degradation of NAD because of inhibition of the glycohydrolase. This explains the old findings of Kaplan et al. (12) and Severin et al. (27). High

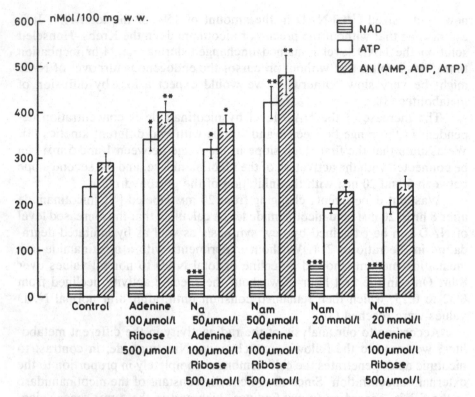

Figure 4.   NAD, ATP, and AN concentrations in spontaneously beating isolated atria of guinea pigs after a 24-hr incubation period under normoxic conditions at 30°C. The incubation was done in Krebs–Henseleit solution plus 15 mM glucose with various precursors of the pyridine and adenine nucleotides. $N = 5$; mean ± S.E.M.; *$P < 0.05$; **$P < 0.01$; ***$P < 0.001$.

concentrations of nicotinic acid in the 20 mM range have negative inotropic effects and show no significant labeling in contrast to the observations with nicotinamide in the same concentration.

The NAD and Adenine Nucleotide Pool in Atria after Normoxic Incubation with Various Precursors.   Since the adenine moiety of the new synthesis in our experiments is from the endogenous AN pool, we determined whether NAD and AN concentrations could be increased under the same conditions by combined incubation of nicotinamide with the AN precursors adenine and ribose for a 24-hr period (Figure 4). We could observe after incubation with 20 mM nicotinamide without AN precursors a 150% increased NAD level with significantly lowered ATP and AN levels, but addition of adenine and ribose did not significantly influence the AN pool, whereas the NAD level was increased as expected.

In contrast to the observations with high nicotinamide concentrations, we observed with low concentrations of 500 μM nicotinamide together with 100 μM adenine and 500 μM ribose significant increases in the ATP concentration (+77%) and the total AN (+60%), whereas with this low nicotinamide concentration, the NAD level was raised to only +23%, in the upper level of the statistical range. We have therefore to assume that high concentrations of nicotinamide (20 mM) which inhibit the glycohydrolase could also inhibit the new aerobic synthesis of AN via the steps of the salvage pathway (16,33). This could explain why we could not find an increased AN synthesis in living guinea pigs after injection of 10 mmol/kg, whereas Severin found with ~4 mmol/kg nicotinamide in rabbits an elevation of the ATP level. Under aerobic conditions for 24 hr, adenine and ribose as the only precursors significantly increase the ATP (+44%) and AN (+32%) levels and at a combined incubation with a small amount (50 μM) of nicotinic acid also increase the NAD level (+72%). The synthesis of AN can be explained by conversion of ribose by the enzyme ribosephosphatase followed by an increase of the PRPP pool. Adenine reacts with PRPP catalyzed by the adenine phosphoribosyl transferase in the AN salvage pathway to produce AMP which, under aerobic conditions, is quickly phosphorylated to ADP and ATP (15,16,32,33). Adenine nucleotide synthesis is, like NAD synthesis, dependent on the PRPP pool and therefore on ATP production.

NAD Synthesis and Degradation in Isolated Atria during Anoxia and Incubation with Nicotinamide in High Concentrations.

We have found that under aerobic conditions 20 mM nicotinamide increases the cardiac NAD level by new synthesis and also by an inhibition of degradation. We determined whether, under anoxic conditions, 20 mM nicotinamide could avoid the loss of NAD in anoxia. We measured under the same conditions (spontaneously beating atria, 30°C) but in different atria the NAD and the NADH concentrations (Table 2). After 8 hr of incubation, we observed a considerably increased NAD concentration and a total of NAD + NADH of 78 nmol/100 mg w.w. After an 8-hr aerobic incubation period, a 3-hr anoxic period was started. At the end, the atria were analyzed , and we observed a loss of total NAD + NADH of 45%. As one could expect, the NADH/NAD quotient was shifted from the aerobic 0.36 to 0.61, in the NADH direction. Therefore, nicotinamide could not completely stop the leakage of anoxic degraded NAD metabolites.

The time course of the NAD concentration (Figure 5A) shows that during

Table 2. Incubation with 20 mM Nicotinamide under Normoxic (8 hr O$_2$) and Anoxic (8 hr O$_2$ + 3 hr N$_2$) Conditions at 30°C[a]

	Normoxic [nmol/100 mg w.w. (%)]	Anoxic [nmol/100 mg w.w. (%)]
NAD$^+$ ($N = 4$)	57.67 ± 4.89 (74%)	26.89 ± 3.28 (62%)
NADH ($N = 3$)	20.79 ± 3.36 (26%)	16.48 ± 1.36 (38%)
NADH/NAD$^+$	0.36	0.61
NAD$^+$ + NADH	78.46 ± 8.25	43.37 ± 4.64*

[a] Means ± S.E.M.; *$P < 0.05$.

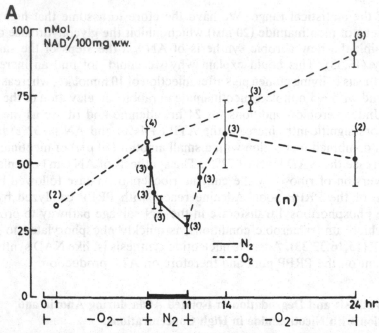

Figure 5. Incubation with unlabeled (A) and ^{14}C-labeled (B) 20 mM nicotinamide under normoxic conditions and under transient anoxic conditions at 30°C. Mean ± S.E.M.; N in parentheses.

a 3-hr anoxic period the aerobically increased NAD concentration declined to normal initial values. After reoxygenation, as a result of the shift from NADH to NAD, the concentration of NAD increased over a 3-hr period, but the further enhancement of the total NAD concentration was inhibited compared with the aerobic control values. This can be explained by the loss of AN in this anoxic period and the lack of the endogenous adenine moiety for a new synthesis of NAD.

In this connection, it is interesting to observe that during anoxia ^{14}C incorporation into [^{14}C]-NAD and therefore new synthesis was stopped (Figure 5B). After 3 hr of anoxia, [^{14}C]-NAD was significantly lowered compared with the aerobically increased value after 8 hr of aerobic incubation.

After reoxygenation, the steep increase in [^{14}C]-NAD can be explained by the shift of [^{14}C]-NADH to [^{14}C]-NAD. The new synthesis and incorporation of [^{14}C]nicotinamide between the 12- and 24-hr incubation period is significantly lowered compared to the aerobic control values.

The question was now whether inhibition of the glycohydrolase by a high concentration of nicotinamide could avoid a decline in the elevated NAD level during anoxia to below the anoxic control values in a nicotinamide-free incubation medium (Table 3). We studied this in our anoxia test (29) with electrically driven left atria and a strongly reduced and metabolically balanced anoxic contractile activity at the higher temperature of 35°C. After 3 hr of incubation under normoxic conditions, we observed an increase of 32.8% in the NAD concentration of atria incubated with 10 mM nicotin-

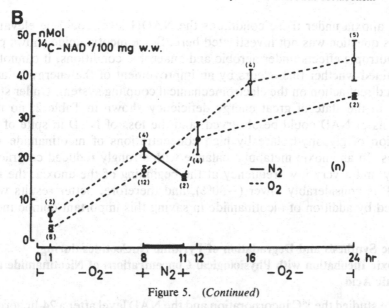

Figure 5. (*Continued*)

amide. We also observed at the end of the anoxia test, after 1 hr of normoxia followed by 2 hr of anoxia, that during this period with nicotinamide, incubated atria had at the end a significantly higher level of NAD (+32%) than the atria in a nicotinamide-free medium. The anoxia-reduced contractile activity was, with nicotinamide, higher than in the control groups. If, after the first hour of anoxia, 10 mM nicotinamide is added to the incubation medium, we observe during the second hour of anoxia a positive inotropic effect. In addition, there was a slightly but significantly higher NAD level 23.6% above that in the control group.

Therefore, we assume that, under anoxia, concentrations of nicotinamide that restrain the degradation of NAD by inhibition of the glycohydrolase cannot completely prevent the loss of intracellular NAD but can provide a higher NAD level compared with the nicotinamide-free medium and can in this way save intracellular NAD to a limited degree. We must also consider

Table 3. Anoxia Test: Content of NAD^+ in the Presence and Absence of Nicotinamide[a]

	NAD^+ (nmol/mg prot.) with 10 mM N_{am}	NAD^+ (nmol/mg prot.) without N_{am}	Difference (%)
Control: 3 hr normoxia	4.73 ± 0.18	3.56 ± 0.22	+32.8%***
Normoxia (1 hr) + 2 hr anoxia	3.20 ± 0.13	2.41 ± 0.13	+32.7%***
Nicotinamide added after first hour of anoxia (1 hr anoxia)	2.98 ± 0.17	2.41 ± 0.13	+23.6%*

[a] Left atria are electrically stimulated at 0.5 Hz and 500 millipond preload in Krebs–Henseleit solution with 15 mM glucose and with or without 10 mM nicotinamide. Means ± S.E.M., $N = 5$: *$P < 0.05$; **$P < 0.01$; ***$P < 0.001$.

that in anoxia under these conditions the NADH level could be elevated, but this question was not investigated here. Since nicotinamide shows positive inotropic effects under aerobic and anaerobic conditions, it cannot be determined whether this occurs by an improvement of the energy balance or by a direct action on the electromechanical coupling system. Under strict anoxia in the state of great energy deficiency shown in Table 2, no new synthesis of NAD could be observed, and the loss of NAD in spite of the inhibition of glycohydrolase by high concentrations of nicotinamide was obvious. In an anoxic metabolic balance with strongly reduced contractile activity and a very low frequency at the beginning of the anoxia, the loss of ATP is considerably lower (-30%), and therefore, better results were obtained by addition of nicotinamide in saving this important compound.

Cardiac Synthesis and Degradation of Pyridine Nucleotides during Normoxic Incubation with Physiological Concentrations of Nicotinamide and Nicotinic Acid

We studied the ^{14}C incorporation and the NAD level after a 24-hr aerobic incubation with 10 μM [^{14}C]nicotinamide, a concentration about 2000-fold lower than that reported above. Here we see a completely different incorporation of nicotinamide into NAD as well as only a slight change of total NAD in the 24-hr incubation period (3).

Incubation with 10 μM Nicotinamide.   No radioactivity could be found in the nicotinic acid spot or in the N$_a$AD spot (Figure 6A). However, in contrast to the results with 20 mM nicotinamide, we observed a small but highly significant incorporation in the NMN spot in a concentration of 0.04 nmol/100 mg w.w. after 24 hr. The incorporation into NAD during this time amounted to only 4.8 nmol/100 mg w.w. It was surprising that the nicotinamidase did not convert nicotinamide to nicotinic acid in this concentration. However, we have seen above that the nicotinamidase must have a Michaelis constant in the 1–5 mM range which is too high for it to operate in micromolar concentrations. We can assume that this small, slow incorporation via NMN synthesis would likely occur in the mitochondrial membrane according to the findings of Severin and co-workers (26,27).

It could be possible that a small amount of NAD synthesis also occurs in the mitochondria as was observed by Grunicke et al. in liver mitochondria (8). But NAD could also be partially synthesized in the nucleus from NMN according to the observation of Severin et al. (27).

Incubation with 10 μM Nicotinic Acid.   In contrast to our experiments with 20 mM nicotinic acid, and also in contrast to the incubation with 10 μM nicotinamide, we have observed an increase of total NAD by 50% as well as a twofold higher ^{14}C incorporation into NAD in comparison with 10 μM nicotinamide if we use 10 μM nicotinic acid as precursor (Figure 6B). In this physiological concentration, nicotinic acid is obviously the favored substrate for NAD synthesis in spite of the fact that nicotinic acid penetrates the cell membrane to a smaller degree than nicotinamide.

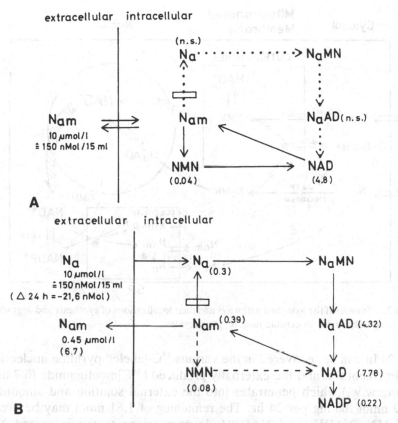

Figure 6.   Incubation with 10 μM [^{14}C]nicotinamide (specific activity: 50 μCi/μmol) (A) or 10 μM [^{14}C]nicotinic acid (100 μCi/μmol) (B) at 30°C. The ^{14}C-labeled nucleotides and metabolites were calculated in nmol/100 mg w.w. per 24 hr (mean in parentheses); $N = 5$; n.s., no significant radioactivity.

We find, over a 24-hr incubation period with nicotinic acid, twice as much [^{14}C]-NAD than after incubation with 10 μM nicotinamide. We also observed that the Preiss–Handler pathway is highly effective in this situation. The degradation of NAD by the glycohydrolase is also working; this is proved by the high concentration of [^{14}C]nicotinamide in atria as well as in the nutrition solution, which can only stem from degraded [^{14}C]-NAD. From our findings with a physiological concentration of 10 μM nicotinamide, we cannot expect deamidation to nicotinic acid under these conditions, but we see a highly significant incorporation into NMN, which proves that the Dietrich pathway is also operating, although, in comparison to the Preiss–Handler pathway, only to a small degree.

Using four atria simultaneously, we checked the balance over a 24-hr incubation period between uptake from external [^{14}C]nicotinic acid (150 nmol in 15 ml Krebs–Henseleit solution) and recovery in atrial [^{14}C]pyridine nucleotides and metabolites and calculated it per 100 mg atrial wet weight. The atrial uptake of 21.6 nmol [^{14}C]nicotinic acid from the nutrition solution

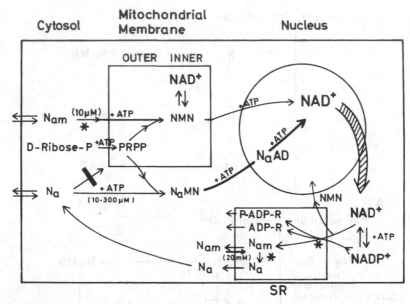

Figure 7.   Scheme of the assumed pathways and their localizations of synthesis and degradation of pyridine nucleotides in cardiac muscle; (*) enzymes.

over 24 hr can be recovered in the various ^{14}C-labeled pyridine nucleotides, [^{14}C]metabolites, and the externally produced [^{14}C]nicotinamide (6.7 nmol/ 100 mg w.w.) which penetrates into the external solution and amounts to 19.79 nmol/100 mg per 24 hr. The remaining of 1.81 nmol may be present in N_aMN, NADH, and NADPH. In comparison to the increased NAD synthesis by 20 mM nicotinamide which uses afterdeamidation to nicotinic acid and also the Preiss–Handler pathway, we can observe here one interesting difference. The ratio of labelled N_aAD to NAD is reversed from 1.32 at incubation with 20 mM nicotinamide to 0.55 after incubation with 10 μM nicotinic acid. We assume that the inhibition of the degradation of NAD by the glycohydrolase with high concentrations of nicotinamide elevates the concentrations in the preceding steps, whereas with low concentrations, the glycohydrolase is active.

We assume, therefore, that at this low, physiological concentration the normal route of synthesis will be the Preiss–Handler pathway from the precursor nicotinic acid. Nicotinamide can, at this concentration, not be deamidated to nicotinic acid and will therefore leave the cell or will be reincorporated via the Dietrich pathway and will here serve for mitochondrial NAD synthesis. In the scheme of Figure 7, the assumed pathways and their localizations of synthesis and degradation of pyridine nucleotides in cardiac muscle under aerobic conditions are summarized.

Physiological concentrations of nicotinic acid in the range between 10 and 300 μM increase the rate of new synthesis of NAD via the Preiss–Handler pathway. NAD is degraded to nicotinamide in an obviously enhanced turnover. Nicotinamide, in these micromolar concentrations, can not be deamidated; it serves as substrate for the Dietrich pathway with a small but significant production of NMN in the mitochondria, which serves for new synthesis of NAD in the inner mitochondrial membrane, or, synthesis can go from NMN to NAD in the nucleus. Nicotinic acid in concentrations of 10–50 μM is the favored precursor for an increased synthesis as well as elevation of the NAD concentration by 50–70%.

Nicotinamide in th 10–20 mM range increases the NAD level to the highest degree (up to 300%) via the Preiss–Handler pathway by new synthesis and by a strongly reduced degradation by inhibition of the glycohydrolase. The anoxic loss of NAD can be lowered significantly. However, these high concentrations of nicotinamide also inhibit the aerobic synthesis of AN from the precursors adenine and ribose.

The question of whether an elevated concentration of cardiac NAD can be effective as coenzyme without new synthesis of the protein moiety of the various dehydrogenases is still open. This can only be answered by experiments in living animals, not in isolated atria. The results of Severin and Tseitlin (26) with the experimental epinephrine myocarditis demonstrated, with increased NAD and AN levels resulting from nicotinamide injection (~4 mmol/kg), beneficial effects in these cases.

The Influence of the Aerobic Contractile Work on the Anoxic Loss of NAD, AN, and CP in Atria Incubated with Various Precursors. The importance of the intensity of aerobic contractile work before the beginning of anoxia is demonstrated in the following experiments. In previous studies (29), it was demonstrated in the anoxia test at 35°C in left atria stimulated at 0.5 Hz and a very low contractile work (30 beats/min) that under these conditions the oxygen consumption exceeds the oxygen need of arrested atria by only 10%. If we start anoxia under these conditions, contractile activity can be observed over 6 hr at a level of 50–80% of the aerobic values. After 2 hr of anoxia, the loss of ATP was observed to be only 30%; however, the CP level decreased by 90%. With a high concentration of 15 mM ribose and 0.1 mM adenine, the anoxic loss of AN and ATP could be avoided (29). In similar experiments illustrated in Table 4, we could find after 2 hr of anoxia concentrations of CP, ATP, and AN in the same range as had been observed previously (A). Under the same conditions of the anoxia test but using spontaneously beating atria at a frequency of ~200 beats/min before anoxia was started, we observed at the end of 2 hr of anoxia a loss of ATP by 77%, of the total AN by 56%, of CP by 94%, and of NAD by 33%. The loss of ATP and AN are therefore, under the same conditions, considerably higher than under the low contractile work at 30 beats/min. If we compare both groups (A and D) at the end of the 2-hr anoxic period, we can observe a considerably higher concentration of ATP and AN in (A) which is highly significant. In NAD and CP levels, however, no difference could be observed. This shows clearly that the anoxic loss of ATP and AN is dependent on the intensity of cardiac work before anoxia was started.

Table 4. Concentrations of NAD and Energy-Rich Phosphates under Anoxic Conditions[a]

	NAD		PCr		ATP		AN	
	Content[b]	Difference	Content[b]	Difference	Content[b]	Difference	Content[b]	Difference
Electrically driven atria[c]								
A. Anoxia control (N = 8)	2.7 ± 0.17	+18% (n.s.)[e]	2.59 ± 0.96	+22% (n.s.)[e]	18.81 ± 0.87	+233%****	28.95 ± 0.73	+122%****[e]
B. Anoxia + 50 μM N$_a$ + 100 μM adenine + 500 μM ribose (N = 9)	2.63 ± 0.1	+8% (n.s.)[f]	3.28 ± 1.12	+5% (n.s.)[f]	21.02 ± 0.93	+163%***[f]	29.91 ± 0.73	+91%***[f]
Spontaneously beating atria[d]								
C. Normoxic control (N = 6)	3.41 ± 0.07		35.58 ± 2.69		24.31 ± 0.7		29.57 ± 0.69	
D. Anoxia control (N = 6)	2.29 ± 0.12	−33%****[g]	2.13 ± 0.34	−94%****[g]	5.65 ± 0.98	−77%****[g]	13.06 ± 1.44	−56%****[g]
E. Anoxia + 50 μM N$_a$ + 100 μM adenine + 500 μM ribose (N = 6)	2.43 ± 0.13	+6% (n.s.)[e]	3.13 ± 0.21	+47%***[e]	8.0 ± 1.64	+42% (n.s.)[e]	15.65 ± 2.01	+20% (n.s.)[e]

F. Anoxia + 500 μM N$_a$ + 100 μM adenine + 500 μM ribose (N = 6)	1.97 ± 0.16	− 14% (n.s.)^c	1.96 ± 0.07	− 8% (n.s.)^c	8.85 ± 1.72	+ 57% (n.s.)^c	17.16 ± 2.57 + 31% (n.s.)^c
G. Anoxia + 5 mM PCr + 100 μM adenine + 500 μM ribose (N = 6)	2.52 ± 0.12	+ 10% (n.s.)^c	14.85 ± 1.42 (see text)		10.8 ± 1.95 + 91%*^{e}		18.65 ± 2.06 + 43% (n.s.)^c
H. Anoxia + 100 μM adenine + 500 μM ribose (N = 6)	2.31 ± 0.25	+ 0.9% (n.s.)^c	2.99 ± 0.54	+ 40% (n.s.)^c	12.8 ± 1.56	+ 127%***^{e}	22.3 ± 2.31 + 71%***^{e}

^{a} Incubation was at 35°C in Krebs–Henseleit solution with 15 mM glucose plus addition of precursors. Anoxia was produced by 2 hr of N$_2$ following 1 hr of O$_2$. The values are determined at the end of each experiment.
^{b} Content is expressed in nmol/mg protein ± S.E.M.
^{c} Atria are driven at 30 beats/min (0.5 Hz) with preload of 500 mp.
^{d} Spontaneously beating atria contract at approximately 200 beats/min.
^{e} Difference vs. D; *P < 0.05; **P < 0.01; ***P < 0.001; n.s., not significant.
^{f} Difference vs. E; significance as above; n.s. vs. A.
^{g} Difference vs. C; significance as above.

It is of interest that with combinations of precursors that lead under aerobic conditions at 30°C after a 24-hr incubation period to considerably increased NAD and AN levels, only a weak protective effect in the concentration on AN can be demonstrated with 100 μM adenine and 500 μM ribose. Also, no protective effect of the NAD levels could be found with low concentrations of nicotinamide (500 μM) and nicotinic acid (50 μM). In contrast to our previous observations in the anoxia test with the protective effects on AN by 15 mM ribose, a concentration of 500 μM ribose shows no difference from control values (A and B).

Therefore, it seems likely that to have protective effects for the anoxic heart the concentration of ribose must be higher than 500 μM which is, however, sufficient for increased aerobic synthesis of AN. In experiment G, we tried to improve the anoxic energy balance with an exogenous concentration of 5 mM CP together with adenine and ribose in 1 hr normoxic and 2 hr anoxic incubation time. The added concentration of 5 mM CP decreased only to 4.84 mM after 3 hr of incubation. By comparing the measured CP concentration of 14.85 nmol/mg protein (G) with that of 35.85 nmol/mg protein (C) found under aerobic conditions, we observe a decrease of only 59% in contrast to the higher decrease of 94% of the anoxic control value (D). If we calculate, however, the values of the atrial extracellular CP, there is a clear decrease of intracellular CP in the same range. In the anoxia test with electrically driven atria, CP shows no protective effect on the anoxic contractile activity in a concentration of 5 or 10 mM; in contrast, it has negative inotropic effects. Up to now we could, therefore, not confirm in our experiments the protective effects of CP reported by Saks and coworkers in frog heart (23). These experiments clearly show the importance of the anoxic deprivation of the ATP and PRPP pool by the intensity of the cardiac work before anoxia was started. With a small ATP and PRPP pool, addition of precursors such as adenine and ribose in low concentrations has only weak effects on the loss of AN and no protective effect on NAD and CP levels.

CONCLUSIONS

It is possible to increase synthesis and concentrations of NAD and AN in cardiac muscle cells by adding precursors under aerobic conditions, thereby providing better initial conditions for anoxic survival. However, the question is open whether an elevated cardiac NAD concentration without newly synthesized protein moieties of the various dehydrogenases has importance for cardiac cell function and cell survival.

It is possible to inhibit by precursors the leakage of NAD and AN in anoxic energy deficiency only if a sufficient anaerobic ATP production with an adequate PRPP pool is provided. Therefore, strongly reduced contractile work or cardiac arrest before anoxic conditions are started may be beneficial as the most energy protective effect combined with the addition of AN and NAD precursors to myocardial perfusion solutions.

ACKNOWLEDGMENTS

The skillful and excellent technical assistance of Mrs. A. Weible and Mr. K. Stieler is gratefully acknowledged.

REFERENCES

1. Collins, P. B., and Chaykin, S. 1972. The management of nicotinamide and nicotinic acid in the mouse. *J. Biol. Chem.* 247:778–783.
2. Delabar, U. 1977. *Die Unterschiedliche Wirkung von Nicotinsäureamid und Nicotinsäure auf die Funktion und auf den Pyridinnukleotidstoffwechsel des Herzmuskels.* Naturwissenschaftliche Dissertation, Fachbereich Pharmazie, Universität Tübingen, Tübingen.
3. Delabar, U., and Siess, M. 1979. Synthesis and degradation of NAD in guinea pig cardiac muscle: I. Dependence upon the extracellular concentration of nicotinamide and nicotinic acid. II. Studies about the different biosynthetic pathways and the corresponding intermediates. *Basic Res. Cardiol.* 74:528–544, 571–593.
4. Dietrich, L. S., Fuller, L., Yero, I. L., and Martinez, L. 1966. Nicotinamide mononucleotide pyrophosphorylase activity in animal tissues. *J.Biol. Chem.* 241:188–191.
5. Dietrich, L. S., Muniz, O., and Powanda, M. 1968. NAD synthesis in animal tissues. *J. Vitaminol.* 14:123–129.
6. Ernster, L., and Kuylenstierna, B. 1969. Structure, composition and function of mitochondrial membranes. In: L. Ernster and Z. Drahota (eds.), *Mitochondria, Structure and Function*, pp. 5–31. Academic Press, London, New York.
7. Ferro, A. M., and Kun, E. 1976. Macromolecular derivatives of NAD in heart nuclei: Poly adenosine diphosphoribose and adenosine diphosphoribose proteins. *Biochem. Biophys. Res. Commun.* 71:150–154.
8. Grunicke, H., Keller, H. J., Puschendorf, B., and Benaguid, A. 1975. Biosynthesis of nicotinamide adenine dinucleotide in mitochondria. *Eur. J. Biochem.* 53:41–45.
9. Gudbjarnasson, S., Mathes, P., and Ravens, R. G. 1970. Functional compartmentation of ATP and creatine phosphate in heart muscle. *J. Mol. Cell. Cardiol.* 1:325–339.
10. Ichiyama, A., Nakamura, S., and Nishizuka, Y. 1967. Studies on the biosynthesis of nicotinamide adenine dinucleotide (NAD) in mammals and its regulatory mechanism, Part I. *Arzneim. Forsch.* 17:1346–1355.
11. Ichiyama, A., Nakamura, S., and Nishizuka, Y. 1967. Studies on the biosynthesis of nicotinamide adenine dinucleotide (NAD) in mammals and its regulatory mechanism, Part II. *Arzneim. Forsch.* 17:1525–1530.
12. Kaplan, N. O., Goldin, A., Humphreys, S. R., Ciotti, M. M., and Stolzenbach, F. E. 1956. Pyridine nucleotide synthesis in the mouse. *J. Biol. Chem.* 219:287–298.
13. Kun, E., Zimber, P. H., Chang, A. C. Y., Puschendorf, B., and Grunicke, H. 1975. Macromolecular enzymatic product of NAD in liver mitochondria. *Proc. Natl. Acad. Sci. U.S.A.* 72:1436–1440.
14. Lowry, O. H., Rosebrough, N. J., Farr, A. L., and Randall, R. J. 1951. Protein measurement with the folin phenol reagent. *J. Biol. Chem.* 193:256–275.
15. Maguire, M. H., Lukas, M. C., and Rettie, J. F. 1972. Adenine nucleotide salvage synthesis in the rat heart; pathways of adenosine salvage. *Biochim. Biophys. Acta* 262:108–115.
16. Namm, D. H. 1973. Myocardial nucleotide synthesis from purine bases and nucleosides. *Circ. Res.* 33:686–695.

17. Neely, J. R., and Morgan, H. E. 1974. Relationship between carbohydrate and lipid metabolism and the energy balance of heart muscle. *Annu. Rev. Physiol.* 36:413–459.
18. Opie, L. H. 1980. Cardiac metabolism. In: M. Tajuddin, P. R. Das, M. Tariq, and N. S. Dhalla (eds.), *Advances in Myocardiology*, Vol. 1, pp. 3–20. University Park Press, Baltimore.
19. Parrat, J. R., and Marshall, R. J. 1974. The response of isolated cardiac muscle to acute anoxia: Protective effect of adenosine triphosphate and creatine phosphate. *J. Pharm. Pharmacol.* 26:427–433.
20. Petrack, B., Greengard, P., Craston, A., and Sheppy, F. 1965. Nicotinamide deamidase from mammalian liver. *J. Biol. Chem.* 240:1725–1730.
21. Preiss, J., and Handler, P. 1958. Biosynthesis of diphosphopyridine nucleotide. I. Identification of intermediates. *J. Biol. Chem.* 233:488–492.
22. Preiss, J., and Handler, P. 1958. Biosynthesis of diphosphopyridine nucleotide. II. Enzymatic aspects. *J. Biol. Chem.* 233:493–500.
23. Saks, V. A., Rosenshtraukh, L. V., Smirnov, V. N., and Chazov, E. I. 1978. Role of creatine phosphokinase in cellular function and metabolism. *Can. J. Physiol. Pharmacol.* 56:691–706.
24. Saks, V. A., Seppet, E. K., and Smirnov, V. N. 1979. Does oxidative phosphorylation increase the rate of creatine phosphate synthesis in heart mitochondria or not? *J. Mol. Cell. Cardiol.* 11:1265–1273.
25. Seifart, H. I., Delabar, U., and Siess, M. 1980. The influence of various precursors on the concentration of energy-rich phosphates and pyridine nucleotides in cardiac tissue and its possible meaning for anoxic survival. *Basic. Res. Cardiol.* 75:57–61.
26. Severin, S. E., and Tseitlin, L. A. 1974. Biosynthesis and degradation of nicotinamide coenzymes in the myocardium. *Circ. Res.* 34–35(Suppl. III):121–128.
27. Severin, S. E., Tseitlin, L. A., and Telepneva, V. I. 1967. [Biosynthesis of nicotinamide mononucleotide in heart muscle.] *Biokhimiia* 32:181–188.
28. Siess, M. 1980. Some aspects on the regulation of carbohydrate and lipid metabolism in cardiac tissue. *Basic Res. Cardiol.* 75:47–56.
29. Siess, M., and Seifart, H. I. 1980. Anoxic energy production and contractile activity in mammalian cardiac muscle. In: M. Tajuddin, B. Bhatia, H. H. Siddiqui, and G. Rona (eds.), *Advances in Myocardiology*, Vol. 2, pp. 295–310. University Park Press, Baltimore.
30. Streffer, C., Brauer, W., and Benes, J. 1971. Levels of pyridine nucleotides after repeated applications of nicotinic acid in animal tissues. In: K. F. Gey and L. A. Carlson (eds.), *Metabolic Effects of Nicotinic Acid and its Derivatives*, pp. 97–114. Hans Huber, Bern.
31. Williamson, J. R. 1979. Mitochondrial function in the heart. *Annu. Rev. Physiol.* 41:485–506.
32. Zimmer, H. G., and Gerlach, E. 1977. Changes of myocardial adenine nucleotide and protein synthesis during development of cardiac hypertrophy. *Basic Res. Cardiol.* 72:241–246.
33. Zimmer, H. G., and Gerlach, E. 1978. Stimulation of myocardial adenine nucleotide biosynthesis by pentoses and pentitols. *Pfluegers Arch.* 376:223–227.
34. Zimmer, H. G., Ibel, H., Steinkopff, G., and Korb, G. 1980. Reduction of the isoproterenol-induced alterations in cardiac adenine nucleotides and morphology by ribose. *Science* 207:319–321.

Effect of Exogenous Amino Acids on the Contractility and Nitrogenous Metabolism of Anoxic Heart

O. I. Pisarenko, E. S. Solomatina, I. M. Studneva, V. E. Ivanov, V. I. Kapelko, and V. N. Smirnov

Department of Experimental Cardiology
USSR Cardiology Research Center
Academy of Medical Sciences
Moscow 101837, USSR

Abstract. The effect of exogenous glutamic acid and arginine on the contractility of isolated perfused rat heart and on the metabolism of some nitrogenous compounds was studied. Sixty-minute anoxic perfusion (95% N_2 + 5% CO_2) led to a fall in developed isovolumic pressure and an elevation in diastolic pressure, to an increase in the production of alanine, glutamine, and ammonia, and to a decrease in the tissue content of aspartate and glutamate. The total pool of free amino acids and taurine under these conditions remained unchanged. Subsequent 40-min reoxygenation partially restored the contractile function. Addition of 3.5 mM glutamic acid or 5 mM arginine into the perfusate before anoxia resulted in a higher level of developed pressure and a lower level of diastolic pressure during anoxia and almost complete recovery of cardiac function after subsequent reoxygenation. Both amino acids had no effect on ammonia formation by the anoxic heart but enhanced its binding in myocardial tissue via formation of glutamine and urea. It is suggested that the exogenous amino acid effect on anoxic heart is mediated by activation of substrate phosphorylation rather than the ability to bind tissue ammonia.

Cardiac contractility is known to be highly dependent on the oxygen supply. Maximal stimulation of glycolysis in anoxic heart does not lead to improvement of contractile function (4,12). Recently it has been demonstrated that some exogenous amino acids including arginine and glutamate are capable of improving contractile function of isolated rabbit interventricular septa during anoxia or ischemia and recovery (14). It is likely that these amino acids can improve energy supply by direct action on ATP synthesis as well as indirectly via the removal of inhibitors of ATP formation. One of the inhibitors may be ammonia which is accumulated in the myocardium during anoxia and ischemia (20,21). It is known that ammonia efflux from myocardium in the free form is insignificant (9). To a large degree, it is bound in cardiac tissue via reactions that lead to the formation of glutamate, glutamine, alanine, and urea (7,13,17); glutamic acid and arginine are the immediate precursors of these compounds.

This work is an attempt to understand whether the protective action of these amino acids on contractile function under anoxic conditions is related to their ability to diminish the toxic effect of ammonia accumulation. For this purpose, we studied the effect of glutamic acid and arginine on the metabolism of ammonia and some other nitrogenous compounds in isovolumic rat heart. It was found that these amino acids diminished the anoxic contracture and enhanced the energy-dependent reactions of ammonia binding but had no effect on ammonia formation.

METHODS

Heart Perfusion

The experiments were carried out using isolated hearts of male Wistar rats weighing from 250 to 300 g. Hearts were removed from urethane-anesthetized animals and perfused at 30°C according to Langendorff with oxygenated (95% O_2 + 5% CO_2) bicarbonate Krebs–Henseleit buffer, pH 7.4, containing 5.5 mM glucose at 60 mm Hg perfusion pressure and stimulation at the frequency of 120 beats per minute. In all experiments, hearts were perfused for 10 min to remove the blood, and then recirculation with 30 ml of buffer was started. Four series of experiments were performed. In the first series, the hearts were perfused for 90 min by oxygenated bicarbonate buffer. In the second series, 30 min of oxygenated perfusion was followed by 60 min of anoxia (95% N_2 + 5% CO_2) and 40 min of reoxygenation. In the third and fourth series of experiments, 3.5 mM glutamic acid or 5 mM arginine was added to the perfusate 5 min before anoxia, respectively, and was present in the perfusate during the anoxia and reoxygenation periods.

Contractility Measurements

In all experiments, a latex balloon of constant volume was inserted into the left ventricular cavity and connected to a pressure transducer (P 50) and monitor (SP 1405, Gould Statham). The following parameters of contractility were measured: systolic pressure ($P_{syst.}$), diastolic pressure ($P_{diast.}$), and the developed pressure [$P_{dev.} = (P_{syst.} - P_{diast.})$/weight of left ventricle].

Biochemical Determinations

After each experiment the weight of the perfused heart as well as the weight of its ventricles was determined. Hearts were quickly frozen in liquid nitrogen and thoroughly ground. Proteins were precipitated with 6% perchloric acid (5 ml/g of tissue, 2.5 ml/ml of perfusate). The concentration of nitrogenous metabolites (aspartic and glutamic acids, glutamine, alanine, and urea) in protein-free tissue extracts and perfusates was determined using an amino acid analyzer (Beckman M-121). In addition to these compounds, in a number of experiments, the content of taurine, phenylalanine, tyrosine, and the total pool of free amino acids were also measured. The analysis was made using one-column method with Li-citrate buffers (8). Norleucine was used as internal standard.

For statistical treatment of the data, Student's *t*-test was used.

RESULTS

The Effect of Glutamic Acid and Arginine on the Contractility of Anoxic Hearts

During 30 min of the preliminary oxygenation, the developed pressure and coronary flow of isolated heart were stabilized at the level of 131 ± 11 hPa and 11 ± 2 ml/min per g, respectively, and maintained practically unchanged for the next 60 min of oxygenated perfusion. The 60 min of anoxic perfusion following stabilization of function led to a threefold drop in the developed pressure with a simultaneous 2.5-fold increase in the diastolic pressure (Table 1, Figure 1). Systolic pressure was decreased by 26% (Table 1), and coronary flow did not change. After subsequent reoxygenation for 40 min, a noticeable restoration of the contractility was found, and the developed pressure increased up to 76% of the initial value. Diastolic pressure increased at the beginning of reoxygenation, then gradually diminished, and at the end of observation was two-fold higher than the initial value (Figure 1).

The addition of 3.5 mM glutamic acid or 5 mM arginine to the perfusate 5 min before anoxic perfusion did not significantly influence the contractility

Table 1. Effect of Glutamic Acid and Arginine on Contractile Function of Isolated Rat Hearts[a]

Perfusion conditions	Number of animals	Systolic pressure (hPa)	Diastolic pressure (hPa)	Developed pressure (hPa/g)
Control				
Oxygenation	20	91 ± 5	16 ± 1	131 ± 11
Anoxia	20	67 ± 4	40 ± 4	44 ± 5
Recovery	10	84 ± 7	32 ± 5	103 ± 9
Glutamic acid, 3.5 mM				
Oxygenation	15	101 ± 5	15 ± 1	162 ± 13
Anoxia	15	65 ± 4	23 ± 3*	79 ± 8*
Recovery	7	84 ± 8	19 ± 4*	139 ± 11*
Arginine, 5 mM				
Oxygenation	15	97 ± 5	16 ± 1	149 ± 15
Anoxia	15	64 ± 3	21 ± 3*	77 ± 9*
Recovery	7	93 ± 5	19 ± 1*	141 ± 9*

[a] Values represent the mean ± S.E.M. *Significantly different from corresponding control values ($P < 0.01$).

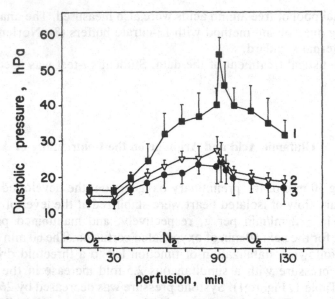

Figure 1.   Effect of exogenous arginine and glutamic acid on diastolic pressure (hPa) changes during perfusion of isolated rat heart. (1) Control (Krebs–Henseleit solution); (2) Krebs–Henseleit solution + 5 mM arginine; (3) Krebs–Henseleit solution + 3.5 mM glutamic acid. Amino acids were administered 5 min before anoxic perfusion. Hearts were perfused at 30°C and stimulated at 120 beats/min.

of oxygenated heart but noticeably preserved the function of anoxic heart. In the presence of these amino acids, the developed pressure of anoxic heart was higher, and during reoxygenation almost complete recovery of function was observed (Table 1). The increase in the diastolic pressure in the presence of amino acids under anoxic conditions was almost twofold lower than without amino acids, and the steep rise in diastolic pressure at the beginning of reoxygenation was practically absent (Figure 1). Thus, the administration of glutamic acid or arginine into the perfusate decreased the impairment of contractility by reducing contracture of the heart muscle.

Content of Nitrogenous Compounds in Tissue and Perfusate of Anoxic Hearts

Changes in the metabolism of a number of nitrogenous compounds were also noticed after anoxic perfusion (Table 2). The most pronounced changes were found for ammonia. Its total content in the heart–perfusate system after anoxic perfusion increased twofold. A parallel increase in alanine and glutamine content was also found in the heart–perfusate system by 81 and 44%, respectively. The opposite effect of anoxia was seen on glutamic and aspartic acids. Their total content in the tissue and perfusate was lower in anoxic than in oxygenated hearts (Table 2).

Anoxic perfusion had no effect on the content of other amino acids in the heart–perfusate system. The taurine pool was also unchanged (Table 3).

Table 2. The Content of Some Nitrogenous Compounds (μmol/g Wet Weight) in Tissue and Perfusate of Isolated Perfused Rat Hearts[a]

Compound	Perfusion conditions	Tissue	Perfusate	Total
Ammonia	Oxygenation	1.87 ± 0.08	2.12 ± 0.15	3.99 ± 0.17
	Anoxia	2.49 ± 0.17*	6.33 ± 1.20*	9.12 ± 1.21*
	Glutamate + anoxia	2.16 ± 0.18	4.61 ± 0.67	6.77 ± 0.70
	Arginine + anoxia	2.59 ± 0.21	6.80 ± 1.13	9.38 ± 1.15
Glutamic acid	Oxygenation	4.12 ± 0.22	0.16 ± 0.03	4.28 ± 0.22
	Anoxia	2.60 ± 0.27*	0.70 ± 0.05*	3.30 ± 0.27*
	Glutamate + anoxia	4.47 ± 0.20**	—	—
	Arginine + anoxia	1.98 ± 0.35	0.46 ± 0.12	3.04 ± 0.37
Aspartic acid	Oxygenation	1.17 ± 0.06	0.11 ± 0.02	1.27 ± 0.06
	Anoxia	0.93 ± 0.06*	0.12 ± 0.03	1.07 ± 0.07*
	Glutamate + anoxia	0.88 ± 0.55	0.39 ± 0.08**	1.27 ± 0.09**
	Arginine + anoxia	0.59 ± 0.08**	0.10 ± 0.01	0.69 ± 0.10**
Glutamine	Oxygenation	5.52 ± 0.77	0.46 ± 0.14	5.98 ± 0.78
	Anoxia	7.20 ± 0.31	1.40 ± 0.12*	8.60 ± 0.33**
	Glutamate + anoxia	10.82 ± 0.59**	—	—
	Arginine + anoxia	6.88 ± 0.44	1.33 ± 0.18	8.21 ± 0.48
Alanine	Oxygenation	2.60 ± 0.22	0.84 ± 0.05	3.44 ± 0.22
	Anoxia	4.04 ± 0.07*	2.12 ± 0.18*	6.22 ± 0.19
	Glutamate + anoxia	3.17 ± 0.22**	1.95 ± 0.28**	5.12 ± 0.36**
	Arginine + anoxia	3.70 ± 0.38**	2.68 ± 0.12**	5.38 ± 0.40

[a] Values represent the mean ± S.E.M.; N = 6–10. Determinations were made after 60 min of anoxic or normal perfusion. *Significantly different from corresponding "oxygenation" value ($P < 0.01$). **Significantly different from corresponding "anoxia" value ($P < 0.01$).

Under the conditions of our experiments, anoxia did not stimulate protein catabolism of the perfused heart: the same amounts of nonmetabolized tyrosine and phenylalanine were found in tissue and perfusate in control and anoxic hearts (Table 3).

The Effect of Glutamic Acid and Arginine on the Metabolism of Some Nitrogenous Compounds during Anoxic Perfusion

To study the effect of glutamic acid on the metabolism of nitrogenous compounds and heart contractility, it was necessary to find a suitable ef-

Table 3. Effect of Anoxia on Total Amino Acid Content (μmol/g Wet Weight) in Tissue and Perfusate of Isolated Rat Heart after 60-min Perfusion

Amino acid	Oxygenation[a]	Anoxia[a]
Taurine	25.62 ± 0.80	24.84 ± 0.89*
Tyrosine	0.13 ± 0.06	0.21 ± 0.04*
Phenylalanine	0.15 ± 0.04	0.20 ± 0.05*
Free amino acid pool	15.48 ± 0.26	16.01 ± 0.57*

[a] Values represent the mean ± S.E.M.; N = 4–6; * not significant.

fective concentration of the compound: 3.5 mM glutamic acid was shown to affect the function of anoxic heart, to change the metabolism of some amino acids and ammonia in the anoxic heart–perfusate system and still to be soluble in the perfusate.

The addition of 3.5 mM glutamic acid to the perfusate stimulated the formation of glutamine, i.e., the reaction by which most of free ammonia is bound (13). Because of the excess of glutamic acid in the perfusate, it was not possible to estimate perfusate glutamine concentration. The tissue concentration of this compound under anoxic conditions increased by 1.5-fold (Table 2). The perfusion of the anoxic heart with glutamic acid maintained the total content of aspartic acid in the tissue and perfusate at the level that was characteristic for oxygenated heart. In the presence of glutamic acid, another product of its transamination, alanine, was accumulated in the heart–perfusate system but at lower level than during anoxia. After addition of glutamic acid, a tendency to a decrease in free ammonia was observed which was more evident for the perfusate.

In addition to glutamic acid, a significant positive effect on heart function was found with arginine perfusion in a concentration of at least 5 mM. The addition of arginine led to a larger decrease in the tissue content of aspartic acid than was typical for anoxic conditions (Table 2). This effect could be caused by the involvement of aspartic acid in the urea synthesis activated by arginine. In fact, after addition of arginine, the total urea content was higher than it is in the oxygenated heart (Table 4). The urea level in the perfusate doubled, and this correlated with an almost twofold decrease in the aspartic acid content. Nevertheless, ammonia formation in the presence of arginine did not change (Table 2).

DISCUSSION

The Nitrogenous Metabolism of Anoxic Heart

Under conditions of anoxic perfusion, the disturbances of heart contractility were accompanied by an increase in the production of ammonia, alanine, and glutamine and a decrease in the level of glutamic and aspartic acids. Glutamic and aspartic acids are usually considered as principle

Table 4. Effect of Arginine on Urea Formation (μmol/g Wet Weight) in Isolated Perfused Rat Hearts[a]

Perfusion conditions	Tissue	Perfusate	Total
Oxygenation	0.57 ± 0.07	0.98 ± 0.15	1.55 ± 0.17
Anoxia	0.95 ± 0.09*	1.03 ± 0.18	1.98 ± 0.20
Arginine + anoxia	1.37 ± 0.07*	1.86 ± 0.15*	3.23 ± 0.17*

[a] Values represent the mean ± S.E.M.; $N = 6$; * significantly different from corresponding "oxygenation" value ($P < 0.01$).

sources of ammonia in muscles (1,11). In our experiments, the decrease in the content of these amino acids, even if it results from their complete deamination, could not compensate for the observed increase in ammonia production (Table 2). The role of amino acids in the formation of ammonia from proteolysis is unlikely since the pool of free amino acids and taurine was not changed, and the content of nonmetabolized tyrosine and phenyl-alanine was not increased during anoxia (Table 3). Glutamine and asparagine deamination could not serve as the source of ammonia formation since during anoxia, the significant accumulation of glutamine in the heart was low (17). At the same time, these data did not rule our possible deamination of glu-tamine and asparagine residues of cardiac proteins (16).

It is quite possible that the increase of ammonia in the anoxic heart–perfusate system could be a result of catabolism of nucleotides. This is indirectly confirmed by the decrease in the level of high-energy phosphates and the increase in their catabolites, inosine and hypoxanthine, and the activation of AMP deaminase in hypoxic myocardium (2,3,6).

During anoxic perfusion, the binding of an excess of free ammonia in the tissue occurs through the formation of nontoxic products, glutamine, alanine, and urea (7,13). The synthesis of glutamine and urea requires ATP, whereas alanine is formed in the reaction of transamination in which no ATP is involved. It is likely that for this reason, under conditions of ATP deficiency during anoxia, the alanine production increased to a larger degree than glutamine synthesis, and the elevation in the formation of urea was negligible (Tables 2,4).

The activation of alanine synthesis under anoxic conditions was prob-ably the result of an increase in stimulation of glycolysis and was the con-sequence of the increase in the concentration of pyruvate, the immediate alanine precursor (19). Lactate, the final product of pyruvate metabolism in muscles, is known to inhibit the glycolytic pathways of energy production. Therefore, alanine synthesis that decreased lactate formation could be con-sidered as an alternative route for pyruvate metabolism. This probably re-flects metabolic adaptation of the myocardium to the inhibition of oxidative processes by anoxia.

The decrease in the content of glutamic and aspartic acids in the anoxic heart–perfusate system could be the result of stimulation of glutamine syn-thesis as well as the use of these amino acids as the source of succinate, the level of succinate being increased under anoxic conditions (15,18,19). The relationship between transamination of these amino acids and succinate production was confirmed by its diminished formation in the presence of aminooxyacetate, the specific inhibitor of cellular and mitochondrial trans-aminases (19).

The Effect of Exogenous Glutamic Acid and Arginine in Anoxia

Anoxic disturbances of contractility were partially compensated by the addition of exogenous glutamic acid and arginine. The ability of these amino acids to decrease the degree of contracture, thus supporting the contractility of hypoxic myocardium at a higher level, could be related to an increase in the energy supply of myofibrils. The changes in the metabolism of nitrogenous compounds after perfusion with these amino acids do not contradict to this view.

Thus, perfusion with glutamic acid prevented the decrease in glutamic and aspartic acids in the anoxic heart–perfusate system observed under anaerobic conditions (Table 2). As a consequence, an increase in intracellular glutamic acid led to a significant increase in the synthesis of glutamine which required ATP. Decrease in alanine formation provided further evidence for the presence of an additional energy source of nonglycolytic origin in the cells of anoxic heart during acid perfusion. However, in spite of intensive formation of glutamine, the ammonia level in the tissue and perfusate was not significantly reduced.

The protective effect of glutamic acid and arginine during anoxia and the improvement of heart function during reoxygenation were similar for both amino acids. However, the effect of arginine on the metabolism of nitrogenous compounds had some peculiarities. In contrast to glutamic acid,

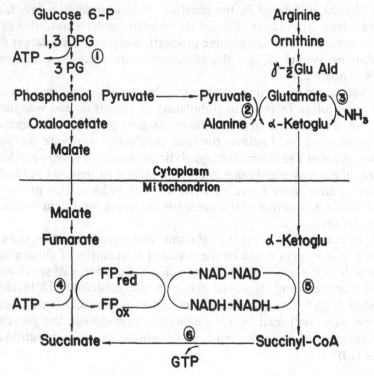

Figure 2. Metabolic pathways demonstrating anaerobic energy production in heart muscle during arginine and glutamate perfusion. (1) 3-Phosphoglycerate kinase; (2) alanine aminotransferase; (3) glutamate dehydrogenase; (4) fumarate reductase; (5) α-ketoglutarate dehydrogenase; (6) succinyl-CoA synthetase. Adapted from Hochachka et al. (5).

arginine perfusion did not lead to significant changes in the metabolism of alanine, glutamic acid, and glutamine during anoxia. At the same time, the perfusion with arginine caused a significant decrease in the tissue level of aspartic acid which was probably related to the activities of urea synthesis requiring ATP (Tables 2 and 4). In spite of the increase in urea synthesis, ammonia accumulated in the tissue and perfusate at the same rate as in the absence of arginine. Probably an additional source of the ammonia that is involved in urea formation was glutamic acid, the product of the arginine oxidation, which would be deaminated in the glutamate dehydrogenase reaction. Figure 2 illustrates possible relationships among amino acid metabolism, glycolysis, and substrate phosphorylation. These reactions could be considered an adaptation for simultaneous mobilization of carbohydrates and amino acids under anoxic conditions. Besides, the mechanism of the stimulation of substrate phosphorylation in the presence of arginine might be related not only to its transformation into glutamic acid but also to the formation of the additional amount of fumarate which was a substrate in reactions leading to ATP synthesis.

Thus, both amino acids had no effect on ammonia formation but stimulated the reaction of its energy-dependent binding and improved the contractile function of hypoxic isolated hearts. The definite improvement after ischemia following intravenous glutamic acid administration was demonstrated in patients (10). These data suggest the use of exogenous amino acids for prevention and treatment of some heart diseases related to the ischemic state of the myocardium. It is also likely that the addition of these amino acids into cardioplegic solutions might have beneficial effect on the state of the myocardium during open heart surgery.

REFERENCES

1. Braunstein, A. E. 1969. Les voies principales de l'assimilation et dissimilation d l'azote chez les animaux. *Adv. Enzymol.* 19:335–389.
2. Deuticke, B., Gerlach, E., and Dierkesmann, K. 1966. Abbau freier Nucleotide im Herz Skelettmusckel, Gehirn und Lebel der Ratte bei Sauerstoffmangel. *Pfluegers Arch.* 292:239–254.
3. Gerlach, E., Deuticke, B., and Dreibach, R. H. 1963. Nucleotid Abbau im Herzmuskel bei Sauerstoffmangel und seine moglicke Bedeutung fur die Coronardurchblutung. *Naturwissenschaften* 50:228–229.
4. Gmeiner, R., Knapp, E., and Dienstl, F. 1974. Effect of insulin on the performance of the hypoxic rat heart. *J. Mol. Cell. Cardiol.* 6:201–206.
5. Hochachka, P., Owen, T. G., Allen, J. F., and Whittow, G. C. 1975. Multiple end products of anaerobiosis in diving vertebrates. *Comp. Biochem. Physiol.* 508:17–22.
6. Imai, S., Riley, A. L., and Berne, R. M. 1964. Effect of ischemia on adenine nucleotides in cardiac and skeletal muscle. *Circ. Res.* 15:443–450.
7. Kato, T. 1968. Myocardial amide nitrogen metabolism with special reference to ammonia metabolism. *Jpn. Circ. J.* 32:1401–1416.
8. Kedenburg, C. P. 1971. A lithium buffer system for accelerated single-column amino acids analysis. *Anal. Biochem.* 40:35–42.

318   O. I. Pisarenko et al.

9. Kobayashi, T. 1967. Myocardial amide–nitrogen metabolism with special reference to ammonia metabolism. *Jpn. Circ. J.* 31:33–38.
10. Kotz, J. L., and Galiautdinov, G. S. 1980. Protection of ischemic myocardium with glutamic acid. *J. Mol. Cell. Cardiol.* 12(Suppl. 1):80.
11. Lowenstein, I. M. 1972. Ammonia production in muscle and other tissues: The purine nucleotide cycle. *Physiol. Rev.* 52:382–414.
12. McLeod, D. P., and Daniel, E. E. 1965. Influence of glucose on the transmembrane action potential of anoxic papillary muscle. *J. Gen. Physiol.* 48:887–899.
13. Pisarenko, O. I., Artemov, A. V., and Smirnov, V. N. 1980. Study of nitrogen metabolism in the cardiac muscle using the isotope ^{15}N. In: *Energy Transport, Protein Synthesis, and Hormonal Control of Heart Metabolism. (Fourth USA–USSR Joint Symposium on Myocardial Metabolism, Tashkent, USSR, Sept. 14–16, 1979)*, pp. 329–351. NIH Publication, Bethesda.
14. Rau, E. E., Shine, K. I., Gervais, A., Douglas, A. M., and Amos, E. C. III. 1979. Enhanced mechanical recovery of anoxic and ischemic myocardium by amino acid perfusion. *Am. J. Physiol.* 236(6):H873–H879.
15. Sanborn, T., Gavin, W., Berkowitz, S., Perille, T., and Lesch, M. 1979. Augmented conversion of aspartate and glutamate to succinate during anoxia in rabbit heart. *Am. J. Physiol.* 237(5):H535–H541.
16. Silakova, A. I., and Yavilyakova, A. 1964. [On participation of protein amide nitrogen in ammonia formation in muscle.] *Vopr. Med. Khim.* 10:40–43.
17. Smirnov, V. N., Asafov, G. B., Cherpachenko, N. M., Chernousova, G. B., Mozzhechkow, V. T., Krivov, V. I., Ovchinnikov, Iu. A., Merimson, V. G., Rozynov, B. G., and Chumachenko, M. T. 1974. Ammonia neutralization and urea synthesis in cardiac muscle. *Circ. Res.* 35:(Suppl. 3):58–69.
18. Taegtmeyer, H. 1978. Metabolic responses to cardiac hypoxia. Increased production of succinate by rabbit papillary muscle. *Circ. Res.* 43:805–815.
19. Taegtmeyer, H., Peterson, M. B., Ragavan, V. V., Ferguson, A. G., and Lesch, M. 1977. De nova alanine synthesis in isolated oxygen-deprived rabbit myocardium. *J. Biol. Chem.* 252:5010–5018.
20. Takahashi, A. 1967. Myocardial protein metabolism following coronary occlusion. *Jpn. Circ. J.* 31:581–600.
21. Thorn, W., and Heimann, J. 1958. Effect of anoxia, ischemia, asphyxia and reduced temperature on the ammonia in the brain and other organs. *J. Neurochem.* 2:166–177.

Regulation of Cardiac Contractility and Glycolysis by Cyclic Nucleotides during Hypoxia

T. Metsä-Ketelä, K. Laustiola, and H. Vapaatalo

Department of Biomedical Sciences
University of Tampere
33101 Tampere 10, Finland

Abstract. It has been suggested that cyclic nucleotides (cAMP and cGMP) participate in the regulation of cardiac contractility and glycolysis. In the present study, this possible involvement was examined in spontaneously beating rat atria during hypoxia (50% oxygen saturation). Thirty seconds after reduction of high oxygen saturation (HiOxSa) in the incubation medium, the contraction amplitude declined to 50% of the initial level. The decline was partly antagonized by norepinephrine (NE) or hypercalcemia. The cAMP level remained unchanged during hypoxia, but the cGMP content gradually increased. Paradoxically, the production of lactate decreased after 30 sec of hypoxia but had increased by 2 min, when depletion of creatine phosphate and ATP stores was also initiated. Sodium nitroprusside (nitroprusside) and NE elevated the cGMP and cAMP, respectively, in both HiOxSa and hypoxia. Nitroprusside and NE also showed a positive inotropic effect in HiOxSa. Verapamil decreased contractility without changing the levels of cAMP or cGMP. In HiOxSa, both nitroprusside and verapamil decreased lactate production but were not able to resist the increase in atrial lactate level brought about by NE. In hypercalcemia the amplitude increased, but lactate production was slightly reduced in HiOxSa. Between 5 and 10 min of hypoxia, ^{45}Ca uptake was reduced to about one-third of that in the control. It is suggested that lack of oxygen has direct and parallel effects on the sarcolemma and the mitochondria. The former induces deterioration of contractility, the latter termination of aerobic energy production. Cyclic nucleotides are not involved in either of these phenomena. However, at a low rate of anaerobic glycolysis, e.g., in HiOxSa or at the very early stage of hypoxia, cGMP could inhibit and cAMP accelerate lactate production.

Both contractility and production of energy in the heart are altered by hypoxia and ischemia. The ATP level remains unaffected during the initial period of hypoxia, although contractility dramatically deteriorates (13). It has therefore been suggested that the functional compartment of ATP is reduced and that this could explain the impaired contractility (10). The response to acidosis mimics the response to hypoxia, and the Ca^{2+}–troponin interaction can be disturbed by a low pH (14). Thus, reduction of intracellular pH may be one of the factors causing the early decline of contractility (23).

The role of adenosine-3′,5′-monophosphate (cAMP) in the regulation of glyogenolysis and positive inotropism is widely accepted (22,24). Cyclic AMP has been assumed to stimulate glycolysis via protein kinases by phosphorylation of phosphorylase kinase and also by a direct stimulatory effect

319

on phosphofructokinase (22). Guanosine-3'-5'-monophosphate (cGMP), according to the yin–yang hypothesis of Goldberg et al. (9), has many antagonistic effects on cAMP. Thus, it decreases phosphofructokinase activity both directly (2) and by reducing the glucose-1,6-diphosphate level (3). Cyclic GMP-dependent protein kinase also phosphorylates several enzymes of carbohydrate metabolism (8). Hypoxia and ischemia have been reported to alter the levels of both cyclic nucleotides (15).

In the present study, we evaluated the effects of hypoxia on glycolysis, contractility, ^{45}Ca uptake, and the levels of cyclic nucleotides in isolated spontaneously beating rat atria. Norepinephrine, nitroprusside, and verapamil, alone and combined with hypoxia, were also used to analyze further the effects mentioned above.

MATERIALS AND METHODS

Spontaneously beating isolated atria of male Wistar rats (200–250 g) were incubated at 30°C in an organ bath (20 ml) with continuous flow of oxygenated Tyrode's solution. The amplitudes of contractions were recorded isometrically. Oxygen saturation was monitored with a Clark's electrode and kept at 95–100% (HiOxSa). Hypoxia was induced after a stabilization period of 45 min by sodium dithionite (2 × 10^{-3} M) and by interrupting oxygenation. The atria were freeze-clamped, powdered, and suspensed in perchloric acid (19). L-Lactate, creatine phosphate (CP), and ATP were determined enzymatically (11,16). The cAMP and cGMP determinations were made by protein-binding assays (4,7). The ^{45}Ca uptake was measured by a modification (19) of the method evolved by Meinertz et al. (18). Student's t-test was used for statistical analysis.

RESULTS

Reduction of oxygen saturation of the incubation medium from HiOxSa to half caused a failure of contractility in a few seconds (Figure 1). The amplitude was about 50% of the control at 30 sec. The decrease in frequency developed more slowly, it being about 70% of the control at 4 min. Hypoxia-induced negative inotropism was resisted by norepinephrine (1 × 10^{-6} M) and hypercalcemia (5.7 × 10^{-3} M) but not by verapamil (5 × 10^{-6} M) or by nitroprusside (1 × 10^{-4} M) (Figure 1). Verapamil itself showed a negative inotropic effect in HiOxSa.

The high-energy phosphates, CP and ATP (Figure 2), were only reduced after 2 min of hypoxia. After 4 min of hypoxia, ATP returned to the control level. The atrial concentration of lactate (Figure 2) was reduced 30 sec after the induction of hypoxia but began gradually to increase thereafter. At 2

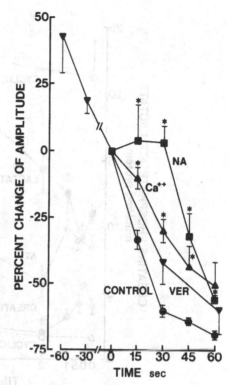

Figure 1. Effects of norepinephrine (NE) (1 × 10⁻⁶ M), hypercalcemia (Ca²⁺) (5.7 × 10⁻³ M instead of 1.9 × 10⁻³ M), and verapamil (Ver) (5 × 10⁻⁶ M) administered 60 sec before hypoxia on hypoxia-induced decline of amplitude in isolated spontaneously beating rat atria. Means ± S.E. of 6–8 preparations. Asterisk indicates statistical significance compared to the control.

min, lactate was already elevated compared to the lowered content at 30 sec and at 4 min compared to the HiOxSa level.

Of cyclic nucleotides only cGMP was influenced by hypoxia, being elevated at 8 min, whereas cAMP remained constant during the observation period of 16 min (not shown in Figure 2). Nitroprusside markedly increased the atrial level of cGMP (Table 1). The effect was additive to that of hypoxia. The level of cAMP was not changed by this drug. Neither verapamil nor

Table 1. Effects of Sodium Nitroprusside (SNP, 1 × 10⁻⁴ M) on Cyclic Nucleotides and Lactate in Isolated Rat Atria at High Oxygen Saturation (100%) and in Hypoxia (50% for 8 min)[a]

Drug	Oxygen saturation (%)	Cyclic AMP (pmol/mg protein)	Cyclic GMP (pmol/mg protein)	Lactate (nmol/mg protein)
Control	100	4.9 ± 0.6	0.27 ± 0.02	36.2 ± 2.7
Control	50	4.8 ± 0.4	0.53 ± 0.07*	59.7 ± 5.6*
SNP (1 × 10⁻⁴ M)	100	5.83 ± 0.6	0.67 ± 0.09*	26.0 ± 1.3*
SNP (1 × 10⁻⁴ M)	50	6.0 ± 0.7	1.15 ± 0.35*	68.3 ± 7.6*

[a] Means ± S.E.M. (N = 7) are given. *P < 0.05 compared to high-oxygen control.

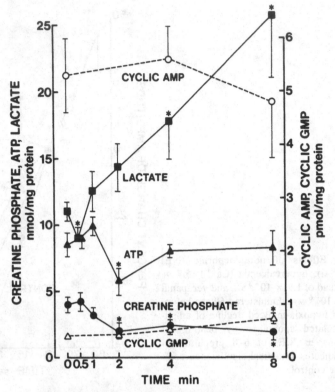

Figure 2.   Effects of hypoxia on the tissue levels of lactate, ATP, creatine phosphate, and cyclic nucleotides in isolated spontaneously beating rat atria. Means ± S.E. of 6–8 preparations are given. Asterisks indicate statistical significance versus the control level (0 value).

hypercalcemia altered the levels of cyclic nucleotides. Norepinephrine enhanced the level of cAMP in both HiOxSa and hypoxia.

In HiOxSa, nitroprusside and verapamil reduced the atrial lactate content (Table 2). Nitroprusside did not influence the rate of lactate generation after 8 min of hypoxia (Table 1). Norepinephrine increased the lactate level at 2 min. Neither nitroprusside nor verapamil could antagonize this increase (Table 2). Verapamil, however, reduced the maximal increase in amplitude caused by norepinephrine (Table 2). Hypercalcemia of 2 min decreased lactate production in HiOxSa.

In HiOxSa, norepinephrine increased ^{45}Ca uptake into atria from 2.03 ± 0.13 pmol/mg protein per 5 min to 2.68 ± 0.34 pmol/mg protein per 5 min ($N = 5$; $P < 0.05$). Hypoxia reduced the uptake to 0.73 ± 0.34 pmol/ mg protein per 5 min ($N = 5$; $P < 0.05$).

DISCUSSION

The role of anaerobic glycolysis in the maintenance of sarcolemmal integrity and preservation of cardiac tissue and contractility in hypoxic or

Table 2. Effects of Various Drugs on Contraction Amplitude and the Production of Lactate in Isolated Rat Atria at High Oxygen Saturation (100%)[a]

Drug	Time of exposure (min)	Amplitude (%)	Lactate (nmol/g protein)
Control	—	100	22.2 ± 1.4
SNP[b] (10^{-4} M)	5	112 ± 6*	16.6 ± 2.0*
NE[c] (10^{-6} M)	2	209 ± 16*[d]	29.8 ± 3.2*
SNP + NE	3 + 2	176 ± 6*[d]	30.4 ± 3.7*
Verapamil (10^{-6} M)	5	48 ± 5*[e]	15.9 ± 0.7*[e]
Verapamil + NE	3 + 2	152 ± 5*[d,e]	27.7 ± 3.8[e]
CaCl$_2$ (5.7 × 10^{-3} M)	2	226 ± 8*	19.0 ± 0.9*

[a] Means ± S.E.M. are given. *$P < 0.05$ compared to control. N = 5–6.
[b] Sodium nitroprusside.
[c] Norepinephrine.
[d] $P < 0.05$ compared with each other.
[e] $P < 0.05$ compared with each other.

ishemic conditions is not exactly known. It has been assumed that ATP generated anaerobically might be critical for the survival of the myocardium in hypoxia. An improvement in the energetic state by anaerobically produced ATP is, however, gained only at the expense of unfavorable changes in the pH (6). It should also be noted that hypoxia causes a strong diminution in contractility which leads to a decreased energy demand in the hypoxic tissue. This could imply that the beneficial effects of the anaerobically produced energy could be overridden by the detrimental effects of simultaneously produced protons. Inhibition of glycolysis has been described in the ischemic heart, but in the case of hypoxia, it was not possible to demonstrate the expected effect.

In spite of the high oxygen saturation of the incubation medium, the energetic state of our preparation was not quite satisfactory. This is indicated by the low CP/ATP ratio. The inability of our atria to meet their energetic requirements could be because of insufficient oxygen diffusion or lack of carbon substrate (20).

Under these conditions, nitroprusside reduced the atrial lactate content with simultaneous doubling of the tissue cGMP content. The slight positive inotropic effect of nitroprusside is not in keeping with the concept of cGMP as a mediator of negative inotropism (5). Nitroglycerin, which also stimulated the formation of cGMP (12), has been shown to prevent ischemic changes in myocardial carbohydrate metabolism in the dog in situ (1). Cyclic GMP inhibits phosphofructokinase (2), especially when the enzyme is partly inhibited by ATP or citrate. We therefore suggest that nitroprusside, as well as nitroglycerin, exerts direct effects on the myocardium. These primarily inhibitory effects on anaerobic glycolysis might be beneficial at an early stage of hypoxia or ischemia in that the fall in intracellular pH is counteracted.

The effect of verapamil on lactate production resembled that of nitroprusside. Verapamil, however, reduced the amplitude but did not increase the cGMP level. The decreased glycolysis and lactate production might consequently be caused by an improvement in phosphate potential which in turn would decrease glycolysis at the level of phosphofructokinase (20). Cyclic AMP could mainly be responsible for the enhanced lactate production caused by norepinephrine. This view is supported by the finding that norepinephrine in the presence of verapamil increased the amplitude by only about 50% without any diminution in lactate production.

The most marked failure of contractility was seen within 30 sec without any changes in CP or ATP. Glycolysis was reduced, which rules out the decrease of pH as a cause of the failure. The atria maintained their responsiveness to norepinephrine and hypercalcemia, which excludes shortage of ATP. Recently, Lebedev et al. (17) demonstrated that calcium permeability through bilayer membranes depends on the amount of primary oxidation products of phospholipids in the membranes. In the present study, the strong inhibition of ^{45}Ca uptake in hypoxia atria could result from a reduction in the lipid hydroperoxides in the membranes. The decline in ^{45}Ca uptake could also partly be caused by decreased frequency (30%), but this hardly explains the whole change (65%) in this parameter. Thus, we would propose that the rapid decline in amplitude is a direct effect of oxygen lack on membrane function rather than a metabolic one. A similar mechanism has been suggested for the increased ^{42}K efflux in hypoxia (21).

In conclusion, we suggest that oxygen shortage directly affects the biological membranes of the heart. Consequently, ion flux through the sarcolemma decreases and causes deterioration of contractility. The termination of oxidative phosphorylation turns the energy production to anaerobic glycolysis and lactate production in 1–2 min. The cyclic nucleotides are not involved in either phenomenon. In light hypoxia, however, cAMP and cGMP might activate or inhibit phosphofructokinase, respectively. Whether the antianginal nitrous compounds exert their beneficial effect partly by a direct inhibitory action of cGMP on anaerobic glycolysis remains to be elucidated.

ACKNOWLEDGMENTS

This study was supported by a grant from the Orion and Medica Scientific Foundation, Finland.

REFERENCES

1. Abiko, Y., Ichihara, K., and Izumi, T. 1979. Effects of antianginal drugs on ischemic myocardial metabolism. In: M. M. Winbury and Y. Abiko (eds.), Perspectives in Cardiovascular Research, Vol. 3, pp. 155–169. Raven Press, New York.
2. Beitner, R., Haberman, S., and Cycowitz, T. 1977. The effect of cyclic GMP on phosphofructokinase from rat tissues. Biochim. Biophys. Acta 482:330–340.

3. Beitner, R., Haberman, S., Nordenberg, J., and Cohen, T. 1978. The levels of cyclic GMP and glucose 1,6-diphosphate, and the activity of phosphofructokinase, in muscle from normal and dystrophic mice. *Biochim. Biophys. Acta* 542:537–541.

4. Dinnendahl, V. A. 1974. A rapid and simple procedure for the determination of guanosine 3′,5′-monophosphate by use of the protein-binding method. *Naunyn Schmiedebergs Arch. Pharmacol.* 284:55–61.

5. George, W. J., Polson, J. B., O'Toole, A. G., and Goldberg, N. D. 1970. Elevation of guanosine 3′,5′-cyclic phosphate in rat heart after perfusion with acetylcholine. *Proc. Natl. Acad. Sci. U.S.A.* 66:398–403.

6. Gevers, W. 1977. Generation of protons by metabolic processes in heart cells. *J. Mol. Cell. Cardiol.* 9:867–874.

7. Gilman, A. G. 1970. A protein-binding assay for adenosine 3′,5′-cyclic monophosphate. *Proc. Natl. Acad. Sci. U.S.A.* 67:305–312.

8. Glass, D. B., and Krebs, E. G. 1980. Protein phosphorylation catalyzed by cyclic AMP-dependent and cyclic GMP-dependent protein kinases. *Annu. Rev. Pharmacol. Toxicol.* 20:363–388.

9. Goldberg, N. D., Haddox, M. K., Nicol, S. E., Glass, D. B., Sanford, C. H., Kuehl, F. A., Jr., and Estensen, R. 1975. Biologic regulation through opposing influences of cyclic GMP and cyclic AMP: The yin yang hypothesis. *Adv. Cyclic Nucleotide Res.* 5:307–330.

10. Gudbjarnason, S., Mathes, P., and Ravens, K. G. 1970. Functional compartmentation of ATP and creatine phosphate in heart muscle. *J. Mol. Cell. Cardiol.* 1:325–339.

11. Hohorst, H.-J. 1970. L-(+)-Lactat. Bestimmung mit Lactat-Dehydrogenase und NAD. In: H. U. Bergmeyer (ed.), *Methoden der Enzymatischen Analyse II*, pp. 1425–1429. Verlag Chemie, Weinheim.

12. Katsuki, S., Arnold, W. P., and Murad, F. 1977. Effects of sodium nitroprusside, nitroglycerin and sodium azide on levels of cyclic nucleotides and mechanical activity of various tissues. *J. Cyclic Nucleotide Res.* 3:239–247.

13. Katz, A. M. 1977. *Physiology of the Heart*, pp. 420–428. Raven Press, New York.

14. Katz, A. M., and Hecht, H. H. 1969. The early "pump" failure of the ischemic heart. *Am. J. Med.* 47:497–501.

15. Krause, E. G., and Wollenberger, A. 1980. Cyclic nucleotides in acute myocardial ischemia and hypoxia. *Adv. Cyclic Nucleotide Res.* 12:49–61.

16. Lambrecht, W., Stein, P., Heinz, F., and Weisser, H. 1970. Creatinphosphat. In: H. U. Bergmeyer (ed.), *Methoden der Enzymatischen Analyse II*, pp. 1729–1733. Verlag Chemie, Weinheim.

17. Lebedev, A. V., Levitsky, D. O., and Loginov, V. A. 1980. Lipid hydroperoxides as indicators of cation permeability through biological membranes (simplest calcium channel). *J. Mol. Cell. Cardiol.* 12(Suppl. 1):92.

18. Meinertz, T., Nawrath, H., and Scholz, H. 1973. Dibutyryl cyclic AMP and adrenaline increase contractile force and ^{45}Ca uptake in mammalian cardiac muscle. *Naunyn Schmiedebergs Arch. Pharmacol.* 277:107–112.

19. Metsä-Ketelä, T., Laustiola, K., Lilius, E.-M., and Vapaatalo, H. 1980. On the role of cyclic nucleotides in the regulation of cardiac contractility and glycolysis during hypoxia. *Acta Pharmacol. Toxicol. (Kbh.)* 48:311–319.

20. Neely, J. R., Whitmer, K. M., and Mochizuki, S. 1976. Effects of mechanical activity and hormones on myocardial glucose and fatty acid utilization. *Circ. Res.* 38(Suppl. I):22–29.

21. Rau, E. E., and Langer, G. A. 1978. Dissociation of energetic state and potassium loss from anoxic myocardium. *Am. J. Physiol.* 235:H537–H543.

22. Robison, G. A., Butcher, R. W., and Sutherland, E. W. 1971. *Cyclic AMP*. Academic Press, New York.

23. Steenbergen, C., Geleew, G., Rich, T., and Williamson, J. R. 1977. Effects of acidosis and ischemia on contractility and intracellular pH of rat heart. *Circ. Res.* 41:849–858.

24. Tsien, R. W. 1977. Cyclic AMP and contractile activity in heart. *Adv. Cycl. Nucl. Res.* 9:363–420.

Hypoxia, Calcium, and Contracture as Mediators of Myocardial Enzyme Release

C. E. Ganote, S. Y. Liu, S. Safavi,
and J. P. Kaltenbach

Department of Pathology
Northwestern University Medical School
Chicago, Illinois 60611, USA

Abstract. During calcium-free perfusion, anoxic contracture of myocardial cells causes cells to separate at intercalated disks and leads to an energy-independent enzyme release in the absence of active transmembrane calcium fluxes. It is proposed that contracture mediates membrane damage and enzyme release in cells sensitized to the calcium paradox.

The mechanism of enzyme release from myocardial cells during irreversible injury has not been established. The enzyme release occurring in both the calcium paradox and on reoxygenation of anoxic myocardium is associated with morphological evidence of abnormal cellular contracture and sarcolemmal membrane injury. The present study was designed to assess the role of calcium and cellular contracture in mediating enzyme release from anoxic hearts. These experiments show that during anoxic perfusions with calcium-free medium, myocardial enzyme release occurs. The results of this study suggest that absence of calcium causes membrane changes in sensitized cells. Anoxic contracture of sensitized cells is associated with cell separations, membrane damage, and enzyme release.

MATERIALS AND METHODS

Hearts were removed from 200- to 300-g Sprague–Dawley rats and cannulated to a Langendorff apparatus for perfusion at 37°C. Perfusion fluid was a Krebs–Henseleit medium containing 2.5 mM calcium and was gassed with 95% O_2, 5% CO_2. Glucose was omitted from the anoxic medium which was gassed with 95% N_2, 5% CO_2. Calcium was omitted from calcium-free media which also contained 0.1 mM EDTA. Creatine kinase activity was measured in heart effluents with an automatic enzyme analyzer. At the end of each experiment, hearts were perfusion-fixed with 1% glutaraldehyde and processed for light and electron microscopy.

327

RESULTS

Hearts perfused with oxygenated but calcium-free medium immediately stopped contractions. No significant enzyme release occurred for a 75-min period. When these hearts were examined by light and electron microscopy, sarcomeres appeared relaxed, with prominent I-bands. The most prominent lesion was clefts in the intercalated disks caused by lysis of macula adherens junctions. Nexus junctions remained intact, and thin membrane protrusions connected cells at nexus junctions.

When hearts were anoxic during calcium-free perfusion, significant enzyme release was observed within 5 min which continued for 75 min but was already declining by 45 min (Figure 1). Microscopy revealed contracted cells which were widely separated at intercalated disks (Figure 2). By electron microscopy sarcolemmal membranes were fragmented, and portons of cell membranes of one cell could be seen attached to nexus junctions of adjacent cells.

Anoxic hearts in the presence of calcium released little enzyme activity by 60 min at which time calcium was removed from the perfusate. After a 2- to 3-min delay, there was a large peak of enzyme release, reaching a maximum by 65 min and declining thereafter (Figure 3). These hearts were morphologically indistinguishable from the hearts in the previous experiment. Cells had undergone contracture and were widely separated one from another. Cell membranes were fragmented, and cellular debris was scattered in the space between cells (Figure 4).

Glucose included in anoxic perfusates largely protected hearts from enzyme release on removal of calcium from the perfusates.

DISCUSSION

An abrupt release of cytoplasmic enzymes and proteins from isolated perfused rat hearts occurs when calcium is readmitted to the perfusate after a brief interval of calcium-free perfusion. This phenomenon, originally described by Zimmerman and Hulsmann (3), is known as the "calcium paradox." It requires about 3 min of calcium-free perfusion to sensitize myocardial cells to calcium. If calcium is reperfused before this critical interval,

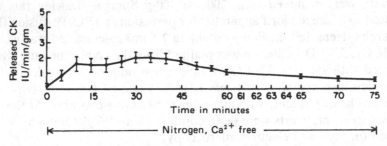

Figure 1. Enzyme release from ten hearts during perfusion with anoxic and calcium-free medium. Values are means ± S.E.M.

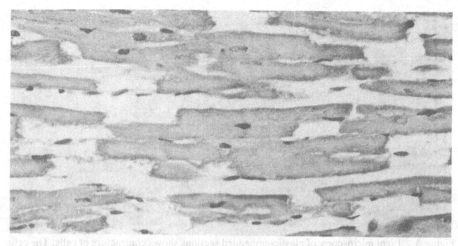

Figure 2. A paraffin-embedded section of a heart perfused with anoxic and calcium-free medium. The cells have undergone contracture and are separated at intercalated disks. Hemotoxylin and eosin. × 200.

cardiac contractions are resumed, and enzyme release is not observed. If calcium is readmitted after 3 min or more of calcium-free perfusion, the calcium paradox occurs with an immediate peak of enzyme release. Histological examination of these hearts reveals that most myocytes are separated from adjacent cells, and each cell is seen to have shortened to form a single contraction band of agglutinated hypercontracted sarcomeres. Sar-

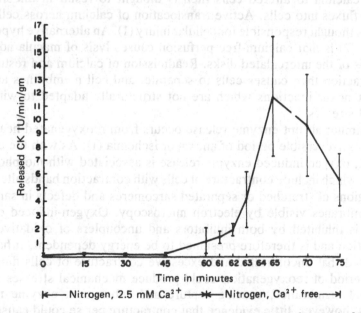

Figure 3. Enzyme release from ten hearts during anoxic perfusion for 60 min followed by anoxic and calcium-free perfusion. After an initial 3-min delay, anoxic hearts rapidly released enzymes during calcium-free perfusion. Values are means ± S.E.M.

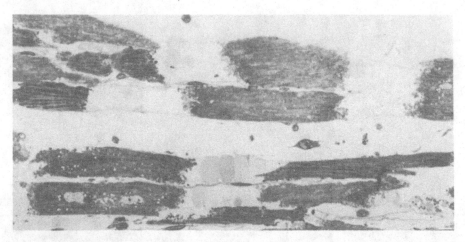

Figure 4.   Light microscopy of plastic-embedded sections shows contracture of cells. The cells have pulled apart at intercalated disks, leaving sarcotubular membranes containing cytoplasmic debris. Toluidine blue. ×600.

colemmal membranes are fragmentated. As little as 50 μM calcium is sufficient to prevent the calcium paradox, and enzyme release in the calcium paradox is energy dependent, not occurring if hearts are depleted of energy supplies prior to readmission of calcium.

Removal of calcium from the extracellular fluid alters sarcolemmal membranes so that calcium permeability is selectively increased. Readmission of calcium to altered cells then is thought to result in uncontrolled calcium fluxes into cells. Active translocation of calcium across cell membranes is thought responsible for cellular injury (1). An alternative hypothesis by Muir (2) is that calcium-free perfusion causes lysis of macula adherens junctions of the intercalated disks. Readmission of calcium and resumption of contraction then causes cells to separate, and cell membranes are torn at intact nexus junctions which are not structurally adapted to withstand physical stresses.

A similar abrupt enzyme release occurs from reoxygenated hearts following an irreversible period of anoxia or ischemia (1). As with the calcium paradox, oxygen-induced enzyme release is associated with morphological changes which include contracture of cells with contraction bands alternating with regions of stretched or separated sarcomeres and defects in sarcolemmal membranes visible by electron microscopy. Oxygen-induced enzyme release is inhibited by both inhibitors and uncouplers of oxidative phosphorylation and is therefore presumed to be energy dependent. It has been postulated that uncontrolled and excessive contracture of cells during the initial period of reoxygenation could produce mechanical stresses on sarcolemmal membranes, causing rupture and subsequent enzyme release. There is, however, little evidence that contracture per se could cause membrane injury in intact hearts.

In the present study we confirmed, in oxygenated hearts, that with calcium-free perfusion, cell sarcomeres remained relaxed. There was breakdown of macula adherens junctions, and clefts appeared in intercalated disk spaces. Many nexus junctions remained intact.

Hearts made anoxic during calcium-free perfusion contained cells with shortened sarcomeres, indicating contracture, and adjacent cells were widely separated at intercalated disks. Fragments of sarcolemmal membranes of one cell could be seen adherent to a nexus junction of adjacent cells. A slow and continuous low level of enzyme release was observed in this experiment.

Hearts made anoxic in the presence of calcium released little enzyme activity during anoxic perfusion but did undergo anoxic contracture. By 60 min of anoxia, these hearts would be largely depleted of energy reserves. Removal of calcium from the perfusion fluid resulted in an abrupt enzyme release which began only after a 2- to 3-min delay. This delay is equivalent to the time required for cells to become sensitized to the calcium paradox. The massive enzyme release under these anoxic conditions occurred both independently of an energy source and in the absence of calcium fluxes into cells. The morphological appearance of these hearts differed from hearts after the calcium paradox. Instead of cells showing single contraction bands, as in the calcium paradox, cells in anoxic hearts were uniformly contracted with distinct sarcomeres equally spaced throughout the cells. Like the calcium paradox, however, cells were widely separated at intercalated disks, and sarcolemmal membranes were fragmented, leaving cellular debris trailing between the separated cells.

A hypothesis to explain these results is that anoxic hearts, during contracture, develop tension which is transmitted between cells by macula adherens junctions across the intercalated disk space. Removal of calcium from the perfusate, after a brief delay, causes lysis of macula adherens junctions and cell separation. As cells separate, sarcolemmal membranes are damaged, perhaps at nexus junctions which are not constructed to withstand contractile forces. Enzyme release from hearts reflects sarcolemmal damage. The slower enzyme release from hearts made anoxic during calcium-free perfusion may indicate membrane injury occurring as cells dehisce during development of anoxic contracture. It is concluded that in some models of irreversible myocardial injury, forces of cellular contracture may cause sarcolemmal membrane injury and enzyme release.

REFERENCES

1. Hearse, D. J., Humphrey, S. M., and Bullock, G. R. 1978. The oxygen paradox and the calcium paradox: Two facets of the same problem? *J. Mol. Cell. Cardiol.* 10:641–668.
2. Muir, A. R. 1967. The effects of divalent cations on the ultrastructure of the perfused rat heart. *J. Anat.* 101:239–261.
3. Zimmerman, A. N. E., and Hulsmann, W. C. 1966. Paradoxical influence of calcium ions on the permeability of the cell membranes of the isolated rat heart. *Nature* 211:646–647.

Cyclic AMP and Early Contractile Failure

D. M. Yellon, A. Boylett, and D. J. Hearse

The Rayne Institute
St. Thomas' Hospital
London, England

Abstract. Cyclic AMP was measured in the isolated rat heart during anoxia in an attempt to demonstrate if this nucleotide is in any way related to the extent and rate of contractile failure. Isolated rat hearts were subjected to 15 min of normoxia followed by periods of between 1 and 300 sec of anoxia. Contractile force and its failure were monitored throughout. Tissue samples were obtained at various times using high-speed freeze-clamping techniques, and the frozen samples were taken for extraction and cAMP analysis. The results showed a significant increase in the levels of cAMP during the first 5 sec of anoxia, followed by a return to control levels as contractile activity fell to 40% of control. A second and significant increase in cAMP occurred during the following 60 sec. These results indicate major changes in cAMP levels during the first minute of anoxia-induced contractile failure and suggest that increases in this nucleotide may be related to extent and rate of contractile failure.

The precise mechanism responsible for early contractile failure observed during the first minute of ischemia or anoxia has been the subject of considerable speculation (4,11,12,15,16,18,22,29). Various theories have been advanced to explain this event. It has been suggested that oxygen deprivation may cause changes in cardiac contractile proteins (16). However, after prolonged ischemia, no irreversible damage has been detected in the myofibrillar adenosine triphosphatase (1) or the contractile proteins (2,13,17). Furthermore, since rapid contractile failure can be reversed, it would seem unlikely that macromolecular changes could occur or account for the early contractile failure.

It has also been suggested (9,16) that reduced intracellular pH may be a possible trigger for contractile failure by reducing the sensitivity of the sarcoplasmic reticulum to local concentrations of calcium, thus affecting the release of this ion. Furthermore, the high concentration of H^+ may compete with calcium for receptor sites on the troponin molecules, reducing contractility (15). However, with the difficulties of measuring intracellular pH (22,23) and thereby actually showing that an increase in H^+ content precedes, let alone triggers, contractile failure, this and other evidence (6,7,11,13,19,21,24–26) may argue against the pH change acting as the primary trigger.

A further theory that has been postulated is that the depletion of high-energy phosphates is responsible for the phenomenon, and in recent studies we (11) have demonstrated for the first time a decline in adenosine triphosphate and creatine phosphate which occurs before the onset of contractile failure.

Since the speculation and controversy into the precise mechanism affecting the onset of failure during the early moments of anoxia and ishemia still continues, and since the involvement of cAMP in the development of cardiac contraction (3,8,27,28) has attracted an equal amount of controversy, it was felt that an investigation into the relationship between this nucleotide and the decline in tension and contractility warranted investigation. The present chapter, therefore, reports preliminary results of a study designed to investigate changes in cAMP during the first minute of anoxia-induced contractile failure.

MATERIALS AND METHODS

Studies were performed on 160 male rats (250–350 g) using the Langendorff isolated perfused rat heart technique. Following ether anesthesia, hearts were removed, immediately mounted, and perfused aerobically at 37°C with Krebs–Henseleit bicarbonate buffer containing 11 mmol glucose/liter. For the measurement of contractile force, a strain gauge was connected to the apex of the left ventricle, and the heart was allowed to work against a preset 10-g load. After a 15-min normoxic period, the hearts were subjected to anoxia by changing from a well-oxygenated perfusion fluid (gassed with 95% O_2 and 5% CO_2) to one that was gassed with 95% N_2 and 5% CO_2. This was accomplished by respectively clamping and unclamping the inflow tubes from each reservoir to the aortic cannula. This crossover period can be accomplished in less than 0.3 sec, thereby permitting a rapid change in the composition of the perfusate.

To facilitate rapid and precise tissue sampling at various times after the changeover to the anoxic perfusion, an electronically and pneumatically operated set of high-speed freeze clamps (11) was used. The principle on which this intrument works is that the clamps are cooled in liquid nitrogen and, immediately prior to use, are attached to the clamp holders. At various time intervals (e.g., 1 sec, 3 sec, 7 sec) after the onset of anoxia, a button is pressed to release an air pressure valve whch causes the clamps to come together at high speed, thereby rapidly freezing the heart tissue at −196°C. Frozen tissue samples are then taken for perchloric acid extraction and metabolic analysis of cAMP using standard protein-binding methods (5,10).

RESULTS

Figure 1 shows the profile for contractile activity during the first 60 sec of anoxia. It reveals that contractile activity remained essentially constant for the first 5 sec of anoxia but that this was followed by a rapid decline to

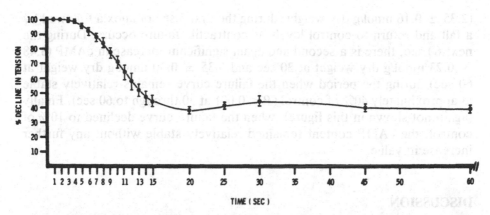

Figure 1.   Contractile failure curve following the onset of anoxia. The decline in contractile activity in the isolated Langendorff heart following the onset of anoxia-induced failure. Each closed circle represents the mean value of a minimum of five hearts, and the bars represent the standard error of the mean. Failure was determined as a percentage decline in tension from control hearts ($N = 13$).

approximately 40% of control during the following 20 sec. During the next 40 sec, contractility was maintained at this level. Although not shown in Figure 1, there was then a slow but steady failure to 10% of control at the end of 5 min of anoxia. Figure 2 shows the parallel changes that occur in the content of cAMP during the first 60 sec of contractile failure. It can be seen that there is a striking and highly significant increase in the content of cAMP (2.87 ± 0.10 nmol/g dry weight at 1 sec, 3.52 ± 0.12 nmol/g dry weight at 3 sec, and 3.49 ± 0.20 nmol/g dry weight at 5 sec) over control

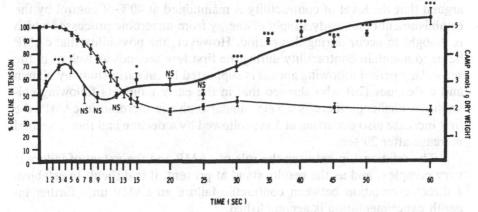

Figure 2.   Changes in the levels of cAMP following the onset of anoxia-induced failure. The relationship between contractile failure (as seen in Figure 1) and changes in the content of cAMP during the same time period. Each point is based on the mean value of a minimum of five hearts, and the bars represent the standard error of the mean. The mean control value for cAMP based on 13 hearts was 2.35 ± 0.16 μmol/g dry weight. Significance of difference from control: $*P < .05$, $**P < .01$, $***P < .001$.

(2.35 ± 0.16 nmol/g dry weight) during the first 5 sec of anoxia followed by a fall and return to control levels as contractile failure occurs. During the next 60 sec, there is a second and again significant increase in cAMP (3.48 ± 0.23 nmol/g dry weight at 30 sec and 5.35 ± 0.30 nmol/g dry weight at 60 sec) during the period when the failure curve remains relatively stable at approximately 40% of control ($P < 0.001$ at 30 through to 60 sec). Finally (again not shown in this figure), when the failure curve declined to 10% of control, the cAMP content remained relatively stable without any further increase in value.

DISCUSSION

Without further detailed investigation, it is difficult to explain why the tissue cAMP content exhibits the biphasic changes shown in Figure 2. However, from these preliminary results, some speculation is possible. The initial increase in cAMP during the first 5 sec while contractility is still stable might be a response to the release of endogenous norepinephrine itself triggered by the onset of anoxia. Such a catecholamine release might act to support contractile activity and thus delay the onset of failure. In other words, whereas in the normoxic heart the release of endogenous norepinephrine would be expected to trigger a positive inotropic response, in the anoxic heart the effect might be to delay the onset of pump failure.

The secondary increase in cAMP that occurs during the first minute of anoxia, at a time when contractile activity has stabilized at a new low level, may in fact contribute to the maintenance of this level, thus delaying the final cardiac failure for some minutes. Alternatively, of course, it could be argued that the level of contractility is maintained at 40% of control by the establishment of a steady supply of energy from anaerobic processes which is thought to occur during this period. However, the possibility that cAMP helps to maintain contractility during the first few seconds as well as in the secondary period following anoxia is supported by an early study by Namm and colleagues (20) who showed that in the early moments following epinephrine challenge there is a very similar biphasic increase in cAMP, the first increase also occurring at 5 sec followed by a decline and then a second increase after 20 sec.

The relationship between the role of cAMP and the extent of failure is very complex, and as the results stand at present, it is difficult to establish a direct correlation between contractile failure an cAMP until further in-depth experimentation is accomplished.

ACKNOWLEDGMENTS

This work was supported by grants from the British Heart Foundation and St. Thomas' Hospital Research Endowments Fund.

REFERENCES

1. Albert, N. R., and Gordon, M. A. 1962. Myofibrillar adenosine triphosphatase activity in congestive heart failure. *Am. J. Physiol.* 202:940–946.
2. Barany, M., Gaetjens, E., Barany, K., and Karp, E. 1964. Comparative studies of rabbit cardiac and skeletal myosins. *Arch. Biochem. Biophys.* 106:280–293.
3. Benfrey, B. B., Kunos, G., and Nickerson, M. 1974. Dissociation of cardiac inotropic and adenylate cyclase activiting adrenoreceptors. *Br. J. Pharmacol.* 51:253–257.
4. Braasch, W., Gudbjarnason, S., Puri, P. S., Ravens, K. G., and Bing, R. J. 1968. Early changes in energy metabolism in the myocardium following acute coronary artery occlusion in anesthetized dogs. *Circ. Res.* 23:429–438.
5. Brown, B. L., Albano, J. D. M., Ekins, R. P., and Scherzi, A. M. 1976. A simple and sensitive saturation assay method for the measurement of adenosine 3',5'-cyclic monophosphate. *Biochem. J.* 121:561–562.
6. Coraboeuf, E., Derouboix, E., and Hoerter, J. 1976. Control of ionic permeabilities in normal and ischemic heart. *Circ. Res.* 38(Suppl. 1):92–98.
7. Danforth, W. H. 1965. Activation of glycolytic pathway in muscle. In: B. Chance, R. W. Eastabrook, and J. R. Williamson (eds.), *Control of Energy Metabolism*, pp. 287–297. Academic Press, New York.
8. Entman, M. L. 1974. The role of cyclic AMP in the modulation of cardiac contractility. *Adv. Cyclic Nucleotide Res.* 4:163–193.
9. Gevers, W. 1977. Generation of protons by metabolic processes in heart cells. *J. Mol. Cell. Cardiol.* 9:867–874.
10. Gilman, A. G. 1970. A protein binding assay for adenosine 3',5'-cyclic monophosphate. *Proc. Natl. Acad. Sci. U.S.A.* 67:305–312.
11. Hearse, D. J. 1979. Oxygen deprivation and early myocardial contractile failure. A reassessment of the possible role of adenosine triphosphate. *Am. J. Cardiol.* 44:1115–1121.
12. Hillis, L. D., and Braunwald, E. 1977. Myocardial ischemia. *N. Engl. J. Med.* 296:971–978.
13. Kako, J., and Bing, R. J. 1958. Contractility of actomyosin bands prepared from normal and failing human hearts. *J. Clin. Invest.* 37:465–470.
14. Katz, A. M. 1968. Effects of interrupted coronary flow upon myocardial metabolism and contractility. *Prog. Cardiovasc. Dis.* 10:450–465.
15. Katz, A. M. 1973. Effects of ischemia on contractile processes of heart muscle. *Am. J. Cardiol.* 32:456–460.
16. Katz, A. M., and Hecht, H. H. 1969. The early pump failure of ischemic heart. *Am. J. Med.* 47:497–502.
17. Katz, A. M., and Maxwell, J. B. 1964. Actin from heart muscle: Sulphydryl groups. *Circ. Res.* 14:345–350.
18. Kubler, W., and Katz, A. M. 1977. Mechanism of early pump failure of the ischemic heart: Possible role of adenosine triphosphate depletion and inorganic phosphate accumulation. *Am. J. Cardiol.* 40:467–471.
19. Nakamura, Y., and Schwartz, A. 1972. The influence of hydrogen ion concentration on calcium binding and release by skeletal muscle sarcoplasmic reticulum. *J. Gen. Physiol.* 59:22–32.
20. Namm, D. H., Mayer, S. E., and Maltbie, M. 1968. The role of potassium and calcium ions in the effect of epinephrine on cardiac cyclic adenosine 3',5'-monophosphate, phosphorylase kinase and phosphorylase. *Mol. Pharmacol.* 4:522–530.
21. Opie, L. H. 1976. Effects of regional ischemia on metabolism of glucose and fatty acids. *Circulation* 38(Suppl. 1):52–68.
22. Poole-Wilson, P. A. 1975. Is early decline of cardiac function in ischemia due to carbon dioxide retention? *Lancet* 2:1285–1287.
23. Poole-Wilson, P. A. 1976. DMO method for intracellular pH. *Circ. Res.* 39:141–142.
24. Poole-Wilson, P. A., Lakatta, E. G., and Nayler, W. G. 1977. The effects of acidosis on myocardial function and the uptake of calcium during and after hypoxia. *Clin. Sci. Mol. Med.* 52:2–3.

338   D. M. Yellon et al.

25. Poole-Wilson, P. A., and Langer, G. A. 1976. The effect of acidosis and manganese on calcium exchange in the myocardium of the rabbit. *J. Physiol. (Lond.)* 265:20–21.
26. Scheuer, J., and Stezoski, S. W. 1972. The effect of alkalosis upon the mechanical and metabolic response of the rat heart to hypoxia. *J. Mol. Cell. Cardiol.* 4:599–510.
27. Sobel, B. A., and Mayer, S. E. 1973. Cyclic adenosine monophosphate and cardiac contractility. *Circ. Res.* 32:407–414.
28. Verma, S. C., and McNeil, J. H. 1976. Actions and interactions of theophylline and imidazole on cardiac contractility, phosphorylase activation and cyclic AMP. *Arch. Int. Pharmacol.* 221:4.
29. Williamson, J. R., Schaffer, S. W., Ford, A., and Safer, B. 1976. The cellular basis of ischemia and infarction, contribution of tissue acidosis to ischemic injury in the perfused rat heart. *Circulation* 53(Suppl. 1):3–14.

Release of Purine Nucleosides and Oxypurines from the Isolated Perfused Rat Heart

J. W. de Jong, E. Harmsen, P. P. de Tombe, and E. Keijzer

Cardiochemical Laboratory
Thoraxcenter
Erasmus University Rotterdam
Rotterdam, The Netherlands

Abstract. In the ischemic heart, high-energy phosphates are rapidly broken down. We studied the release of AMP catabolites from the isolated perfused rat heart which was temporarily made ischemic or anoxic. We measured the concentration of purine nucleosides and oxypurines with a novel high-pressure liquid chromatographic technique. The postischemic working heart released adenosine, inosine, hypoxanthine, and also substantial amounts of xanthine. The latter could indicate that xanthine oxidase is present in rat heart. Further evidence for the myocardial occurrence of this enzyme was obtained from experiments with hearts perfused retrogradely with allopurinol, an inhibitor of xanthine oxidase. This drug greatly enhanced the release of hypoxanthine, both during normoxic and anoxic perfusions. We conclude that xanthine oxidase could play an essential role in the myocardial breakdown of AMP catabolites.

The myocardial cell needs a variety of nucleotides as precursors of nucleic acids and the nucleotide coenzymes for group transfer and bioenergetic processes. ATP plays a special role in heart muscle because it is the fuel for the pump. Large amounts of oxygen are permanently needed for the production of ATP through oxidative phosphorylation. There is a delicate equilibrium between synthesis and breakdown of ATP. During hypoxia ATP is rapidly dephosphorylated, and adenosine and its catabolites are released from the heart (for review, see ref. 3). We used inosine and hypoxanthine as markers for ischemia in animal models such as the isolated perfused rat heart (12) and the open-chested pig heart preparation (4) and in the clinical setting, during an atrial pacing stress test (11). In these instances, inosine and the combination of hypoxanthine and xanthine were measured with Olsson's enzymological method (9). We assumed that hypoxanthine was the end product of myocardial adenine nucleotide metabolism.

With a novel high-pressure liquid chromatographic method, we are now able to distinguish between xanthine and hypoxanthine (6) and report here the production of adenosine, inosine, hypoxanthine, and xanthine from the isolated perfused rat heart. Studies with allopurinol indicate that xanthine oxidase (E.C. 1.2.3.2) is present in rat heart.

MATERIALS AND METHODS

The experiments were performed with F_1 hybrid male rats (250–440 g) obtained from two inbred Wistar substrains. The animals were anesthetized with 30 mg pentobarbital i.p. Hearts were quickly excised and arrested in cold perfusion medium, a modified Tyrode solution (2). For our first set of experiments, the working heart preparation developed by Neely and Rovetto (8) was used. For the induction of ischemia, a one-way ball valve was placed in the aortic outflow tract (8). In a second series of experiments,

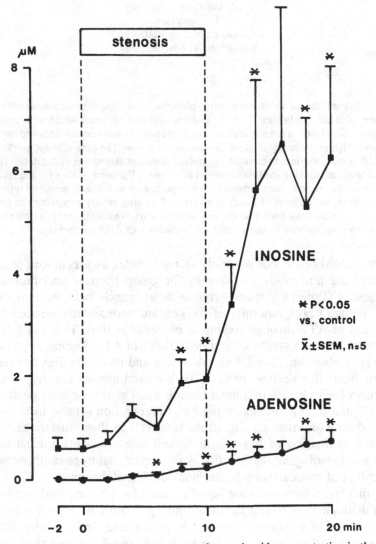

Figure 1.   Ischemia-induced rise in coronary purine nucleoside concentration in the isolated working rat heart.

the Langendorff preparation was used (2). In this case hearts were made temporarily anoxic by replacing the oxygen in the perfusion fluid by nitrogen. The latter perfusions were performed in the presence or absence of 100 μM allopurinol [4-hydroxypyrazolo(3,4-d)pyrimidine] purchased from Burroughs Wellcome, London.

The analysis of AMP catabolites was performed with a high-pressure liquid chromatograph (Varian 8520, Palo Alto, California) as described briefly before (6). Essentially, a 200-μl sample of perfusate was put on a C_{18} μBondapak® column (Waters, Milford, Mass.; 0.4 × 30 cm) and eluted isocratically with 10 mM ammonium phosphate/methanol (10 + 1), pH 5.50, at a rate of 60 ml/hr. The retention times of hypoxanthine, xanthine, inosine, and adenosine (detected at 254 nm) were 5.2, 5.4, 6.8, and 15 min, respectively.

Values are presented as means ± S.E.M. Statistical analysis was performed with Student's t-test. $P > 0.05$ was considered not significant.

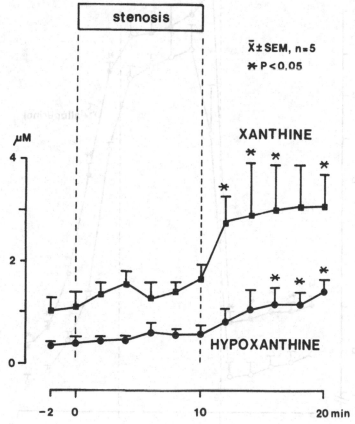

Figure 2.   Rise in coronary oxypurine content following ischemia and "reperfusion" of the isolated working rat heart.

RESULTS

Working Heart

After a 10-min period of control perfusion (coronary flow 69 ± 4 ml/min per g dry weight), the hearts were made ischemic for 10 min. At the end of this period, coronary flow was only 5 ± 2 ml/min per g dry weight (dwt) ($P < 0.001$ vs. control), and aortic flow had ceased. The concentration of purine nucleosides (Figure 1) and oxypurines (Figure 2) in the coronary effluent was increased, but high concentrations of these compounds were observed during "reperfusion." Coronary flow recovered only partially

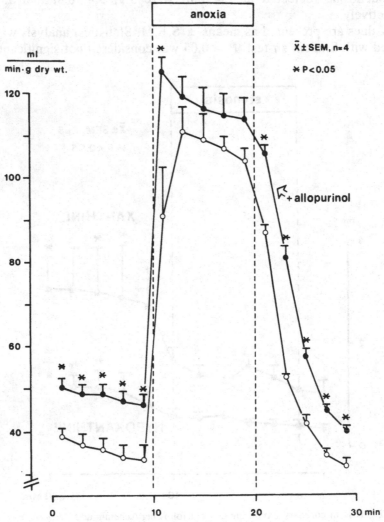

Figure 3. Influence of 100 μM allopurinol on the coronary flow of the retrogradely perfused rat heart.

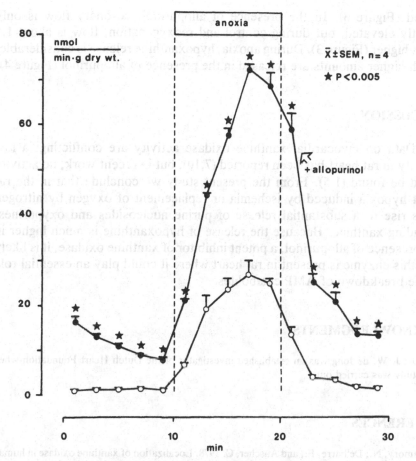

Figure 4.   Release of hypoxanthine from the retrogradely perfused rat heart in the absence or presence of 100 μM allopurinol.

when the constriction was removed. The 10-min post-ischemia coronary flow was only 19 ± 10 ml/min per g dwt ($P < 0.01$ vs. control). From the large standard error of the mean, it is clear that there is a large variation: some hearts regain their control flow, others do not. It is noteworthy that the hearts released substantial amounts of xanthine, indicating the possible presence of xanthine oxidase in rat heart. With allopurinol, an inhibitor of this enzyme, we obtained further evidence that xanthine oxidase is indeed present in rat heart.

Retrogradely Perfused Heart

After a 10-min control perfusion period, hearts were made anoxic for the same period and reoxygenated for 10 min. Coronary flow increased during anoxia, presumably because adenosine, a potent vasodilator, is released (Figure 3). In the presence of allopurinol, coronary flow is only slightly elevated, but during control and reoxygenation, flow is about 1.5 times higher (Figure 3). During anoxia, hypoxanthine release is considerable. Much higher amounts are released in the presence of allopurinol (Figure 4).

DISCUSSION

Data on myocardial xanthine oxidase activity are conflicting: a low activity in rat heart has been reported (7,10), but in recent work, no activity could be found (1,5). From the present study we conclude that in the rat heart hypoxia induced by ischemia or replacement of oxygen by nitrogen gives rise to a substantial release of purine nucleosides and oxypurines, including xanthine. Because the release of hypoxanthine is much higher in the presence of allopurinol, a potent inhibitor of xanthine oxidase, it is likely that this enzyme is present in rat heart where it could play an essential role in the breakdown of AMP catabolites.

ACKNOWLEDGMENTS

Dr. J. W. de Jong was an established investigator of the Dutch Heart Foundation when this study was carried out.

REFERENCES

1. Amory, N., Delbarre, F., and Auscher, C. 1978. Localization of xanthine oxidase in human and rat tissues. A histochemical study. *C. R. Acad. Sci. [D] (Paris)* 287:1007–1009.
2. De Jong, J. W. 1972. Phosphorylation and deamination of adenosine by the isolated perfused rat heart. *Biochim. Biophys. Acta* 286:252–259.
3. De Jong, J. W. 1979. Biochemistry of acutely ischemic myocardium. In: W. Schaper (ed.), *The Pathophysiology of Myocardial Perfusion*, pp. 719–750. Elsevier/North-Holland, Amsterdam.
4. De Jong, J. W., Verdouw, P. D., and Remme, W. J. 1977. Myocardial nucleoside and carbohydrate metabolism and hemodynamics during partial occlusion and reperfusion of pig coronary artery. *J. Mol. Cell. Cardiol.* 9:297–312.
5. Gandhi, M. P. S., and Ahuja, S. P. 1979. Absorption of xanthine oxidase from the intestines of rats and rabbits and its role in initiation of atherosclerosis. *Zentralbl. Veterinaermed.* 26:635–642.
6. Harmsen, E., De Jong, J. W., Keijzer, E., and Uitendaal, M. P. 1980. Assay of whole blood (hypo)xanthine and its precursors. *J. Mol. Cell. Cardiol.* 12(Suppl. 1):54.
7. Maguire, M. H., Lukas, M. C., and Rettie, J. F. 1972. Adenine nucleotide salvage synthesis in the rat heart; pathways of adenosine salvage. *Biochim. Biophys. Acta* 262:108–115.
8. Neely, J. R., and Rovetto, M. J. 1975. Techniques for perfusing isolated rat hearts. *Methods Enzymol.* 39:43–60.
9. Olsson, R. A. 1970. Changes in content of purine nucleoside in canine myocardium during coronary occlusion. *Circ. Res.* 26:301–306.

10. Ramboer, C. R. H. 1969. A sensitive and nonradioactive assay for serum and tissue xanthine oxidase. *J. Lab. Clin. Med.* 74:828–835.
11. Remme, W. J., De Jong, J. W., and Verdouw, P. D. 1977. Effects of pacing-induced myocardial ischemia on hypoxanthine efflux from the human heart. *Am. J. Cardiol.* 40:55–62.
12. Stam, H., and De Jong, J. W. 1977. Sephadex-induced reduction of coronary flow in the isolated rat heart: A model for ischemic heart disease. *J. Mol. Cell. Cardiol.* 9:633–650.

Pathophysiology of Irreversible Ischemic Injury
The Border Zone Controversy

D. J. Hearse and D. M. Yellon

The Rayne Institute
St. Thomas' Hospital
London, England

Abstract. At the present time our experimental findings plus the weight of other experimental evidence suggest that there is unlikely to be a quantitatively significant border zone in the lateral plane. The transition from normal to ischemic tissue is likely to be accomplished over a distance of 1.0 mm or less and possibly in as little as the dimensions of one cell. The situation in the transmural plane is less well established, but if the same situation occurs, then the absence of a spatially indentifiable border zone of intermediate injury will require a major reappraisal, although not an abandonment, of concepts for the therapeutic limitation of infarct size. Any extrapolation of the observations, comments, and conclusions made in this paper to the human heart should be made with extreme caution. Major species differences exist, particularly in relation to the characteristics of collateral flow. Most experimental studies have involved single or multiple coronary artery ligation, a situation that generates large areas of sharply demarcated ischemia. These areas are very severely ischemic and short of reperfusion, which is hardly a practical consideration in the early phases of evolving myocardial infarction; the affected tissue is inevitably condemned to cell death and necrosis. The situation prevailing in man with partial coronary artery occlusion or diffuse ischemic heart disease may well be be very different and is clearly in urgent need of investigation.

The object of this chapter is to present a spatial consideration of the pathophysiology of irreversible injury with particular reference to regional ischemia and some of the three-dimensional factors that may determine whether infarct size limitation is really possible.

The ultimate size of an evolving infarct is determined by the mass of affected tissue, the severity of the ischemia withn that tissue, and, in particular, the number of cells that undergo the critical transition from reversible to irreversible injury. Conventionally it has been thought that our ability to use therapeutic agents to prevent this critical transition is dependent on the existence of some "border zone" of intermediate injury (19,43).

Recently, however, the traditional concept of a relatively static border zone of intermediate injury has been challenged on the grounds that it gives an oversimplified view that fails to take adequate account of such factors as the anatomy of the coronary circulation, the dynamic nature of the ischemic process, and the practical realities of tissue salvage.

347

THE BORDER ZONE CONTROVERSY

The starting point of this controversy is the nature of the interface between normal and ischemic tissue. If we traverse an area of regional ischemia in either the lateral or the transmural plane, we may observe one of several situations. We may, for example, observe an abrupt transition such that sharp interfaces of flow and metabolism may result in normal tissue lying adjacent to severely ischemic tissue, with the ishemic injury being relatively homogeneous throughout the affected area. If such a situation prevailed, then there would be no spatially identifiable zone of intermediate injury.

The alternative viewpoint is that the transition between normal and ischemic tissue is charaterized by a gradual progression of flow, metabolism, and injury, thus creating a border zone of intermediate damage which would represent the target tissue for protective interventions. Clearly, the determining factor in this controversy is the nature and distribution of the coronary circulation.

Role of the Coronary Circulation

If the tissue bed supplied by a specific coronary artery is sharply differentiated from adjacent coronary beds, then the occlusion or constriction of one artery, as shown in Figure 1A, should lead to a relatively uniform reduction of flow throughout its bed without any great effect on adjoining tissue. Such a situation would generate sharp interfaces of flow and hence metabolism, and with the possible exception of an extremely narrow band of cells between the tissue beds, there would be no spatially distinct border zone of intermediate injury. From a therapeutic viewpoint, the only option would be to attempt to increase or restore flow to the entire ischemic mass.

An alternative viewpoint stems from the known existence of coronary artery anastamoses and an element of interdigitation between coronary beds. Figure 1B shows how anastamoses of the subendocardial plexus and intramural vessels, together with some merging of coronary beds, could generate a distinct zone of intermediate perfusion where the progression of tissue injury would be considerably slower than that at the core of the ischemic mass. In this model many more options are available for therapeutic salvage. Figure 1B shows how a lateral border zone might arise; Figure 1C shows how collateral flow might generate a similar zone of intermediate injury but this time in the transmural plane.

Temporal Considerations

The models illustrated in Figures 1A–C give a static representation of myocardial injury. In order to take into account the dynamic nature of the ischemic process, a temporal component should be added to any model. By way of example, a consideration of the time and space relationships for adenosine triphosphate (ATP) depletion during evolving myocardial infarction provides a good example of the importance of time in determining our view of the genesis of a border zone of intermediate injury. If, for the sake of argument, one assumes that cellular ATP content is a determinant of the severity of tissue injury (16,26) and that the transition from reversible to irreversible injury injury occurs when the mean tissue content falls below 12 μmol/g dry wt., then two possible situations might arise. At the moment of the onset of ischemia, as shown in Figures 2A and B, all tissue, including that within the area of cyanosis, will have a normal content of, say, 30 μmol/g dry wt. If there is a sharp interface of flow between normal and ischemic tissue with little or no flow invading the periphery of the ischemic area (Figure 2A), then the relatively homogeneous reduction of flow throughout the ischemic area should lead to a relatively uniform rate of depletion of ATP throughout the affected tissue, and thus, the ATP content might fall to indicated levels after 5, 15, and 30 min. In this way, for up to 30 min, the entire ischemic area can be considered as a potentially salvageable border zone of jeopardized cells. However, within the next few minutes, as the ATP content of most cells falls below 12 μmol/g dry wt., the entire ischemic area will undergo the transition from reversible to irreversible injury, and thus, by 45 min, the border zone will have disappeared. In this model with sharp interfaces of flow, the border zone does not represent a spatially distinct subfraction of the ischemic mass but rather a time-dependent phase through which the tissue passes.

Figure 2B illustrates an opposing view that accounts for the existence of a spatially identifiable zone of jeopardized cells within the ischemic mass; however, this border zone will move with time. This model relies on the existence of substantial gradients of flow or diffusion across the ischemic zone. Under these conditions, a nonuniform depletion of ATP should occur, and peripheral tissue will take far longer to reach the point of transition to irreversible injury. Thus, as before, for up to 30 min, the entire ischemic area will represent a potentially salvageable border zone, but beyond that time cells in the center of the infarct first undergo the transition. In this way, a central zone of infarction would be initiated, and this would radiate outwards with time. In such a model, the border zone would consist of an annulus of tissue which shrinks in a time-dependent manner from its inner surface towards the boundary of the ischemic area. Such a situation would correspond very closely to the transmural wave front of ischemic death that has been proposed by Reimer and Jennings (37,38).

In terms of tissue salvage, the two views of a temporal border zone are very different. In the first example, early intervention would be critical, whereas in the second situation, protective procedures are likely to be effective for much longer, but the quantity of target tissue available would diminish with time.

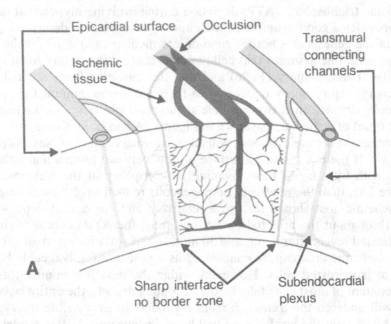

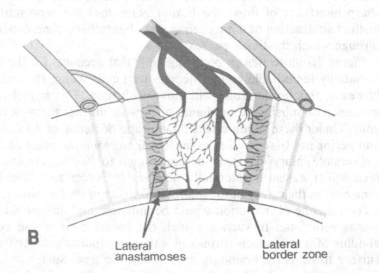

Figure 1.   Coronary artery anatomy. (A) Diagrammatic representation of sharp interfaces of flow where a discrete demarcation of coronary bed could, on occlusion of one artery, lead to sharply differentiated zones of perfusion. In such a model there would be no border zone of intermediate perfusion, and the transition from normal to ischemic tissue would be characterized by sharp interfaces of flow and metabolism. (B) Lateral gradients of flow where coronary anastamoses of the subendocardial plexus and intramural vessels, together with an element of interdigitation between adjacent coronary beds, could generate a lateral zone of intermediate perfusion where relatively wide gradients of flow and metabolism would characterize the transition from normal to ischemic tissue.

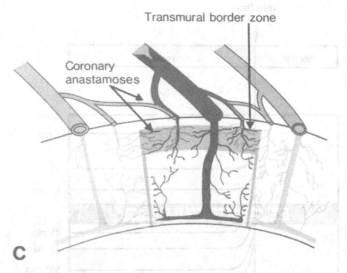

(C) Transmural gradients of flow where coronary anastamoses could generate a transmural zone of intermediate perfusion. Relatively wide gradients of flow and metabolism would characterize the transition from normal to ischemic tissue.

REVIEW OF THE LITERATURE

Clearly, it is vital to establish whether sharp interfaces or progressive gradients characterize the transition between normal and ischemic tissue. During the last 10 to 15 years, there have been many studies in which the results have been presented as supportive of a border zone of intermediate injury. In a number of instances, however, these studies have been subject to misquotation and misinterpretation. More recently there have been an increasing number of reports that have been supportive of the concept of sharp interfaces. For clarity of review, the various studies have been divided on the basis of their visualization technique. These include polarographic studies and studies of surface fluorescence, histochemical and ultrastructural studies, and investigations involving the measurement of changes in flow distribution, the electrocardiogram, or the metabolism of the heart.

Polarographic and Surface Fluorescence Studies

The simplest and most striking evidence for a sharp interface is the very clearly defined edge of visible cyanosis (40) that develops immediately after the occlusion of a coronary artery and indicates a very sharp gradient for oxygen availability. Complementing this oldest piece of evidence are the recent studies by Barlow, Chance, Harken, and colleagues (2,14,15,42,44). Using surface fluorescence techniques to visualize lateral and transmural gradients for NAD reduction in a number of species, these workers dem-

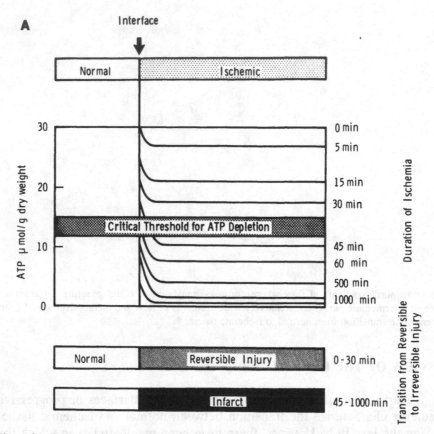

Figure 2.   Temporal border zones: transition states. Time–space relationship for the decline of ATP at various sites in normal and ischemic tissue. For the sake of argument the transition from reversible to irreversible injury is marked by the depletion of myocardial ATP below a critical value of 12 μmol/g dry wt. (A) A sharp interface of flow between the normal and ischemic tissue together with a relatively uniform reduction of flow throughout the ischemic zone will result in a relatively uniform, time-dependent reduction in ATP content throughout the ischemic zone. For up to 30 min, all tissue is potentially salvageable, but in the following minutes the entire zone will become irreversibly injured. In this model, with the possible exception of a small shell of tissue at the edge of the infarct, the border zone does not represent a spatially distinct subfraction of the ischemic mass but a time-dependent phase through which the tissue passes. (B) Gradients of flow across the ischemic area result in a nonuniform depletion of ATP. A spatially identifiable border zone of intermediate injury exists, and this would comprise an annulus of reversibly injured tissue which shrinks in a time-dependent manner from its inner surface towards the boundary of the ischemic area. These figures are speculative but are likely to represent the time course of events occurring during severe myocardial ischemia in the dog heart.

onstrated sharp fluorescence interfaces. However, before taking these findings as conclusive evidence against the border zone, two cautions should be considered. First, the very sharp boundaries of fluorescence only identify an abrupt gradient for NAD reduction—they do not necessarily identify a boundary between reversible and irreversible injury, nor do they necessarily

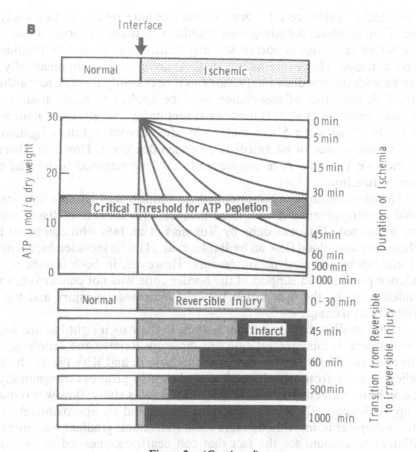

Figure 2. (*Continued*)

identify the location of gradients for diffusable metabolites or substrates. Second, the transition of NAD from a state of predominate oxidation to one of predominant reduction occurs over a very narrow (45) P_{O_2} range, and thus, fluorescence studies could artificially sharpen an apparent oxygen gradient.

Histochemical and Ultrastructural Studies

Rather like polarographic and surface fluorescence studies, microscopic investigations (1,9,10,22,37,38,46) tend to indicate a very sharp interface of injury. However, unlike the former, these studies are often carried out at postmortem or at least 24 hr after the onset of ischemia and must therefore suffer the criticism that even if a border zone had existed, it would probably have disappeared by this time. However, not at all histochemical studies deny the border zone. Thus, the early dog heart study by Cox et al. (8) is often cited as evidence for a zone of intermediate injury. In this study, a zone of intermediate dehydrogenase staining was found to persist for several days before reverting to normal staining characteristics or deteriorating to necrotic tissue. However, intermediate staining cannot automatically be equated with intermediate injury, nor can it necessarily identify jeopardized cells. This limitation of association must be applied to many studies, for example, Fishbein et al. (11) used serial sectioning and glycogen staining in the rat heart between 5 min and 72 hr after coronary artery ligation to demonstrate a zone of intermediate glycogen depletion. However, there is no evidence that this zone subsequently died or returned to normal mechanical function.

The association between intermediate staining and intermediate injury would be strengthened if additional independent markers of tissue injury were measured. This was done by Vokonas et al. (46) who combined histochemistry and blood flow an by Banka et al. (1) who included biochemical and electrophysiological measurements. However, in both instances, the evidence presented in support of the border zone was not conclusive, since it failed to make the association between intermediate injury and the reversibility of damage.

Three studies that are very important in their own right but are sometimes subject to misinterpretation are those by Reimer and Jennings, and Reimer et al. (37,38) and by Factor, Sonnenblick, and Kirk (9). In the first studies, a wave front of cell death was shown to progress transmurally in the dog heart with circumflex artery ligation. In this study, flow was reduced by approximately 97% in the subendocardium and by approximately 83% in the subepicardium. Although this small transmural gradient was probably sufficient to account for the fact that cell death commenced in the endocardial region, it does not really indicate that tissue distal to the wave front of death can be truly designated as a salvageable border zone, since the reduction of flow throughout the ischemic area was so severe that all tissue must be considered as condemned: other than very early reperfusion, no intervention could be expected to do more than delay inevitable cell death. In addition to clarifying the concept of the wave front of cell death, the studies by Reimer and Jennings and Reimer et al. (37,38) illustrate very clearly the importance of coronary bed size and distribution in the determination of patterns of tissue injury.

The elegant dog heart study by Factor et al. (9), in which serial sectioning techniques were used to reconstruct the three-dimensional geometry of the zone of change, is often cited as evidence against the border zone. However, since the study was 24 hr post-ligation, a border zone might easily have been missed. What this study does, however, show is the extent to which interdigitating peninsulas of normal tissue invade the ischemic zone. Under these conditions, it is quite clear that conventional biopsy samples obtained from the zone of change, on homogenization and analysis, could lead to the incorrect interpretation of intermediate injury.

Coronary Flow Studies

As already stressed, coronary flow and its distribution are the ultimate determinants of tissue injury, and there have been many studies (3,5,13,20,28,30,31,37,38,41,46), usually with radioactive microspheres, that have been cited as evidence for a zone of intermediate flow. In all of these investigations, for example, the one by Schaper and Pasyk (41) shown in Figure 3, the myocardium was sectioned into blocks after a relatively short duration of ischemia. Transition zones with intermediate degrees of radio-activity were observed. However, this cannot be used as evidence for in-termediate tissue flow since the random nature of sampling and the size of the tissue blocks would almost inevitably lead to the retrieval of mixed tissue. In fact, a careful consideration of these results can argue strongly against the border zone. Consider, for example, that if a border zone of similar width to the tissue sections had actually existed, then in view of the random nature of sampling, it would be most likely to have been retrieved over two adjacent biopsies. Thus, the transition from predominantly normal to predominantly ischemic would usually involve two intermediate meas-urements. The regular observation that the transition involved just one in-termediate value is very strong evidence for a sharp interface which lies somewhere in the intermediate biopsy.

Electrocardiographic Studies

Numerous electrocardiographic studies (1,4,6,7,12,17,20,22,28,32,33, 34,36,39) have claimed to have detected the presence of a border zone of in-

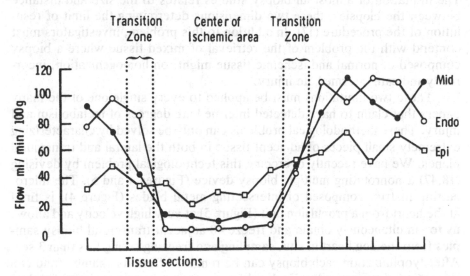

Figure 3. Transition zones in the ischemic myocardium. Profiles of the distribution of coronary flow in the myocardium with acute regional ischemia. Adapted from Schaper et al. (23) with permission of the American Heart Association.

termediate injury. Two strong cautions must, however, be considered. First, the electrocardiographic signal is the sum of that generated throughout the myocardium, and thus, even sharp conduction interfaces may be blurred by signals from surrounding tissue. Second, electrocardiographic changes are usually based on ST segment shifts which are influenced not only by the severity but also the duration of ischemia. ST segment changes evolve with time, and their disappearance from one zone may well represent recovery or advanced injury (12,39).

A particularly notable electrocardiographic study has been reported by Janse and colleagues (22). In this study, electrocardiographic recordings from several electrodes, each with multiple transmural detecting sites, were related to biochemical and histochemical changes measured in the pig heart over a 2-hr period of ischemia. The results indicated that for all variables the transition from near normal to maximally ischemic occurred over the distance of one or two sampling sites. Janse interpreted these findings against a border zone of intermediate injury, suggesting that the zone of change was composed of interdigitating normal and ischemic zones sharply demarcated from each other.

Metabolic Studies

Biochemical studies (18,20,22, 23,24,25,27,29,32,35,36,48) of lateral and transmural gradients have mostly been based on rapid sequential or simultaneous multiple biopsies followed by the analysis of conventional markers of ischemic injury such as ATP, CP, lactate, glycogen, and creatine kinase. The limitation of almost all biopsy studies relates to the size and distance between the biopsies, these two dimensions determining the limit of resolution of the procedure (17). In addition to this problem, investigators must contend with the problem of the retrieval of mixed tissue where a biopsy composed of normal and ischemic tissue might, on homogenization, incorrectly indicate intermediate injury.

These two limitations must be applied to every single one of the many papers that claim to have detected intermediate degrees of metabolism and injury. These methodological problems can only be solved by characterizing extremely small pieces of adjacent tissue in both the lateral and transmural planes. We have recently overcome this technological problem by devising (18,47) a nonrotating multiple biopsy device (Figures 4 and 5). The microcutting matrix, composed of intersecting metal blades (Figure 4), is fired at the heart from a propulsion unit (Figure 5) at very high velocity and allows us to simultaneously obtain and freeze 40 adjacent transmural biopsy samples from the dog heart in situ, sampling and freezing taking less than 3 sec. After lyophilization each biopsy can be removed from its chamber and can be sectioned transmurally. Each subfragment can then be analyzed for flow and a number of metabolites such as ATP, creatine phosphate, and lactate.

Figure 6 shows a three-dimensional representation of the creatine phos-

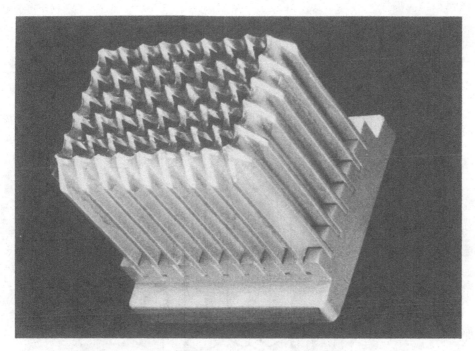

Figure 4.   Multiple biopsy cutter. Metal cutter capable of sampling 40 adjacent biopsies, each 4 mm × 4 mm in cross section.

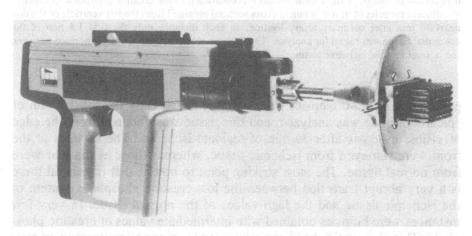

Figure 5.   Propulsion unit for high-velocity impact biopsy. The unit uses explosive cartridges to propel a drive shaft carrying the biopsy cutter over a restricted distance (50 mm) at high velocity (10^5 mm/sec).

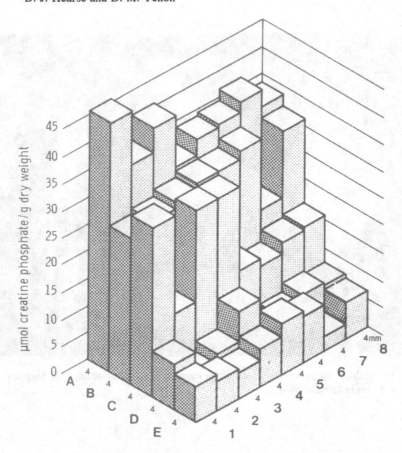

Figure 6.   Three-dimensional representation of the creatine phosphate content in regional myocardial ischemia. A three-dimensional representation of the creatine phosphate content of 40 adjacent biopsies (4 mm × 4 mm in cross section) obtained from the left ventricle of the dog heart 30 min after coronary artery ligation. In each instance only the first 1.8 mm of the epicardial tissue was taken for analysis. The findings would suggest a sharp interface between the normal and the ischemic tissue.

phate content of 40 biopsies from one dog heart. Only the top 1.8 mm of epicardial tissue was analyzed, and this tissue was obtained from the edge of visible cyanosis after 30 min of regional ischemia. The samples at the front were retrieved from ischemic tissue, whereas those at the rear were from normal tissue. The most striking point to note is that in general there is a very abrupt transition between the low creatine phosphate content of the ischemic tissue and the high values of the normal tissue. In very few instances were biopsies obtained with intermediate values of creatine phosphate. This observation had been reinforced from our measurements of over 200 biopsies which have also shown sharp interfaces for flow, ATP, and lactate in the lateral plane of the epicardium (48).

ACKNOWLEDGMENTS

This work was supported by grants from the British Heart Foundation and St. Thomas' Hospital Research Endowments Fund.

REFERENCES

1. Banka, VV. S., Bodenheimer, M. M., Ramanathan, K. B., Hermann, G. A., and Helfant, R. H. 1978. Progressive transmural electrographic, myocardial potassium ion/sodium ion ratio and ultrastructural changes as a function of time after acute coronary occlusion. *Am. J. Cardiol.* 42:429–443.
2. Barlow, C. H., and Chance, B. 1976. Ischemic areas in perfused rat hearts: Mesurement by NADH fluorescence photography. *Science* 193:909–910.
3. Becker, L. C., Ferreira, R., and Thomas, M. 1973. Mapping of left ventricular blood flow with radioactive microspheres in experimental coronary artery occulsion. *Cardiovasc. Res.* 7:391–400.
4. Beller, G. A., Smith, T. W., and Hood, B. W., Jr. 1972. Altered distribution of tritiated digoxin in the infarcted canine left ventricle . *Circulation* 46:572–579.
5. Bishop, S. P., White, F. C., and Bloor, C. M. 1976. Regional myocardial blood flow during acute myocardial infarction in the conscious dog. *Circ. Res.* 38:429–438.
6. Braunwald, E., Maroko, P. R., and Libby, P. 1974. Reduction of infarct size following coronary occlusion. *Circ. Res.* 35(Suppl. 3):192–201.
7. Bruyneel, K. J. J. 1975. Use of moving epicardial electrodes in defining ST-segment changes after acute coronary occlusion in the baboon. Relations to primary ventricular fibrillation. *Am. Heart J.* 89:731–741.
8. Cox, J. L., McLaughlin, V. W., Flowers, N. C., and Horan, L. G. 1968. The ischemic zone surrounding acute myocardial infarction. Its morphology as detected by dehydrogenase staining. *Am. Heart J.* 76:650–659.
9. Factor, S. M., Sonnenblick, E. H., and Kirk, E. S. 1978. The histologic border zone of acute myocardial infarction—islands or peninsulas. *Am. J. Pathol* 92:111–120.
10. Farrer-Brown, G. 1976. *A Colour Atlas of Cardiac pathology,* p. 78. Wolf Medical, London.
11. Fishbein, M. C., Hare, C. A., Gissen, S. A., Spadaro, J., Maclean, D., and Moroko, P. R. 1980. Identification and quantification of histochemical border zones during the evolution of myocardial infarction in the rat. *Cardiovasc. Res.* 14:41–49.
12. Fozzard, H. A., and Das Gupta, D. S. 1976. ST-segment potentials and mapping. Theory and experiments. *Circulation* 54:533–537.
13. Fulton, W. F. M. 1965. *The Coronary Arteries.* Charles C Thomas, Springfield, Illinois.
14. Harden, W. R., Simson, M. B., Barlow, C. H., Soriano, R., and Harkens, A. H. 1978. Display of epicardial ischemia by reduced nicotinamide adenine dinucleotide fluorescence photography, electron microscopy and ST segment mapping. *Surgery* 83:732–740.
15. Harken, A. J., Barlow, C. H., Harden, W. R., and Chance, B. 1978. Two and three dimensional display of myocardial ischemic "border zone" in dogs. *Am. J. Cardiol.* 42:954–959.
16. Hearse, D. J., Garlick, P. M., and Humphrey, S. M. 1977. Ischemic contracture of the myocardium: Mechanisms and prevention. *Am. J. Cardiol.* 39:986–993.
17. Hearse, D. J., Opie, L. H., Katzeff, I. E., Lubbe, W. F., Van der Werff, T. J., Peisach, M., and Boulle, G. 1977. Characterization of the "border zone" in acute regional ischemia in the dog. *Am. J. Cardiol.* 40:716–726.
18. Hearse, D. J., Yellon, D. M., Chappell, D. A., Wyse, R. K. H., and Ball, G. R. 1981. A high velocity impact device for obtaining multiple, contiguous myocardial biopsies. *J. Mol. Cell. Cardiol.* 13:197–206.
19. Helfant, R. H., Banka, V. S., and Bodenheimer, M. M. 1978. Perplexities and complexities

concerning the myocardial infarction border zone and its salvage. *Am. J. Cardiol.* 41:345–347.

20. Hillis, L. D., Askenazi, J., Braunwald, E. Radvany, P., Muller, J. E., Fishbein, M. C., and Moroko, P. R. 1976. Use of changes in the epicardial QRS complex to assess interventions which modify the extent of myocardial necrosis following coronary artery occlusion. *Circulation* 54:591–598.

21. Hirzel, H. O., Sonnenblick, E. H., and Kirk, E. S. 1977. Absence of a lateral border zone of intermediate creatine phosphokinase depletion surrounding a central infarct 24 hours after acute coronary occlusion in the dog. *Circ. Res.* 41:673–683.

22. Janse, M. J., Cinca, J., Morena, H., Fiolet, J. W. T., Kléber, A. G., De Vries, G. P., Becker, A. E., and Durrer, D. 1979. The "border zone" in myocardial ischemia. An electrophysiological, metabolic and histochemical correlation in the pig heart. *Circ. Res.* 44:576–588.

23. Kjekshus, J. K. 1976. Assessment of myocardial injury with creatine phosphokinase (CPK). *Circulation* 53(Suppl. 1):106–108.

24. Kjekshus, J. K., Maroko, P. R., and Sobel, B. E. 1972. Distribution of myocardial injury and its relation to epicardial ST-segment changes after coronary artery occlusion in the dog. *Cardiovasc. Res.* 6:490–499.

25. Kjekshus, J. K., and Sobel, B. E. 1970. Depressed myocardial creatine phosphokinase activity following experimental myocardial infarction in rabbit. *Cir. Res.* 27:403–414.

26. Kubler, W., and Spieckermann, P. G. 1970. Regulation of glycolysis in the ischemic and anoxic myocardium. *J. Mol. Cell. Cardiol.* 1:351–377.

27. Lie, J. T., Pairoleno, P. C., and Holley, K. E. 1975. Time course and zonal variations of ischemia-induced myocardial cationic electrolyte derangements. *Circulation* 51:860–866.

28. Lubbe, W. F., Peisach, M., Pretorius, R., Bruyneel, K. J. J., and Opie, L. H. 1974. Distribution of myocardial blood flow before and after coronary artery ligation in the baboon. Relation to early ventricular fibrillation. *Cardiovasc. Res.* 8:478–487.

29. Maclean, D., Fishbein, M. C., Braunwald, E., and Moroko, P. R. 1978. Long term preservation of ischemic myocardium after experimental coronary artery occlusion. *J. Clin. Invest.* 61:541–551.

30. Malsky, P. M., Vokonas, P. S., Paul, S. J., Robbins, S. L., and Hood, W. B. 1977. Autoradiographic measurement of regional blood flow in normal and ischemic myocardium. *Am. J. Physiol.* 232:576–583.

31. Marcus, M. L., Kerber, R. E., Ehrhardt, J., and Abboud, F. M. 1975. Three dimensional geometry of acutely ischemic myocardium. *Circulation* 52:254–263.

32. Maroko, P. R., Bernstein, E. F., Libby, P., De Laria, G. A., Covell, J. W., Ross, J., Jr., and Braunwald, E. 1972. Effects of intraaortic balloon counterpulsation on the severity of myocardial ischemic injury following acute coronary occlusion. *Circulation* 45:1150–1159.

33. Maroko, P. R., Hillis, L. D., and Muller, J. E. 1977. Favourable effects of hyaluronidase on electrocardiographic evidence of necrosis in patients with acute myocardial infarction. *N. Engl. J. Med.* 296:898–903.

34. Maroko, P. R., Kjekshus, J. K., Sobel, B. E., Watanabe, T., Covell, J. W., Ross, J., Jr, and Braunwald, E. 1971. Factors influencing infarct size following experimental coronary artery occlusions. *Circulation* 43:67–82.

35. Opie, L. H., Bruyneel, K., and Owen, P. 1975. Effects of glucose, insulin and potassium infusion on tissue metabolic changes within first hour of myocardial infarction in the baboon. *Circulation* 52:49–57.

36. Opie, L. H., and Owen, P. 1976. Effect of glucose–insulin–potassium infusions on arteriovenous differences of glucose and of free fatty acids and on tissue metabolic changes in dogs with developing myocardial infarction. *Am. J. Cardiol.* 38:310–321.

37. Reimer, K. A., and Jenning, R. B. 1979. The "wavefront" of myocardial ischemic cell death. 11. Transmural progression of necrosis within the framework of ischemic bed size (myocardium at risk) and collateral flow. *Lab. Invest.* 40:633–644.

38. Reimer, K. A., Lowe, J. E., Rasmussen, M. M., and Jennings, R. B. 1977. The wavefront phenomenon of ischemic cell death. 1) Myocardial infarct size vs duration of coronary occlusion in dogs. *Circulation* 56:786–798.

39. Ross, J., Jr. 1976. Electrocardiograph ST-segment analysis in the characterization of myocardial ischemia and infarction. *Circulation* 53(Suppl. 1):73–81.

40. Sayen, J. J., Sheldon, W. F., Horwitz, O., Kuo, P. T., Peirce, G., Zinsser, H. F., and Mead, J., Jr. 1952. Studies of coronary disease in the experimental animal. 11. Polarographic determinations of local oxygen availability in the dogs left ventricle during coronary occlusion and pure oxygen breathing. *J. Clin. Invest.* 30:932–940.

41. Schaper, W., and Pasyk, S. 1976. Influence of collateral flow on the ischemic tolerance of the heart following acute and subacute coronary occlusion. *Circulation* 53(Suppl. 1):57–65.

42. Simson, M. B., Harden, W., Barlow, C. H., and Harken, A. H. 1979. Visualization of the distance between perfusion and anoxia along an ischemic border. *Circulation* 60:1151–1155.

43. Sobel, B. E., and Shell, W. E. 1973. Jeopardized, blighted and necrotic myocardium. *Circulation* 47:215–216.

44. Steenbergen, C., Deeleeuw, G., Barlow, C. H., Chance, B., and Williamson, J. R. 1977. Heterogeneity of the hypoxic state of perfused rat heart. *Circ. Res.* 41:606–615.

45. Sugano, S., Oshino, N., and Chance, B. 1974. Mitochondrial functions under hypoxic conditions: The steady states of cytochrome c reduction and of energy metabolism. *Biochim. Biophys. Acta.* 347:340–358.

46. Vokonas, P. S., Malsky, P. M., Paul, S. J., Robbins, S. L., and Hood, W. B. 1978. Radioautographic studies in experimental myocardial infarction: Profiles of ischemic blood flow and quantification of infarct size in relation to magnitude of ischemic zone. *Am. J. Cardiol* 42:67–75.

47. Yellon, D. M. 1979. A multiple biopsy gun for the study of three dimensional metabolic geometry. *J. Physiol. (Lond.)* 293:5–6.

48. Yellon, D. M., Hearse, D. J., Crome, R., Grannell, J., and Wyse, R. K. M. 1981. Characterization of the lateral interface between normal and ischemic tissue during acute myocardial infarction. *Am. J. Cardiol* 47:1233–1239.

Acid Hydrolases in the Initiation of Ischemic Myocardial Necrosis

T. Katagiri, Y. Sasai, N. Nakamura,
H. Minatoguchi, M. Yokoyama, Y. Kobayashi,
Y. Takeyama, K. Ozawa, and H. Niitani

The Third Department of Internal Medicine
Showa University School of Medicine
Tokyo 142, Japan

Abstract. Alterations in myocardial acid hydrolases in acute ischemia were studied in relation to the evolution of cardiac cellular necrosis by the determination of cathepsin D, acid phosphatase (AcPase), and β-glucuronidase activities of the myocardial fractions and by electron microscopic cytochemical studies on AcPase in the canine heart. In the normal myocardium, the same level of activity of acid hydrolases was found in sarcoplasmic reticulum (SR) as in the lysosome fraction. In electron microscopy, AcPase reaction products were observed markedly in SR and moderately in lysosomes, in residual bodies, and in Golgi apparatus. In the ischemic myocardium, at 20 to 30 min after coronary ligation, activation of these enzymes was observed in both SR and lysosomes, and at 60 to 90 min they were decreased in the particles and, in turn, increased in the cytoplasm accompanying the ischemic fine structural changes. At 2 to 3 hr those acid hydrolase activities in the cytosol were decreased, indicating the loss of enzymes from necrotic myocardial cells. Acid hydrolases are the most important factor for the evolution of ischemic myocardial necrosis by being activated not only in lysosomes but also in SR and by being released to the cytoplasm to disintegrate the cellular structures.

The process of myocardial cellular injury to necrosis in the acute ischemic state has not yet been fully elucidated. Among the theories reported in many previous articles, the participation of acid hydrolases has been proposed as the primary factor for the evolution of ischemic myocardial necrosis. Formerly, these enzymes were considered to be located mainly in lysosomes and lysosomal changes have been studied for a long time (3,7–9,11). However, recently, distribution of cardiac acid hydrolases in the sarcoplasmic reticulum (SR) has been reported (5,6) in relation to cardiac cellular necrosis. We previously have reported the degradation of ATPase protein of SR in the early stage of myocardial infarction (10). From these viewpoints, we studied the alterations in the activities and the intracellular redistribution of cardiac acid hydrolases in the acute ischemic state by means of comparative biochemical and electron microscopic investigations.

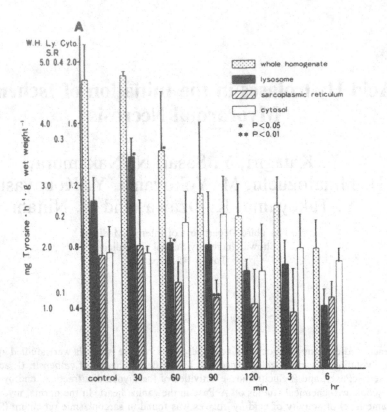

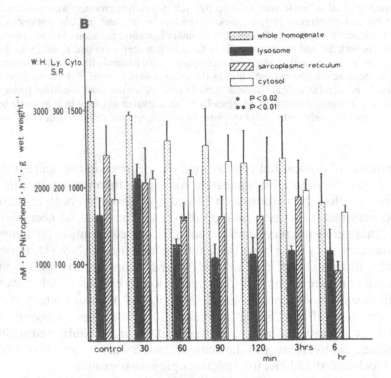

Figure 1. Acid hydrolase activities in myocardial fractions in acute ischemia in the canine heart. (A) Cathepsin D; (B) acid phosphatase; (C) β-glucuronidase.

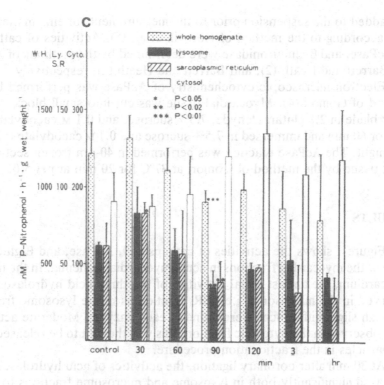

Figure 1. (*Continued*)

MATERIALS AND METHODS

Ligation of the left anterior decending coronary artery was performed in 55 adult mongrel dogs (10 to 25 kg) under anesthesia with sodium pentobarbital. Production of acute transmural ischemia was confirmed by typical ST–T elevation in the electrocardiogram. At 20, 30, 60, and 90 min, and at 2, 3, and 6 hr after coronary ligation, at least four dogs in each period were slaughtered; the beating heart was taken out immediately, and the central ischemic subendocardial portion was removed. As control experiments, seven sham-operated dogs in which the coronary artery was only isolated but not ligated were treated in the same manner.

Myocardial tissues were chopped into small pieces with scissors and then with a razor blade and homogenized in 9 volumes of 0.25 M sucrose, 0.1 M KCl, 0.001 M EDTA, 0.01 M imadazole-Cl (pH 7.4) with a Teflon–glass homogenizer. The homogenate was spun at 600 × g for 10 min. Fractionation of the 600 × g supernatant was performed by differential centrifugation to produce precipitates of centrifugations at 5000 × g for 10 min, at 15,000 × g for 20 min, at 120,000 × g for 30 min, and the final supernatant, regarded as the fractions of mitochondria, lysosomes, microsomes, and cytosol, respectively. Each precipitate was resuspended in the same buffer, and the protein concentration was determined by biuret procedure. Triton X-100 was added to the suspension prior to the measurements of enzymatic activities according to the method of Gottwik et al. (5). Activities of cathepsin D, AcPase, and β-glucuronidase were determined by the methods of Anson (1), Barrett and Heath (2), and Barrett and Heath (2), respectively.

Electron microscopic cytochemistry of AcPase was performed by the method of Gomori (4). Myocardial tissue was cut into small blocks with a razor blade in 2% glutaraldehyde, 7.5% sucrose, and 0.1 M cacodylate (pH 7.2) for 60 min and immersed in 7.5% sucrose and 0.1 M cacodylate (pH 7.2) overnight. The AcPase reaction was performed in 40-μm frozen sections of heart tissue by the method of Gomori at 37°C for 20 min at pH 5.0.

RESULTS

Figure 1 shows the activities of cathepsin D, AcPase, and β-glucuronidase of the myocardial fractions in acute myocardial ischemia. In the normal myocardium, the almost equal activities of the three acid hydrolases were observed in the microsome, i.e., SR, fraction as in the lysosome fraction, although slight differences were found in each enzyme. Moderate activities were observed in the cytosolic fraction; this was thought to be released from the particles in the fractionation procedure.

At 30 min after coronary ligation, the activities of acid hydrolases were increased significantly both in lysosome and microsome fractions to about 30% of the control values. At 60 to 90 min, they were decreased in the particle fractions, and the activities in the cytosol were increased, conversely. At 2 to 3 hr, the cytosolic activities were decreased together with a reduction in the activities in the whole homogenate, indicating the loss of enzymes from the ischemically injured sarcolemma.

Figure 2 shows electron micrographs of cardiac cells with the AcPase reaction. In the normal myocardium the AcPase reaction products were observed intensely in the terminal cisternae (TC) and longitudinal tubules of SR and moderately in primary and secondary lysosomes, in residual bodies, and in Golgi apparatus.

At 20 to 30 min after coronary ligation, the AcPase reaction products were increased in lysosomes with depletion of glycogen and slight margination of nuclear chromatin. The fine deposits of the reaction products were found around lysosomes and SR. At 60 to 90 min, the morphological changes in mitochondria such as the appearance of dense deposits and swelling and disruption of cristae were apparent. Swelling of SR, intracellular edema, and overstretch of the I-band were also found. The AcPase reaction products were decreased moderately in SR and in lysosomes but, in turn, increased in number in the cytoplasm. At 2 to 6 hr, mitochondrial dense deposits were increased in number and size, and ruptures of TC and sarcolemma and disruption of myofilaments were observed in places. The reaction products in SR and lysosomes were further decreased, and those in the cytoplasm were released. The changing patterns of reaction and leakage of hydrolase enzymes as observed by electron microscope findings were seen in parallel biochemically and quantitatively.

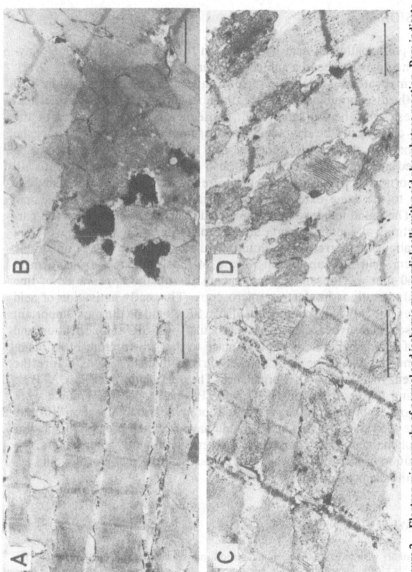

Figure 2. Electron micrographs of normal and ischemic myocardial cells with acid phosphatase reaction. Bars indicate 1 μm. (A) The normal myocardial cell. Acid phosphatase reaction products in SR and in lysosomes. (B) At 20 min after coronary ligation. Activation of acid phosphatase in lysosomes. (C) At 60 min after coronary ligation. Appearance of dense deposits in mitochondria and leakage of reaction products from lysosomes and from SR. (D) At 3 hr after coronary ligation. Severe fine structural changes and reaction products on myofilaments.

were also lessened. The changing patterns of the biochemical acid hydrolase activities and those of the electron microscopic findings seemed to be in parallel chronologically and quantitatively.

DISCUSSION

The participation of acid hydrolases in the evolution of ischemic myocardial necrosis has been a subject of interest in recent decades (5–9,11). In acute myocardial ishemia the regional myocardium becomes acidic as a result of the discontinuance of aerobic metabolism, and intramyocardial acid hydrolases would be activated, and, consequently, the structures of the involved cells would be degraded. This assumption was expressed as the "lysosomal hypothesis" (7). Recently, acid hydrolases were reported to be distributed not only in lysosomes but also in SR (5,6). In agreement with those reports, acid hydrolase activities were found in both lysosome and SR fractions to the same extent in biochemical and in electron microscopic studies. The initial increase in multiple acid hydrolase activities in the particle fractions at around 30 min after coronary ligation would have been brought about by the reduction in intracardiac pH as a result of anaerobic metabolism, and the subsequent release of those enzymes from them at around 60 min was observed simultaneously with the appearance of fine structural alterations in electron microscopy. This early activation of acid hydrolases not only in lysosomes but also in SR would be the most important step in ischemic myocardial injury, particularly in SR; the activation and release of enzymes per se indicate damage to the substructure of its membrane, and this would be indicative of early irreversible signs before the released enzymes attack other organelles. The degradation of SR = ATPase protein and the decreases in Ca^{2+} = ATPase and Ca^{2+} = uptake were found in our laboratory in the early stages of myocardial infarction (10); the activation of acid hydrolases in SR should have been the precipitating factor for this phenomenon. In complete agreement with many other papers, the redistribution of acid hydrolases from particles to the cytoplasm would accelerate the damages further.

ACKNOWLEDGMENTS

The authors wish to express sincere thanks to Professor Yasumitsu Nakai of Showa University for his kind guidance in electron microscopy.

REFERENCES

1. Anson, M. L. 1937. The estimation of cathepsin with hemoglobin and the partial purification of cathepsin. *J. Gen. Physiol.* 20:565–574.

2. Barrett, A. J., and Heath, M. F. 1977. Assay methods of lysosomal enzymes. In: J. T. Dingle (ed.), *Lysosomes*, pp. 110–127. North-Holland, Amsterdam.
3. Decker, R. S., and Wildenthal, K. 1978. Sequential lysosomal alterations during cardiac ischemia. II. Ultrastructural and cytochemical changes. *Lab. Invest.* 38:662–673.
4. Gomori, G. 1950. An improved histochemical technic for acid phosphatase. *Stain Technol.* 25:81–85.
5. Gottwik, M. G., Kirk, E. S., Hoffstein, S., and Weglicki, W. B. 1975. Effects of collateral flow on epicardial and endocardial lysosomal hydrolases in acute myocardial ischemia. *J. Clin. Invest.* 56:914–923.
6. Hoffstein, S., Gennaro, D. E., Weissman, G., Hirsch, J., Streuli, F., and Fox, A. C. 1975. Cytochemical localization of lysosomal enzyme activity in normal and ischemic dog myocardium. *Am. J. Pathol.* 79:193–206.
7. Okuda, M., and Lefer, A. M. 1979. Lysosomal hypothesis in evolution of myocardial infarction. Subcellular fractionation and electron microscopic cytochemical study. *Jpn. Heart J.* 20:643–656.
8. Ravens, K. G., and Gudbjarnason, S. 1969. Changes in the activities of lysosomal enzymes in infarcted canine heart muscle. *Circ. Res.* 24:851–856.
9. Ricciutti, M. A. 1972. Myocardial lysosome stability in the early stage of acute ischemic injury. *Am. J. Cardiol.* 30:492–497.
10. Toba, K., Katagiri, T., and Takeyama, Y. 1978. Studies on the cardiac sarcoplasmic reticulum in myocardial infarction. *Jpn. Circ. J.* 42:447–453.
11. Wildenthal, K., Decker, R. S., Poole, A. R., Griffin, E. E., and Dingle, J. T. 1978. Sequential lysosomal alterations during cardiac ischemia. I. Biochemical and immunohistochemical changes. *Lab. Invest.* 38:656–661.

Release of Prostacyclin into the Coronary Venous Blood in Patients with Coronary Arterial Disease

L. Kaijser, J. Nowak, C. Patrono, and Å. Wennmalm

Department of Clinical Physiology
Huddinge Hospital, Karolinska Hospital; and St. Erik's Hospital
Stockholm, Sweden
and
Department of Pharmacology
Catholic University
Rome, Italy

Abstract. Voluntary patients with a history of myocardial infarction and with typical effort angina underwent catheterization of the coronary sinus and a brachial artery. Healthy young males, serving as controls, were subjected to the same procedure. Arterial and coronary venous blood was drawn at rest and during atrial pacing to angina (patients) or to a heart rate of 140 beats/min (healthy volunteers) for analysis of 6-ketoprostaglandin $F_{1\alpha}$ (6-keto-PGF$_{1\alpha}$) and prostacyclin-like activity (PILA). 6-Keto-PGF$_{1\alpha}$ levels were measured using radioimmunoassay; PILA in the blood was assayed by rapid preparation of platelet-rich plasma followed by determination of the ADP-induced platelet aggregation. Increased arterial levels of PILA and of radioimmunoactive 6-keto-PGF$_{1\alpha}$ (RIA-6-keto-PGF$_{1\alpha}$) were observed in the patients at rest as well as during pacing. No obvious release of RIA-6-keto-PGF$_{1\alpha}$ occurred at rest, either in the patients or in the controls. However, during pacing, increased amounts of RIA-6-keto-PGF$_{1\alpha}$ appeared in the coronary venous blood of the patients. The results demonstrate that an increased cardiac prostacyclin formation prevails in patients with signs of impaired coronary flow and suggest that ischemic heart disease is characterized by an insufficient vascular response to this vasodilator prostaglandin rather than by its insufficient endogenous production.

In recent years, much interest has been focused on the possible role of endogenous prostaglandins (PGs) in the mediation of coronary vascular phenomena. It has been demonstrated in several studies that hypoxia is a powerful stimulus for cardiac PG release and that the vasodilation following coronary occlusion can be markedly reduced by inhibitors of PG synthesis (1–3,5,7,20,21,29); these data suggest that PGs play an essential part in coronary vasoregulation. On the other hand, contradictory results showing a failure of PG synthesis inhibitors to influence the coronary blood flow and reactive hyperemia have also been reported (9,14,25). At present, no clear evidence is available for any major role of endogenous PGs in the control of coronary blood flow under physiological conditions. Nevertheless, the vasodilator PGs, possibly interacting with purine nucleotides, can still be of importance in the relaxation of the coronary vasculature under conditions of more severe myocardial ischemia.

Only limited data have been presented on the release of prostaglandins in patients with impaired coronary blood flow. Release of prostaglandins E and F into the coronary venous blood has been reported in patients with coronary arterial disease during pacing to angina (4), but prostacyclin (PGI_2) levels were not assayed. Therefore, the aim of the present investigation was to study whether myocardial ischemia resulting from impaired coronary flow in patients with coronary arterial disease is accompanied by an increased cardiac release of prostacyclin.

MATERIALS AND METHODS

Five males, aged 48 to 62 years, with a history of myocardial infarction and with subsequent typical stable agina with tolerance level at 100 to 110 beats/min were studied. Each of them showed evidence of transient ischemia during exercise by generally accepted criteria (electrocardiographic ST changes). Three additional males, aged 23 to 36 years, all volunteers without any history of cardiovascular disease, served as controls. All studies were performed in the morning with the subject in supine position.

A Teflon® catheter was inserted percutaneously into one of the brachial arteries. A second Teflon® catheter was introduced similarly into a cubital vein and advanced under fluoroscopic guidance 4 to 8 cm into the coronary sinus. Its position was checked initially by determining the oxygen saturation in the blood sampled from the catheter and subsequently by repeated fluoroscopy during the investigation. A bipolar pacemaker electrode was introduced via one of the femoral veins and passed in position in the right atrium under fluroscopic control. Atrial pacing was performed using an external generator (EM 145, Siemens-Elema, Sweden). The frequency of stimulation was increased by 10 impulses/min starting from a rate 10 impulses/min higher than the spontaneous heart rate. The increase in pacing frequency was continued until chest pain, described by the patients as "rather severe pain" (grade 6–7 on a ten-grade scale) was achieved and then maintained at this level until blood sampling was completed. Using this technique, all the patients experienced characteristic anginal pain, associated with electrocardiographic changes consistent with myocardial ischemia, during the entire pacing. The controls were paced similarly to a heart rate level of 140 beats/min.

Blood samples were drawn simultaneously from the coronary sinus and from the brachial artery at rest and during pacing: 10-ml portions of blood were collected in polypropylene tubes containing 1/10 vol of 3.8% sodium citrate. The blood was then immediately centrifuged at $200 \times g$ for 4 min. The platelet-rich plasma (PRP) thus obtained was separated and transferred in 0.5-ml portions into aggregometer cuvettes containing 0.5 ml isotonic Tris buffer (pH 7.4). Platelet aggregation recordings for assessment of prostacyclin-like activity (PILA) in the plasma were performed within 8 min after blood collection. Aggregation was induced by the addition of 2 μg of ADP (Sigma Chemical Co.) to the PRP–Tris buffer mixture. Aggregation was recorded as an increase in light transmission in a Vitatron UC 200 photometer connected to a linear ink recorder. After separation of PRP, the remaining blood was recentrifuged at 2000 × g for 15 min at +4°C. The plasma was then separated and stored at −80°C until radioimmunoassay (RIA) of 6-ketoprostaglandin $F_{1\alpha}$ (6-keto-$PGF_{1\alpha}$) was performed. The RIA of plasma 6-keto-$PGF_{1\alpha}$ was performed in triplicate in 150-μl aliquots of unextracted arterial and coronary venous samples at 1:10 dilution of 0.02 M phosphate buffer (pH 7.4) as described elsewhere (26). Standard curves were prepared similarly in 1:10 dilution of PG-free plasma (peripheral venous plasma obtained from an aspirin-treated subject.)

RESULTS

At rest, a decreased platelet aggregability in comparison to controls was observed in PRP separated from the coronary venous as well as from the arterial blood of the patients (Figure 1), thus indicating increased levels of PILA in the patients' blood. In the coronary venous PRP of the patients, platelet aggregation was often almost completely inhibited. In the controls, no antiaggregatory activity was observed, either in the arterial or in the coronary venous plasma. As also seen from Figure 1, PILA in the arterial and coronary sinus blood of the controls remained undetectable during pacing, whereas in the patients platelet aggregation in the coronary venous PRP remained markedly, and often almost completely, inhibited. The resting arterial and coronary venous plasma levels of RIA-6-keto-$PGF_{1\alpha}$ were 104 ± 36 and 125 ± 29 pg/ml, respectively, which is considerably higher that the corresponding levels in the controls (8 ± 4 and 14 ± 8 pg/ml, respectively). No obvious release of RIA-6-keto-$PGF_{1\alpha}$ into the coronary circulation occurred at rest, either in patients or in controls (Figure 2). Atrial pacing slightly lowered the arterial RIA-6-keto-$PGF_{1\alpha}$ in the patients but not in the controls, the levels being 81 ± 28 and 10 ± 10 pg/ml, respectively.

During pacing, increased amounts of RIA-6-keto-$PGF_{1\alpha}$ appeared in the coronary venous plasma of the patients, indicating a release of prostacyclin into the coronary circulation (Figure 2). In contrast, no release of RIA-6-keto-$PGF_{1\alpha}$ was observed during pacing in controls.

DISCUSSION

In the present study, the release of prostacyclin into the coronary venous blood was investigated at rest and during atrial pacing in patients with

coronary arterial disease and in healthy volunteers. The aim of the study
was to elucidate whether myocardial ischemia in man is accompanied by an
enhanced local formation of this vasodilator prostaglandin. Such increased
release of prostacyclin into the coronary circulation can be an early response
to myocardial ischemia and can represent a naturally arising protective

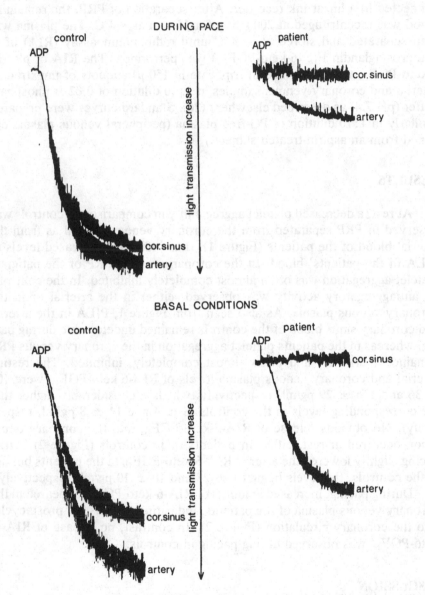

Figure 1. Typical recordings of ADP-induced aggregation in platelet-rich plasma collected
from an artery and from the coronary sinus of controls and patients. Note that PRP of the
controls contains no apparent platelet-antiaggregating activity in contrast to the patients, in
whom platelet aggregation in both arterial and coronary sinus blood is inhibited.

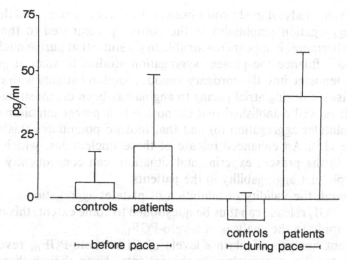

Figure 2.   Veno–arterial plasma concentration differences of RIA-6-keto-PGF$_{1\alpha}$ in patients and controls at rest and during atrial pacing. Note the increased amounts of RIA-6-keto-PGF$_{1\alpha}$ in the coronary venous plasma of the patients during pacing.

mechanism directed to preserve coronary blood flow and to prevent myo-cardial injury.

Prostacyclin in the plasma was measured by radioimmunoassay of its stable metabolite, 6-keto-PGF$_{1\alpha}$, and its activity was also estimated by ag-gregometry. Regarding the validity of the results obtained by aggregometry, some methodological considerations must be kept in mind. First, the an-tiaggregatory activity of prostacyclin declines rather rapidly after blood sam-pling, thereby restricting the time during which satisfactory results can be obtained. Second, the method does not rule out the possibility for other naturally occurring compounds with antiaggregatory action to influence platelet aggregation. Finally, platelet aggregation is, in addition to such factors as pH and temperature of the suspending medium, influenced also by platelet count.

Regarding these methodological considerations, it is necessary to stress that in the current study aggregometry was performed within 8 min after blood sampling. It is known that prostacyclin decomposes spontaneously in aqueous solutions to inactive 6-keto-PGF$_{1\alpha}$ within 10 min at 37°C (10,16), but it is, on the other hand, considerably more stable in plasma (17). It is therefore unlikely that spontaneous decomposition and subsequent inacti-vation of prostacyclin could have influenced the results of the present ag-gregation studies to any serious extent. All current platelet aggregations were recorded in medium of the same temperature and pH, but the platelet count in the plasma samples was not estimated because of the obvious shortage of time. Low platelet counts in coronary venous blood have been observed earlier in patients with coronary arterial disease (22). If the platelet count in the coronary sinus blood were also lower in the patients participating in the present study, it might contribute to the currently observed decreased platelet aggregation amplitudes in the coronary compared to the arterial PRP. Furthermore, it appears reasonable to presume that purine nucleotides, too, could influence the present aggregation studies to some degree. Release of adenosine into the coronary venous blood in patients with coronary arterial disease during atrial pacing to angina has been demonstrated earlier (8), and it is well established that adenosine is a potent inhibitor of ADP-induced platelet aggregation (6) and that inosine potentiates this effect of adenosine (15). An enhanced release of these nucleotides, which is to be expected in the present experimental situation, can consequently have influenced platelet aggregability in the patients.

Although the validity of inhibition of platelet aggregation as indicator of cardiac PGI_2 release can thus be questioned to some extent, this objection does not apply to the analysis of 6-keto-$PGF_{1\alpha}$.

Current analysis of plasma levels of RIA-6-keto-$PGF_{1\alpha}$ revealed increased arterial concentrations in the patients. Even though these results accord well with the data from aggregation studies, the finding is somewhat puzzling. It has been reported earlier that human atherosclerotic arteries exhibit a decreased capacity to synthesize prostacyclin (27), and a hypothesis has been put forward that atherosclerosis is a disease caused by deficiency of PGI_2 (11). According to this hypothesis, the arterial levels of 6-keto-$PGF_{1\alpha}$ in the patients with coronary arterial disease should be low. The present data demonstrate, however, completely contradictory results. Although there is at present no apparent explanation for the observed high arterial plasma levels of RIA-6-keto-$PGF_{1\alpha}$ in our patients, a possible effect of some drugs usually used by this patient category, e.g., nitroglycerin and its derivatives, cannot be excluded. In fact, it has been shown recently that nitroglycerin stimulates myocardial prostaglandin E release (24). On the other hand, the present finding leads to a tempting speculation that the higher arterial levels of RIA-6-keto-$PGF_{1\alpha}$ in the patients may reflect an enhanced release of PGI_2 from the lungs—a compensatory mechanism subsequent to an increased need for prostacyclin in other vascular regions more severely affected by the atherosclerotic process. Lungs have been proposed as "endocrine" organs generating circulating "hormonal" prostacyclin (12,13,23). Normally, only small amounts of prostacyclin are released from the lungs, but the pulmonary PGI_2 generation can be greatly increased by some stimuli, e.g., hyperventilation or angiotensin II (13,28). If a possibly increased local need for prostacyclin in occlusive arterial disease is able to activate the mechanisms controlling pulmonary PGI_2 release, it may then explain the currently observed higher arterial levels of RIA-6-keto-$PGF_{1\alpha}$ in the patients.

Atrial pacing in the patients resulted in increased amounts of RIA-6-keto-$PGF_{1\alpha}$ in the coronary sinus blood. This finding accords well with the earlier animal experiments in which increased cardiac PG release was observed during myocardial ischemia (2,3,5,19,29), thus suggesting that the enhanced PG formation can be an early response to ischemic myocardial injury. The mechanism behind such an increased coronary formation of PGI_2 is probably a stimulated endothelial production of the compound as a response to impaired local oxygen supply. This assumption is based on earlier findings in animals showing that hypoxia is a potent stimulus for PG synthesis in coronary arteries (18). The enhanced generation of PGI_2 in the coronary circulation of the patients paced to angina can thus be an important mechanism triggered to preserve myocardial perfusion.

Summing up, the results of this study demonstrate that an increased cardiac formation of prostacyclin prevails in patients with coronary arterial disease paced to a level at which clinical signs of impaired coronary flow arise. We propose that this increase represents the activation of a myocardial defense mechanism against an insufficient tissue oxygen supply. The increased formation of prostacyclin suggests that ischemic heart disease is characterized by an impaired vascular response to this prostaglandin rather than by its insufficient endogenous synthesis.

ACKNOWLEDGMENTS

This study was supported by grants from The Swedish National Association Against Heart and Chest Diseases and by the Swedish Medical Research Council (project 04X-4341).

REFERENCES

1. Afonso, S., Bandow, G. T., and Rowe, G. G. 1974. Indomethacin and the prostaglandin hypothesis of coronary blood flow regulation. *J. Physiol. (Lond).* 241:299–308.
2. Alexander, R. W., Kent, K. M., Pisano, J. J., Keiser, H. R., and Cooper, T. 1975. Regulation of post-occlusive hyperemia by endogenously synthesized prostaglandins in the dog heart. *J. Clin. Invest.* 55:1174–1181.
3. Berger, H. J., Zaret, B. L., Speroff, L., Cohen, L. S., and Wolfson, S. 1976. Regional cardiac prostaglandin release during myocardial ischemia in anesthetized dogs. *Circ. Res.* 38:566–571.
4. Berger, H. J., Zaret, B. L., Speroff, L., Cohen, L. S., and Wolfson, S. 1977. Cardiac prostaglandin release during myocardial ischemia induced by atrial pacing in patients with coronary artery disease. *Am. J. Cardiol.* 30:481–486.
5. Block, A. J., Feinberg, H., Herbaczynska-Cedro, K., and Vane, J. R. 1975. Anoxia-induced release of prostaglandins in rabbit isolated hearts. *Circ. Res.* 36:34–42.
6. Born, G. V. R., and Cross, M. J. 1963. Inhibition of the aggregation of blood platelets by substances related to adenosine diphosphate. *J. Physiol. (Lond.)* 166:29P–30P.
7. De Deckere, E. A. M., Nugteren, D. H., and Ten Hoor, F. 1977. Prostacyclin is the major prostaglandin released from the isolated perfused rabbit and rat heart. *Nature* 268:160–163.
8. Fox, A. C., Reed, G. E., Glassman, E., Kaltman, A. J., and Silk, B. B. 1974. Release of adenosine from human hearts during angina induced by rapid atrial pacing. *J. Clin. Invest.* 53:1447–1457.
9. Giles, R. W., and Wilcken, D. E. 1977. Reactive hyperaemia in the dog heart: Inter-relations between adenosine, ATP, and aminophylline and the effect of indomethacin. *Cardiovasc. Res.* 11:113–121.

10. Gryglewski, R. J., Bunting, S., Moncada, S., Flower, R. J., and Vane, J. R. 1976. Arterial walls are protected against deposition of platelet thrombi by a substance (prostaglandin X) which they make from prostaglandin endoperoxides. *Prostaglandins* 12:685–715.

11. Gryglewski, R., Dembinska-Kiec, A., Zmuda, A., and Gryglewska, T. 1978. Prostacyclin and thromboxane A_2 biosynthesis capacities of heart, arteries and platelets at various stages of experimental artherosclerosis. *Atherosclerosis* 31:385–394.

12. Gryglewski, R., Korbut, R., and Ocetkiewicz, A. 1978. Generation of prostacyclin by lungs in vivo and its release into the arterial circulation. *Nature* 273:765–766.

13. Gryglewski, R., Korbut, R., Ocetkiewicz, A., Splawinski, J., Wojtaszek, B., and Swies, J. 1978. Lungs as a generator of prostacyclin—hypothesis on physiological significance. *Naunyn Schmiedebergs Arch. Pharmacol.* 304:45–50.

14. Hintze, T. H., and Kaley, G. 1977. Prostaglandins and the control of blood flow in the canine myocardium. *Circ. Res.* 40:313–320.

15. Jenkins, C. S. P., Caen, J. P., Vainer, H., and Pokutecky, J. 1972. Inhibition of adenosine uptake by platelets. *Nature [New Biol.]* 23:210–211.

16. Johnson, R. A., Morton, D. R., Kinner, J. H., Gorman, R. R., McGuire, J. C., and Sun, F. F. 1976. The chemical structure of prostaglandin X (prostacyclin). *Prostaglandins* 12:915–928.

17. Jørgensen, M. A., Stoffersen, E., and Dyerberg, J. 1979. Stability of prostacyclin in plasma. *Lancet* 1:1352.

18. Kalsner, S. 1977. The effect of hypoxia on prostaglandin output and tone in isolated coronary arteries. *Can. J. Physiol. Pharmacol.* 55:882–887.

19. Kent, K. M., Alexander, R. W., Pisano, J. J., Keiser, H. R., and Cooper, T. 1973. Prostaglandin dependent coronary vasodilator responses. *Physiologist* 16:361.

20. Kraemer, R. J., and Folts, J. D. 1973. Release of prostaglandin following temporary occlusion of the coronary artery. *Fed. Proc.* 32:454.

21. Kraemer, R. J., Phernetton, T. M., and Folts, J. D., 1976. Prostaglandin-like substances in coronary venous blood following myocardial ischemia. *J. Pharmacol. Exp. Ther.* 199:611–619.

22. Metha, J., Metha, P., and Pepine, C. J. 1978. Platelet aggregation in aortic and coronary venous blood in patients with and without coronary disease. 3. Role of tachycardia stress and propranolol. *Circulation* 58:881–886.

23. Moncada, S., Korbut, R., Bunting, S., and Vane, J. R. 1978. Prostacyclin is a circulating hormone. *Nature* 273:767–768.

24. Morcillio, E., Reid, P. R., Dubin, N., Ghodgaonkar, R., and Pitt, B. 1980. Myocardial prostaglandin E release by nitroglycerin and modification by indomethacin. *Am. J. Cardiol.* 45:53–57.

25. Owen, T. L., Ehrhart, I. C., Weidner, W. J., Scott, J. B., and Haddy, F. J. 1975. Effect of indomethacin on local blood flow regulation in canine heart and kidney. *Proc. Soc. Exp. Biol. Med.* 149:871–876.

26. Patrono, C., Wennmalm, A., Ciabattoni, G., Nowak, J., Pugliese, F., and Cinotti, G. A. 1979. Evidence for an extra-renal origin of urinary prostaglandin E_2 in healthy men. *Prostaglandins* 18:623–629.

27. Sinzinger, H., Silberbauer, K., Wagner, O., Winter, M., and Auerswald, W. 1978. Prostacyclin—preliminary results with vascular tissue of various species and its importance for atherosclerotic involvement. *Atherogenesis* 3:123–136.

28. Swies, J., Radomski, M., and Gryglewski, R. J. 1979. Angiotensin-induced release of prostacyclin (PGI_2) into circulation of anaesthetized cats. *Pharmacol. Res. Commun.* 11:649–655.

29. Wennmalm, A., Pham-Huu-Chanh, and Junstad, M. 1974. Hypoxia causes prostaglandin release from perfused rabbit hearts. *Acta Physiol. Scand.* 91:133–135.

The Effects of Systole on Left Ventricular Blood Flow

J. B. Caulfield, T. K. Borg, and F. L. Abel

Departments of Pathology and Physiology
USC School of Medicine
Columbia, South Carolina 29208, USA

Abstract. Coronary artery flow is complex. Flow in this system is divided into systolic and diastolic. However, systolic flow should be divided into two phases, isovolumetric and the ejection phase, since these two components are determined by completely different parameters. Flow through the myocardium is affected by the close mechanical coupling between myocytes and capillaries effected by the array of collagen struts and their disposition. This latter provides the anatomic arrangement that makes possible the integrated "massaging" effect postulated by Wiggers (26).

Blood flow through the myocardium is governed by a number of factors that can be divided into vascular components and extravascular components (21). The unique and overriding extravascular component is the phasic contraction of the myocardium. This cyclic phenomenon alters ventricular wall pressure from a low of 5–10 mm Hg to a high of 120–150 mm Hg in the normal heart (16). Further, the pressure at any time in systole varies from the endocardium to the epicardium over a range of intracavitary pressure at the endocardium to near thoracic pressure at the epicardium. This combination of pressure differences has led to the development of the "waterfall" theory to explain systolic flow (11). If simple compressive effects on otherwise unrestrained blood vessels are the only contribution of systole to coronary flow, one would expect a decrease in systolic flow as the force of contraction (i.e., increase in wall tension) occurs, other factors being constant. In recent work, this did not seem to be the case; rather, as wall tension increased, systolic flow increased (1,2).

A possible explanation for this phenomenon is present in the extracellular collagen network of the heart (7). This complex system consists of, among other components, an extensive array of collagen struts that extend from the basal laminae of all capillaries to all contiguous myocytes. The distribution of this array is such that during systole, tension would be placed on the capillaries as a result of shortening and thickening of the myocytes (7). To test this hypothesis, an in vivo isolated dog heart preparation that permitted measurement of systolic and diastolic coronary arterial flow as well as independent variation of afterload and coronary perfusion pressure was developed (3). The results of these experiments indicate a direct correlation between wall tension and systolic flow that is best explained by assuming that during systole vascular patency is maintained in the presence of marked compressive forces.

MATERIALS AND METHODS

Physiological Data

The experiments were performed in 17 adult male mongrel dogs following anesthetization with sodium pentobarbital (30 mg/kg intravenously). Surgery consisted of isolation of the superior and inferior vena cava, azygos vein, aorta, and pulmonary, brachiocephalic, and left subclavian arteries. A large glass cannula was inserted into the left subclavian artery or the brachiocephalic artery and connected to an open reservoir chamber (coronary reservoir) which could be raised or lowered. A second reservoir, one-way ball valve, and electromagnetic flow probe were connected to the left ventricle by means of a cannula inserted into the apex and retained by a purse-string suture. A reversible pump connected the two reservoirs. A cannulating electromagnetic flow probe and one-way valve were also incorporated in the connecting tubing from the coronary reservoir. Bypass tubing around the valve permitted the use of the coronary reservoir as an outflow reservoir until the preparation had been completed. A T-tube connected the second reservoir to a pump oxygenator and heat exchanger. The output of the pump, after oxygenating, warming, and debubbling of the blood, was returned to the heart through a Bardic catheter inserted into the anterior aspect of the right ventricle. A polyethylene catheter inserted into the right atrium permitted continuous sampling of the right atrial inflow for oxygen saturation using a Waters oximeter. That catheter, or a second catheter in the right atrium, was also connected to a Statham pressure transducer for right atrial pressure measurement. A side arm from the subclavian cannula was connected to a Statham transducer to monitor the coronary reservoir pressure. A catheter-tipped transducer (Millar) was inserted into the left ventricle through a pulmonary vein for recording left ventricular pressure; a pressure gauge was also attached to the outflow cannula to record the simulated systemic arterial pressure. A Walton–Brodie circumferential-type strain gauge was inserted into the anterior aspect of the left ventricle for monitoring ventricular wall tension (12; obtained courtesy Dr. W. H. Newman, Medical University of South Carolina).

The superior and inferior vena cava, azygos vein, aorta, and brachiocephalic arteries were ligated in a sequence to prevent damage to the left ventrical from increased afterload. This consisted of bleeding the animal into the subclavian reservoir and then gradually occluding the aorta followed by ligating the veins. The resultant heart–lung preparation is thus totally isolated from the remainder of the animal as evidenced by the maintenance of a constant reservoir volume. Shortly after occluding the aorta and brachiocephalic arteries, brain death occurs, and neural outflow is assumed to become nonexistent. No additional adrenal secretions can enter the system, and no further anesthesia was given. The blood volume obtained was usually sufficient to fill the system, thereby eliminating the need for using a cross-matched animal or colloid solutions. The heat exchanger maintained temperature constant at 37°C.

The second reservoir was connected to the left ventricle after the preparation was stabilized, and the bypasss tubing around the valve in the subclavian reservoir was clamped to provide independent control of coronary pressure. The reversible pump connecting the two reservoirs now pumped from the ventricular reservoir into the coronary reservoir. Electrodes in the latter switched the pump on and off to maintain the fluid level constant.

The data were A-to-D converted at a rate of 200 samples/sec per channel and processed on line by a minicomputer (Nova 1200). The variables of interest were calculated and stored for later analysis on a flexible disk file. Final grouping for statistical analysis was by coronary flow levels. The primary variables consisted of aortic (coronary) pressure, afterload (apex reservoir) pressure, right atrial pressure, left ventricular pressure, left ventricular tension, output flow (into apex reservoir), and coronary flow (out of subclavian reservoir). From these were obtained aortic systolic pressure, mean ventricular pressure in systole, systolic time, diastolic time, maximal *dp/dt*, time to peak ventricular pressure, end-diastolic pressure, heart rate, stroke volume, stroke work (from the ventricular pressure and stroke volume), the integral of ventricular pressure, cardiac output, cardiac work, and tension–time index. The computer programs used to obtain these variables have been previously published (4). The ventricular wall tension was used to obtain peak tension, mean systolic tension, and mean isovolumetric tension. Because of drift of the gauge unit, diastolic readings were set equal to zero, and only relative tension magnitudes were obtained. Consequently, the gauge was not usually calibrated in absolute units except for a few of the pictorial records where a 100-g weight was hung on the suspended gauge at the end of the experiment. This provides only an amplitude calibration; true zero while in the ventricle was not obtained. The Millar transducer was precalibrated with a known force. Prior to insertion, it was balanced and zeroed in a water bath at 37°C. The zero pressure value was rechecked at the end of the experiment. The flowmeter probes were calibrated by pumping blood of equivalent hematocrit through them.

Coronary flows were divided into systolic, diastolic, and isovolumetric contraction flows. The isovolumetric contraction phase was calculated from the time of beginning of the rise in ventricular pressure until the apex flowmeter registered an outflow. With the onset of ventricular contraction, flow usually entered the lower-pressure apex reservoir. However, if flow into the aorta began to occur, the one-way valve system caused the aortic pressure to rapidly rise, thereby preventing significant outflow. To the extent that such outflow did occur, our systolic coronary flow valves are underestimated; this error appeared to be small based on the usual pressure gradients used, the coronary reservoir pressure tracings (short increase in pressure only at peak ventricular pressures), and several attempts to completely block the aortic valve using an intraventricular balloon.

Morphological Data

Inasmuch as cardiac muscle contracts when placed in contact with most fixatives, it is necessary to counteract the resultant displacement if structural parameters are to be related to functional states. This has been successfully accomplished using both isolated papillary muscle and intact ventricles (22). The data in this chapter are based on a variety of methods for obtaining heart muscle at systolic and diastolic lengths. The methods used to obtain diastolic or systolic lengths provided essentially identical data with regard to the distribution of the extracellular collagen struts. The length of the muscle, i.e., diastolic or systolic, was the determining factor for the collagen strut distribution.

Hearts from 12 dogs were fixed by various techniques. These included instillation of 5% buffered glutaraldehyde into the left and right coronary arteries to fix the hearts in a contracted state. Some hearts were removed and sliced perpendicular to the long axis, and the segments fixed by immersion, resulting in marked contraction. Samples of the left ventricle and papillary muscle were removed from the heart to provide cross or longitudinal surfaces of both papillary muscle and circumferentially oriented ventricular wall muscle. The samples were transferred to fresh glutaraldehyde, then to buffered osmium tetroxide, dehydrated in graded acetones, and subjected to critical point drying. After critical point drying, samples were placed in liquid nitrogen, fractured with a precooled razor blade, mounted on specimen stubs for SEM, and coated with gold.

Initial fixation was obtained using a buffered glutaraldehyde with a total tonicity of 590 mOsmol. The osmolarity of the vehicle, 290, seems to be the most important factor (6). Using this fixative and subsequent appropriate fixiation and dehydration techniques, minimal evidence of cell damage was noted by either transmission or scanning electron microscopy (7).

Two papillary muscles were removed from 12 rabbits and placed in 30 ml of Krebs bicarbonate buffer gassed with 95% O_2 and 5% CO_2 (15). After 30 min of equilibration, muscle preparations were adjusted to maximal contraction length or rest length and stimulated 12 times per minute using 4-msec duration impulses. The muscles were allowed to equilibrate under these conditions for 15 min. With 12 of the preparations, the bathing medium was replaced with 5% buffered glutaraldehyde, resulting in fixation at rest length or maximal contraction length. With 12 papillary muscles equilibrated at rest or maximal contraction length, the bathing medium was replaced with one containing ethylenediaminetetraacetic acid (EDTA), and stimulations continued for 20 min past the last recorded contraction. At this time, the EDTA-containing bathing medium was replaced with 5% buffered glutaraldehyde. One-half (six) of the muscles were fixed at rest length, and one-half at maximal contraction length as determined previously.

RESULTS

The results of the hemodynamic studies are presented in Table 1, and those values with significant correlations are presented with their correlation coefficient in Table 2. Total systolic flow is strongly correlated with cardiac work, peak ventricular pressure, tension–time index, etc. This would suggest that metabolic factors predominate in determining systolic flow, although probably not on a beat-to-beat basis. Systolic flow accounts for about 30% of total coronary flow and is thus a significant factor in myocardial metabolism. Systolic flow can be divided into two components, that occurring during isovolumetric contraction and that during the remainder of systole.

Isovolumetric flow, as visualized in Figure 1, occurs as a rise in flow at the time of increase in ventricular pressure. This flow is closely correlated with isovolumetric tension: the higher the isovolumetric tension, the greater the isovolumetric flow. This portion of systolic flow varies from about 20% to 50% of total systolic flow yet does not correlate with work parameters of the heart, suggesting that is is not subject to autoregulation but simply to the level of tension during this phase of contraction.

The pertinent morphological studies are presented in Figures 2 and 3 and summarized in Figure 4. The capillaries are parallel to each other and parallel to the adjacent myocytes (13). There is an extensive network of collagen struts that extend from the basal lamina of each capillary to all contiguous myocytes. These struts insert near perpendicular to the capillary myocyte and extend for a way around the contiguous myocytes to insert into the basal lamina tangentially. With this arrangement, as the myocytes shorten, their radii increase. This increase in radius would stretch the collagen struts and place tension on the basal lamina of the capillary (7). Figure 2, a stereo pair, depicts the struts in diastole as determined by a length–tension curve. The struts are curved, not straight. In Figure 3, a stereo pair taken from a heart fixed at systolic length, the struts are straight, consistent with the notion of tension transmission.

DISCUSSION

The observation that blood flow occurs through the heart during systole has been made repeatedly (14,18,19). This somewhat anomalous situation

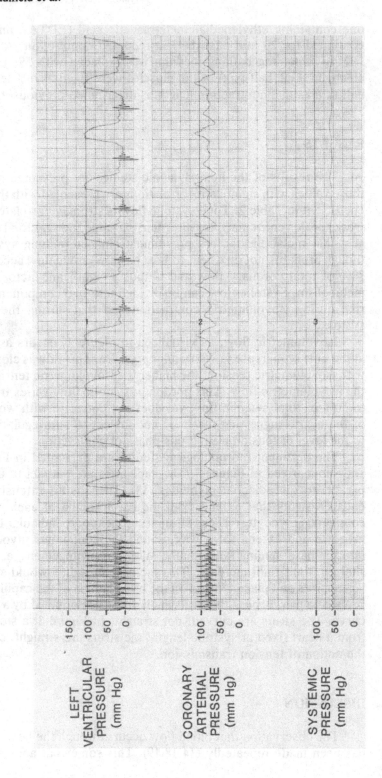

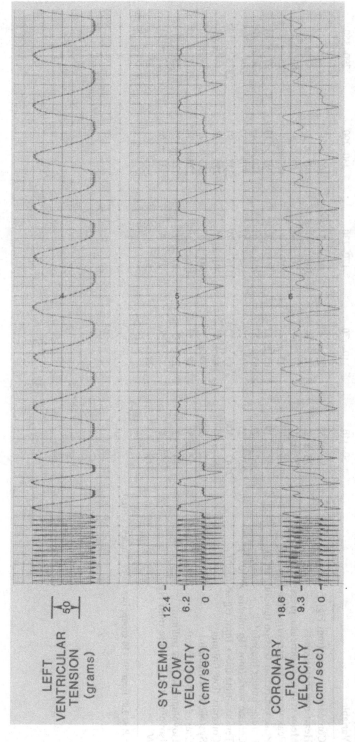

Figure 1. Tracing demonstrates pulsatile coronary flow as correlated with ECG, pressure, tension, and ventricular outflow recordings. The onset of isovolumetric contraction is indicated by the heavy line. The oscillations in the left ventricular tracing are caused by a ball valve in the outflow tract.

Table 1.   Data Grouped by Coronary Flow (ml/min)

Variable	50–110	110–170	170–230	230–290	290–350
Coronary pressure (mm Hg)	86 ± 5	100 ± 4	94 ± 3	102 ± 4	114 ± 2
Heart rate (beats/min)	126 ± 2	121 ± 3	103 ± 1	109 ± 3	112 ± 3
Mean systolic ventricular pressure (mm Hg)	77 ± 5	77 ± 4	76 ± 4	84 ± 4	84 ± 5
Peak ventricular pressure (mm Hg)	115 ± 3	123 ± 4	125 ± 4	125 ± 4	125 ± 3
Peak ventricular tension (uncalibrated)	137 ± 10	103 ± 12	99 ± 7	91 ± 17	97 ± 14
Cardiac output (ml/min)	365 ± 71	363 ± 57	461 ± 61	420 ± 49	530 ± 105
Cardiac work (mm Hg·ml/min × 10^{-2})	271 ± 25	271 ± 22	334 ± 27	370 ± 37	449 ± 36[a]
Tension–time index (mm Hg·sec/min)	2147 ± 100	2108 ± 158	2115 ± 79	2235 ± 91	2373 ± 102
Coronary flow (ml/min)	84 ± 4	148 ± 4[a]	201 ± 2[a]	255 ± 3[a]	316 ± 3[a]
Systolic flow (ml/min)	22 ± 3	49 ± 4[a]	80 ± 5[a]	103 ± 7[a]	139 ± 10[a]
Diastolic flow (ml/min)	62 ± 3	98 ± 5[a]	196 ± 18[a]	223 ± 34[a]	177 ± 10[a]
Isovolumetric flow (ml/min)	14 ± 2	23 ± 2	27 ± 1	22 ± 2[a]	23 ± 6
Isovolumetric pressure (mm Hg)	35 ± 8	32 ± 5	25 ± 4	31 ± 6	27 ± 11
N	19	21	51	32	27

[a] $P \leq 0.05$ from 50–110 group, two-tailed Student's t-test.

Table 2.   Correlation Coefficients

Variable	Total flow	Systolic flow	Diastolic flow	Isovolumetric flow
Systolic flow	0.827[a]	1.000	0.566[a]	0.369[a]
Diastolic flow	0.914[a]	0.566[a]	1.000	0.325[a]
Isovolumetric flow	0.332[a]	0.369[a]	0.325[a]	1.000
Cardiac work	0.338[a]	0.498[a]	0.109	−0.104
Tension–time index	0.257[a]	0.426[a]	0.098	−0.064
Peak ventricular pressure	0.306[a]	0.370[a]	0.197[a]	0.100
Mean ventricular pressure	0.306[a]	0.422[a]	0.156	0.073
Peak ventricular tension	−0.249	−0.150	−0.268	0.172
Systolic time	0.428[a]	0.494[a]	0.319[a]	−0.129
Diastolic time	0.203[a]	0.057	0.275[a]	0.095
PVP time	0.276[a]	0.402	0.171	−0.103
Coronary systolic pressure	0.063	0.513[a]	−0.253[a]	0.012
Coronary mean pressure	0.059	0.371[a]	−0.147	−0.269[a]
Cardiac output	0.276[a]	0.487[a]	0.040	−0.203
Isovolumetric pressure	−0.124	−0.133	−0.117	0.631[a]

[a] $P \leq 0.01$; significance level computed for number of pairs of matched data in each case.

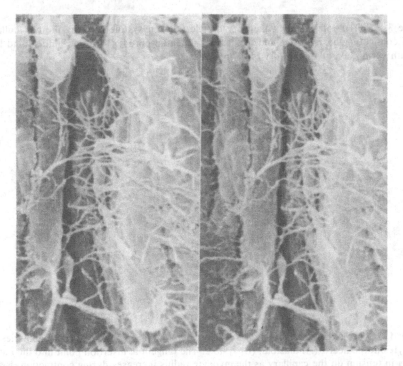

Figure 2.   Stereo pair of rabbit papillary muscle fixed in diastole showing the wavy collagen fibers connecting myocytes and the capillary . ×5.500. Reproduced from Caulfield and Borg (7) with permission of *Laboratory Investigation*.

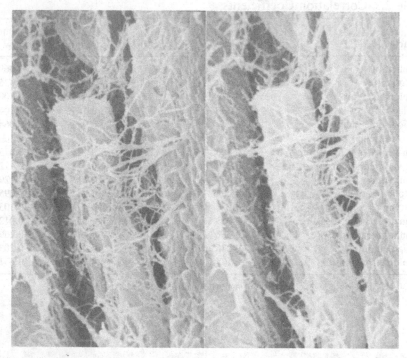

Figure 3. Stereo pair of rabbit papillary muscle fixed in systole showing the taut collagen struts connecting the myocytes and capillaries . ×5,500. Reproduced from Caulfield and Borg (7) with permission of *Laboratory Investigation*.

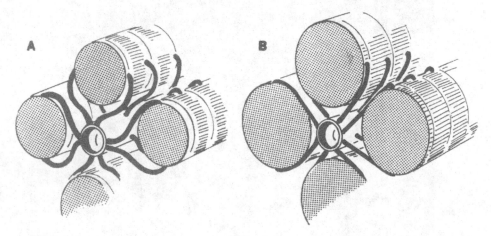

Figure 4. Schematic demonstrating the distribution of collagen struts between capillaries and myocytes in the heart; (A) diastole, (B) systole. The tangential insertion point into the muscle results in tension on the capillary as the myocyte radius increases·during contraction. Reproduced from Borg and Caulfield (27) with permission of the Federation of American Societies for Experimental Biology.

of flow through vessels subjected to external stresses of 150 mm Hg has provoked numerous investigations, yet a clear understanding of myocardial flow is not at hand. This is in part because the small vessels in the mid-myocardial region are not visible, and measurements of flow are made quite distant from these sites, and extrapolations need be made.

On the basis of our finding that systolic flow is divisible into two segments, isovolumetric and the reminder of systole, certain hypotheses can be made relative to flow, and these related to various phenomena. During isovolumetric contraction, an increase in coronary flow occurs as measured near the origin of the left circumflex artery. This flow is directly related to the wall tension: the higher the tension, the greater the flow. Probably the simplest explanation of this phenomenon is that during isovolumetric contraction, the struts from the myocytes place tension on the walls of the capillaries and hold them open, permitting easy egress of blood from arterioles to capillaries. It would seem that this may occur, since, during systole, the epicardial arteries, arterioles, and capillaries can be seen to decrease in diameter 15–20% (23,24). If this occurs in the epicardial vessels with little external pressure, it is reasonable to assume that the intramyocardial vessels do not dilate. Therefore, the increased flow measured in the circumflex artery enters vessels that are decreasing in diameter, indicating that flow during isovolumetric contraction at least must enter capillaries in the myocardium and is not a result of increased vascular compliance. Since the tension on the struts from the myocytes to the capillaries is dependent on the increase in diameter of the myocytes, little tension would occur except in those regions in which actual motion occurs. During isovolumetric contraction, this is probably limited to the subendocardial region where some contraction occurs, resulting in alteration of ventricular geometry from an ellipsoid to a more globular shape.

During the ejection phase of systole, left circumflex flow decreases markedly. However, flow velocity in capillaries and venules near the surface of the heart increase (24). During late ejection, there is a marked increase in coronary sinus flow (5).

During the ejection phase of systole, the struts connecting myocytes to the adjacent capillaries which are parallel to the myocytes will not only place tension on the capillary to maintain patency but will shorten the capillary consonant with myocyte shortening. This shortening will decrease the length of the capillary by about 20%, decreasing the volume of the capillary by 20%. There is not likely to be an increase in capillary radius since wall pressures are 120–150 mm Hg, whereas coronary sinus pressures are 5 mm Hg late in ventricular systole. Thus, with the struts maintaining capillary patency, very high wall pressures, capillary volume decreasing, and a low outflow pressure one could expect rapid translocation of the blood from capillaries and venules during systole. This has been reported for the capillaries and venules on the epicardial surface (24).

The decrease in volume of the capillaries even with rapid outflow would increase the intracapillary pressure and affect outflow from the arterioles. This is reflected in the fact that total systolic flow is closely correlated with coronary systolic pressure and coronary mean pressure. At some driving forces, systolic flow is high and, in all probability, forward in arterioles. On the other hand, isovolumetric flow does not show a correlation with coronary systolic pressure, suggesting that outflow pressure from the arterioles is into a low-pressure vessel during isovolumetric contraction and that limitations of flow secondary to driving pressure occur below the levels we used (60–120 mm Hg). This is similar to the situation during diastolic flow, there being no correlation between it and the driving pressures that we used. This is reasonable in view of the fact that precapillary pressures are about 15 mm Hg during diastole (9).

Thus, we propose that the myocyte-to-capillary struts maintain capillary patency during isovolumetric contraction and that flow is high during this brief phase. During ejection, the capillary volume decreases because of the shortening of the myoctyes and the tight coupling of the myocytes to capillaries via the struts causing shortening of the capillaries. Flow rate increases in the capillaries and venules secondary to the volume decrease. This notion of tightly coupling myocardial flow to contraction was made by Wiggers (26). This hypothesis can be used to explain two observations, the "no-reflow" phenomenon and subendocardial ischemia.

When a coronary artery is ligated for 30–40 min and then released, reactive hyperemia occurs (17). If the ligature is left in place 90–120 min, rather than reactive hyperemia, there is failure of flow into the central ischemic portion of myocardium. Three things occur between 40 and 90 min that may relate to this. In the central ischemic area, most of the cells are reversibly damaged at 40 min, whereas most are irreversibly damaged at 90 min. Secondly, at 40 min, although there is some bulging and stretching of the ischemic area, it is not severe, whereas at 2 hr, there is marked bulging and excessive stretching of sarcomeres to lengths of 3.5 μm (10). Clearly, some structure alterations have occurred. The third aberration is that the point of maximum vascular resistance at 2 hr post-occlusion is no longer the arteriole but the capillary (13).

An explanation of reactive hyperemia is the presence of metabolites causing maximal dilatation of the arteriolar sphincters, and upon reinstitution of flow, myocyte contraction occurs, insuring capillary patency and forward flow, However, after 2 hr of ischemia, there is overstretching of some myocytes. In these regions, the capillaries would also be overstretched because of numerous struts that interconnect myocytes and capillaries. Since myocardial capillaries are in the range of 4–5 μm in diameter, a stretch from sarcomere lengths of 2.2 μm to 3.5 μm would result in a diameter reduction to the range of 3 μm, a diameter that prohibits red cell passage (8). Since these myocytes are irreversibly damaged, during systole with no myocyte thickening, the capillaries would be subjected to wall tension effectively blocking flow in the presence of maximal systolic coronary artery pressure which is still below intracavity pressure. During diastole, with lower coronary artery perfusion pressures (15 mm Hg) and low wall tension, flow would be prohibited by excessively linearly stretched segments of capillaries with lumena in the vicinity of 3 μm which would block red cell entry.

That something external to the vessels must occur is suggested by the fact that the "no-reflow" phenomenon does not occur after periods of total ischemia varying from 1 to 18 hr in skeletal muscle. At each interval of ischemia between 1 and 18 hr, on reestablishment of arterial flow, good pulsation occurred throughout the ischemic limb in dogs (20). One must conclude from this that either the metabolism of the small vessels of the heart is markedly dissimilar from those in skeletal muscle or factors external to the small vessels results in the "no-reflow" phenomenon in the heart. It appears to us that structural alterations and lack of contraction in the necrotic zone of the heart are a more likely probability.

A drop in perfusion pressure does not affect diastolic flow in the ranges that we used, suggesting very low resistance of the myocardium during this phase of the cardiac cycle. However, systolic flow is very dependent on coronary driving pressure, and any drop would decrease systolic flow. This decrease would appear in the subendocardial region, the point farthest from the source, which also has the highest extravascular tension. This decrease in flow should be accompanied by altered contraction, and, in fact, when coronary perfusion is lowered by about 7%, there is a decrease in wall motion in the subendocardial region (25). This decrease in motion will have two effects: a decrease in myocyte contraction, hence smaller myocyte diameters, because the myocyte-to-capillary strut arrangement will cause a decrease in capillary diameter and decreased flow; and a second effect resulting from decreased myocyte shortening and reflected in failure of the capillaries to shorten and loss of this propulsive effect on the column of blood. Thus, during diastole, as the capillaries should be lengthened and should have expelled their contents of blood, they in fact are not lengthening, and their contents have not been expelled, thus increasing the resistance to diastolic flow and further aggravating the subendocardial ischemia.

ACKNOWLEDGMENTS

This work was partially supported by a grant in aid from the American Heart Association and with funds contributed in part by the American Heart Association, Palm Beach County Chapter (Florida), and by NIH Grant HL-24935.

REFERENCES

1. Abel, F. L. 1980. Direct effects of ethanol on myocardial performance and coronary resistance. *J. Pharmacol. Exp. Ther.* 212:28–33.
2. Abel, F. L. 1980. The effects of acetylstrophanthidin and glucocorticoids on canine left ventricular performance and coronary hemodynamics. *Circ. Shock* 7:265–276.

3. Abel, F. L., Borg, T. K., and Caulfield, J. B. 1980. The effects of left ventricular systole on coronary blood flow. In: *28th International Congress of Physiological Sciences, Budapest, July, 1980*, p. 289. Hungarian Physiological Society, Budapest.

4. Abel, F. L., and McCutcheon, E. P. 1979. *Cardiovascular Function: Principles and Applications*, pp. 396–408. Little, Brown, Boston.

5. Anrep, G. V. 1945. Quoted in: C. H. Best and N. B. Taylor (eds.), *The Physiological Basis of Medical Practice*, 4th ed., p. 278. Williams & Wilkins, Baltimore.

6. Arborgh, B., Bell, P., Brunk, V., and Collins, V. P. 1976. The osmotic effect of glutaraldehyde during fixation: A transmission electron microscopy, scanning electron microscopy, and cytochemical study. *J. Ultrastruct. Res.* 56:339–350.

7. Caulfield, J. B., and Borg, T. K. 1979. The collagen network of the heart. *Lab. Invest.* 40:364–372.

8. Charm, S. E., and Kurland, G. S. 1974. *Blood Flow and Microcirculation*, pp. 138–139. John Wiley & Sons, New York.

9. Coulson, R. L., Grayson, J., and Irvin, M. 1970. Observations on the coronary collateral communications and the control of flow in the coronary circulation in dogs. *J. Physiol. (Lond.)* 208:563–581.

10. Crozatier, B., Ashrof, M., Franklin, D., and Ross, J. 1977. Sarcomere length in experimental myocardial infarction: Evidence for sarcomere overstretch in dyskinetic ventricular regions. *J. Mol. Cell. Cardiol.* 9:785–797.

11. Downey, J. M., and Kirk, E. S. 1975. Inhibition of coronary blood flow by a vascular waterfall mechanism. *Circ. Res.* 36:753–760.

12. Feigl, E. O. 1966. I. Mechanical force measurement in biology. In: R. F. Rushmer, (ed.), *Methods in Medical Research*, Vol. 11, pp. 122–136. Year Book Medical Publishers, Chicago.

13. Grayson, J., Davidson, J. W., Fitzgerald-Finch, A., and Scott, C. 1974. The functional morphology of the coronary microcirculation in the dog. *Microvasc. Res.* 8:20–43.

14. Hess, D. S., and Bache, R. J. 1976. Transmural distribution of myocardial blood flow during systole in the awake dog. *Circ. Res.* 38:5–15.

15. Ingebretsen, W. R., Jr., Becker, E., Friedman, W. F., and Mayer, S. E. 1977. Contractile responses of cardiac and skeletal muscle to isoproteronal covalently linked to glass beads. *Circ. Res.* 40:474–484.

16. Kittleson, M. D., Hamilin, R. L., Levesque, M. J., and Muir, W. W. III. 1980. Transmural myocardial blood flow and pressure in systole and in diastole in the horse. *Fed. Proc.* 39:1107.

17. Kloner, R. A., Ganote, C. E., and Jennings, R. B. 1974. The "No-Reflow" phenomenon of the temporary coronary occlusion in the dog. *J. Clin. Invest.* 54:1496–1508.

18. Kreuzer, H., and Schoeppe, W. 1963. Das Verhalten des Bruckes in der Herzewand. *Pfluegers Arch.* 278:181–198.

19. Kreuzer, H., and Schoeppe, W. 1963. Fur Entstehung der Differenz zwischen systolischem Myokard und Ventrikeldruck. *Pfluegers Arch.* 278:199–208.

20. Miller, H. H., and Welch, C. S. 1949. Quantitative studies on the time factors in arterial injuries. *Ann. Surg.* 130:428–438.

21. Shkhvatsabaya, I. K. 1979. *Ischemic Heart Disease.* translated by U. N. Bobrov and G. S. Vats, pp. 24–26. C. V. Mosy, St. Louis.

22. Spotnitz, H. M., Sonnerblick, E. H., and Spiro, D. 1966. Relation of ultrastructure to function in the intact heart: Sarcomere structure relative to pressure volume curves of intact left ventricles of dog and cat. *Circ. Res.* 18:49–66.

23. Tillmans, H., Ikeda, S., Hansen, H., Sarma, J. S. M., Fauvel, J. M., and Bing, R. J. 1974. Microcirculation in the ventricle of the dog and turtle. *Circ. Res.* 34:561–569.

24. Tillmans, H., Leinberger, H., Thederon, H., Steinhausen, M., and Kubler, W. 1981. Pressure–velocity–diameter relations in the microvessels of the heart. In: P. Gaehtgens (ed.), *Abstracts of XI European Conference for Microcirculation*, Bibliotheca Anatomica No. 20, pp. 484–489, S. Karger, Basel.

25. Vatner, S., Manders, T., and Baig, H. 1979. Correlation between ischemia induced reductions in regional myocardial blood flow and function in conscious dogs. *Circulation* 60(Suppl. II):29.
26. Wiggers, C. J. 1954. The interplay of coronary vascular resistance and myocardial compression in regulating coronary flow. *Circ. Res.* 2:271–279.
27. T. K. Borg, and J. B. Caulfield, 1981, The collagen matrix of the heart, *Fed. Proc.* 40:2037–2041.

Prolonged Depletion of ATP Because of Delayed Repletion of the Adenine Nucleotide Pool following Reversible Myocardial Ischemic Injury in Dogs

K. A. Reimer, M. L. Hill, and R. B. Jennings

Department of Pathology
Duke University Medical Center
Durham, North Carolina 27710, USA

Abstract. Sixty-five percent of the ATP and 50% of the total adenine nucleotide (ΣAd) pool is lost from the subendocardial myocardium after 15 min of severe ischemia induced by circumflex artery occlusion in open-chest dogs (12). In the present experiment, we assessed the effects of various periods of arterial reflow following 15 min of ischemic injury on resynthesis of ATP and ΣAd. The circumflex artery was occluded for 15 min and reperfused for 20 or 60 min or 24 or 96 hr. The mean ATP after 15 min of ischemia was reduced 62% from 5.42 ± 0.33 to 2.08 ± 0.21 μmol/g; and the total nucleotide content was reduced by 50%. ATP content recovered slightly during the first 20 min of reperfusion but remained markedly depressed for at least 24 hr because of the initial depletion of adenine nucleotides and because minimal salvage of de novo repletion occurred in the injured muscle during this time period. By 4 days, ATP and total adenine nucleotides were still slightly depressed but had recovered to 88% and 91% of control. Electrolyte changes and an increased inulin-diffusible space, which are characteristic of irreversibly injured myocardium, reperfused for 20 or 60 min, were not observed. Also, tissue necrosis was absent in the hearts reperfused for 24 or 96 hr. These observations indicate that the marked depression of ATP and adenine nucleotides and the slow recovery of these metabolites occurred in myocardium that nevertheless was reversibly injured in terms of cellular viability.

Fifteen minutes of severe myocardial ischemia in dogs causes reversible cell injury in the sense that cell death does not develop if reperfusion is established at this time (14). Nevertheless, a number of recent studies have found prolonged abnormalities of contractile function following brief periods of ischemia (6–8,28,31). The cause of the prolonged contractile dysfunction has not been established but potentially could be related to depressed levels of adenosine triphosphate (ATP).

We showed recently that only 15 min of severe myocardial ischemia in dogs caused a 65% decrease in tissue ATP content (12). Furthermore, catabolism of adenine nucleotides to nucleosides and bases occurred so that half of the total pool of adenine nucleotides (ΣAd) was lost. Consequently, restoration of ATP content following reperfusion would require resynthesis of adenine nucleotides as well as restoration of oxidative phosphorylation.

395

However, the rate of adenine nucleotide synthesis by either de novo or salvage pathways has been found to be slow relative to the size of the total adenine nucleotide pool (20,33). The purpose of the present study was to determine the rate of net ATP and adenine nucleotide repletion following a 15-min period of severe myocardial ischemia induced by circumflex occlusion in dogs.

METHODS

Experimental Design

Forty-two healthy mongrel dogs of either sex and weighing 30–40 lb were used. Each dog was anesthetized with 30–40 mg/kg of sodium pentobarbital and was intubated and ventilated on a Harvard respirator at a rate of 200 ml/kg per min. The respirator rate was adjusted, and supplemental oxygen was given if necessary to maintain arterial blood gases at physiological levels. Lead II of the ECG was monitored, and peripheral blood pressure was recorded through a catheter in the right femoral artery. A left thoracotomy was done using aseptic techniques, and the circumflex artery was isolated beneath the left atrial appendage.

All dogs were subjected to 15 min of ischemia which was induced by occluding the circumflex artery with a silk snare. Thirty-seven dogs survived occlusion and were assigned to one of five groups. Ten were studied immediately without reperfusion. In the other 27 dogs, the snare was released to allow reperfusion. Reperfusion at this time resulted in ventricular fibrillation within the first 2 min in 15 of these dogs. Five were quickly defibrillated using external paddles, but the other ten were lost to the study. The 17 dogs surviving reperfusion were assigned to groups studied after 20 or 60 min or 24 or 96 hr after reperfusion. In the 24- and 96-hr groups, incisions were closed, and animals recovered from anethesia until reanesthetized the following day. The number of dogs in each group is indicated in Table 1. One dog with 4 days of reperfusion had developed focal subendocardial necrosis and was excluded.

Sampling Techniques

In order to identify areas that were severely ischemic or had been severely ischemic, the fluorescent dye thioflavin S (TS) was injected intravenously (1.0 ml/kg of a 4% solution of normal saline). In the reperfusion groups, the circumflex artery was reoccluded just prior to administration of the dye. Ten seconds after TS injection, each heart was quickly excised and rapidly cooled with stirring in 750 ml of 0° isotonic KCl. The atria and ventricles were opened widely after the first minute of cooling in order to insure rapid cooling of the endocardial regions. After complete cooling, the

Table 1. Water, IDS, and Electrolytes of Nonischemic and Ischemic (or Previously Ischemic) Myocardium[a]

Group	N	TTW		IDS		Na$^+$		K$^+$		Ca^{2+}		Mg^{2+}	
		NI	I	NI	I	NI	I	NI	I	NI	I	NI	I
15 + 0 min	10	355 ± 7.0	368 ± 4.9*	82 ± 3.3	82 ± 2.6	17.3 ± 1.3	18.4 ± 1.9	38.2 ± 1.3	36.2 ± 1.5	0.57 ± 0.05	0.63 ± 0.05*	5.1 ± 0.10	5.2 ± 0.09
15 + 20 min	4	363 ± 5.4	399 ± 6.8***	91 ± 6.7	99 ± 12.1	19.3 ± 1.7	21.5 ± 1.6*	37.8 ± 1.4	44.7 ± 0.8**	0.43 ± 0.04	0.53 ± 0.07	5.0 ± 0.25	4.6 ± 0.11
15 + 60 min	4	356 ± 4.5	381 ± 3.3***	79 ± 5.0	97 ± 3.4	18.2 ± 1.0	20.5 ± 2.7	38.4 ± 1.1	43.3 ± 0.6*	0.47 ± 0.07	0.50 ± 0.03	4.3 ± 0.30	3.6 ± 0.24*
15 min + 24 hr	5	363 ± 5.5	380 ± 1.2*	96 ± 6.7	102 ± 2.3	21.4 ± 1.7	20.9 ± 1.0	35.8 ± 1.0	35.9 ± 2.2	0.38 ± 0.01	0.61 ± 0.08	4.6 ± 0.25	3.7 ± 0.51*
15 min + 96 hr	3	353 ± 2.7	372 ± 8.7	84 ± 7.8	96 ± 9.2	21.8 ± 0.5	21.7 ± 1.4	37.7 ± 0.3	37.3 ± 0.9	0.75 ± 0.02	0.67 ± 0.03	5.1 ± 0.44	5.0 ± 0.36

[a] This table lists the effects of 15 min of ischemia plus 0, 20, or 60 min or 24 or 96 hr of reperfusion on the total tissue water (TTW), inulin-diffusible space (IDS), and electrolytes. Group means and standard errors of the means are shown for nonischemic (NI) and ischemic (or previously ischemic) (I) myocardium. Units are ml/100 g dry tissue for the TTW and IDS and mmol/100 g dry tissue for all electrolytes. Statistical comparisons were made between nonischemic and ischemic samples using paired t analysis. *$P < 0.05$, **$P < 0.01$, ***$P < 0.001$. Reproduced from ref. 23 with permission of the publisher from the Journal of Molecular and Cellular Cardiology.

heart was removed from the cold KCl and placed under ultraviolet light to identify nonischemic (TS fluorescent) and severely ischemic (nonfluorescent) areas of the anterior and posterior papillary muscles, respectively. Areas of the posterior papillary muscle with some collateral perfusion were fluorescent, and these areas were excluded. The ischemic and nonischemic samples were transferred to 0° Krebs Ringer's phosphate (KRP) and were kept cool until processed. First, the ischemic posterior papillary muscle and then the nonischemic anterior papillary muscle were cut into a minimum of 6 thin slices weighing 30–150 mg each. These were used to measure, in duplicate, (1) adenine nucleotides, (2) total tissue water (TTW) and electrolytes, or (3) the TTW and inulin-diffusible space.

Adenine Nucleotides

Two slices from each papillary muscle were used for adenine nucleotide assays and were quickly weighed on a Cahn Model DTL microbalance and transferred to 3.6% ice-cold (0°C) perchloric acid. The entire process of slicing and weighing took 30–60 sec. These slices were homogenized with a Tri-R homogenizer and brought to pH 5.0–6.0 with K_2CO_3 and KOH. Extracts were centrifuged to remove $KClO_4$, and the supernatant was frozen. Samples were later assayed either by enzymatic methods or by high-pressure liquid chromatography (HPLC). The enzymatic methods used to measure ATP were those of Lamprecht and Trautschold (17) and for adenosine diphosphate (ADP) and adenosine monophosphate (AMP) were those of Jawouk et al. (10). The same nucleotides were assayed in some cases by HPLC using the method of Anderson and Murphy (1). A Waters model 6000-A solvent delivery system, model U6K sample injector system, and a model 440 absorbance detector and data module were used to separate peaks and to quantitate peak area against standard solutions of the same nulceotides. An ammonium dihydrogen phosphate isocratic buffer (0.05 M, pH = 6.0) containing the samples was passed through a μ-Bondapak® reverse-phase C_{18} column (Waters) at a flow rate of 2 ml/min, and the nucleotides were measured at a wavelength of 254 Å. The concentration of each standard was assayed in a Gilford Model 250 spectrophotometer by UV absorption at the wavelength of the molar extinction coefficient of the nucleotides. Tissue nucleotide contents were expressed as μmol/g wet weight, and ΣAd was calculated as the sum of ATP, ADP, and AMP content.

Electrolytes, Total Tissue Water, and Inulin-Diffusible Space

Water and electrolytes were measured in two additional slices from each papillary muscle. These slices were weighed and then dried overnight at 105°C. The dry slices were reweighed, and the TTW was calculated as ml H_2O/100 g dry tissue.

Electrolytes were extracted from each dried slice in 5 ml of 0.75 N

HNO_3, according to techniques described previously (11–13). Briefly, Mg^{2+}, Na^+, and K^+ were determined in a dilution containing 5000 ppm of RbCl of each HNO_3 extract. The Ca^{2+} was determined in a 1:10 dilution containing 10,000 ppm La^{3+}. These dilutions were done in ion-free glassware verified prior to use to have no detectable sodium. All four electrolytes were measured in an IL 351 atomic absorption spectophotometer interfaced with a Tektronix Model 31 computer calculator. Standard curves were prepared for all four ions, and two standards and two reagent blanks were analyzed with every series of unknowns. Electrolyte contents were calculated as mmol/100 g dry tissue.

The inulin-diffusible space (IDS) was measured in a third pair of slices by incubating them for 60 min in oxygenated KRP medium containing trace quantities of [^{14}C]hydroxymethylinulin. The slices were then quickly rinsed in isotonic sucrose to remove excess KRP and were blotted on Whatman #1 filter paper, weighed, and dried.

The dry slices were weighed and then rehydrated by adding one or two drops of deionized water and solubilized in Soluene 350 (Packard). The ^{14}C activity was counted in a Packard liquid scintillation counter. The IDS was calculated as ml H_2O/100 g dry tissue.

RESULTS

Adenine Nucleotide Loss during Ischemia

The ATP and ΣAd contents of nonischemic myocardium in all groups were similar to values reported by others (3,4) using quick freezing techniques. Fifteen minutes of ischemia caused a loss of 40% of the tissue ATP (Figure 1). At this time, ADP also was slightly reduced, evidently by conversion to ATP and AMP through the adenylate kinase (myokinase) reaction. AMP was significantly increased, but this increase was small compared to the marked loss of ATP. These changes together resulted in a 50% decrease in total adenine nucleotides.

Net ATP and Adenine Nucleotide Resynthesis during Reperfusion

Twenty minutes of reperfusion following an initial 15-min period of ischemia caused a significant increase in ATP (Figure 2) which could be accounted for by a rapid resumption of oxidative phosphorylation and recharging of accumulated AMP. Nevertheless, after 20 min of reperfusion, the ATP still was depressed significantly and was only half of the normal value. No further increase in ATP was detected even after 24 hr of reperfusion (Figure 2). By 4 days, ATP was nearly normal but still significantly depressed compared to the nonischemic region. The prolonged depression in the level of ATP did not result from an increase in the ADP or AMP pools

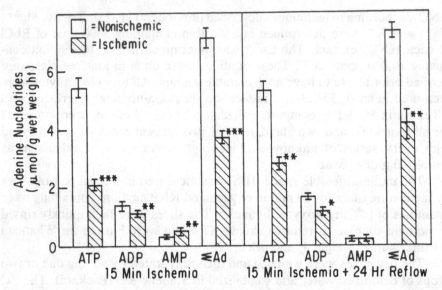

Figure 1.   The effects of 15 min of ischemia without reperfusion or with 24 hr of reperfusion on total adenine nucleotides are compared. Following ischemia, ATP was reduced 60%; ADP was also reduced, and although AMP was increased, the total adenine nucleotide content was decreased 50%. After 24 hr of reperfusion, ATP was still reduced nearly 50%, associated with over 40% decrease in total adenine nucleotides. Brackets indicate 1 standard error of the mean. Nonischemic and ischemic samples from each dog were compared by paired t statistical analysis. *$P < 0.05$, **$P < 0.01$, ***$P < 0.001$. Comparison between groups using a nonpaired t test showed less AMP ($P < 0.05$) but no other significant differences between 15 min of ischemia and ischemia plus 24 hr of reperfusion. (Reproduced from ref. 23 with the permission of the publisher from the *Journal of Molecular and Cellular Cardiology*.)

but rather reflected the fact that the ΣAd pool remained unchanged during the first 24 hr of reperfusion (Figure 1). By 4 days, adenosine nucleotides had returned to nearly normal levels but were still significantly reduced (Figure 3).

Evidence of Myocardial Viability in the Ischemic Region

The validity of these results rests on the assumptions that blood flow was restored and the injury was truly reversible. Previous studies have shown that 15 min of severe ischemia in this model causes reversible cell injury in that no necrosis develops if blood flow is restored (14). This was confirmed in the seven dogs studied at 24 to 96 hr in the present study. However, one dog with 15 min of ischemia and 4 days of reperfusion did have small foci of subendocardial necrosis and was excluded from the study. Reperfusion for only 20 or 60 min would have been too short a time period in which to detect infarction by either gross or histological techniques. Nevertheless, cell death can be detected this early because characteristic electrolyte changes, termed "explosive cell swelling," do occur within minutes after reperfusion of irreversibly injured myocardium (29) (see Discussion).

Electrolyte changes observed in the present study were not indicative of irreversible ischemic injury (Table 1) and provide direct evidence in all groups that blood flow was restored and cellular viability preserved. Statistically significant but quantitatively small increases in TTW occurred at all time periods, indicating mild edema of the ischemic region. The IDS remained in the normal range in all samples, however, providing no evidence for increased membrane permeability to inulin which is chracteristic of irreversibly injured myocytes. Tissue sodium content was increased slightly after 20 min of reperfusion but returned to normal thereafter. Potassium, which washes out of dying myocardium, was actually increased at 20 and

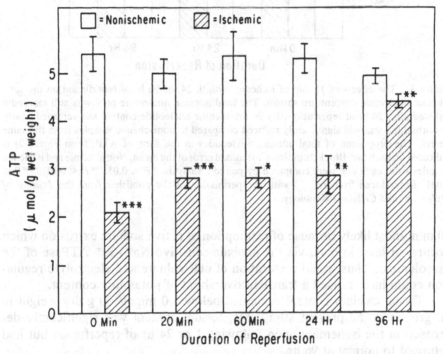

Figure 2.   The effects of 15 min of ischemia with 0, 20, or 60 min or 24 or 96 hr of reperfusion on ATP content are shown. ATP was markedly reduced in ischemic samples without reperfusion. ATP content increased slightly during the first 20 min of reperfusion, most likely because of rephosphorylation of ADP and AMP, but showed no additional increase over the next 24 hr. By 96 hr, ATP was nearly normal but was still significantly reduced compared to corresponding samples from the nonischemic region. Brackets indicate 1 standard error of the mean. Nonischemic and ischemic samples from each dog were compared by paired t statistical analysis. *$P < 0.05$, **$P < 0.01$, ***$P < 0.001$. Comparison between groups using a nonpaired t test showed significant increases in ATP with all times of reperfusion compared to no reperfusion ($P < 0.05$). Reproduced from ref. 23 with the permission of the publisher from the *Journal of Molecular and Cellular Cardiology*.

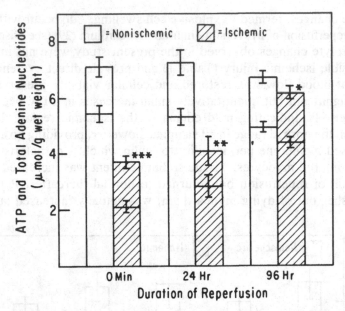

Figure 3.   The effects of 15 min of ischemia with 0, 24, or 96 hr of reperfusion on the total adenine nucleotide content are shown. The total adenine nucleotide pool was still markedly reduced after 24 hr of reperfusion. By 96 hr, adenine nucleotide content had returned nearly to normal but was still significantly reduced compared to nonischemic samples from the same hearts. The proportion of total adenine nucleotides in the form of ATP (from Figure 2) is indicated on each bar. Brackets indicate 1 standard error of the mean. Nonischemic and ischemic samples from each dog were compared by paired t analysis. *$P < 0.05$, **$P < 0.01$, ***$P < 0.001$. Reproduced from ref. 23 with the permission of the publisher from the *Journal of Molecular and Cellular Cardiology*.

60 min, most likely because of resumption of active sodium extrusion which occurs, at least in part, via the ouabain-sensitive $Na^+ - K^+$ ATPase of the sarcolemma. Thus, rapid restoration of cell volume and electrolyte regulation could have caused a transient overshoot of potassium content.

Tissue calcium content remained below 1.0 mmol/100 g dry weight in all groups in the present study. Magnesium content was significantly decreased in the ischemic region following 1 or 24 hr of reperfusion but had returned to normal at 96 hr.

DISCUSSION

The results show that 15 min of severe myocardial ischemia is associated with prolonged depletion of ATP, even though this brief period of ischemia is reversible in the sense that cell death is prevented by reperfusion.

The method of sampling employed in the present study deserves further comment. Because of the 1 to 3 min required to cool the heart before sampling, creatine phosphate stores always were partially degraded. Thus, measurements of this metabolite were artifactually low and are not included in this report. We accepted the loss of CP data, which were not critical for the aims of the present study, because our sampling techniques permitted us to study pure samples of severely ischemic myocardium using the fluorescent dye, thioflavin S, to identify and exclude areas with significant collateral blood flow. This method of sampling provided measurements of ATP and total adenine nucleotides in nonischemic samples that were equivalent to those measured by quick freezing techniques (3,4). Also, purine nucleosides and bases were measured by HPLC techniques in some of the samples in order to detect adenine nucleotide catabolism during sampling. If degradation of the adenine nucleotide pool had occurred during sampling, inosine, hypoxanthine, and xanthine would have been detected in the samples (R. B. Jennings and M. L. Hill, unpublished data). However, these products were not detected either in samples of nonischemic or ishemic–reperfused myocardium. Presumably, ATP was preserved during the initial cooling period by the rephosphorylation of the ADP produced by continued metabolism, at the expense of CP (the creatine kinase reaction). Because creatine is not lost from myocardium after sublethal periods of ischemia (24) and because CP is resynthesized when ischemic but viable myocardium is reoxygenated (9,12,27), the creatine kinase reaction also should have preserved existing ATP levels in ischemic–reperfused myocardium.

The validity of the conclusion that adenine nucleotide repletion is slow following reperfusion of reversibly injured myocardium also is dependent on the assumptions that blood flow was actually restored and that the injury was, in fact reversible. Previous studies have shown areas of vascular damage and "no reflow" after 90 min but not after 40 min of temporary ischemia (16). Thus, existence of areas of inadequate reperfusion at 15 min seems unlikely. If persistent ischemia had occurred in the present study, further depletion of ATP and total adenine nucleotides (12) and cell death would have been expected. However, in all instances, reperfusion arrested the progressive depletion of adenine nucleotides and allowed some resynthesis of AMP and ADP to ATP.

Evidence that the injury was reversible in terms of cellular viability is twofold. (1) Previous studies have established that 15 min of temporary ischemia is seldom associated with necrosis in this model. No necrosis was present in those dogs studied at 24 or 96 hr. On the other hand, 20 to 60 min of reperfusion is too short for necrosis to be detectable by gross or histological techniques. (2) Nevertheless, characteristic electrolyte changes do occur rapidly during reperfusion of irreversibly injured myocardium (27). For example, 40 min of ischemia followed by only 10 min of reperfusion was associated with explosive cell swelling characterized by loss of K^+, influx of Na^+ and water (29), and massive Ca^{2+} overload (25). Total tissue Ca^{2+} increases from about 0.5 to as much as 5.0 mmol/100 g dry tissue (25). Moreover, membrane damage is detectable in incubated slices of such tissue by an increased inulin-diffusible space (12). These parameters were assessed in the present study to detect irreversibly injured myocytes, if present. Tissue Na^+ was not increased, nor was K^+ decreased. In fact, K^+ was increased early, most likely because of overshoot as cell volume regulation and active Na^+ extrusion resumed. Massive Ca^{2+} loading was not detected in any dog; Mg^{2+} was decreased following reperfusion, but this loss is not indicative of cell death. Much of the myocardial Mg^{2+} is normally complexed with the ATP and ADP of the cell, and the decrease in Mg^{2+} content is most likely a manifestation of the low adenine nucleotide content of ischemic–reperfused tissue (12).

Other studies also have shown rapid adenine nucleotide depletion and failure of repletion following 5 to 15 min of global myocardial ischemia induced by cardiac arrest in dogs (21) or following as little as 5 min of myocardial hypoxia induced by asphysia in rabbits (9). In addition, Vial et al. (27) have recently shown a 30% reduction in ATP and ΣAd following 15 min of ischemia induced by occlusion of the anterior descending artery in open-chest dogs. Resynthesis of either ATP or ΣAd was negligible during a 1-hr period of reperfusion. The present study showed a more rapid depletion of ATP and ΣAd during ischemia, a difference that can best be explained by our use of thioflavin S to identify and sample only severely ischemic myocardium. In addition, the present study confirmed the slow recovery of adenine nucleotide content and demonstrated that even 24 hr later, little net resynthesis of adenine nucleotides had occurred.

Adenine nulceotide synthesis can occur either through de novo pathways or through "salvage" pathways. De novo synthesis is a costly process in terms of myocardial energetics because it takes six high-energy phosphate bonds to manufacture one molecule of inosine monophosphate (IMP) from the initial precursor, ribose-5-phosphate (19). This pathway is slow in myocardium, occurring at a rate of only 0.016 μmol/g per hr in rat hearts in vivo even when stimulated by a brief period of ischemia (33). The rate-limiting factor is the availability of 5-phosphoribosyl-1-pyrophosphate which is limited by the rate of production of ribose-5-phosphate in the hexose monophosphate shunt (32). If the rate of adenine nucleotide synthesis observed in rats (33) is similar in dogs, and if this pathway were the only means of net adenine nucleotide resynthesis, it would have required at least (7.08 − 3.71)/0.016 = 211 hr or 9 days to restore normal ΣAd content.

However, myocardium also is capable of manufacturing adenine nucleotides from purine nucleosides and bases via various salvage pathways (2,26). Adenosine is converted directly to AMP by adenosine kinase, and inosine is largely converted to hypoxanthine which then is converted to IMP by hypoxanthine phosphoribosyl transferase (30). Flux through these pathways is 10–20 times faster than de novo synthesis in isolated rat hearts supplied with adenosine, inosine, or hypoxanthine (20). Nevertheless, these rates also are slow relative to the magnitude of adenine nucleotide loss we observed in the present study. In isolated rat hearts, 5 hr of perfusion with adenosine was required to replete the adenine nucleotides lost during 30 min of ischemia (22).

Several studies have shown that functional recovery following brief periods of ischemia is slow (6–8,28,31). This delayed functional recovery has been associated with decreased Ca^{2+} uptake by the sarcoplasmic reticulum and decreased myofibrillar ATPase activity (6), loss of glycogen and phosphorylase activity and depressed mitochondrial function (31), and persistence of mildly reduced blood flow to the previously ischemic region (7). However, the mechanism(s) for this prolonged functional recovery period has not been established. The delayed resynthesis of adenine nucleotides and the prolonged depletion of ATP demonstrated in the present study comprise another potential mechanism of the delayed functional recovery.

These experimental studies have direct clinical relevance in that cardiac surgical procedures frequently require periods of myocardial ischemia. The delayed cardiac functional recovery observed in some patients postoperatively may reflect a delayed resynthesis of ATP. If ΣAd depletion is the cause of prolonged mechanical depression following ischemia, both abnormalities might theoretically be ameliorated by infusion of ribose (32) and/or purine nucleosides or bases to enhance de novo and/or salvage (22) resynthesis of adenine nucleotides.

The results of the present study have an additional practical implication which is that sequential brief coronary occlusions probably will result in a cumulative depression in the adenine nucleotide content of the heart. Thus, experimental studies utilizing two or more occlusions to compare various interventions on parameters of ischemic injury need to be interpreted with caution. It seems likely that repeat occlusions will not be comparable metabolically because the high-energy phosphate pool will be lower at the onset of the second occlusion then it was initially. In addition, the limited benefit from intermittent reperfusion during myocardial ischemia (5,18) also may be explained by a cumulative reduction in ATP and ΣAd because of the slow resynthesis of this pool.

ACKNOWLEDGMENTS

The authors express appreciation to Ms. Nancy J. Kramer for the assistance in the conduct of these animal experiments and to Ms. Diane Magnuson for the electrolyte measurements. This research was supported in part by NIH Grant HL-23138.

REFERENCES

1. Anderson, F. S., and Murphy, R. C. 1976. Isocratic separation of some purine nucleotide, nucleoside, and base metabolites from biological extracts by high-performance liquid chromatography. *J. Chromatog.* 121:251–262.
2. Bartlett, G. R. 1977. Biology of free and combined adenine; distribution and metabolism. *Transfusion* 17:339–350.

3. Braasch, W., Gudbjarnason, S., Puri, P. S., Ravens, K. G., and Bing, R. J. 1977. Early changes in energy metabolism in the myocardium following acute coronary artery occlusion in anesthetized dogs. *Circ. Res.* 23:429–438.

4. Dunn, R. B., and Griggs, D. M., Jr. 1975. Transmural gradients in ventricular tissue metabolites produced by stopping coronary blood flow in the dog. *Circ. Res.* 37:438–445.

5. Follette, D. M., Mulder, D. G., Maloney, J. V., Jr., and Buckberg, G. D. 1978. Advantages of blood cardioplegia over continuous coronary perfusion or intermittent ischemia. *J. Thorac. Cardiovasc. Surg.* 76:604–617.

6. Hess, M. L., Barnhart, G. R., Crute, S., Komwatana, P., Krause, S., and Greenfield, L. J. 1979. Mechanical and biochemical effects of transient myocardial ischemia. *J. Surg. Res.* 26:175–184.

7. Heyndrickx, G. R., Baig, H., Nellens, P., Leusen, I., Fishbein, M. C., and Vatner, S. F. 1978. Depression of regional blood flow and wall thickening after brief coronary occlusions. *Am. J. Physiol.* 234(6):H653–H659.

8. Heyndrickx, G. R., Millard, R. W., McRitchie, R. J., Maroko, P. R., and Vatner, S. F. 1975. Regional myocardial functional and electrophysiological alterations after brief coronary artery occlusion in conscious dogs. *J. Clin. Invest.* 56:978–985.

9. Isselhard, W. 1968. Metabolism and function of the heart during acute asphyxia and in postasphyxial recovery. *Acta Anaesthesiol. Scand.* [*Suppl.*] 29:203–216.

10. Jawouk, D., Gruber, W., and Bergmeyer, H. U. 1974. Adenosine-5'-diphosphate and adenosine-5'-monophosphate. In: H. U. Bergmeyer (ed.), *Methods of Enzymatic Analysis,* pp. 2127–2131. Academic Press, New York.

11. Jennings, R. B., Crout, J. R., and Smetters, G. W. 1957. Studies on distribution and localization of potassium in early myocardial ischemic injury. *Arch. Pathol.* 63:586–592.

12. Jennings, R. B., Hawkins, H. K., Lowe, J. E., Hill, M. L., Klotman, S., and Reimer, K. A. 1978. Relation between high energy phosphate and lethal injury in myocardial ischemia in the dog. *Am. J. Pathol.* 92:187–214.

13. Jennings, R. B., Sommers, H. M., Kaltenbach, J. P., and West, J. J. 1964. Electrolyte alterations in acute myocardial ischemic injury. *Circ. Res.* 14:260–269.

14. Jennings, R. B., Sommers, H. M., Smyth, G. A., Flack, H. A., and Linn, H. 1960. Myocardial necrosis induced by temporary occlusion of a coronary artery in the dog. *Arch. Pathol.* 70:68–78.

15. Jones, R. N., Hill, M. L., Reimer, K. A., Wechsler, A. S., and Jennings, R. B. 1980. Effect of hypothermia on the rate of myocardial ATP and adenine nucleotide degradation in total ischemia. *Fed. Proc.* 39:1111.

16. Kloner, R. A., Ganote, C. E., and Jennings, R. B. 1974. The "no-reflow" phenomenon after temporary coronary occlusion in the dog. *J. Clin. Invest.* 54:1496–1508.

17. Lamprecht, W., and Trautschold, I. 1974. Determination of ATP with hexokinase and glucose-6-phosphate dehydrogenase. In: H. U. Bergmeyer (ed.), *Methods of Enzymatic Analysis,* pp. 2101–2110. Academic Press, New York.

18. Levitzky, S., Wright, R. N., Rao, K. S., Holland, C., Roper, K., Engelman, R., and Feinberg, H. 1977. Does intermittent coronary perfusion offer greater myocardial protection than continuous aortic cross-clamping? *Surgery* 82:51–58.

19. Murray, A. W. 1971. The biological significance of purine salvage. *Annu. Rev. Biochem.* 40:773–826.

20. Namm, D. H. 1973. Myocardial nucleotide synthesis from purine bases and nucleosides. Comparison of the rates of formation of purine nucleotides from various precursors and identification of the enzymatic routes for nucleotide formation in the isolated rat heart. *Circ. Res.* 33:686–695.

21. Parker, J. C., Smith, E. E., and Jones, C. E. 1976. The role of nucleoside and nucleobase metabolism in myocardial adenine nucleotide regeneration after cardiac arrest. *Circ. Shock* 3:11–20.

22. Reibel, D. K., and Rovetto, M. J. 1979. Myocardial adenosine salvage rates and restoration of ATP content following ischemia. *Am. J. Physiol.* 237:H247–H252.

23. Reimer, K. A., Hill, M. L., and Jennings, R. B. 1981. Prolonged depletion of ATP and of the adenine nucleotide pool due to delayed resynthesis of adenine nucleotides following reversible myocardial ischemic injury in dogs. *J. Mol. Cell. Cardiol.* 13:229–239.
24. Reimer, K. A., Jennings, R. B., and Hill, M. L. 1981. Total ischemia in dog hearts in vitro. 2. High energy phosphate depletion and associated defects in energy metabolism, cell volume regulation, and sarcolemmal integrity. *Circ. Res.* 49:901–911.
25. Shen, A. C., and Jennings, R. B. 1972. Myocardial calcium and magnesium in acute ischemic injury. *Am. J. Pathol.* 67:417–440.
26. Tsuboi, K. K., and Buckley, N. M. 1965. Metabolism of perfused C^{14}-labeled nucleosides and bases by the isolated heart. *Circ. Res.* 16:343–352.
27. Vial, C., Font, B., Goldschmidt, D., Pearlman, A. S., and Delaye, J. 1978. Regional myocardial energetics during brief periods of coronary occlusion and reperfusion: Comparison with ST-segment changes. *Cardiovasc. Res.* 12:470–476.
28. Weiner, J. M., Apstein, C. S., Arthur, J. H., Pirzada, F. A., and Hood, W. B. 1976. Persistence of myocardial injury following brief periods of coronary occlusion. *Cardiovasc. Res.* 10:678–686.
29. Whalen, D. A., Jr., Hamilton, D. G., Ganote, C. E., and Jennings, R. B. 1974. Effect of a transient period of ischemia on myocardial cells. I. Effects on cell volume regulation. *Am. J. Pathol.* 74:381–398.
30. Wiedmeier, V. T., Rubio, R., and Berne, R. M. 1972. Inosine incorporation into myocardial nucleotides. *J. Mol. Cell. Cardiol.* 4:445–452.
31. Wood, J. M., Hanley, H. G., Entman, M. L., Hartley, C. J., Swain, J. A., Busch, U., Chang, C., Lewis, R. M., Morgan, W. J., and Schwartz, A. 1979. Biochemical and morphological correlates of acute experimental myocardial ischemia in the dog. IV. Energy mechanisms during very early ischemia. *Circ. Res.* 44:52–61.
32. Zimmer, H., and Gerlach, E. 1978. Stimulation of myocardial adenine nucleotide biosynthesis by pentoses and pentitols. *Pfluegers Arch.* 376:223–227.
33. Zimmer, H., Trendelenburg, C., Kammermeier, H., and Gerlach, E. 1973. De novo synthesis of myocardial adenine nucleotides in the rat. *Circ. Res.* 32:635–642.

Cytochrome Oxidase Activity of Mitochondria from Ischemic and Reperfused Myocardium

A. Toleikis

Laboratory of Metabolism
Institute for Cardiovascular Research
Kaunas, Lithuanian SSR, USSR

Abstract. Polarographic measurements show that activity of cytochrome oxidase (CO), assayed as ascorbate plus TMPD oxidase, is decreased in the mitochondria (M) from postischemic areas of rabbit heart 1, 6, and 9 days after temporary (1-hr) coronary artery occlusion (CAO). This effect is observable only in the absence of added cytochrome c. Cytochrome oxidase activity in the cytochrome c-containing medium was not different from the control level. Levels of cytochromes $c + c_1$ and a were substantially lower in tissue from postischemic areas and elevated in the intact tissue 1 and 6 days after temporary CAO as compared with control hearts. Stoichiometry of the cytochromes was not changed. After 1 or 4 hr of permanent CAO, CO activity (plus cytochrome c) of ischemic M was equal to that of M from intact area; CO activity (with or without cytochrome c) was reduced after 0.5 and 1 hr but elevated after 3 or 4 hr of in vitro ischemia as compared with control. The changes of CO activity in infarcted human heart M were similar to those in rabbits after temporary CAO; CO activity was restored after addition of cytocrome c. The data suggest that leakage of cytochrome c occurs during isolation of M and is more pronounced in ischemia-damaged M.

Cytochrome c oxidase (CO) (E.C. 1.9.3.1)—the terminal member of the electron-transport chain and an integral part of the mitochondrial inner membrane—is responsible for catalyzing the reduction of dioxygen to water. Under coupled conditions, the free energy released in this reaction may be converted to membrane potential (24) which subsequently may be used by the ATP synthetase complex to make ATP. Especially high levels of CO have been observed in heart muscle (4) where the energy requirements are very high. It is estimated that 90% of the energy for heart muscle contraction is provided through aerobic metabolism via CO (4), through which 90% of biological oxygen consumption is directed (see ref. 3 for review).

Despite its importance in the energetics of the myocardial cell, little attention has been paid to studies of the influence of permanent and transient ischemia on this oxidase in isolated cardiac mitochondria. It was established that neither ligation of coronary arteries (7) nor perfusion of isolated heart under ischemic conditions (14) for 20 min produced an alteration of CO activity measured both in isolated mitochondria (7,14) and homogenates (14). Severe ischemia produced by 60 min of left circumflex artery occlusion resulted in a small decrease of CO activity in isolated mitochondria (22).

But in the work of Constatinescu et al. (6), a significant decrease of enzyme activity was observed within 10 min after coronary occlusion; this progressed with time and reached a 70% reduction after 40 min. It was also found that restoration of circulation in the ischemic area did not improve CO activity. Anoxic perfusion for 5 hr (2) or permanent coronary artery occlusion for 1–180 days (9) caused significant decreases in CO activity in heart tissue.

Most of the above mentioned investigations were performed using spectrophotometric methods. As striking differences have been found under some experimental conditions between spectrophotometric and polarographic measurements of CO activity (25), it was of interest to investigate the effect of ischemia on CO activity by the polarographic method.

In the present work, mitochondrial CO activity was investigated using different models of ischemia as well as in myocardial infarction. An attempt was also made to elucidate some factors responsible for the observed decrease of enzyme activity.

MATERIALS AND METHODS

Animal experiments were performed on rabbits weighing 2.5 to 3.5 kg. Temporary (60 min) as well as permanent coronary artery occlusion and autolysis were used as ischemia models in this work. Occlusion of the left anterior descending branch of the coronary artery was achieved by a method described previously (29).

The effect of ischemia in situ (autolysis) was examined in samples of myocardium removed 0.5, 1, 1.5, 2, 3, and 4 hr after killing of the rabbits. The bodies after killing were left at room temperature.

Another series of experiments was performed on hearts of humans who died from myocardial infarction.

Isolation of Mitochondria

The mitochondrial isolation procedure was similar to that already described (29). Homogenization was performed in a Teflon®–glass homogenizer with 10 volumes of 0.3 M sucrose and 10 mM EDTA, pH 7.5.

Assay Methods

Cytochrome c oxidase (ascorbate plus TMPD oxidase) activity of isolated mitochondria was measured polarographically under the conditions described in the text or legends to the figures and tables.

Difference spectrum analysis of the cytochromes in myocardial homogenates was carried out according to the methods of Mokhova and coworkers (8,20) in a medium containing 0.3 M sucrose and 5 mM KH_2PO_4, pH 7.5 Amobarbital (4.8 mM) and 2,4-dinitrophenol (240 μM) were added to one of the cuvettes to oxidize cytochromes, and succinate (5 mM), 2,4-dinitrophenol (40 μM) and potassium cyanide (3 mM) to another to reduce them. Both cuvettes contained 20 mg of rabbit heart tissue (wet weight). Measurements were standardized with a known concentration of cytochrome c.

Mitochondrial protein concentration was determined by the biuret method (12) in the presence of 0.25% deoxycholate, with human serum albumin as a standard. In the autolysis experiments, the extraction of mitochondrial lipids with diethylether was performed (after development of color).

The Student's t-test was used to determine statistical significance of the results. Differences were considered significant, if $P < 0.05$.

RESULTS AND DISCUSSION

In the first series of polarographic measurements of cytochrome oxidase (ascorbate plus TMPD oxidase) activity, which were performed in isotonic medium without added cytochrome c, the following control values were obtained (mean ± S.E.M.): 96 ± 6, 180 ± 10, 378 ± 25 natoms O/min per mg mitochondrial protein with 25, 50, and 100 μM of TMPD, respectively. As can be seen from Figure 1, CO activity clearly decreases in mitochondria from the postischemic area of rabbit heart 1, 6, and 9 days after temporary (1-hr) coronary artery occlusion (TCAO) in comparison with control. All differences were statistically significant as compared with control mitochondria. Changes observed in mitochondria from nonischemic areas (data not shown), although similar in character, were less pronounced, although they were statistically significant 1 and 6 days postoperatively.

One can assume that the changes observed may be caused by decrease of activity and/or level of CO as well as more pronounced leakage of cytochrome c from ischemia-damaged mitochondria in comparison with control ones.

It is well established that the ultrastructure of cardiac mitochondria is rapidly altered during ischemia (11,15,16,18), with marked changes in the

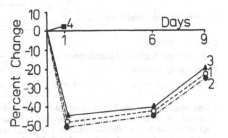

Figure 1. Effect of temporary coronary artery occlusion on cytochrome oxidase activity of mitochondria isolated from postischemic area of the rabbit heart. Incubation medium contained 0.3 M sucrose, 5 mM KCl, 5 mM KH₂PO₄, pH 7.5 (curves 1, 2, 3) or 5 mM KCl, 5 mM KH₂PO₄, pH 7.5 (curve 4). Additions: ascorbate, 8 mM (1–3) or 5 mM (4); TMPD, 25 μM (1), 50 μM (2), 100 μM (3), 1 mM (4); antimycin A, 0.2–1.8 μM; 2,4-DNP, 100 μM (1–3); ClCCP, 0.4 μM (4); cytochrome c, 20 μM (4); temperature, 23–25°C. Changes in experiments 1–3 were statistically significant at all periods of TCAO.

intactness of the outer membrane (11,18)—a barrier for cytochrome c (34)–and an increase in their fragility (15). On the other hand, significant damage to the intactness of the outer membrane of mitochondria, especially cardiac mitochondria, occur during the isolation procedure (33,35). Therefore, it seems reasonable to assume that mitochondria isolated from a postischemic area should be deficient in cytochrome c (in comparison with control mitochondria) which is loosely bound to the outer surface of inner mitochondrial membrane (21). Loss of cytochrome c was observed in cardiac mitochondria isolated from the damaged area of the heart after 7 days of permanent ischemia (23) as well as in liver mitochondria after 3 hr of ischemia (19). In both of these studies, loss of cytochrome a (aa_3) was also observed.

The following series of experiments was designed to evaluate the possibility of reconstitution of CO activity with added cytochrome c. In these experiments, CO activity was measured in isotonic and hypotonic medium simultaneously. Pretreatment of mitochondria in hypotonic conditions was considered necessary for better penetration of exogenous cytochrome c to its binding sites. Hypoosmotic shock for 2–3 min (in a polarographic cuvet) led to significantly greater activation of CO by added cytochrome c in comparison with measurements in isotonic medium. In the absence of cytochrome c, CO activities were not significantly different, but they were in most cases slightly lower in hypotonic medium. The following control activities were obtained in this series in isotonic medium (mean values of seven experiments): 101, 131, 293, and 585 natoms O/min per mg protein with 25, 50, 200, and 600 μM TMPD, respectively. Corresponding values in hypotonic medium were 95, 121, 255, and 495 natoms O/min per mg protein.

As shown in Table 1, CO activity of mitochondria from a postischemic area of the heart 1 day after TCAO is significantly decreased compared with controls in the isotonic medium without and with added cytochrome c; this confirms the abovementioned findings (see Figure 1, curves 1, 2, 3). It is

Table 1. Effect of Temporary Coronary Artery Occlusion[a] on Cytochrome Oxidase Activity of Mitochondria Isolated from a Postischemic Area of the Rabbit Heart

Experimental conditions[b]	TMPD μM			
	25	50	200	600
Isotonic medium	− 19*	− 23*	− 32**	− 40**
Isotonic medium + cytochrome c	− 22	− 24*	− 37**	− 45***
Hypotonic medium	− 23	− 17	− 15	− 29*
Hypotonic medium + cytochrome c	+ 5	+ 1	− 2	− 24

[a] One hour of ischemia followed by 24 hr of reperfusion.
[b] Isotonic medium: 0.3 M sucrose, 5 mM KCl, 5 mM KH$_2$PO$_4$, pH 7.5. Hypotonic medium: 5 mM KCl, 5 mM KH$_2$PO$_4$, pH 7.5. Additions: ascorbate, 8 mM; TMPD, concentrations as indicated in the table; cytochrome c, 20 μM; antimycin A, 1.8 μM; 2,4-DNP, 100 μM. Temperature, 23–25°C. Differences were statistically significant with respect to control at *$P < 0.05$; **$P < 0.01$; ***$P < 0.001$. Percentage changes are given with respect to control.

interesting to note that the effect of TCAO was more pronounced at higher TMPD concentrations, which is difficult to explain. This observation stresses the methodological problems in the investigation of oxidase activity changes during ischemia. However, in hypotonic medium plus cytochrome c, CO activity of postischemic mitochondria was not statistically different from control. This observation was also confirmed in a separate series of experiments with different experimental conditions and higher TMPD concentration (1 mm) (see Figure 1, curve 4). Control activity of CO (hypotonic medium plus cytochrome c) in this series ($N = 5$) was equal to 1418 ± 96 natoms O/min per mg protein, and that of mitochondria from nonischemic and postischemic area 1 day after TCAO ($N = 6$) 1461 ± 130 and 1449 ± 158, respectively (means ± S.E.M.).

In summary, all of those experiments show clearly that reduced CO activity of mitochondria isolated from a postischemic area 1 day after TCAO is completely restored in hypotonic but not in isotonic medium after simple addition of cytochrome c. Accordingly, this suggests that the apparent decrease of CO activity may simply reflect loss of endogenous cytochrome c. It seems likely, too, that the binding to as well as reactivity with CO of added cytochrome c do not change during TCAO.

Whether or not this reduction of cytochrome c results from degenerative changes within the damaged cardiac muscle cell or loss during isolation of the mitochondria remains unclear.

The following experiments were designed as an attempt to elucidate this problem. With this purpose, difference spectrum analysis of the cytochromes in myocardial homogenates was performed.

As can be seen from Table 2, the level of cytochromes a and $c + c_1$ 1 and 6 days after TCAO was signficantly lower in tissue from a postischemic area and higher in an intact one compared with hearts of control or sham-operated rabbits (latter data not shown). The stoichiometry of the cytochromes in the postischemic tissue was not changed, which indicates the

Table 2.   Effect of Temporary Coronary Artery Occlusion on the Content of Cytochromes in Myocardial Tissue[a]

	N	Area	Cytochromes $c + c_1$	Cytochrome a	$(c + c_1)/a$
Control	7	Nonischemic	39.2 ± 1.9	30.6 ± 1.7	1.28
	7	Postischemic	42.5 ± 3.2	33.1 ± 3.1	1.29
Days after TCAO					
1	7	Nonischemic	49.6 ± 1.9***	35.7 ± 1.0*	1.39
	7	Postischemic	34.8 ± 1.3*	25.5 ± 0.7*	1.37
6	9	Nonischemic	45.7 ± 1.3**	35.7 ± 0.9*	1.28
	9	Postischemic	31.5 ± 1.3**	23.9 ± 1.5*	1.32

[a] Experimental conditions as described in Materials and Methods. Values are given in nmol/g fresh tissue as mean ± S.E.M. Differences were statistically significant with respect to corresponding area of control heart at *$P < 0.05$; **$P < 0.01$; ***$P < 0.001$.

consistency of composition of this part of the mitochondrial respiratory chain. On the basis of data obtained, the decrease of mitochondrial CO activity observed after TCAO was interpreted to be a result of more pronounced cytochrome c leakage from ischemia-damaged mitochondria during the isolation procedure. If the leakage of cytochromes from mitochondria occurred in the ischemic myocardial cell, it would be reasonable to assume that loosely bound cytochrome c had to leak out first of all. Subsequently, it would pass the ischemia-damaged cell membrane, as occurs with cytoplasmic and mitochondrial creatine phosphokinase, malate dehydrogenase, lactate dehydrogenase, and aspartate aminotransferase during anoxia (ischemia) and postanoxic (postischemic) reperfusion (10,13,27,32); these are enzymes with molecular weights 3–11 times higher than that of cytochrome c. As a consequence, the ratio of cytochromes $c + c_1$ to cytochrome a should be decreased, but this was not the case in our experiments. Undoubtedly, more detailed investigations of this problem must be performed.

In the following groups of experiments, the effects of permanent coronary artery occlusion (PCAO) and autolysis were investigated.

As shown in Figure 2, curves 1, 2, the changes in CO activity of mitochondria isolated from an ischemic area of heart 1 and 4 hr after PCAO were negligible and statistically insignificant in comparison with a nonischemic zone despite the presence or absence of cytochrome c in the medium (hypotonic in these experiments). When mitochondria were isolated in the presence of rotenone (100 µg/g of heart), and CO activity was measured in hypotonic medium plus cytochrome c, an average ($N = 5$) 23.8% decrease of activity in mitochondria from the ischemic area was observed relative to the nonischemic one 1 hr after PCAO (Figure 2, curve 3). Control activity in this series was equal to 3429 ± 528 natoms O/min per mg protein. Whether the effect of ischemia in this case results from an increase of long-chain fatty acyl-CoA, which occurs in rotenone-isolated ischemic mitochondria (14), remains to be determined.

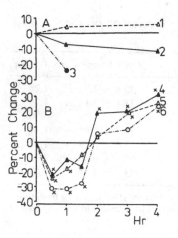

Figure 2.   Effect of permanent coronary artery occlusion (A) and autolysis (B) on cytochrome oxidase activity of isolated rabbit heart mitochondria. Incubation medium contained 10 mM KCl, 5 mM KH$_2$PO$_4$, 1 mM EDTA, pH 7.2 (1,2); 0.1 M KCl, 5 mM KH$_2$PO$_4$, 1 mM EDTA, pH 7.5 (3); 5 mM KCl, 5 mM KH$_2$PO$_4$, pH 7.5 (4,5); 0.25 M sucrose, 10 mM KCl, 5 mM KH$_2$PO$_4$, 1 mM EDTA, pH 7.2 (6). Additions: ascorbate, 5 mM (1–6), TMPD, 0.5 mM (1,2), 1.2 mM (3), 0.2 mM (4–6); antimycin A, 0.2 µM (1,2,4–6), 0.43 µM (3); ClCCP, 0.8 µM (1,2), 0.4 µM (4–6); polysorbate 80, 0.12% (3); cytochrome c, 20 µM (1,3,5). Temperature, 25°C (1,2,4–6), 37°C (3); in experiment 3, mitochondria were isolated with rotenone (100 µg/g fresh tissue). *Statistically significant changes, $P < 0.05$, with respect to control group (B, 4–6) or nonischemic area (A, 1–3).

Comparison of the effects of permanent and temporary coronary occlusion on the activity of CO allows us to suggest that postischemic reperfusion extends the alteration in mitochondrial ultrastructure and loss of cytochrome c but not the loss of CO activity.

It is known that ligation of coronary arteries or ischemic perfusion produces partial as well as heterogeneous hypoxia of myocardium. Therefore, a series of experiments was performed on the model of total ischemia—autolysis of the heart.

As Figure 2 shows (see curves 4–6), a statistically significant fall of CO activity was already seen 0.5 hr later. After 1–1.5 hr of autolysis, CO activity started to increase progressively with time, and after 3–4 hr, it exceeded control values by some 20–31%. Despite the differences in tonicity of incubation medium and the presence or absence of exogenous cytochrome c, similar changes were seen. The activation of CO by added cytochrome c was expressed equally in both control (2.3 times) and autolysis (from 2.03 to 2.52 times).

These findings permit one to conclude that decrease of mitochondrial CO activity in the case of total ischemia can not be explained by the loss of cytochrome c. However, we have no explanation for the observed change of inhibition to activation of the enzyme. It is known that removal of phospholipids from a CO preparation decreases its activity (for review, see 1,3,17). On the other hand, degradation of phospholipids was observed during ischemia in the heart (5,28) and liver (19) as well as in heart mitochondria (31). An increased content of lysophospholipids in the myocardium was observed in our laboratory after 30 min of autolysis (30). Content of lysophospholipids increased, and that of cardiolipin decreased in rabbit heart mitochondria in early periods of autolysis (unpublished data). It is not clear, however, whether these changes may cause the observed decrease of CO activity during autolysis.

Cytochrome oxidase activity of human heart mitochondria (see Table 3) isolated from an infarcted area 1.5–6.5 hr after death from myocardial infarction of various durations was significantly lower (from 65 to 93%) than that from a noninfarcted area when measured in the absence of added cytochrome c (all measurements were performed in isotonic medium). Addition of cytochrome c clearly but not completely reduced this difference. This fact suggests that the main cause of decline of CO activity is a reduction of mitochondrial cytochrome c content, as was the case in TCAO. It is of interest that in the case of rabbit TCAO, a similar effect on cytochrome c was achieved in the hypotonic medium only. Most probably, the reason for this discrepancy is more pronounced alteration of the intactness, and consequently increased permeability to cytochrome c, of the outer membrane of infarcted human heart mitochondria as compared with that of the rabbit.

As this work developed, the choice of more optimal experimental conditions for CO activity measurement caused their variability, which to some extent complicated the comparison of different models of ischemia. Despite

Table 3. Effect of Myocardial Infarction on Cytochrome Oxidase
Activity (natoms O/min per mg) of Human Heart Mitochondria[a]

Time after death (hr)	Area	Without cytochrome c	With added cytochrome c	Effect of cytochrome c (%)
1.5	Control	420	560	+33
	Infarcted	30 (−93%)[b]	403 (−28%)	+1243
3	Control	280	320	+14
	Infarcted	50 (−82%)	260 (−19%)	+420
6.5	Control	345	490	+42
	Infarcted	121 (−65%)	397 (−19%)	+228

[a] Incubation medium contained 0.25 M sucrose, 10 mM KCl, 5 mM KH₂PO₄, 1 mM EDTA, pH 7.2. Additions: ascorbate, 5 mM; TMPD, 0.2 mM; ClCCP, 0.4 μM; antimycin A, 0.2 μM; cytochrome c, 20 μM; mitochondria, 0.15–0.20 mg/ml. Temperature, −25°C.
[b] Percentage change is with respect to control (noninfarcted) area.

this fact, some similarities as well as differences between them were discovered.

The problem of comparability of CO activity measurements in different laboratories was stressed by Lemberg (17). The same conclusion can be made from the studies of Smith et al. (25,26). One must admit, therefore, that closer standardization of investigations in this field is needed.

REFERENCES

1. Capaldi, R. A., and Briggs, M. 1976. The structure of cytochrome oxidase. In: A. Martonosi (ed.), *The Enzymes of Biological Membranes*, Volume 4, pp. 87–102. Plenum Press, New York.
2. Carroll, B. J., and Welman, E. 1979. Loss of respiratory enzyme activity in anoxic myocardium. Effect of propranolol. *J. Mol. Cell. Cardiol.* 11:1209–1214.
3. Caughey, W. S., Wallace, W. J., Volpe, J. A., and Yoshikawa, S. 1976. Cytochrome c oxidase. In: P. Boyer (ed.), *The Enzymes*, Volume 13, Part C, 3rd ed. pp. 299–344. Academic Press, New York.
4. Challoner, D. R. 1968. Respiration in myocardium, *Nature* 217:78–79.
5. Chien, K. R., Pfau, R. G., and Farber, J. L. 1979. Ischemic myocardial cell injury. *Am. J. Pathol.* 97:505–530.
6. Constatinescu, S., Filipescu, G., Laky, D., Constantinesku, N. M., Ratea, E., and Halalau, F. 1978. Biochemical and ultrastructural alterations of the mitochondrial fraction in experimental acute ischemia. *Rev. Roum. Biochim.* 15:189–195.
7. Ekholm, R., Kerstell, J., Olson, R., Rudenstam, C.-M., and Svanborg, A. 1968. Morphologic and biochemical studies of dog heart mitochondria after short periods of ischemia. *Am. J. Cardiol.* 22:312–318.
8. Evtodienko, J. V., and Mokhova, E. N. 1967. [Quantitative measurements of cytochromes in mitochondria.] In: V. A. Yakovleva (ed.), [*Mechanisms of Respiration, Photosynthesis and Nitrogen Fixation*,] pp. 35–40. Nauka, Moscow.
9. Fetisova, T. V., Frolkis, R. A., Tsiomik, V. A., Smirnova, I. P., and Likhtenstein, I. E. 1976. [Activity of enzymes in heart and serum at the experimental myocardial infarction.] *Kardiologiia* 16:110–116.

10. Gebhard, M. M., Denkhaus, H., Sakai, K., and Spieckermann, P. G. 1977. Energy metabolism and enzyme release. *J. Mol. Med.* 2:271–283.
11. Glagoleva, V. V., and Chechulin, J. S. 1968. [*Ultrastructural Basis of Heart Muscle Function Alterations. Atlas.*] Nauka, Moscow.
12. Gornall, A. G., Bardavill, C. J., and David, M. M. 1949. Determination of serum proteins by means of the biuret reaction. *J. Biol. Chem.* 177:751–766.
13. Hearse, D. J., Humphrey, S. M., Feuvray, D., and deLeiris, J. 1976. A biochemical and ultrastructural study of the species variation in myocardial cell damage. *J. Mol. Cell. Cardiol.* 8:759–778.
14. Idell-Wenger, J. A., Grotyohann, L. W., and Neely, J. R. 1978. Coenzyme A and carnitine distribution in normal and ischemic hearts. *J. Biol. Chem.* 253:4310–4318.
15. Jennings, R. B., and Ganote, C. E. 1976. Mitochondrial structure and funtion in acute myocardial ischemic injury. *Circ. Res.* 38(Suppl. I):80–89.
16. Jennings, R. B., Herdson, P. B., and Sommers, H. M. 1969. Structural and functional abnormalities in mitochondria isolated from ischemic dog myocardium. *Lab. Invest.* 20:548–557.
17. Lemberg, M. R. 1969. Cytochrome oxidase. *Physiol. Rev.* 49:48–121.
18. Mitin, K. S. 1974. [*Electron-Microscopic Analysis of Heart at Myocardial Infarction.*] Medicine, Moscow.
19. Mittnacht, S., Sherman, S., Jr., and Farber, J. L. 1979. Reversal of ischemic mitochondrial dysfunction. *J. Biol. Chem.* 254:9871–9878.
20. Mokhova, E. N., and Zhigacheva, I. V. 1977. [Content of cytochromes in liver mitochondria and homogenate during adaptation to cold.] In: S. E. Severin (ed.), [*Mitochondria. Energy Accumulation and Regulation of Enzymatic Reactions*], pp. 138–143. Nauka, Moscow.
21. Nicholls, P. 1974. Cytochrome *c* binding to enzymes and membranes. *Biochem. Biophys. Acta* 346:261–310.
22. Rouslin, W., and Millard, R. W. 1980. Canine myocardial ischemia: Defect in mitochondrial electron transfer complex I. *J. Mol. Cell. Cardiol.* 12:639–645.
23. Schwartz, A., Wood, J. M., Allen, J. C., Bornet, E. P., Entman, M. L., Goldstein, M. A., Sordahl, L. A., and Suzuki, M. 1973. Biochemical and morphologic correlates of cardiac ischemia. *Am. J. Cardiol.* 32:46–61.
24. Skulachev, V. P. 1974. [Mechanism of oxidative phosphorylation and some principles of bioenergetics.] *Adv. Mod. Biol.* 77:125–154.
25. Smith, L., Davies, H. C., and Nava, M. E. 1979. Studies of the kinetics of oxidation of cytochrome *c* by cytochrome *c* oxidase: Comparison of spectrophotometric and polarographic assays. *Biochemistry* 18:3140–3146.
26. Smith, L., Davies, H. C., and Nava, M. E. 1980. Effect of adenosine 5'-triphosphate and adenosine 5'-diphosphate on the oxidation of cytochrome *c* by cytochrome *c* oxidase. *Biochemistry* 19:1613–1617.
27. Smith, A. F., Wong, P. C.-P., and Oliver, M. F. 1977. Release of mitochondrial enzymes in acute myocardial infarction. *J. Mol. Med.* 2:265–269.
28. Sobel, B. E., Corr, P. B., Robison, A. K., Goldstein, R. A., Witkowski, F. X., and Klein, M. S. 1978. Accumulation of lysophosphoglycerides with arrhythmogenic properties in ischemic myocardium. *J. Clin. Invest.* 62:546–553.
29. Toleikis, A., Džėja, P., Praškevičius, A., and Jasaitis, A. 1979. Mitochondrial functions in ischemic myocardium. I. Proton electrochemical gradient, inner membrane permeability, calcium transport and oxidative phosphorylation in isolated mitochondria. *J. Mol. Cell. Cardiol.* 11:57–76.
30. Toleikis, A., Trumpickas, A., Dagys, A., and Džėja, P., 1979. Studies on mitochondrial function and myocardial lipid changes in ischemic rabbit heart. In: *Abstracts, 8th International Colloquium on Bioenergetics and Mitochondria. Smolenice Castle, Czechoslovakia,* p. 78.
31. Vasdev, S. C., Kako, K. J., and Biro, G. P. 1979. Phospholipid composition of cardiac

mitochondria and lysosomes in experimental myocardial ischemia in the dog. *J. Mol. Cell. Cardiol.* 11:1195–1200.

32. Waldenström, A. P., Hjalmarson, A. C., Jodal, M., and Waldenström, J. 1977. Significance of enzyme release from ischemic isolated rat heart. *Acta Med. Scand.* 201:525–532.

33. Wojtczak, L. 1974. Permeability and other properties of the outer mitochondrial membrane. *Rev. Roum. Physiol.* 11:173–185.

34. Wojtczak, L., and Zaluska, H. 1969. On the impermeability of the outer mitochondrial membrane to cytochrome *c*. *Biochim. Biophys. Acta* 193:64–72.

35. Wojtczak, L., Zaluska, H., Wroniszewska, A., and Wojtczak, A. B. 1972. Assay for the intactiness of the outer membrane in isolated mitochondria. *Acta Biochim. Pol.* 19:227–234.

The Effect of Experimentally Induced Myocardial Ischemia on the Norepinephrine Metabolism of the Dog Heart

I. Préda, P. Kárpáti, M. Sebeszta, and Z. Antalóczy

Second Medical Clinic of Postgraduate Medical School
H-1389 Budapest, Hungary

Abstract. Myocardial ischemia is known to provoke an excess in circularing norepinephrine and thus be related to an increased irritability of the heart. In the present experiments, we studied the norepinephrine and potassium content, oxygen tension, and pH values of the effluent of coronary sinus after thoracotomy and catheter placement into the coronary sinus. Once a steady state was reaached, the measurements were repeated in the fifth, tenth, 20th, and 60th minutes of experimental myocardial ischemia provoked by coronary ligation of the left anterior descending coronary artery. The parameters obtained were compared to the corresponding values measured in the peripheral vessels. The results indicate an increased release and probably an increased turnover of norepinephrine in the ischemic myocardium. The role of metabolism acidosis in the changes in norepinephrine metabolism was suggested. It is assumed that intracellular acidosis is involved in the enhanced accumulation and release of norepinephrine in the damaged myocardium and that an increase of norepinephrine concentration in the myocardium may be considered a risk factor in supporting heart function.

Numerous experimental and clinical observations have shown an increased sympathetic–adrenal activity during the early stage of myocardial infarction (9,14,31). Blood catecholamine concentration is significantly increased on the first 2 days following coronary occlusion and is accompanied by an increased catecholamine excretion (19,23,32). Similarly, it was shown that catecholamine concentration is elevated within the first 10 min after coronary ligation in dogs (28). The role of catecholaminemia in the development of arrhythmias has been suggested by several authors, and a beneficial effect of cardioselective β-receptor-blocking agents seems to support this assumption (2,13).

A high concentration of catecholamines in the heart was recorded by a number of investigators, and the norepinephrine content was found to exceed that of epinephrine and dopamine (3,4,12,14). Regional distribution of catecholamine content in the atria and ventricular muscle as well as its localization in the neuronal and nonneuronal elements is widely discussed in the literature (4).

In the present investigation, we have studied the role of experimentally induced myocardial ischemia on norepinephrine metabolism in the dog heart.

MATERIALS AND METHODS

Twelve mongrel dogs weighing 8–17 kg were used in the study. General anesthesia was introduced by intravenous administration of pentobarbital (25 mg/kg body weight), and artificial respiration with a gas mixture of N_2O and O_2 (2:1) was performed. The chest was opened at the fourth left intercostal space; the pericardium was incised, and the heart was exposed. The coronary sinus was cannulated by a polyethylene catheter inserted through the right auricular appendage and introduced into the sinus from 6–8 cm distal to its orifice, and then the catheter position was lightly fixed, not interfering with the normal coronary sinus blood flow. Arterial and venous cannulas were than placed into the right femoral artery and vein for peripherial blood sampling. After the chest had been open 60 min, and the animal was assumed to have reached a steady state (17), a coronary ligature was taken around the proximal part of the left anterior descending coronary artery, and the resultant myocardial ischemia was estimated by serial epicardial electrograms and mechanograms. For blood norepinephrine, pH, and oxygen tension determinations, blood samples were taken in the fifth, tenth, 20th, and 60th minutes of experimental myocardial ischemia from the coronary sinus as well as from the femoral artery and vein.

RESULTS

A marked decrease of coronary blood flow was observed as a consequence of coronary ligation. As is shown in Figure 1, a significant increase in the norepinephrine content of the coronary sinus may be detected as early as 5 min after coronary occlusion and reaches its highest value after 20 min of experimental ischemia. Similar trends of changes in norepinephrine content but to a lesser degree were observed in the peripheral venous samples.

Figure 2 illustrates the changes in potassium content of the coronary sinus blood after coronary ligation. The potassium content increased slightly but significantly in the first 5 min of myocardial ischemia, and this higher extracellular potassium level persisted during the whole observation period. Parallel potassium determinations in the peripheral blood revealed no significant changes from the basal value.

The alterations of oxygen tension and pH in the coronary sinus blood are summarized in Figure 3. As shown, marked decreases in both oxygen tension and pH were observed following coronary ligation; each parameter remained significantly different from the control group after 10 min following the ligature.

DISCUSSION

Preliminary studies suggested that the myocardial norepinephrine concentration was markedly increased in acidotic animals (15) and that meta-

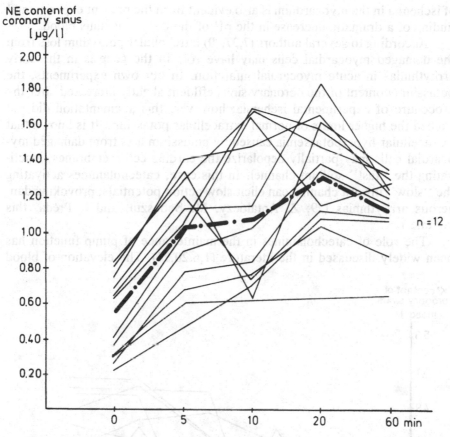

Figure 1.   Changes in norepinephrine (NE) content of the coronary sinus blood after coronary ligature.

bolic acidosis associated with heart failure in coronary-ligated animals had a role in the increased uptake of circulating catecholamines (16). According to the data accumulated in the literature, biochemical analysis of the sinus coronary effluent blood provides a method to permit a finer distinction to be made metabolic alterations in the ischemic myocardium (5,8,11,22,24, 30), but the question arises whether the changes observed represent ischemic, periischemic, or nonischemic heart tissue.

Our own results show that the norephinephrine concentration of the sinus coronary blood is significantly elevated in the early stage of experimental myocardial ischemia, which may result not only from the catecholamine release of peripheral stores (16) but also from a higher norepinephrine turnover of the ischemic heart. There is also evidence of a markedly increased uptake of labeled norepinephrine in experimental coronary occlusion in rats, and intracellular acidosis has been suggested to be a causative factor in the enhanced norepinephrine accumulation in the damaged myocardium (25,26). A possible severe intracellular acidosis as a consequence

of ischemia in the myocardium is also evident from the present experimental
finding of a dramatic decrease in the pH of the coronary sinus blood.

According to several authors (7,27,29) intracellular potassium loss from
the damaged myocardial cells may have role in the genesis in the early
arrhythmias in acute myocardial infarction. In our own experiments, the
potassium content of the coronary sinus effluent slightly increased after the
procedure of experimental ischemia; however, this augmentation did not
exceed the higher limits of normal extracellular potassium. It is known that
extracellular hyperpotassemia caused by potassium loss from damaged myocardial cells may partially depolarize the cardiac cell membranes, inacti-
vating the "fast" sodium channel. In this case, catecholamines activating
the "slow" inward channel can elicit slow action potentials, provoking dangerous arrhythmias (29; Z. Antalóczy, M. Sebeszta, and I. Préda, this
volume.)

The role of catecholamines in the maintenance of pump function has
been widely discussed in the literature (1,6,20,21). The elevation of blood

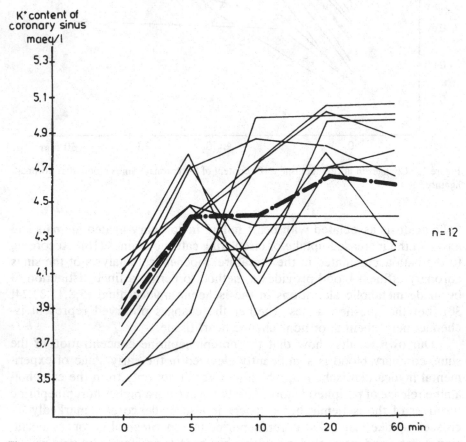

Figure 2.   Changes of extracellular potassium concentration in the coronary sinus blood after
coronary ligature.

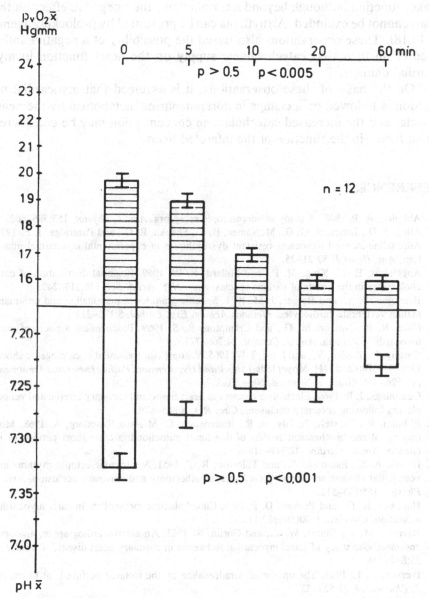

Figure 3. Modifications in oxygen tension and pH in coronary sinus blood after experimental coronary occlusion.

catecholamines level as well as the increased norepinephrine accumulation in the heart muscle after coronary occlusion must not be interpreted exclusively as positive effects on heart function. There are numerous observations to show that the catecholamines at physiological concentrations exert a positive influence on coronary blood flow, muscular contractility, and pacemaker function, although beyond a certain limit, their negative effect on the heart cannot be excluded. Arrhythmia can be prevented by β-blocking agents (2,10,18). These observations also raised the possibility of a negative influence of an increased catecholamine supply on the heart function in myocardial damage.

On the basis of these observations, it is assumed that myocardial infarction is followed by a change in norepinephrine metabolism by the heart muscle, and the increased catecholamine concentration may be considered a risk factor in the function of the infarcted heart.

REFERENCES

1. Ahlquist, R. P. 1948. A study of adrenotropic receptors. *Am. J. Physiol.* 153:586–600.
2. Allen, J. D., James, R. G. G., McNamee, B. T., Shanks, R. G., and Pantridge, J. F. 1974. Adrenaline-induced lignocaine-resistant dysrhythmias in experimental myocardial infarction. *Am. Heart J.* 87:21–25.
3. Angelakos, E. T., King, M. P., and Millard, R. W. 1969. Regional distribution of catecholamines in the hearts of various species. *Ann. N.Y. Acad. Sci.* 156:219–240.
4. Bensome, S. A., and Berger, J. M. 1971. Specific granules in mammalian and non-mammalian vertebrate cardiocytes. *Methods Achiev. Exp. Pathol.* 5:173–213.
5. Case, R. B., Nasser, M. G., and Crampton, R. S. 1969. Biochemical aspects of early myocardial ischemia. *Am. J. Cardiol.* 24:766–775.
6. Corday, E., Basiko, V., and Lang, T-W. 1965. Vasopressor treatment of cardiogenic shock. In: L. E. Mills and J. H. Moyer (eds.) *Shock and Hypotension; Pathogenesis and Treatment,* pp. 526–536. Grune & Stratton, New York.
7. Cummings, J. R. 1960. Electrolyte changes in heart tissue and coronary arterial and venous plasma following coronary occlusion. *Circ. Res.* 8:865–870.
8. Ekholm, R., Kerstell, J., Olsson, R., Rudenstam, C. M., and Svandorg, A. 1968. Morphological and biochemical studies of dog heart mitochondria after short periods of ischemia. *Am. J. Cardiol.* 22:312–318.
9. Harris, A. S., Estandia, A., and Tillotson, R. F. 1951. Ventricular ectopic rhythms and ventricular fibrillation following cardiac sympathectomy and coronary occlusion. *Am. J. Physiol.* 165:505–512.
10. Hayasky, K. D., and Penney, D. P. 1969. Catecholamine metabolism in early myocardial infarction. *Circulation* 40(Suppl.):113.
11. Herman, M. V., Elliott, W. C., and Gorlin, R. 1967. An electrocardiographic, anatomic and metabolic study of zonal myocardial ischaemia in coronary heart disease. *Circulation* 35:834–846.
12. Iversen, L. L. 1963. The uptake of noradrenaline by the isolated perfused rat heart. *Br. J. Pharmacol.* 21:523–537.
13. Jewitt, D. E., and Croxon, R. 1971. Practolol in the management of cardiac dysrhythmias following myocardial infarction and cardiac surgery. *Postgrad. Med. J.* 47(Suppl.):25–29.
14. Jewitt, D. E., Mercer, C. J., Ried, D., Valori, C., Thomas, M., and Shillingford, F. P. 1969. Free noradrenaline and adrenaline excretion in relation to the development of cardiac arrhythmias and heart failure in patients with acute myocardial infarction. *Lancet* 1:635–641.
15. Kárpáti, P., Préda, I., and Endröczi, E. 1973. Norepinephrine metabolism of heart and hypothalamic tissue in acidosis of the rat. *Acta Physiol. Acad. Sci. Hung.* 43:315–320.
16. Kárpáti, P., Préda, I., and Endröczi, E. 1974. Effect of acidosis and noradrenaline infusion on ^{14}C noradrenaline uptake by the rat myocardium. *Acta Physiol. Acad. Sci. Hung.* 45:109–114.

17. Kárpáti, P., Préda, I., Kenedi, P., Kékes, E., and Langermann, J. 1972. Acid-base and blood gas examinations after experimental coronary ligature. *Cardiol. Hung.* 1:59–63.
18. Khan, M., Hamilton, J. T., and Manning, G. W. 1972. Protective effect of beta adreno-receptor blockade in experimental coronary occlusion in conscious dogs. *Am. J. Cardiol.* 30:832–837.
19. Lukomsky, P. E., and Oganov, R. G. 1972. Blood plasma catecholamines and their urinary excretion in patients with acute myocardial infarction. *Am. Heart J.* 83:182–188.
20. Maroko, P. R., Kjekshus, J. K., Sobel, B. E., Watanabe, T., Covell, J. W., Ross, J., and Braunwald, E., 1971. Factors influencing infarct size following experimental coronary artery occlusions. *Circulation* 43:67–82.
21. Marshall, R. J., Parrat, J. R., and Pharm, B. 1973. The effect of noradrenaline on blood flow and oxygen consumption in normal and ischaemic areas of myocardium. *Am. Heart J.* 86:653–662.
22. Moore, R. M., and Greenberg, M. M. 1937. Acid production in the functioning heart under conditions of ischemia and of congestion. *Am. J. Physiol.* 118:217–224.
23. Nelson, P. G. 1970. Effect of heparin on serum free fatty acids, plasma catecholamines and the incidence of arrhythmias following acute myocardial infarction. *Br. Med. J.* 3:735–737.
24. Obeid, A., Smulyan, H., Gilbert, R., and Eich, R. 1972. Regional metabolic changes in the myocardium following coronary ligation in dogs. *Am. Heart J.* 83:189–196.
25. Préda, I., Kárpáti, P., and Endröczi, E., 1975. Myocardial noradrenaline uptake after coronary occlusion in the rat. *Acta Physiol. Acad. Sci. Hung.* 46:99–106.
26. Préda, I., Kárpáti, P., and Endröczi, E. 1980. The effect of acidosis and coronary occlusion on the noradrenaline uptake of the rat heart. In: *Proceedings of the International Union of Physiological Sciences, Budapest*, Volume 14, p. 649.
27. Regan, T. J., Harman, M. A., Lehan, P. H., Burke, W. M., and Oldewurten, H. A. 1967. Ventricular arrhythmias and K transfer during myocardial ischemia and intervention with procaine amide, insulin or glucose solution. *J. Clin. Invest.* 46:1657–1668.
28. Richardson, J. A. 1963. Plasma catecholamine concentrations in acute infarction. In: W. Lihoff and J. H. Moyer (eds.) *Coronary Heart Disease.* pp. 273–277. Grune & Stratton, New York.
29. Sebeszta, M., and Coraboeuf, E. 1980. The importance of potassium conductance in the initiation of slow action potentials in guinea-pig papillary muscle. In: *Proceedings of the International Union of Physiological Sciences, Budapest*, Vol. 14, p. 691.
30. Shea, T. M., Watson, E., Piotrowski, S. F., Dermaksian, G., and Case, R. B. 1962. Anaerobe myocardial metabolism. *Am. J. Physiol.* 203:463.
31. Staszewska-Barczak, J., and Ceremuzynsky, L. 1968. The continuous estimation of catecholamine release in the early stages of myocardial infarction. *Clin. Sci.* 34:531–539.
32. Valori, C., Thomas, M., and Shillingford, J. P. 1967. Free noradrenaline and adrenaline excretion in relation to clinical syndromes following myocardial infarction. *Am. J. Cardiol.* 20:605–617.

Reperfusion Injury
A Possible Link between Catecholamine-Induced and Ischemic Myocardial Alterations

G. Rona, M. Boutet, and I. Hüttner

Department of Pathology
McGill University
Montreal, Quebec H3A 2B4, Canada

Abstract. In this study we have compared myocardial lesions induced by catecholamines and coronary occlusion and reperfusion injuries in rats. Although microcirculatory factors were found to play an important role in catecholamine-induced cardiac muscle cell injury, alterations in sarcolemmal membrane permeability suggest a direct cardiotoxic effect. Cardiac muscle cells damaged irreversibly by ischemia reveal sarcomeres in extreme relaxation and mitochondria with floccular densities; cardiac muscle cells that die following reperfusion exhibit contraction band formation and mitochondria with calcium phosphate deposits. The ultrastructural appearance of reperfused ischemic cardiac muscle cells was similar to that observed following administration of catecholamines. These morphological similarities suggest a common causal pathway for stress-induced and ischemic heart diseases.

Ischemic heart disease and its complications constitute the most common cause of death in the industrialized countries. Although the cause of myocardial ischemia in clinical medicine is most frequently coronary artery narrowing or occlusion, the correlation between the severity of coronary artery disease and myocardial damage is not always evident (11).

Early experimental work by Franz Büchner and co-workers focused attention on various forms of coronary circulatory disturbances that without coronary artery occlusion may produce acute myocardial hypoxia and disseminated myocardial necrosis (15,16,56). Wilhelm Raab, who pioneered similar clinical studies, proposed that following stress, overstimulation of the sympathetic nervous system results in catecholamine release which in turn disproportionately increases myocardial oxygen consumption in comparison with augmentation in work performance; subsequently, coronary insufficiency and myocardial necrosis ensue (60–62). Although it was demonstrated by Josué (46) and Anitschkow (3) early in this century and later by Vishnevskaja (78) that epinephrine (E) produces focal myocardial necrosis, and similar disseminated myocardial lesions were also reported following norepinephrine (NE) administration in experimental animals (42,77), the fact that catecholamines also elicit massive infarctlike myocardial necrosis in the presence of patent coronary arteries was not appreciated until 1959 (68).

427

The availability of a well-defined and standardized animal model, the isoproterenol (ISO)-induced infarctlike myocardial necrosis, stimulated great interest. In the Soviet Union, Amelin et al. (1,2), Anshelevitch and associates (4,5), Cellarius, Semenova, and Eriskovskaja (20,21,72), and Meerson (55) have contributed important observations to the pathogenesis, morphology, evolution, and functional aspects of this model. Experimental observations with catecholamines provided impetus to investigate the myocardial injury in humans that develops in the face of non-occluded coronary arteries (8). This led to differentiation of coronarogenic and nonconarogenic myocardial necrosis (7,63).

The objective of this chapter is to illuminate some of the mechanisms responsible for the discrepancy between coronary artery pathology and the extent of myocardial necrosis by using the catecholamine-induced and is-chemic myocardial injuries as models.

EXPERIMENTAL STUDIES WITH CATECHOLAMINES

The role of coronary microcirculation in the catecholamine-induced myocardial lesion was studied by using the extracellular fine structural protein tracer horseradish peroxidase (HRP) (12–14).

As compared with control rat myocardium (Figure 1), following administration of ISO, the appearance of HRP was delayed in the myocardial interstitium, whereas following NE and E infusion, the tracer appeared earlier (69). As early as 10 min following NE infusion, some cardiac muscle cells with intact ultrastructure showed sarcolemmal permeability alteration as indicated by the intrasarcoplasmic presence of the tracer (14). The same phenomenon was observed in the ISO model following return of blood pressure to normotensive level and the concurrent appearnce of tracer in the myocardial interstitium (Figure 2).

The divergence of results is related to the pressor and depressor effect of the catecholamines and the subsequent influence on the coronary microculation. Although NE and E constrict the large coronary vessels, they dilate small coronary branches. In conjunction with their pressor effect, coronary blood flow is improved. The latter is demonstrated by the increased passage of the tracer through the coronary vasculature. In contrast, however the depressor effect of ISO in the crucial early period precludes such compensation despite coronary dilatation which is produced both directly and indirectly through increased metabolic demand (see ref. 69 for review). Coronary injection studies by Handforth (33) have indicated that ISO dilates preexisting communication channels between coronary arteries and veins, thereby causing blood to bypass the capillary bed in the myocardium. Somani et al. (75), using ^{86}Rb extraction in the isolated supported heart preparation, demonstrated that ISO decreased coronary pressure, effective coronary capillary flow (nutritional blood flow), and, hence, myocardial perfusion.

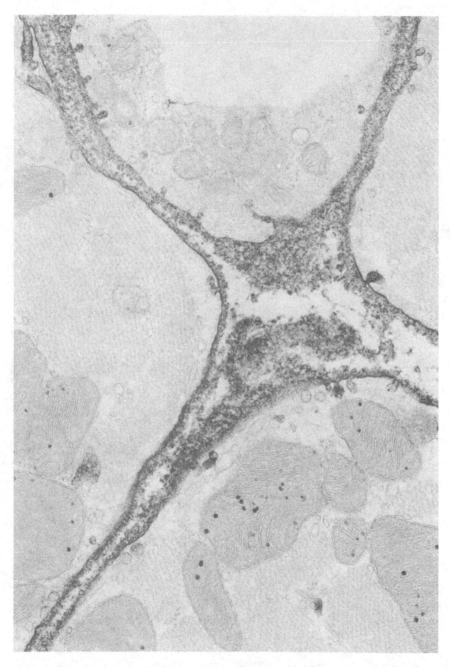

Figure 1.   Electron microscopy of control rat myocardium following i.v. injection of horse-radish peroxidase (HRP). The extracellular diffusion tracer outlines intact cardiac muscle cells. Top, coronary capillary. Lead citrate. × 30,000.

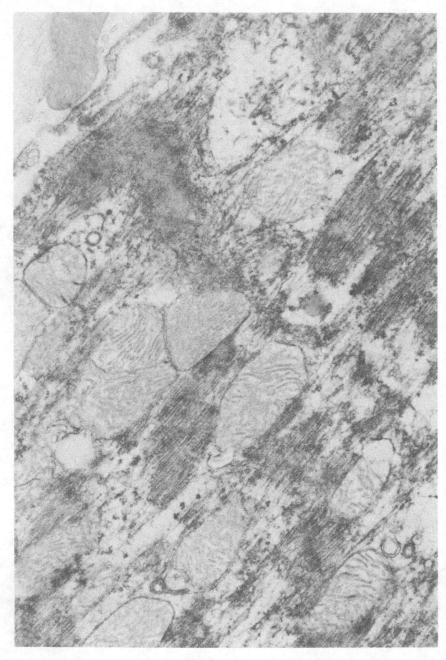

Figure 2.   Cardiac muscle cell with contraction band necrosis. Rat was killed 90 min following s.c. injection of 85 mg/kg isoproterenol; 30 min HRP circulation time. The tracer is selectively bound to hypercontracted myofilaments. Lead citrate. ×28,000.

Although coronary microcirculatory factors certainly have a major role in the evolution of catecholamine-induced cardiac muscle cell injury, the early sarcolemmal membrane permeability alteration visualized in the NE model suggests a direct cardiotoxic effect. Membrane permeability alterations were also detected in the ISO model following return of blood pressure toward normal level and subsequent resumption of macromolecular transport through coronary capillaries. Catecholamines exercise their effect through receptors situated on cell membrane (6,40), which may suggest that alteration of the sarcolemma results from a direct overstimulation of β receptors. This potentiates Ca^{2+} influx and increases contractile force and oxygen requirement (27,28,30). Each of these mechanisms, and possibly also some other factors (67,81), may be instrumental in cell injury (70).

EXPERIMENTAL ISCHEMIC MYOCARDIAL INJURY WITH AND WITHOUT REPERFUSION

Coronary artery ligation was carried out by the method of Selye (71). The coronary microcirculation and the myocardial ultrastructure were studied under conditions of varying periods of no flow and reflow, applying the tracer technique as outlined in the catecholamine model (69).

After 20 min of coronary ligation, the central ischemic zone demonstrated HRP in some capillary lumina, indicating open circulation in some vessels in the ischemic myocardium. Following 60-min ischemia, in some of the "closed" or nonperfused capillaries, the lumen was compromised by the ballooning of endothelial cells and/or platelet thrombi. By this time, cardiac muscle cells showed ultrastructural signs of irreversible damage. In some cells with hyperrelaxed sarcomeres, the tracer appeared in the sarcolemma where it was not associated with myofilaments but apparently deposited around mitochondria, sarcoplasmic tubules, and ribosomes.

Cardiac muscle reperfused following 20 min of ischemia showed HRP in the sarcoplasm of occasional cardiac muscle cells. Reperfusion following 60-min ischemia resulted in striking differences in the ultrastructural alteration of the cardiac muscle cells as well as in the pattern of tracer localization. Cardiac muscle cells following reperfusion demonstrated contraction band necrosis, and there was heavy deposition of HRP on the hypercontracted myofilaments (Figure 3).

Sarcolemmal membrane permeability alterations as well as binding of tracer to hypercontracted myofilaments following reperfusion of the ischemic myocardium can be correlated with observations obtained in the catecholamine models. The sarcolemmal permeability alteration has been shown to be an early event following NE infusion in which overstimulated cardiac muscle cells are permanently exposed to constituents of circulating blood and Ca^{2+}. The findings with HRP following 60-min ischemia and reperfusion resemble those obtained in the ISO-induced injury in which

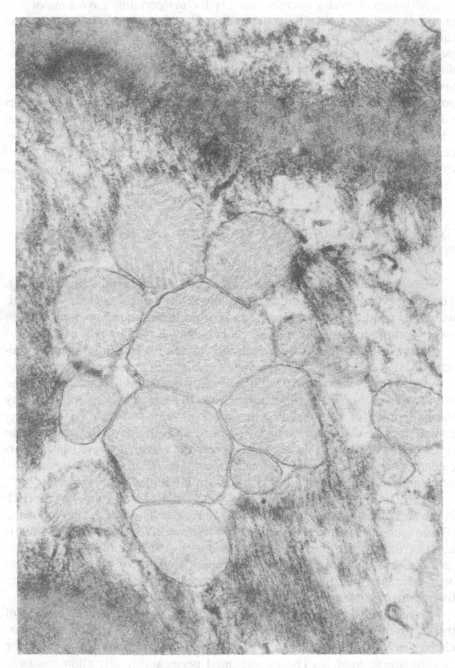

Figure 3. Contraction band necrosis with HRP deposition similar to that shown in Figure 2 following reperfusion of ischemic rat myocardium. Calcium phosphate deposits in mitochondria, another pertinent feature of this lesion, are not conspicuous because of lack of uranyl acetate staining. ×30,000.

tracer studies disclosed a permeability alteration of the membranes of the cardial muscle cell only following return of blood pressure toward normal levels and resumption of coronary perfusion.

Sarcolemmal alteration may also allow leaking of intracellular constituents including enzymes necessary for cellular reconstitution. The studies of Sharma and associates (73) disclosed a dramatic severalfold rise in enzyme activity levels following reperfusion. Our experiments demonstrate a complete disappearance of enzyme activity from myocardium ischemic for 60 min followed by 15 min of reperfusion (C. B. Bier, unpublished data). Furthermore, the intrasarcoplasmic deposition and binding of macromolecules to contractile proteins could impede the myofilament reassembly and thus contribute to an irreversible cardiac muscle cell injury.

THE LINK BETWEEN CATECHOLAMINE-INDUCED AND REPERFUSION MYOCARDIAL INJURY

In recent years, a great deal of information has accumulated on interventions designed to salvage ischemic myocardium and to reduce infarct size (35,44). Among the protective interactions, the most important is the reestablishment of blood flow to the ischemic myocardium. Although the beneficial effect of reperfusion is well established (10,36,66), there are experimental data (18,43,57,80) and human observations (17,32,37,38) that reperfusion under certain conditions fails to protect ischemic myocardium and even produces a deleterious effect.

The failure of reperfusion has been attributed to coronary capillary collapse, endothelial swelling, and thrombosis. The loss of volume regulation of impaired myocardial cells, accompanied by swelling and interstitial edema, results in compression of the capillaries, further inhibiting flow (48). Thus, ischemia initiates a chain of events that, even upon reperfusion, may hinder normal circulation of arterial blood to the previously occluded area. It has been suggested that this no-reflow phenomenon depends on the duration of ischemia (49,66) and that ischemic cell death is the direct consequence of high-energy phosphate depletion in cardiac muscle cell (45). However, it was also shown that the no-reflow phenomenon does not determine the critical time for salvageability of myocardium by revascularization (24). Furthermore, the cell death following reperfusion is more rapid, and the morphology is entirely different from that of ischemic cell injury, thus suggesting different mechanisms (50–52,57). Whereas cardiac muscle cells damaged irreversibly by ischemia reveal sarcomeres in extreme relaxation and mitochondria with floccular densities, cardiac muscle cells that die following reperfusion exhibit contraction band formation and mitochondria with calcium phosphate deposits.

An extreme example of severe reperfusion injury in humans is concentric hemorrhagic necrosis following aorto–coronary bypass surgery (Figure 4A,B). The hemorrhagic character of the myocardial lesion and the con-

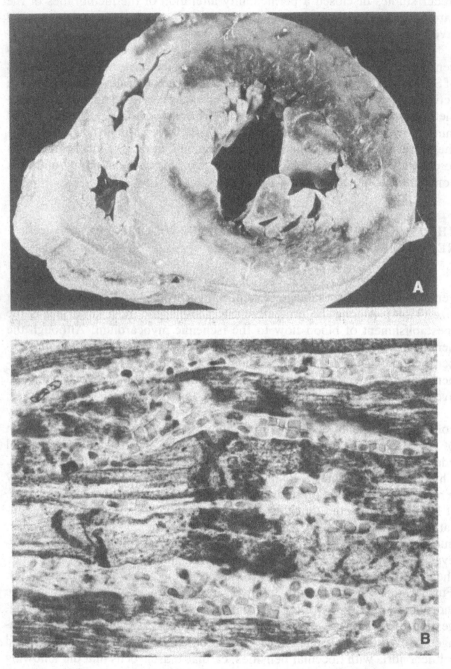

Figure 4. (A) Concentric hemorrhagic necrosis of human left ventricle following open-heart surgery. (B) Light microscopy from the same case showing contraction band necrosis and extravasation of red blood cells from dilated capillaries. HPS staining. ×680.

traction band necrosis indicate both microcirculatory damage and excessive cardiac muscle cell stimulation. Similar mechanisms may operate in a number of clinical conditions such as coronary spasm (25,54), acute intermittent coronary insufficiency (59), cardiac resuscitation (39), shock (53), hypertension (41), and sudden death (65).

The ultrastructural presentation of reperfused ischemic cardiac muscle cells is similar to that observed following administration of catecholamines (22). There are clinical observations that release of endogenous catecholamines following stress (19,63,64,79) and massive pulmonary embolism (23) lead not only to similar myocardial injury but also to hemorrhagic lesions of other organs (76). This morphological similarity could suggest a common causal pathway. As indicated by Fleckenstein, stimulation of Ca^{2+}-dependent ATPase and Ca^{2+} release would serve as the ultimate biochemical link for both myofilament overstimulation and Ca^{2+} overload of the mitochondria (29). This assumption is supported by experimental and clinical observations that show myocardial protection using β blockers (9,31,42,57) and Ca^{2+}-antagonistic compounds (26,34,58,74).

ACKNOWLEDGMENT

The authors are grateful to Mrs. S. Mongeau and Mrs. S. Sauvé for their cooperation in the typing of the manuscript.

REFERENCES

1. Amelin, A., Anshelevich, Yu. V., and Dombrovskaya, L. 1966. Reproduction of necrosis of myocardium and of aorta in dogs by isadrin (isopropylnoradrenalin). *Latv. Acad. Sci. News* 228:115–119.
2. Amelin, A. Z., Anshelevich, Yu. V., and Melzobs, M. Ya. 1963. [Experimental infarction-like changes of the myocardium under isadrin (isopropylnoradrenalin) action.] *Arkh. Patol.* 1:25–29.
3. Anitschkow, N. 1913. Uber die Histogenese der Myokardveränderungen bei einigen Intoxikationen. *Arch. Pathol. Anat.* 211:193.
4. Anshelevitch, Y., Amelin, A., and Melzobs, M. 1961. Reproduction of necrosis in the myocardium of rabbits by isadrine (isopropylnoradrenalin). *Latv. Acad. Sci. News* 173:91–94.
5. Anshelevitch, Y., Vuskalne, L., and Kartashova, O. 1964. Histochemical investigation of the myocardium in experiments with application of isopropylnoradrenalin. *Latv. Acad. Sci. News*. 203:87–91.
6. Axelrod, J., and Weinshilboum, R. 1972. Catecholamines. *Physiol. Med.* 287:237–242.
7. Baroldi, G. 1972. Human myocardial infarction: Coronarogenic or noncoronarogenic coagulation necrosis? In: E. Bajusz and G. Rona (eds.), *Recent Advances in Studies on Cardiac Structure and Metabolism*. Vol. 1: *Myocardiology*, pp. 399–413. University Park Press, Baltimore.
8. Baroldi, G., and Scomazzoni, G. 1967. Coronary Circulation in the Normal and the Pathologic Heart. Office of the Surgeon General, Department of the Army, Washington.
9. Baroldi, G., Silver, M. D., Lixfeld, W., and McGregor, D. C. 1977. Irreversible myocardial

damage resembling catecholamine necrosis secondary to acute coronary occlusion in dogs: Its prevention by propranolol. *J. Mol. Cell. Cardiol.* 9:687–691.

10. Baughman, K. L., Maroko, P. R., and Vatner, S. F. 1981. Effects of coronary artery reperfusion on myocardial infarct size and survival in conscious dogs. *Circulation* 63:317–323.

11. Boor, P. J., and Reynolds, E. S. 1977. Myocardial infarct size: Clinicopathologic agreement and discordance. *Hum. Pathol.* 8:685–695.

12. Boutet, M., Hüttner, I., and Rona, G. 1973. Aspect microcirculatoire des lésions myocardiques provoquées par l'infusion de catécholamines. Etude ultrastructurale à l'aide de traceurs de diffusion. I. Isoprotérénol. *Pathol. Biol. (Paris)* 21:811–825.

13. Boutet, M., Hüttner, I., and Rona, G. 1974. Aspect microcirculatoire des lésions myocardiques provoquées par l'infusion de catécholamines. Etude ultrastructurale à l'aide de traceurs de diffusion. II. Norépinéphrine. *Pathol. Biol. (Paris)* 22:377–387.

14. Boutet, M., Hüttner, I., and Rona, G. 1976. Permeability alteration of sarcolemmal membrane in catecholamine induced cardiac muscle cell injury. *Lab. Invest.* 34:482–488.

15. Büchner, F. 1932. Die Rolle des Herzmuskels bei der Angina Pectoris. *Beitr. Pathol. Anat. (Stuttgart)* 89:644–667.

16. Büchner, F. 1933. Das morphologische Substrat der Angina Pectoris in Tierexperiment. *Beitr. Pathol. Anat. (Stuttgart)* 92:311–328.

17. Bulkley, B. H., and Hutchins, G. M. 1977. Myocardial consequences of coronary artery bypass graft surgery. *Circulation* 56:906–913.

18. Bush, L. R., Shlafer, M., Haack, D. W., and Lucchesi, B. R. 1980. Time-dependent changes in canine cardiac mitochondrial function and ultrastructure resulting from coronary occlusion and reperfusion. *Basic Res. Cardiol.* 75:555–571.

19. Cebelin, M. S., and Hirsch, C. S. 1980. Human stress cardiomyopathy. *Hum. Pathol.* 11:123–132.

20. Cellarius, Yu. G., and Semenova, L. A. 1971. [Changes in the myocardial stroma in adrenaline injuries of the heart.] *Arkh. Pathol* 33:43–49.

21. Cellarius, Yu. G., and Semenova, L. A. 1972. *Histopathology of Focal Metabolic Lesions of the Myocardium.* Nauka Siberian Branch, Novosibirsk.

22. Csapo, Z., Dusek, J., and Rona, G. 1972. Early alterations of the cardiac muscle cells in isoproterenol-induced necrosis. *Arch. Pathol.* 93:356–365.

23. Cuénoud, H. F., Joris, I., and Majno, G. 1978. Ultrastructure of the myocardium after pulmonary embolism. *Am. J. Pathol.* 92:421–458.

24. Darsee, J. R., and Kloner, R. A. 1980. The no reflow phenomenon: A time-limiting factor for reperfusion after coronary occlusion? *Am. J. Cardiol.* 46:800–806.

25. Ellis, E. F., Oelz, O., Roberts II, L. J., Payne, N. A., Sweetman, B. J., Nies, A. S., and Oates, J. A. 1976. Coronary arterial smooth muscle contraction by a substance released from platelets: Evidence that it is thromboxane A_2. *Science* 193:1135–1137.

26. Fleckenstein, A. 1971. Specific inhibitors and promotors of calcium action in the excitation–contraction coupling of heart muscle and their role in the prevention or production of myocardial lesion. In: P. Harris and L. Opie (eds.), *Calcium and the Heart*, pp. 135–188. Academic Press, New York, London.

27. Fleckenstein, A., Janke, J., Doring, H. J., and Leder, O. 1971. Die intrazellüläre Überladung mit Kalzium als entscheidender Kausalfaktor bei der Entstehung nicht-coronarogener Myokard-nekrosen. *Verh. Dtsch. Ges. Kreislauffforsch.* 37:345–353.

28. Fleckenstein, A., Janke, J., Doring, H. J., and Leder, O. 1974. Myocardial fibre necrosis due to intracellular Ca^{2+} overload—a new principle in cardiac pathophysiology. In: N. S. Dhalla (ed.), *Recent Advances in Studies on Cardiac Structure and Metabolism*. Vol. 4: *Myocardial Biology*, pp. 563–580. University Park Press, Baltimore.

29. Fleckenstein, A., Janke, J., Doring, H. J., and Leder, O. 1975. Key role of Ca in the production of noncoronarogenic myocardial necroses. In: A. Fleckenstein and G. Rona (eds.), *Recent Advances in Studies on Cardiac Structure and Metabolism*. Vol. 6: *Path-*

ophysiology and Morphology of Myocardial Cell Alteration, pp. 21–32. University Park Press, Baltimore.

30. Fleckenstein, A., Janke, J., Doring, H. J., and Pachinger, O. 1973. Ca overload as the determinant factor in the production of catecholamine-induced myocardial lesions. In: E. Bajusz and G. Rona (eds.), *Recent Advances in Studies on Cardiac Structure and Metabolism*. Vol. 2: *Cardiomyopathies*, pp. 455–466. University Park Press, Baltimore.

31. Gold, H. K., Leinback, R. C., and Maroko, P. R. 1976. Propranolol-induced reduction of signs of ischemic injury during acute myocardial infarction. *Am. J. Cardiol.* 38:689–695.

32. Gotlieb, A., Masse, S., Allard, J., Dobell, A., and Huang, S.-N. 1977. Concentric hemorrhagic necrosis of the myocardium. *Hum. Pathol.* 8:27–37.

33. Handforth, C. P., 1962. Isoproterenol-induced myocardial infarction in animals. *Arch. Pathol.* 73:161–165.

34. Hearse, D. J., Baker, J. E., and Humphrey, S. M. 1980. Verapamil and the calcium paradox. *J. Mol. Cell. Cardiol.* 12:733–739.

35. Hillis, L. D., and Braunwald, E. 1977. Myocardial ischemia. *N. Engl. J. Med.* 296:971–978, 1034–1044, 1093–1096.

36. Hofmann, M., Hofmann, M., Genth, K., and Schaper, W. 1980. The influence of reperfusion on infarct size after experimental coronary artery occlusion. *Basic Res. Cardiol.* 75:572–582.

37. Hultgren, H. N., Miyagawa, M., Busch, W., and Angell, W. W. 1973. Ischemic myocardial injury during cardiopulmonary bypass surgery. *Am. Heart J.* 85:167–176.

38. Hutchins, G. M., and Bulkley, B. H. 1977. Correlation of myocardial contraction band necrosis and vascular patency. *Lab. Invest.* 36:642–648.

39. Hutchins, G. M., and Silverman, K. H. 1979. Pathology of the stone heart syndrome. Massive myocardial contraction band necrosis and widely patent coronary arteries. *Am. J. Pathol.* 95:745–750.

40. Hüttner, I. 1980. The sarcolemma. In: M. R. Bristow (ed.), *Drug-Induced Heart Disease*, pp. 3–37. Elsevier/North Holland Biomedical Press, Amsterdam.

41. Hüttner, I., Rona, G., and More, R. H. 1971. Fibrin deposition within cardiac muscle cells in malignant hypertension. An electron microscopic study. *Arch. Pathol.* 91:19–28.

42. Jellinek, H., Hüttner, I., and Kerényi, T. 1963. Pathohistologische Veränderungen im Myocard bei mit Noradrenalin behandelten Hunden. In: G. Gottsegen (ed.), *Acta Secundi Conventus Medicinae Internae Hungarici Cardiologia*, pp. 338–339. Hungarian Society for Cardiology, Budapest.

43. Jennings, R. B., Ganote, C. E., and Reimer, K. A. 1975. Ischemic tissue injury. *Am. J. Pathol.* 81:179–198.

44. Jennings, R. B., and Reimer, K. A. 1974. Salvage of ischemic myocardium. *Mod. Concepts Cardiovasc. Dis.* 43:125.

45. Jennings, R. B., and Reimer, K. A. 1981. Lethal myocardial ischemic injury. *Am. J. Pathol.* 102:241–255.

46. Josué, O. 1907. Hypertrophie cardiaque causée par l'adrénaline et la toxine typhique. *C. R. Soc. Biol. (Paris)* 63:285–286.

47. Kloner, R. A., Fishbein, M. C., Cotran, R. S., Braunwald, E., and Maroko, P. R. 1977. The effect of propranolol on microvascular injury in acute myocardial ischemia. *Circulation* 55:872–879.

48. Kloner, R. A., Ganote, C. E., and Jennings, R. B. 1974. The "no-reflow" phenomenon after temporary coronary occlusion in the dog. *J. Clin. Invest.* 54:1496–1508.

49. Kloner, R. A., Rude, R. E., Carlson, N., Maroko, P. R., DeBoer, L. W. V, and Braunwald, E. 1980. Ultrastructural evidence of microvascular damage and myocardial cell injury after coronary artery occlusion: Which comes first? *Circulation* 62:945–952.

50. Korb, G., and Totovic, V. 1969. Electron microscopical studies on experimental ischemic lesions of the heart. *Ann. N.Y. Acad. Sci.* 156:48–59.

51. Krug, A., du Mesnil de Rochemont, W., and Korb, G. 1966. Blood supply of the myocardium after temporary coronary occlusion. *Circ. Res.* 19:57–62.

52. Long, R., Symes, J., Allard, J., Burdon, T., Lisbona, R, Hüttner, I., and Sniderman, A. 1980. Differentiation between reperfusion and occlusion myocardial necrosis with technetium-99m pyrophosphate scans. *Am. J. Cardiol.* 46:413–418.

53. Martin, A. M., Jr., Hackel, D. B., and Kurtz, S. M. 1964. The ultrastructure of zonal lesions of the myocardium in hemorrhagic shock. *Am. J. Pathol.* 44:124–140.

54. Maseri, A., Severi, S., DeNes, M., L'Abbate, A., Chierchia, S., Marzilli, M., Ballestra, A.-M., Parodi, O., Biagini, A., and Distante, A. 1978. "Variant" angina: One aspect of a continuous spectrum of vasopastic myocardial ischemia. Pathogenetic mechanisms, estimated incidence, clinical and coronarographic findings in 138 patients. *Am. J. Cardiol.* 42:1019–1035.

55. Meerson, F. Z. 1980. Disturbances of metabolism and cardiac function under the action of emotional painful stress and their prophylaxis. *Basic Res. Cardiol.* 75:479–500.

56. Meessen, H. 1939. Experimentelle Untersuchungen zum Collapsproblem. *Beitr. Pathol. Anat. (Stuttgart)* 102:191–267.

57. Mickleborough, L., Hüttner, I., Symes, J., Poirier, N., and Sniderman, A. D. 1978. Significance of epicardial Q waves as an acute marker of myocardial necrosis in dogs. *Cardiovas. Res.* 12:376–386.

58. Nayler, W. G., Ferrari, R., and Williams, A. 1980. Protective effect of pretreatment with verapamil, nifedipine and propronolol on mitochondrial function in the ischemic and reperfused myocardium. *Am. J. Cardiol.* 46:242–248.

59. Neill, W. A., Wharton, T. P., Fluri-Lundeen, J., and Cohen, I. S. 1980. Acute coronary insufficiency—coronary occlusion after intermittent ischemic attacks. *N. Engl. J. Med.* 302:1157–1162.

60. Raab, W. 1960. Key position of catecholamine in functional and degenerative cardiovascular pathology. *Am. J. Cardiol.* 5:571–578.

61. Raab, W., Stark, E., MacMilan, W. H., and Gigee, W. R. 1961. Sympathogenic origin and antiadrenergic prevention of stress-induced myocardial lesions. *Am. J. Cardiol.* 8:203–211.

62. Raab, W., Van Lith, P., Lepeschkin, E., and Herrlich, H. C. 1962. Catecholamine-induced myocardial hypoxia in the presence of impaired coronary dilatability independent of external cardiac work. *Am. J. Cardiol.* 9:455–570.

63. Reichenbach, D., and Benditt, E. P. 1968. Myofibrillar degeneration: A response of the myocardial cell to injury. *Arch. Pathol.* 85:189–199.

64. Reichenbach, D. D., and Benditt, E. P. 1970. Catecholamines and cardiomyopathy: The pathogenesis and potential importance of myofibrillar degeneration. *Hum. Pathol.* 1:125–150.

65. Reichenbach, D., Moss, N., and Meyer, E. 1977. Pathology of the heart in sudden cardiac death. *Am. J. Cardiol* 39:865–872.

66. Reimer, K. A., and Jennings, R. B. 1979. The "wavefront phenomenon" of myocardial ischemic cell death. II. Transmural progression of necrosis within the framework of ischemic bed size (myocardium at risk) and collateral flow. *Lab. Invest.* 40:633–644.

67. Rona, G., Boutet, M., Hüttner, I., and Peters, H. 1973. Pathogenesis of isoproterenol-induced myocardial alterations. Functional and morphological correlates. In: N. Dhalla (ed.), *Recent Advances in Studies on Cardiac Structure and Metabolism.* Vol. 3: *Myocardial Metabolism*, pp. 507–525. University Park Press, Baltimore.

68. Rona, G., Chappel, C. I., Balazs, T., and Gaudry, R. 1959. An infarct-like myocardial lesion and other toxic manifestations produced by isoproterenol in the rat. *Arch. Pathol.* 67:443–455.

69. Rona, G., Hüttner, I, and Boutet, M., 1977. Microcirculatory changes in myocardium with particular reference to catecholamine-induced cardiac muscle cell injury. In: H. Meessen (ed.), *Handbuch der Allgemeinen Pathologie.* III/7: *Microcirculation*, pp. 791–888. Springer-Verlag, Berlin, Heidelberg, New York.

70. Schanne, F. A. X., Kane, A. B., Young, E. E., and Farber, J. L. 1979. Calcium dependence of toxic cell death: A final common pathway. *Science* 206:700–702.

71. Selye, H., Bajusz, E., Grasso, S., and Mendell, P. 1960. Simple techniques for the surgical occlusion of coronary vessels in the rat. *Angiology* 2:398–407.
72. Semenova, L. A., Eriskovskaja, N. K., and Cellarius, Y. G. 1971. Polarization and electron microscopic investigations of intracellular regeneration of the myocardium after myocytolysis. *Morphol. Pathomorphol.* 3:102–105.
73. Sharma, G. O., Varley, K. G., Kim, S. W., Barwinsky, J., Cohen, M., and Dhalla, N. Alterations in energy metabolism and ultrastructure upon reperfusion of the ischemic myocardium after coronary occlusion. *Am. J. Cardiol.* 36:233–243.
74. Siegel, H., Janke, J., and Fleckenstein, A. 1975. Restriction of isoproterenol-induced myocardial Ca^{2+} uptake and necrotization in rats by a new Ca^{2+} antagonistic compound [ethyl-4-(3,4,5-trimethoxycinnamoyl)piperazinyl acetate (Vascoril).] In: A. Fleckenstein and G. Rona (eds.), *Recent Advances in Studies on Cardiac Structure and Metabolism.* Vol. 6: *Pathophysiology and Morphology of Myocardial Cell Alteration*, pp. 121–126. University Park Press, Baltimore.
75. Somani, P., Laddu, A. R., and Hardman, H. R. 1970. Nutritional circulation in the heart. III. Effect of isoproterenol and beta adrenergic blockage on myocardial hemodynamics and rubidium-86 extraction in the isolated supported heart preparation. *J. Pharmacol. Exp. Ther.* 175:577–592.
76. Szabo, S., Hüttner, I., Kovacs, K., Horvath, E., Szabo, D., and Horner, H. C. 1980. Pathogenesis of experimental adrenal hemmorhagic necrosis "apoplexy." Ultrastructural, biochemical, neuropharmacologic and blood coagulation studies with acrylonitrile in the rat. *Lab. Invest.* 42:533–546.
77. Szakacs, J. E., and Cannon, A. 1958. *l*-Norepinephrine myocarditis. *Am. J. Clin. Pathol.* 30:425–430.
78. Vishnevskaja, O. P. 1956. [Reflex mechanisms in the pathogenesis of adrenalin myocarditis.] *Bull. Eksp. Biol. Med.* 41:307–310.
79. Waagstein, F., Hjalmarson, A., Swedberg, K., and Waldenstrom, A. 1979. The role of catecholamines in the development of heart disease. In: S. Hayase and S. Murao (eds.), *Cardiology*, pp. 644–650. Excerpta Medica, Amsterdam.
80. Weishaar, R., Tschurtschenthaler, G. V., Ashikawa, K., and Bing, R. J. 1979. The relationship of regional coronary blood flow to mitochondrial function during reperfusion of the ischemic myocardium. *Cardiology* 64:350–364.
81. Yates, J. C., Taam, G. M. L., Singal, P. K., Beamish, R. E., and Dhalla, N. S. 1980. Modification of adrenochrome-induced cardiac contractile failure and cell damage by changes in cation concentrations. *Lab. Invest.* 43:316–326.

Ultrastructural, Functional, and Metabolic Correlates in the Ischemic Rat Heart

Effects of Free Fatty Acid

D. Feuvray

Laboratory of Comparative Physiology
University of Paris-Sud
91405 Orsay, France

Abstract. A study correlating functional, metabolic, and ultrastructural changes in the ischemic myocardium was conducted on isolated working rat hearts, both in the presence and absence of fatty acid. Glucose alone (11 mM) or glucose plus palmitic acid (1.5 mM) were used as metabolic substrates. A 60-min period of whole-heart ischemia resulted in a more dramatic morphological alteration in those hearts receiving palmitate than in those receiving no palmitate. In ischemic hearts receiving palmitate, intramitochondrial amorphous densities of both rounded and elongated types were observed. These densities did not develop in hearts receiving glucose alone over the same period of ischemia. Such morphological alterations were associated with a more severe deterioration of mechanical function in the presence of palmitate. Biochemical determinations of fatty acid derivatives showed increased tissue levels of acyl esters of CoA and carnitine in ischemic hearts, but levels of long-chain acyl carnitine were much higher in those ischemic hearts receiving palmitate. Furthermore, from the data obtained on isolated mitochondria, it appeared that the mitochondrial level of long-chain acyl carnitine was approximately four times higher in the ischemic hearts receiving palmitate than in those receiving no palmitate. This great rise in mitochondrial levels of long-chain acyl carnitine correlated with modifications of the mitochondrial structure and with the appearance of amorphous densities.

Among the fine structural changes occurring during myocardial ischemia in vivo, the development of intramitochondrial amorphous densities is a characteristic feature of severe injury (5–7). The nature of the amorphous densities is not clear. It has been suggested (6) that they could represent accumulated lipids as a result of their decreased metabolism.

We observed in previous studies (8) similar amorphous densities in the isolated working rat heart after coronary artery ligation. However, intramitochondrial amorphous densities developed in our experiments, only when long-chain fatty acids were provided in the perfusate.

Recently, it has been shown that the inhibition of fatty acid oxidation during ischemia results in increased tissue levels of long-chain acyl CoA (18,20) and long-chain acyl carnitine derivatives. The increase in acyl carnitine is proportional to the amount of exogenous fatty acid available (20).

The purpose of the present study was to determine the role of fatty acids in the development of amorphous densities. Experiments were carried

441

out on the isolated whole-ischemic rat heart model which made it possible to correlate tissue levels of lipid metabolites with mitochondrial structural alterations, both in the presence and absence of fatty acid.

MATERIALS AND METHODS

Hearts from male Wistar rats weighing 280–320 g were removed and perfused by the working-heart technique of Neely et al. (13) under aerobic control or ischemic conditions. Whole-heart ischemia was induced by use of a one-way aortic valve that reduced coronary diastolic perfusion (14). The perfusate was Krebs bicarbonate buffer containing either 11 mM glucose plus 3% bovine serum albumin or 11 mM glucose and 1.5 mM palmitate bound to 3% bovine serum albumin (1).

At the end of perfusion, hearts were used either to determine levels of metabolic intermediates or for electron microscopy. Tissue levels of long-chain acyl CoA and acyl carnitine were assayed as CoA (3) and carnitine (12) following separation and hydrolysis of the esters. For electron microscopy, hearts were perfusion-fixed, dehydrated, and embedded in resin as previously described (8). Thin sections were cut in samples taken from the subendocardial part of the left ventricular wall and stained before examination with the electron microscope. Mitochondria containing amorphous densities were counted on a large number of electron micrographs randomly selected from each tissue sample.

In other series of experiments, hearts from each group were used immediately after perfusion for isolation of mitochondria (4). Mitochondrial levels of long-chain acyl CoA and acyl carnitine were measured as described above for the tissue. Aliquots of mitochondrial suspensions were fixed (19) and treated for electron microscopy.

RESULTS

The functional response of both groups of hearts, i.e., those perfused in the presence or absence of palmitate, to the same reduction in coronary flow is shown in Table 1. Ventricular function was slightly affected in hearts receiving glucose alone (no palmitate) as the exogenous substrate. Reduced function resulted from decrease in both heart rate and peak systolic pressure. In the presence of palmitate, in contrast, the rate of decline in pressure development was faster. The decline in pressure reduced coronary flow further, and function continued to deteriorate. The difference in function between hearts receiving palmitate or no palmitate was evident throughout 60 min of ischemic perfusion.

Tissue levels of long-chain fatty acyl CoA and fatty acyl carnitine measured after 60 min of perfusion are shown in Table 1. Sixty minutes of ischemia resulted in about the same increase in levels of long-chain acyl CoA in hearts

Table 1. Effects of Palmitate and Ischemia on Ventricular Function and Tissue Levels of Long-Chain Acyl CoA and Acyl Carnitine Derivatives in Isolated Perfused Hearts[a]

Condition		CF (ml/min)	PSP × HR (mm Hg/min × 10³)	Acyl CoA[b] (nmol/g dry wt.)	Acyl carnitine[b] (nmol/g dry wt.)
Control	+ palmitate	18.4 ± 0.6	24.9 ± 1.0	129 ± 4	1647 ± 148
	− palmitate	18.5 ± 0.6	25.0 ± 1.2	107 ± 6	416 ± 15
Ischemic	+ palmitate	2.2 ± 0.9	3.9 ± 2.3	237 ± 5	2950 ± 216
	− palmitate	4.9 ± 0.8	14.3 ± 1.9	208 ± 20	767 ± 49

[a] Hearts were perfused for 10 min as Langendorff preparations with buffer containing glucose (11 mM). They were then switched to the working preparation with a left atrial pressure of 10 cm H_2O and perfused with buffer containing glucose alone or glucose plus palmitate (1.5 mM) as described earlier (1). Ventricular function was estimated by the product of peak systolic pressure (PSP) and heart rate (HR). Ventricular function and coronary flow (CF) remained constant throughout 60 min of control perfusion. Ischemic values given for ventricular function and coronary flow are those obtained at the end of the 60-min period of ischemia. The hearts were frozen at 60 min and used for tissue assays. Long-chain acyl CoA and acyl carnitine levels were determined on the perchloric acid precipitate as free CoA and carnitine released after alkaline hydrolysis. The values represent the mean ± S.E.M. for six determinations.
[b] Reproduced with permission by American Journal of Physiology (ref. 1).

either receiving or not receiving palmitate. Long-chain acyl carnitine also increased with both substrate conditions, but the levels were much higher in those hearts receiving palmitate. The levels of total CoA and total carnitine remained essentially the same in all conditions used over the 60 min of perfusion. Table 2 shows mitochondrial levels of long-chain acyl CoA and acyl carnitine. Levels of long-chain acyl CoA in mitochondria isolated from hearts receiving no palmitate were practically the same for control and ischemic hearts and were only slightly increased in mitochondria of ischemic hearts receiving palmitate. On the other hand, levels of long-chain acyl carnitine in mitochondria of ischemic hearts were double those found in control hearts. Moreover, the mitochondrial level of long-chain acyl car-

Table 2. Effects of Palmitate and Ischemia on Mitochondrial Levels of Long-Chain Acyl CoA and Acyl Carnitine Derivatives[a]

Condition		Acyl CoA[b]	Acyl carnitine[b]
Control	+ palmitate	0.87 ± 0.11	0.259 ± 0.030
	− palmitate	0.35 ± 0.04	0.066 ± 0.003
Ischemic	+ palmitate	1.03 ± 0.08	0.498 ± 0.047
	− palmitate	0.49 ± 0.04	0.136 ± 0.021

[a] Hearts were perfused 60 min under control or ischemic conditions before being homogenized and mitochondria isolated in MSE buffer containing 1 mM cyanide. Cyanide was added to prevent oxidation of the long-chain acyl derivatives during the isolation procedure. Long-chain acyl esters were determined as described for the tissue. Each group includes five to seven hearts.
[b] Expressed as nmol/mg mitochondrial protein. Reproduced with permission from Circulation Research (ref. 2).

nitine was approximately four times higher in the ischemic hearts receiving palmitate than in those receiving no palmitate. Thus, 60 min of ischemia in vitro resulted in a large increase in tissue levels of acyl carnitine in the presence of palmitate in the perfusate. A large rise in long-chain acyl carnitine levels was also found in the mitochondria isolated from those ischemic hearts receiving palmitate.

The mitochondrial structure observed after 60 min of ischemia was noticeably different depending on whether palmitate or no palmitate was provided in the perfusate. In ischemic hearts receiving no palmitate, ultra-structural alterations were very slight. The changes mainly included enlargements of the unspecialized regions of the intercalated disks and the presence of autophagic vacuoles containing myelin structures and mitochondrial remnants (1). All mitochondria had slightly clear matrices but no amorphous densities were observed. In ischemic hearts receiving palmitate, most of the cells appeared dramatically damaged, with contracted myofibrils, marginal clumping of nuclear chromatin, disorganization of the tubular systems, depletion of glycogen, and defects in the sarcolemma. Mitochondria (Figure 1) appeared swollen, they had clearing of the matrix, partial fragmentation of the cristae, and occasionally broken external membranes. Seventy-five percent of the mitochondria contained two types of amorphous densities: (1) large rounded amorphous densities as previously described and (2) finger-shape amorphous densities of different lengths. Either or both types were encountered in any mitochondrion. Mitochondria isolated from ischemic hearts receiving palmitate are shown in Figure 2 for comparison. Numerous intramitochondrial densely staining bodies were observed. This densely staining material looked very similar to the amorphous densities seen in the intact tissue (Figure 1) under comparable situations.

DISCUSSION

It has generally been observed that high levels of fatty acids cause more rapid or more severe deterioration of ischemic myocardium (9,10,11,15). In the present study, the more marked decrease in ventricular function in ischemic hearts perfused with 1.5 mM palmitate than in those perfused with glucose alone was associated with more marked ultrastructural damages. In this regard, the appearance of numerous intramitochondrial amorphous densities is particularly striking. Most previous studies (5,7,17) describing the development of amorphous densities have utilized blood-perfused hearts where fatty acids were always present. In the present study using the isolated heart, the development of amorphous densities was related to the supply of fatty acid. From the results obtained on the intact ischemic tissue, there is a good correlation between the presence of a large number of intramito-chondrial densities and the great increase in levels of acyl carnitine. Both long-chain acyl CoA and acyl carnitine increase in ischemic rat hearts

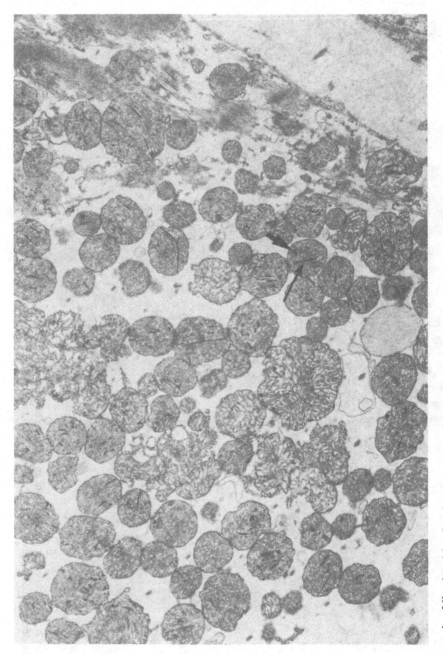

Figure 1. Mitochondria of an ischemic heart receiving 1.5 mM palmitate. A portion of ischemic myocardial cell illustrating the two types of intramitochondrial amorphous densities that developed when palmitate was provided in the perfusate: rounded (thick arrow) and finger-shape (thin arrow). × 10,000.

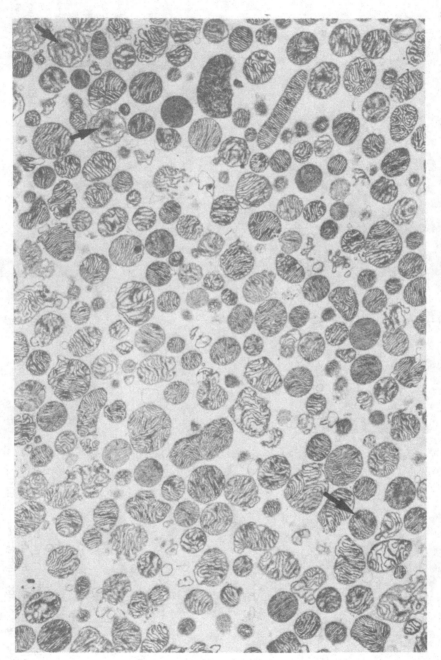

Figure 2. Mitochondria isolated from an ischemic heart receiving 1.5 mM palmitate (perfusion conditions similar to those in Figure 1). Many densely staining areas (amorphous densities) are present (arrows) in both the more and less damaged mitochondria. ×8000.

(18,20). High tissue levels of these long-chain acyl esters have been shown to affect several enzymatic reactions (16,18,21), and they are active detergent agents.

The existence of an association between the presence of palmitate in the perfusate, high tissue levels of acyl carnitine, and development of amorphous densities is further supported by the data obtained on isolated mitochondria. Indeed, these data clearly indicate that palmitate perfusion during ischemia results in formation of mitochondrial amorphous densities associated with increased mitochondrial levels of long-chain acyl carnitine.

Our data, as well as previous work in this field (4,8), suggest that under extreme conditions of fatty acid supply, enough acyl carnitine may accumulate on the mitochondrial membrane (4) to cause structural alterations. In our isolated mitochondria, the amorphous densities appear to be bound to the inner membrane (2). They may represent rearrangement of lipids from mitochondrial membranes as a result of the detergent action of acyl carnitine. Binding of acyl carnitine may disrupt the membrane sufficiently to cause melting of adjacent cristae membranes and/or rearrangement of membrane components and may contribute to loss of cellular function during ischemia.

ACKNOWLEDGMENTS

This work was supported by grants from INSERM and DGRST.

REFERENCES

1. Feuvray, D. 1981. Structural, functional and metabolic correlates in ischemic hearts: Effects of substrates. *Am. J. Physiol.* 240:H391–398.
2. Feuvray, D., and Plouet, J. 1981. Relationship between structure and fatty acid metabolism in mitochondria isolated from ischemic rat hearts. *Circ. Res.* 48:740–747.
3. Garland, P. B., Shepherd, D., and Yates, D. W. 1965. Steady state concentrations of coenzyme A, acetyl coenzyme A and long-chain fatty acyl coenzyme A in rat liver mitochondria oxidizing palmitate. *Biochem. J.* 97:587–594.
4. Idell-Wenger, J. A., Grotyohann, L. W., and Neely, J. R. 1978. Coenzyme A and carnitine distribution in normal and ischemic hearts. *J. Biol. Chem.* 253:4310–4318.
5. Jennings, R. B., and Ganote, C. E. 1972. Ultrastructural changes in acute myocardial ischemia. In: M. F. Oliver, D. G. Julian, and K. W. Donald (eds.), *Effects of Acute Ischaemia on Myocardial Function,* pp. 50–74. Churchill Livingstone, Edinburgh.
6. Jennings, R. B., and Ganote, C. E. 1976. Mitochondrial structure and function in acute myocardial ischemic injury. *Circ. Res.* 38:80–91.
7. Jennings, R. B., and Herdson, P. B. 1965. Fine structural changes in myocardial ischemic injury. *Arch. Pathol.* 79:135–143.
8. Leiris, J. de, and Feuvray, D. 1977. Ischaemia-induced damaged in the working rat heart preparation: The effect of perfusate substrate composition upon subendocardial ultrastructure of the ischaemic left ventricular wall. *J. Mol. Cell. Cardiol.* 9:365–373.
9. Leiris, J. de, and Opie, L. H. 1978. Effect of substrates and of coronary artery ligation on mechanical performance and on release of lactate dehydrogenase and creatine phosphokinase in isolated working rat hearts. *Cardiovasc. Res.* 12:585–596.

10. Leiris, J. de, Opie, L. H., and Feuvray, D. 1975. Effect of substrate on enzyme release and electron microscopic appearances after coronary artery ligation in isolated rat heart. *Acta Med. Scand.* 587:137–139.
11. Liedtke, A. J., Nellis, S., and Neely, J. R. 1978. Effects of excess free fatty acids on mechanical and metabolic function in normal and ischemic myocardium in swine. *Circ. Res.* 43:652–661.
12. McGarry, J. D., and Foster, D. W. 1976. An improved and simplified radioisotope assay for the determination of free and esterified carnitine. *J. Lipid Res.* 17:277–281.
13. Neely, J. R., Liebermeister, H., Battersby, E. J., and Morgan, H. E. 1967. Effect of pressure development on oxygen consumption by isolated rat heart. *Am. J. Physiol.* 212:804–814.
14. Neely, J. R., Rovetto, M. J., Whitmer, J. T., and Morgan, H. E. 1973. Effects of ischemia on ventricular function and metabolism in the isolated working rat heart. *Am. J. Physiol.* 225:651–658.
15. Opie, L. H. 1972. Metabolic response during impending myocardial infarction. I. Relevance of studies of glucose and fatty acid metabolism in animals. *Circulation* 45:483–489.
16. Pitts, B. J. R., Tate, C. A., Van Winkle, W. B., Wood, J. M., and Entman, M. L. 1978. Palmityl carnitine inhibition of the calcium pump in cardiac sarcoplasmic reticulum. A possible role in myocardial ischemia. *Life Sci.* 23:391–402.
17. Schaper, J., Mulch, J., Winkler, B., and Schaper, W. 1979. Ultrastructural, functional and biochemical criteria for estimation of reversibility of ischemic injury: A study on the effects of global ischemia on the isolated dog heart. *J. Mol. Cell. Cardiol.* 11:521–541.
18. Shug, A. L., Shrago, E., Bittar, N., Folts, J. D., and Kokes, J. R. 1975. Acyl CoA inhibition of adenine nucleotide translocation in ischemic myocardium. *Am. J. Physiol.* 228:689–692.
19. Sordahl, L. A., Johnson, C., Blailock, Z. R., and Schwartz, A. 1971. In: A. Schwartz (ed.), *Methods in Pharmacology* Vol. 1, pp. 247–286. Appleton Century Crofts, New York.
20. Whitmer, J. T., Idell-Wenger, J. A., Rovetto, M. J., and Neely, J. R. 1978. Control of fatty acid metabolism in ischemic and hypoxic hearts, *J. Biol. Chem.* 253:4305–4309.
21. Wood, J. M., Busch, B., Pitts, B. J. R., and Schwartz, A. 1977. Inhibition of bovine heart Na^+,K^+-ATPase by palmityl carnitine and palmityl CoA. *Biochem. Biophys. Res. Commun.* 74:677–684.

Detection of Intracellular Anoxia and Its Relationship to Onset of Hemodynamic Dysfunction and ST-Segment Elevation in the Intact Dog Heart

D. W. Baron and C. E. Harrison

Cardiac Muscle Research Laboratory
Mayo Clinic and Mayo Foundation
Rochester, Minnesota 55905, USA

Abstract. The temporal relationships among onset of cellular anoxia after coronary artery occlusion, contractile dysfunction, and electrocardiographic ischemia were studied in dogs with an intact circulation. Nicotinamide adenine dinucleotide (NADH) fluorescence was used to detect intracellular anoxia, using a fiber-optic method. Paired NADH concentrations from ischemic (394 ± 10 µmol/g) and normoxic (285 ± 11 µmol/g) regions of the heart were obtained, and the differences ($\Delta[NADH]$) were correlated with compensated fluorescence ($r = 0.76$, $P < 0.01$). Onset of fluorescence occurred 1 to 2 sec after coronary artery occlusion, followed by hemodynamic (5 sec) and electrocardiographic (13 sec) changes. These data indicate that intracellular anoxia, with alterations in redox potential, is not synchronous with the onset of contractile failure and provide indirect support for intracellular acidosis as the likely mediator of contractile failure.

In 1935, Tennant and Wiggers (15) first described the onset of myocardial contraction abnormalities after coronary artery occlusion. The series of events whereby reduction in oxygen and substrate delivery leads to reduced myocardial contractility is unclear. During the early stages of ischemia, persistently normal levels of myocardial adenosine triphosphate (ATP) have been found (7,16), long after the onset of contractile dysfunction. Normal levels of creatine phosphate also have been found early after the onset of contractile failure (7), although the levels decline sharply shortly thereafter (1,10,16).

Based on known fluorometric patterns of nicotinamide adenine dinucleotide (NADH), Chance and Baltscheffsky (4), in 1958, using isolated mitochondria from the rat liver, first described NADH fluorescence as a means of monitoring tissue ischemia at the subcellular level. NADH is a coenzyme essentially localized to mitochondria which accumulates in anoxic conditions owing to failure of electron transport with the consequent failure of oxidative phosphorylation and production of high-energy phosphates (9).

To date, NADH fluorescence in various forms has been applied to the study of various tissues and organs, including liver, kidney, brain, skeletal muscle, and, more recently, the isolated heart. Fluorometry of the intact heart may provide a sensitive, continuous, real-time technique of monitoring the cardiac mitochondrial NAD–NADH redox levels and therefore the adequacy of high-energy phosphate production (3).

This study characterizes the temporal relationships among myocardial cell anoxia, ventricular hemodynamic dysfunction, and epicardial ST-segment elevation by analyzing NADH fluorescence in the in situ heart during regional ischemia.

MATERIALS AND METHODS

Experimental Model

Mongrel dogs (N = 12) weighing 10–12 kg were anesthetized with sodium pentobarbital, 30 mg/kg intravenously, and ventilated to maintain normal arterial pH and gases. The heart was exposed by a lateral thoracotomy and suspended in a pericardial cradle. The proximal anterior descending coronary artery was isolated and snared at a point 1 to 2 cm from its origin. Teflon® 14-gauge end-hole cannulas were used to record pressures directly from the right femoral artery, left atrium, and left ventricle. Cardiac output was measured in triplicate using the dye-dilution method. Regional myocardial blood flows (2) were measured using carbonized plastic 9-μm radiospheres of ^{85}Sr and ^{46}Sc before and during coronary artery constriction.

NADH Fluorescence

A trifurcated fiber-optic probe simultaneously recorded epicardial fluorescence (F), reflectance (R), and compensated fluorescence (CF) in millivolts (Figure 1). The technique, in which CF = kF − R (k being a correction coefficient), is similar to that described by Chance et al. (5). Briefly, fiber-optic bundles transmit excitation light of wavelength 366 ± 10 nm via a probe, which has a 4-mm field of view, positioned distal to the anterior descending coronary artery in an area of potential ischemia. Fiber-optic bundles randomly distributed with the probe transmit both reflectance light (λ 366 nm) and fluorescent light (λ 465 nm). In normoxic myocardium, compensated fluorescence is set at zero. Fluorescent peak readings were taken at 60 sec of occlusion, as this represented virtually 100% ischemia (Figure 2). Measurements were repeated at least six times. Paired NADH assays (12) were then performed from ischemic (underlying the light guide) and nonischemic myocardia. Increase in NADH concentration (Δ[NADH]) was defined as: Δ[NADH] = ischemic [NADH] − nonischemic [NADH].

RESULTS

During coronary artery ligation, myocardial blood flow decreased from 122 ± 12 (mean ± S.E.) to 7 ± 5 ml/min per 100 g tissue (Table 1). After

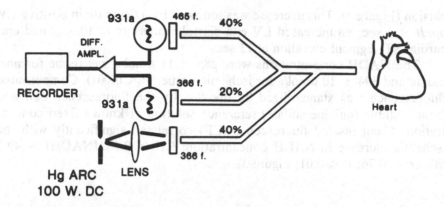

Figure 1.   Schematic diagram of the trifurcated compensated fluorometer. Excitation light is produced from a 100-watt direct-current mercury arc lamp and filtered (f) to obtain a wavelength of 366 nm. Forty percent of fiber-optic bundles conduct fluorescent light (465 nm) from the epicardial surface of the heart, and 20% reflected light (366 nm) to matched (931a) photomultiplier tubes.

coronary artery constriction, there was an average delay of 1.3 ± 0.1 sec before the onset of NADH fluorescence. Fluorescence increased exponentially, reaching half-maximum at 8.8 ± 0.5 sec, after which it increased slowly, with a 95% peak at 26.8 ± 1.6 sec and a constant plateau usually by 60 sec. Occlusion of the coronary artery repeated six times with adequate reperfusion intervals (approximately 2 to 3 min) demonstrated the reproducibility of the procedure (Figure 3). With release of the occlusion, fluorescence decreased rapidly, with half-maximal recovery at 15.3 ± 1.6 sec, and 98% recovery by 54.8 ± 2.9 sec.

The earliest significant hemodynamic change was in the negative LV dp/dt which decreased from control values 5 sec after coronary artery oc-

Table 1.   Resting (Control) and Ischemic Hemodynamics, Epicardial Blood Flow, ST-Segment Elevation, and Myocardial Blood Flow

Parameter	Control[a]	Ischemic[a]
Heart rate (beats/min)	158 ± 5	161 ± 5
Cardiac output (ml/min per kg)	162 ± 23	116 ± 12[b]
LV end-diastolic pressure (mm Hg)	4.2 ± 0.5	7.1 ± 0.6[b]
LV systolic pressure (mm Hg)	119 ± 7	110 ± 10[b]
LV dp/dt_{max} (mm Hg/sec)	1535 ± 81	1049 ± 70[b]
LV dp/dt_{min} (mm Hg/sec)	1635 ± 104	1066 ± 68[b]
ST-segment (mm)	1.0 ± 0.3	3.2 ± 0.6[b]
Myocardial blood flow (ml/min per 100 g)	122 ± 12	7 ± 5[b]

[a] Mean ± S.E. ($N = 12$).
[b] Significantly different from corresponding control value ($P < 0.05$).

clusion (Figure 4). This decrease was followed by a decrease in positive LV *dp/dt* at 7 sec, an increased LV end-diastolic pressure at 10 sec, and epicardial ST-segment elevation at 13 sec.

The NADH concentrations were 285 ± 11 μmol/g wet tissue for normoxic and 394 ± 10 μmol/g for ischemic tissue ($P < 0.001$). Compensated fluorescence was standardized by dividing by the fluorescence obtained from a stable (quinine sulfate) reference solution of known fixed concentration. Compensated fluorescence (CF) correlated significantly with the ischemic increase in NADH concentration: CF = 0.68Δ[NADH] + 49.2 mV ($r = 0.76$; $P < 0.01$; Figure 5).

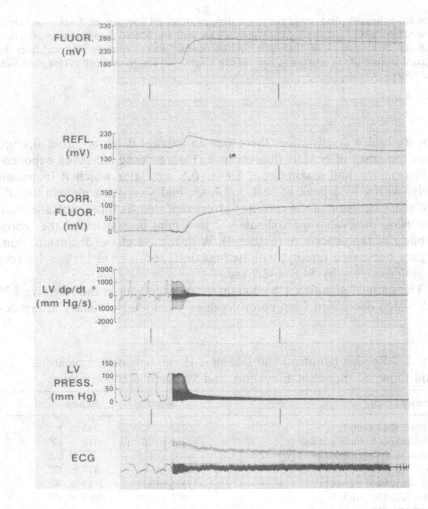

Figure 2.   Corrected myocardial fluorescence (third tracing) induced by lethal overdose of sodium pentobarbital. Onset of fluorescence is rapid, with plateau by 60 sec. Paper speed is 2 mm/sec.

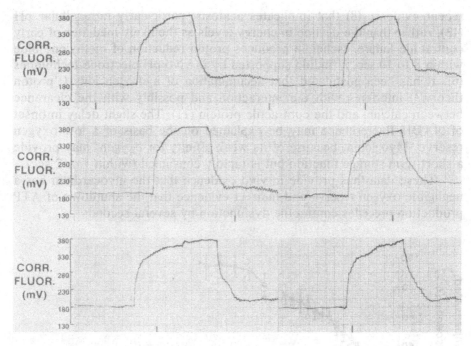

Figure 3.   Series of six sequential fluorescence traces from a dog during anterior descending coronary artery ligations with adequate (2 to 3 min) reperfusion intervals. Note similarity among trials in shape and peak of corrected fluorescence.

DISCUSSION

Myocardial ischemia produces a complex series of interrelated events, including altered glycolytic flux, inhibition of oxidative phosphorylation, inhibition of Krebs cycle and fatty acid oxidations, decreased glycogen stores, abnormal cation fluxes, and tissue acidosis. However, the relationship of these events to the cause of contractile failure is unclear. By its characteristic fluorescent responses to ultraviolet light, NADH provides a sensitive index of the mitochondrial redox potential (14). More than 90% of the oxygen consumption by mammalian tissues occurs via cytochrome a_3 at the terminal end of the electron transport system (9), so that, theoretically at least, the state of the redox potential should provide a reliable indirect assessment of the phosphorylative activity within the mitochondrion. Myocardial NADH fluorescence is responsive to oxygen tension that is less than 0.07 mm Hg (3). As oxygen concentration decreases from 10^{-7} to 10^{-8} M, NAD converts from being 80% oxidized to 70% reduced.

The data indicate that NADH fluorescence afforded the earliest evidence of tissue anoxia, within 1 to 2 sec after coronary artery occlusion. The onset of hemodynamic dysfunction, evidenced by decreased LV *dp/dt* and increased LV end-diastolic pressure, occurred 5 to 10 sec later, followed by epicardial ST-segment elevation at 13 sec. This is in agreement with recent evidence (8) that implicates acidosis, particularly intracellular pH (13), rather than the decline in energy levels as the likely mediator of early contractile failure. Ischemia produces proton reduction of methylene blue within 8 to 10 sec, a finding supported by in vivo pH electrode techniques (6). It has been postulated that accumulation of hydrogen ions ("proton theory") interferes with the interaction and possibly with the clearance between calcium and the contractile protein (11). The slight delay in onset of NADH fluorescence may be explained on the basis of a low oxygen reserve. Myoglobin, because of its weak affinity for oxygen, may provide a short-term storage function but is rapidly consumed (within 1 or 2 sec).

These data thus provide in vivo evidence that the myocardium has a negligible oxygen reserve and indirect evidence that the shutdown of ATP production precedes contractile dysfunction by several seconds.

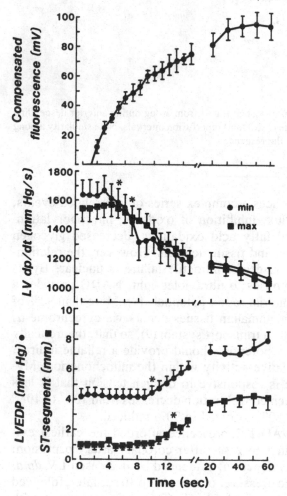

Figure 4. Relationships among compensated fluorescence, LV *dp/dt*, LV end-diastolic pressure, and epicardial ST-segment during 60-sec coronary artery occlusion. Onset of occlusion is at time zero. Values are means ± S.E. Significant (*P* < 0.05) difference from control indicated by asterisk.

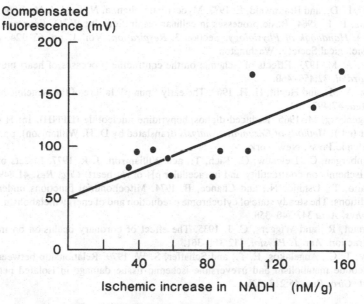

Figure 5. Relationship between compensated fluorescence and increase in NADH concentration during myocardial ischemia ($r = +0.76$).

ACKNOWLEDGMENTS

The authors gratefully acknowledge the technical assistance of Jerry D. Dewey, B.S. This investigation was supported in part by Research Grant HL-12997 from the National Institutes of Health, U.S. Public Health Service.

REFERENCES

1. Braasch, W., Gudbjarnason, S., Puri, P. S., Ravens, K. G., and Bing, R. J. 1968. Early changes in energy metabolism in the myocardium following acute coronary artery occlusion in anesthetized dogs. *Circ. Res.* 23:429–438.
2. Buckberg, G. D., Luck, J. C., Payne, D. B., Hoffman, J. I. E., Archie, J. P., and Fixler, D. E. 1971. Some sources of error in measuring regional blood flow with radioactive microspheres. *J. Appl. Physiol.* 31:598–604.
3. Chance, B. 1976. Pyridine nucleotide as an indicator of the oxygen requirements for energy-linked functions of mitochondria. *Circ. Res.* 38(Suppl. 1):31–38.
4. Chance, B., and Baltscheffsky, H. 1958. Respiratory enzymes in oxidative phosphorylation. VII. Binding of intramitochondrial reduced pyridine nucleotide. *J. Biol. Chem.* 233:736–739.
5. Chance, B., Legallis, V., Sorge, J., and Graham, N. 1975. A versatile time-sharing multichannel spectrophotometer, reflectometer, and fluorometer. *Anal. Biochem.* 66:498–514.
6. Cobbe, S. M., and Poole-Wilson, P. A. 1979. Onset and severity of tissue acidosis in myocardial ischemia and hypoxia. *Circulation* 60(Suppl. 2):11.
7. Covell, J. W., Pool, P. E., and Braunwald, E. 1967. Effects of acutely induced ischemic heart failure on myocardial high energy phosphate stores. *Proc. Soc. Exp. Biol. Med.* 124:126–131.

8. Hillis, L. D., and Braunwald, E. 1977. Myocardial ischemia. *N. Engl. J. Med.* 296:971–978.
9. Jöbsis, F. F. 1964. Basic processes in cellular respiration. In: W. O. Fenn and H. Rahn (eds.), *Handbook of Physiology*. Section 3: *Respiration*, Vol. 1, pp. 63–124. American Physiological Society, Washington.
10. Katz, A. M. 1973. Effects of ischemia on the contractile processes of heart muscle. *Am. J. Cardiol.* 32:456–460.
11. Katz, A. M., and Hecht, H. H. 1969. The early "pump" failure of the ischemic heart. *Am. J. Med.* 47:497–502.
12. Klingenberg, M. 1965. Reduced diphosphopyridine nucleotide (DPNH). In: H.-U. Bergmyer (ed.), *Methods of Enzymatic Analysis* (translated by D. H. Williamson), pp. 531–534. Academic Press, New York.
13. Steenbergen, C., Deleeuw, G., Rich, T., and Williamson, J. R. 1977. Effects of acidosis and ischemia on contractility and intracellular pH of rat heart. *Circ. Res.* 41:849–858.
14. Sugano, T., Oshino, N., and Chance, B. 1974. Mitochondrial functions under hypoxic conditions: The steady state of cytochrome c reduction and of energy metabolism. *Biochim. Biophys. Acta* 347:340–358.
15. Tennant, R., and Wiggers, C. J. 1935. The effect of coronary occlusion on myocardial contraction. *Am. J. Physiol.* 112:351–361.
16. Vary, T. C., Angelakos, E. T., and Schaffer, S. W. 1979. Relationship between adenine nucleotide metabolism and irreversible ischemic tissue damage in isolated perfused rat heart. *Circ. Res.* 45:218–225.

The Relationship between Glucose Utilization during Ischemia and Ventricular Fibrillation during Early Reperfusion

Evidence for Two Populations of Guinea Pig Hearts

S. C. Dennis,* D. J. Hearse, and D. J. Coltart

The Myocardial Metabolism and Cardiac Pharmacology Units
The Rayne Institute
St. Thomas' Hospital
London, England

Abstract. Guinea pig hearts perfused in the presence of 9 mM glucose were subjected to 30 min of ischemia (coronary flow reduced to 6%) and were then reperfused. During reperfusion, 18 of the 34 hearts studied (first subgroup) exhibited irreversible ventricular fibrillation. The remaining 16 hearts (second subgroup) exhibited serious rhythm disturbances but did not fibrillate. Attempts to identify critical factors that might precipitate fibrillation led to an observation that hearts that fibrillated during reperfusion were characterized by low rates of glucose utilization (0.6 ± 0.8 μmol/min per g dry wt. and low lactate plus pyruvate production (2.5 ± 0.32 μmol/min per g dry wt.) during ischemia. In addition, these hearts had a low calculated cytplasmic ATP-to-ADP ratio (10.0) and low residential glycogen levels (55 ± 7.0 μmol glucose equivalents/g dry wt.) at the end of the ischemic period. In contrast, in hearts that did not fibrillate (group 2), glucose utilization (2.5 ± 0.12 μmol/min per g dry wt.) was higher, lactate plus pyruvate production was higher (7.4 ± 0.03 μmol/min per g dry wt.), cytoplasmic ATP-to-ADP ratio was higher (36.0), and residual glycogen levels were higher (163 ± 23 μmol glucose equivalents/g dry wt.). Thus, two distinct populations of guinea pig hearts were apparent, and comparison between the two groups indicated an association among glucose utilization, cytoplasmic energy status, and myocardial electrical stability.

There have been a number of studies involving manipulation of patterns of substrate utilization that support the thesis that there is an inverse relationship between glycolytic flux and ischemic injury. Thus, for example, glucose has been shown to reduce ischemic damage (2,3,16,17,24) and the incidence of postischemic reperfusion arrhythmias (2–4,15,21,23,24). To explain this effect, it has been proposed that ATP, produced in the cytoplasm from glycolysis, may play some special role in the maintenance of cellular membrane integrity and function (2,3,15,16). In the study detailed below, glucose utilization and myocardial cytoplasmic energy status during ischemia have

* Present address: The Likoff Cardiovascular Institute, The Hahnemann Medical College, Philadelphia, Pennsylvania 19102, U.S.A.

458   S. C. Dennis et al.

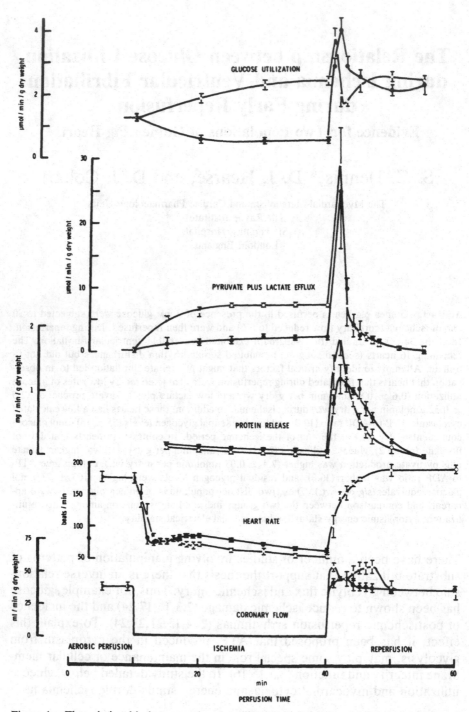

Figure 1. The relationship between glucose utilization during ischemia and the incidence of ventricular fibrillation during reperfusion. Hearts were subjected to aerobic perfusion, ischemia, and reperfusion as shown in the figure and detailed in the text. Heart rate and cardiac rhythm

been investigated in relation to the incidence of ventricular fibrillation during early reperfusion.

MATERIALS AND METHODS

Hearts (1.5–2.2 g wet wt.) from male guinea pigs (350–500 g) of the Duncan Hartley strain were subjected to a 10-min period of aerobic Langendorff perfusion (11) at 37°C with a modified (6) Krebs–Henseleit bicarbonate buffer containing 8 mM [5-³H]glucose. Tritium-labeled glucose was present to permit the measurement (20) of glucose utilization. During this period of aerobic perfusion, coronary flow was 6.6 ± 0.4 ml/min per g wet wt. The hearts were then made ischemic for 30 min. This was accomplished by reducing coronary flow to 0.37 ± 0.01 ml/min per g wet wt. To insure adequate temperature control and oxygenation during this period of low-flow perfusion, the fluid was oxygenated via a hollow fiber membrane oxygenator which was attached directly to a thermostatically controlled (37°C) aortic cannula (13). At the end of the ischemic period, coronary flow was restored to its previous level for 20 min during which time cardiac rhythm was monitored, and disturbances of rhythm were quantitated (5,7).

In some experiments, hearts were freeze-clamped either just before or at the end of the ischemic period. Measurements of creatine phosphate, ATP, ADP, AMP, and glycogen were made using conventional spectrophotometric enzymatic assays (1). Adenine nucleotide compartmentation was calculated using the creatine phosphokinase equilibrium constant of 10^2 at a free 0.5 mM Mg^{2+} and 22% of the adenine nucleotides in the mitochondrial space.

Results presented are means and standard errors. Statistical significance of differences was assessed using the nonpaired Student's t-test as a correction for unequal variances.

RESULTS

Thirty-four hearts were studied, and we were interested to observe that the results fell into two distinct groups. Thus, during the reperfusion period, 18 hearts (first subgroup, represented as closed circles in Figure 1) fibrillated. The remaining 16 hearts (second subgroup, represented as open circles in Figure 1), although exhibiting serious disturbances of rhythm (25 ± 2.3

---

were monitored (5,7), and, in aliquots of coronary effluent, measurements (8) were made of protein release, pyruvate plus lactate efflux (1), and glucose utilization (20). The results shown are the means and standard errors of values obtained from 18 hearts that fibrillated (●—●, group 1) during reflow and from 16 hearts that did not fibrillate during reperfusion (○—○, group 2)

rhythm disturbance units), did not fibrillate at any time during the reperfusion period. In an attempt to distinguish between these two groups and identify any critical factors that might precipitate ventricular fibrillation, a number of comparisons were made between the two groups. It was clear that the occurrence of ventricular fibrillation was not explicable in terms of sex, weight, age, source of the animals, or diet. Furthermore, during aerobic perfusion and ischemia, heart rates (Figure 1) in the two groups did not differ significantly ($P > 0.05$). Similarly, the occurrence of ventricular fibrillation could not be attributed to differing degrees of ischemic injury, since protein leakage (Figure 1), which can be equated with enzyme leakage (8) during ischemia and reperfusion, was essentially the same in both groups. Thus, during the 20-min reperfusion period, the total protein leakage was 7.6 ± 0.6 mg/g dry wt. in the first group and 6.8 ± 1.0 mg/g dry wt. in the second group.

Striking differences ($P < 0.001$), however, were apparent at the metabolic level, in the anaerobic energy-producing capacity of the hearts. Hearts that fibrillated during reperfusion (closed circles in Figure 1) were characterized by low rates of glucose utilization (0.6 ± 0.08 μmol/min per g dry wt.) and low lactate plus pyruvate production (2.5 ± 0.32 μmol/min per g dry wt.) during the preceding ischemic period. In contrast, hearts that did not fibrillate (open circles in Figure 1) had high rates of glucose utilization and lactate plus pyruvate production (2.5 ± 0.12 and 7.4 ± 0.03 μmol/min/ g dry wt., respectively). Thus, two distinct populations were apparent: those in which glucose utilization during ischemia declined to almost half that observed during the preceding aerobic period—these hearts fibrillated during reperfusion—and those in which anaerobic energy production was almost doubled during ischemia—these hearts did not fibrillate during reperfusion.

Further investigating a possible association between the capacity for glucose utilization during ischemia and the incidence of fibrillation during reperfusion, we repeated the experiments, but this time the hearts were freeze-clamped either immediately prior to or at the end of the ischemic period. The frozen tissue was taken for measurements (1) of creatine, creatine phosphate, ATP, ADP, AMP, and glycogen. The results were then used to establish the energy status of the myocardium at the time of sampling. It was revealed (Table 1) that in both groups cellular energy production during ischemia was unable to meet cellular energy requirements. Creatine phosphate-to-creatine and ATP-to-ADP ratios fell, glycogen was depleted, and there was a similar decline in both groups in the total tissue content of creatine plus creatine phosphate (18% reduction) and ATP plus ADP plus AMP (40% reduction).

Despite the similarities between the two groups, marked differences were also apparent, particularly in relation to the degree of glycogen depletion and the extent of decline in the ratios of whole-cell creatine phosphate to creatine and ATP and ADP. Thus, in group 1 hearts during ischemia,

Table 1.   The Relationship between Anaerobic Energy Production and Ischemic Tissue Energy Status[a]

	Metabolite levels (μmol/g dry weight)			
	Aerobic control hearts (6)	Ischemic group 1 hearts (5)	Ischemic group 2 hearts (5)	P[b]
Creatine phosphate	54 ± 2.6	11 ± 0.5	28 ± 1.9	<0.001
Creatine	79 ± 5.9	109 ± 8.5	77 ± 3.2	<0.01
Creatine phosphate/creatine	0.7 ± 0.03	0.1 ± 0.01	0.4 ± 0.02	<0.001
ATP	36 ± 1.4	16 ± 1.3	21 ± 1.1	<0.02
Mitochondrial	1.5	0.4	0.9	
Cytoplasmic	34.5	15.6	20.1	
ADP	8.6 ± 0.4	6.1 ± 0.7	5.5 ± 0.3	NS
Mitochondrial	8.1	4.5	4.9	
Cytoplasmic	0.5	1.6	0.6	
AMP	2.0 ± 0.1	4.4 ± 0.2	2.1 ± 0.2	<0.001
ATP/ADP	4.2 ± 0.2	2.5 ± 0.2	3.9 ± 0.2	<0.001
Mitochondrial	0.2	0.1	0.2	
Cytoplasmic	69	10	36	
Glycogen (glucose equivalents)	215 ± 14	55 ± 7.0	163 ± 23	<0.001

[a] Experimental conditions were as described in the text. Metabolite levels determined in hearts freeze-clamped either just prior to ischemia (aerobic control hearts) or at the end of ischemia (ischemic hearts) are the means and standard errors of the results from a number (shown in parentheses) of hearts. Ischemic hearts were subdivided into groups 1 and 2 on the basis of whether glucose utilization [measured (20) as ^3H_2O release from 8 mM [5-^{3}H]glucose, 0.02 μCi/μmol] declined (group 1) or accelerated (group 2) during ischemia. Adenine nucleotide compartmentation was calculated using the creatine phosphokinase equilibrium constant 10^2 at a free 0.5 mM Mg^{2+} concentration, pH 7.0 (25), and 22% of the adenine nucleotides in the mitochondrial space (12).
[b] Statistical significance (nonpaired Student's t-test) of the difference between groups 1 and 2.

glycogen levels fell from 215 ± 14 to 55 ± 7.0 μmol glucose equivalents/g dry wt., and the ratios of creatine phosphate to creatine and ATP to ADP declined from 0.7 ± 0.03 and 4.2 ± 0.2 to 0.1 ± 0.01 and 2.5 ± 0.2, respectively, whereas in group 2 hearts high rates of anaerobic energy production from glucose during ischemia maintained higher levels of glycogen (163 ± 23 μmol glucose equivalents/g dry wt.), possibly as a consequence of glucose-6-phosphate inhibition of phosphorylase b (14) and high ratios of creatine phosphate to creatine and ATP to ADP (0.4 ± 0.02 and 3.9 ± 0.2, respectively).

In addition to providing the above assessments of myocardial energy status based on whole-cell data, the metabolic measurements were also used to calculate the distribution of adenine nucleotides in the cytoplasmic and mitochondrial compartments. This was felt to be important for a number of reasons. First, whereas creatine and creatine phosphate are essentially restricted to the cytoplasmic space, 20% of the total adenine nucleotide content of the heart is mitochondrial (12). Second, because of the electrogenic nature of the adenine nucleotide translocase, extramitochondrial ATP-to-ADP ratios are considerably greater than the intramitochondrial ATP-to-ADP ratios (25). Therefore, in order to avoid error in interpretation introduced when there is a large concentration gradient across the mitochondrial membrane, and because we were interested in electrophysiological events that may be influenced by ATP availability in the cytoplasm, the phosphorylation state of adenine nucleotides in this compartment was estimated using the creatine phosphokinase equilibrium (Table 1). In hearts in which glucose utilization was high during ischemia (group 2), the cytoplasmic ATP-to-ADP ratio of 36 was almost fourfold higher than the value of 10 calculated in group 1. The results may thus indicate that the association between glucose utilization and myocardial electrical stability might involve or reflect some aspect of the cytoplasmic energy status and thus provide support for the proposition (2,3,15,16,18) that ATP produced from glycolytic flux may play some special role in the maintenance of membrane function.

DISCUSSION

In addition to seeking to explain an association between cytoplasmic energy status and electrical instability, we also felt it to be important to question why some hearts had a low status during ischemia and why the segregation between the groups was so sharp. With reference to the last point, it has been our increasing impression that in a number of species hearts often fall into two distinct groups. Thus, in 1976, Hearse et al. (9), studying the ability of glucose to protect the anoxic myocardium, reported two distinct populations of rabbit hearts—those that appeared to be resistant to anoxia and those that exhibited early and extensive biochemical and ultrastructural injury. The latter group were characterized by a low glycolytic capacity. More recently, a reassessment (D. J. Hearse, unpublished observations) of several hundred rat heart perfusion studies has indicated that postischemic or postanoxic functional recoveries very often fall into two clearly defined groups—those that recover well and those that fail to recover; rarely are intermediate recoveries observed. Thus, in three species, a bimodal response has been observed, and in each instance there was some association between the response and glycolytic activity.

In view of the possible connection between anaerobic energy production capacity and the appearance of two groups, we have examined the results of our guinea pig heart studies in order to compare the capacity for glycolytic flux in the two groups in terms of the input to and the output from the glycolytic pathway. Thus, in group 2 hearts (where glucose utilization was increased during ischemia), net glucose utilization during the 30 min of ischemia was calculated to be 119 μmol glucose/g dry wt., this figure being derived from 52 μmol glucose equivalents from glycogen degradation plus 67 μmol glucose from the perfusate. This value accounted almost exactly for the total production of lactate and pyruvate (245 μmol/g dry wt.). In groups 1 hearts (where glucose utilization declined during ischemia), this equation did not balance. Increased glycogen utilization (160 μmol glucose equivalents/30 min per g dry wt.), which more than compensated for reduced glucose utilization (18 μmol/30 min per g dry wt.), created a net input into glycolysis of 178 μmol/30 min per g dry wt. Output from glycolysis (lactate plus pyruvate efflux), however, was only 70 μmol/30 min per g dry wt. Since both the release of end products of glycolysis and the generation of cytoplasmic high-energy phosphate were depressed in these hearts, it must be presumed that some rate-limiting step exists in this subgroup of hearts in the metabolic sequence of the glycolytic pathway.

To substantiate such an impression, the activities of all of the glycolytic enzymes and the levels of their reactants in the two subgroups would need to be compared. Such a study might reveal an altered activity of one or more of the glycolytic enzymes which could account for the intraspecies variation in anaerobic energy production capacity. Although such a proposition is clearly highly speculative, enzyme-based individual-to-individual variations of this type are by no means uncommon (10) and often have a genetic basis. We are currently considering this possibility which, if proven, could shed new light on the study of hereditary factors in human susceptibility to ischemic heart disease (19,22).

ACKNOWLEDGMENTS

This work was supported in part by grants from the British Heart Foundation, the St. Thomas' Hospital Research Endowment Fund, and Stuart Pharmaceuticals.

REFERENCES

1. Bergmeyer, H. U. 1965. *Methods of Enzymatic Analysis*. Academic Press, New York.
2. Bricknell, O. L., and Opie, L. H. 1978. Effect of substrates on tissue metabolic changes in the isolated rat heart during underperfusion and on release of lactate dehydrogenase and arrhythmias during reperfusion. *Circ. Res.* 43:102–115.
3. Bricknell, O. L., and Opie, L. H. 1978. Glycolytic ATP and its production during ischaemia in isolated Langendorff-perfused rat hearts. In: T. Kobayashi, T. Sano, and N. S. Dhalla (eds.), *Recent Advances in Studies on Cardiac Structure and Metabolism*. Vol. 11: *Heart Function and Metabollism*, pp. 509–518. University Park Press, Baltimore.
4. Dennis, S. C., Hearse, D. J., and Coltart, D. J. 1979. Reperfusion arrhythmias: The role of glycolysis. *J. Mol. Cell. Cardiol.* 11(Suppl. 2):10.
5. Dennis, S. C., Hearse, D. J., and Coltart, D. J. 1980. Quantitation of ventricular arrhythmias. *Eur. J. Cardiol.* 12:15–23.
6. Dennis, S. C., Manning, A. S., Hearse, D. J., and Coltart, D. J. 1980. Myocardial electrical instability after abrupt withdrawal of long-term administration of propranolol to guinea-pigs. *Clin. Sci.* 59:207–209.
7. Dennis, S. C., Stoate, M. W., and Waldron, C. B. 1979. A technique for quantitation of cardiac arrhythmias. *J. Physiol.* (*Lond.*) 293:2–3.
8. Hearse, D. J., and Baker, J. E. 1980. Verapamil and the calcium paradox. *J. Mol. Cell. Cardiol.* 12:733–739.

464   S. C. Dennis et al.

9. Hearse, D. J., Humphrey, S. M., Feuvray, D., and De Leiris, J. 1976. A biochemical and ultrastructural study of the species variation in myocardial cell damage. *J. Mol. Cell. Cardiol.* 8:759–778.
10. La Du, B. N. 1971. Genetic factors modifying drug metabolism and drug response. In: B. N. La Du (ed.), *Fundamentals of Drug Metabolism and Drug Disposition,* p. 308. Williams & Wilkins, Baltimore.
11. Langendorff, O. 1895. Untersuchungen am uber lebenden Saugethier Herzen. *Pfluegers Arch.* 61:291–332.
12. La Noue, K. F., Bryla, J., and Williamson, J. R. 1972. Feedback interactions in the control of citric acid cycle activity in rat heart mitochondria. *J. Biol. Chem.* 247:667–679.
13. Manning, A. S., Hearse, D. J., Dennis, S. C., Bullock, G. R., and Coltart, D. J. 1980. Myocardial ischaemia: An isolated, globally perfused rat heart model for metabolic and pharmacological studies. *Eur. J. Cardiol.* 11:1–21.
14. Morgan, H. E., and Parmeggiani, A. 1964. Regulation of glycogenolysis in muscle. III: Control of glycogen phosphorylase activity. *J. Biol. Chem.* 239:2440–2445.
15. Opie, L. H. 1976. Glycolysis and electrogenesis. *Am. J. Cardiol.* 38:388–400.
16. Opie, L. H., and Bricknell, O. L. 1979. Role of glycolytic flux in effect of glucose in decreasing fatty acid induced release of lactate dehydrogenase from isolated coronary ligated rat heart. *Cardiovasc. Res.* 13:693–702.
17. Opie, L. H., and De Leiris, J. 1979. Metabolic manipulations: Tissue damage and enzyme leakage. In: D. J. Hearse and J. De Leiris (eds.), *Enzymes in Cardiology Diagnosis and Research,* pp. 481–502. John Wiley & Sons, New York.
18. Opie, L. H., Nathan, D., and Lubbe, W. F. 1979. Biochemical aspects of arrhythmogenesis and ventricular fibrillation. *Am. J. Cardiol.* 43:131–148.
19. Rose, G. 1964. Familial patterns in ischaemic heart diease. *Br. J. Prev. Soc. Med.* 18:75–80.
20. Rovetto, M. J., Lamberton, W. F., and Neely, J. R. 1975. Mechanisms of glycolytic inhibition in ischaemic rat hearts. *Circ. Res.* 37:742–751.
21. Russel, D. C., and Oliver, M. F. 1979. Effect of intravenous glucose on ventricular vulnerability following acute coronary artery occlusion in the dog. *J. Mol. Cell. Cardiol.* 11:31–44.
22. Slack, J., and Evans, K. A. 1966. The increased risk of death from ischaemic heart disease in first degree relatives of 121 men and 96 women with ischaemic heart disease. *J. Med. Genet.* 3:239–257.
23. Surer, J. R., Urshcel, C. W., Sonnenblick, E. G., and La Raia, P. J. 1976. Experimental myocardial ischaemia. III: Protective effect of glucose on myocardial function. *J. Mol. Cell. Cardiol.* 8:521–531.
24. Willebrands, A. F., Tasseron, S. J. A., ter Welle, H. F., and Van Dam, T. R. 1976. Effects of oleic acid and oxygen restriction followed by reoxygenation on rhythm and contractile activity of the isolated rat heart: Protective action of glucose. *J. Mol. Cell. Cardiol.* 8:375–388.
25. Williamson, J. R., Ford, C., Illingworth, J., and Safer, B. 1976. Co-ordination of citric acid cycle activity with electron transport flux. *Circ. Res.* 38(Suppl. 1):39–51.

Correlation among Water Content, Left Ventricular Function, Coronary Blood Flow, and Myocardial Metabolism after Hypothermic Ischemic Cardiac Arrest

J. Amano, M. Sunamori, T. Kameda, T. Okamura, and A. Suzuki

Department of Cardiothoracic Surgery
Juntendo University School of Medicine
Tokyo, Japan

Abstract. Subendocardial ischemia is a common cause of death following ischemic cardiac arrest. We studied relationships among myocardial water content (WC), left ventricular function, coronary blood flow, and myocardial metabolism following ischemic cardiac arrest. Under cardiopulmonary bypass with hypothermia, 120 min of aortic occlusion was employed, and myocardial temperature was kept around 20°C in 10 mongrel dogs. Left ventricular function (peak LVP, max dp/dt, LVEDP, LVSWI), coronary blood flow, myocardial enzymes (m-GOT, total CPK, MB-CPK), myocardial ATP and creatine phosphate (CP), and WC of the subendocardium of the left ventricle were measured. Data were obtained in the control state and immediately and 30 and 60 min after aortic unclamping. Significant negative correlations were obtained between WC and max dp/dt ($r = -0.8384$), coronary blood flow ($r = -0.9928$), ATP ($r = -0.7038$), and CP ($r = -0.7835$). Significant positive correlations were obtained between WC and LVEDP ($r = 0.7525$), m-GOT ($r = 0.7638$), and total CPK ($r = 0.7079$). These data suggest that myocardial edema results in depression of left ventricular function and metabolism.

Myocardial edema is not uncommon subsequent to cardiopulmonary bypass by the currently used methods (1–3,5,6,11). It is known that an increase in myocardial edema resulting from shock or anoxia is responsible for depression of cardiac function (7,8,12). We have already demonstrated that myocardial edema is sometimes a cause of subendocardial ischemia subsequent to ischemic cardioplegia and is linked to the no-reflow phenomenon (10). Accumulated evidence regarding myocardial edema suggests that a disturbance in myocardial flow distribution as a result of edema may be related to recovery of cardiac function and metabolism following ischemic cardioplegia (10,13). Thus, this study was undertaken to characterize the relationships of water content to left ventricular function, coronary blood flow, and myocardial metabolism following 2 hr of ischemic cardiac arrest under hypothermia.

465

MATERIALS AND METHODS

Ten mongrel dogs were used in this investigation. All dogs were anesthetized with sodium pentobarbital, 30 mg/kg, and respiration was controlled by a positive-pressure ventilator with oxygen supplement to maintain arterial oxygen pressure about 100 mm Hg. Left thoracotomy was performed for exposure of the heart. Arterial pressure, left ventricular pressure, and electrocardiogram were recorded using pressure transducers and a polygraph. Cardiac output was measured by a thermodilution method using a Swan–Ganz catheter. Coronary blood flow was measured at the proximal portion of the left anterior descending coronary artery and at the left circumflex coronary artery by electromagnetic flow meters. A coronary sinus catheter was inserted via the left external jugular vein for sampling of coronary venous blood.

Cardiopulmonary bypass was instituted at a flow rate of 80 ml/kg per min with left femoral arterial cannulation and right atrial venous cannulation. The pump oxygenator was primed with 1000 ml canine blood, 200 ml of mannitol, and 60 ml of 7% sodium bicarbonate. Moderate hemodilution to a hematocrit around 25% was employed.

Systemic hypothermia was employed using a heat exchanger. The aorta was cross clamped when myocardial temperature reached 20°C, and the same temperature was maintained during global ischemia of the heart.

After 2 hr of ischemia, the aorta was unclamped and rewarmed about 15 min to reach a 36°C myocardial temperature. Defibrillation was done at 34–36°C of myocardial temperature, and cardiopulmonary bypass was weaned when esophageal temperature reached 36°C.

Hemodynamic parameters such as arterial pressure, left ventricular pressure, left ventricular end-diastolic pressure, left ventricular max dp/dt, cardiac output, and coronary blood flow were measured before cardiopulmonary bypass and 30 and 60 min after unclamping of the aorta.

At the end of the experiment, after 60 min following unclamping, endocardium of the left ventricle was excised for measurement of tissue high-energy phosphate such as adenosine triphosphate (ATP) and creatine phosphate (CP) by Bergmeyer's method.

The left ventricular endocardium was dried in the oven at 180°C for 4 hr immediately after excision. The water content was calculated by the following formula and expressed as a percentage of the wet weight.

$$\left(\frac{\text{Wet weight} - \text{dry weight}}{\text{Wet weight}} \right) \times 100$$

Coronary sinus blood was withdrawn for measuring serum creatine phosphokinase (CPK) activity and mitochondrial glutamic oxaloacetic transaminase (m-GOT) activity in the control period, immediately after unclamping, and 60 min following unclamping. Serum CPK was measured by a UV method, and CPK isozyme was measured by immunoelectrophoresis. Serum m-GOT was measured by a column UV method.

RESULTS

Hemodynamically, peak left ventricular pressure, left ventricular end-diastolic pressure, left ventricular max dp/dt, and left ventricular stroke work index are significantly depressed during reperfusion. Coronary blood flow decreased significantly at 30 min of the reperfusion period ($P < 0.05$) and returned to control level at 60 min of reperfusion (Table 1).

Myocardial enzymes such as total CPK, MB-CPK, and m-GOT in the coronary sinus blood increased after unclamping. Serum m-GOT level increased significantly from control level (8.78 ± 1.88 Karmen U) to 23.65 ± 4.74 ($P < 0.01$) at 30 min of reperfusion and to 33.17 ± 5.28 ($P < 0.01$) at 60 min of reperfusion.

Myocardial ATP and CP were 2.279 ± 0.182 μmol/g and 0.4632 ± 0.0776 μmol/g, respectively, after 60 min of reperfusion. The water content of the left ventricular endocardium was 82.3 ± 0.77%.

From these data, the following correlations were drawn concerning 60 min of reperfusion.

Table 1. Correlations between Water Content and Various Parameters

Parameter[a]	r	Significance
Hemodynamics		
Peak LVP	−0.5760	n.s.
LVEDP	0.7525	$P < 0.05$
LV max dp/dt	−0.8384	$P < 0.05$
LVSWI	−0.3581	n.s.
CBF	−0.9928	$P < 0.001$
Myocardial enzymes		
Total CPK	0.7079	$P < 0.05$
MB-CPK	0.0665	n.s.
m-GOT	0.7638	$P < 0.05$
High-energy phosphate		
ATP	−0.7038	$P < 0.01$
CP	−0.7835	$P < 0.02$

[a] Peak LVP, peak left ventricular pressure; LVEDP, left ventricular end-diastolic pressure; LV max dp/dt, left ventricular maximal rate of rise of pressure; LVSWI, left ventricular stroke work index; CBF, coronary blood flow; ATP, adenosine triphosphate; CP, creatine phosphate; n.s., not significant.

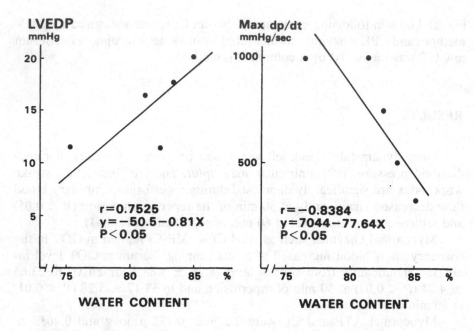

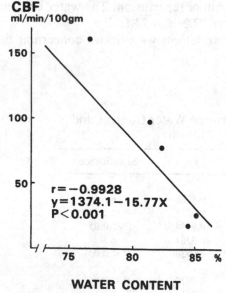

Figure 1. Correlation between water content and left ventricular end-diastolic pressure (LVEDP), left ventricular maximal rate of rise of pressure (max *dp/dt*), and coronary blood flow (CBF).

Hemodynamics

Water content was correlated with LVEDP [correlation coefficient *r* = 0.7525 (*P* < 0.05), and *Y* = −50.5 − 0.81*X* (*N* = 5)] (Figure 1). Also, water content was correlated with LV max *dp/dt* [correlation coefficient *r* = −0.8384 (*P* < 0.05), and *Y* = 7044 − 77.64*X* (*N* = 5)] (Figure 1). However, there was a poor correlation between water content and peak LVP (*r* = −0.5760) as well as LVSWI (*r* = −0.3581).

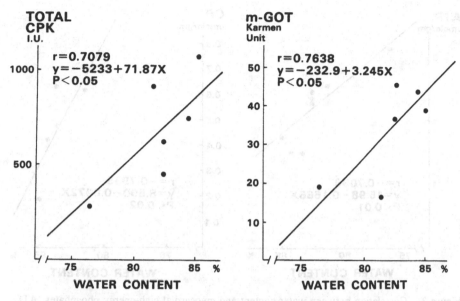

Figure 2.   Correlation between water content and myocardial enzymes in the coronary sinus blood. CPK, creatine phosphokinase; m-GOT, mitochondrial glutamic oxaloacetic transaminase.

Coronary Blood Flow

Coronary blood flow showed a negative correlation with water content at 60 min of reperfusion [correlation coefficient $r = -0.9923$ ($P < 0.001$), and $Y = 1374.1 - 15.77X$ ($N = 5$)] (Figure 1).

Myocardial Enzymes

Water content showed a positive correlation to total CPK at 60 min of reperfusion [correlation coefficient $r = 0.7079$ ($P < 0.05$), and $Y = -5233 + 71.87X$ ($N = 6$)] (Figure 2).

There was also the same positive correlation between water content and m-GOT [correlation coefficient $r = 0.7638$ ($P < 0.05$), and $Y = -232.9 \pm 3.245X$ ($N = 6$)] (Figure 2).

However, no significant correlation was demonstrated between water content and MB-CPK ($r = 0.0665$).

Myocardial High-Energy Phosphate

Water content was correlated to myocardial ATP [correlation coefficient $r = -0.7038$ ($P < 0.01$), and $Y = 15.98 - 0.1665X$ ($N = 9$)] (Figure 3). Also, water content was correlated to myocardial CP [correlation coefficient $r = -0.7835$ ($P < 0.02$), and $Y = 8.590 - 0.0972X$ ($N = 5$)] (Figure 3).

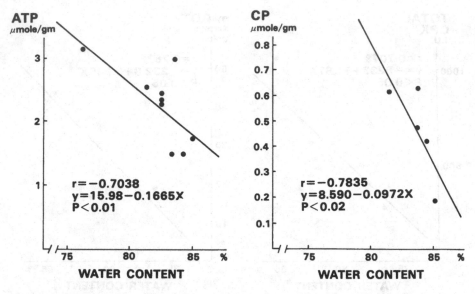

Figure 3.   Correlation between water content and myocardial high-energy phosphates. ATP, adenosine triphosphate; CP, creatine phosphate.

DISCUSSION

This study appraised the significant increment of myocardial edema in the endocardium of the left ventricle following ischemic cardioplegia associated with hypothermia. Furthermore, it is clearly demonstrated that the water content of the endocardium after 2 hr of ischemia under hypothermia and 60 min of reperfusion showed a positive correlation to LVEDP, m-GOT, and total CPK but, in contrast, showed a negative correlation to left ventricular max dp/dt, adenosine triphosphate, creatine phosphate, and coronary blood flow.

Myocardial edema associated with ischemic cardioplegia reflects intracellular and extracellular fluid retension (4,5,7,10). If normal metabolic processes are restored in reversible tissue after ischemic injury, swollen cells and increased interstitial edema, which may occur in the reperfusion period, will return to normal (7). But once myocardium is severely damaged, swollen myocordial cells and increased interstitial pressure may cause vascular compression and distortion of the small vessels, and swollen capillary endothelium may provoke vascular stenosis or obstruction (7,10). These secondary changes caused by myocardial edema, which are considered part of the no-reflow phenomenon, inhibit the recovery of production of myocardial high-energy phosphate (ATP and CP). Furthermore, in addition to the delayed recovery of the myocardial high-energy store, decreased CBF and decreased mechanical distensibility caused by the myocardial edema itself prevent recovery of left ventricular function, structure, and metabolism (1,7,9,10,13).

From these points, it is concluded that myocardial edema is a result of ischemia and in turn causes depression of left ventricular performance and deteriorates myocardial metabolic recovery during reperfusion.

REFERENCES

1. Allen, W. B., Blackstone, E. H., and Kouchoukos, N. T. 1974. Effects of cardiopulmonary bypass and ischemic cardioplegia on the diastolic pressure–volume relationship and water content of the canine left ventricle. *Circulation* 49/50(Suppl.):III-19.
2. Buckberg, G. D., Fixler, D. E., Archie, J. P., and Hoffman, J. I. E. 1972. Experimental subendocardial ischemia in dogs with normal coronary arteries. *Circ. Res.* 30:67–81.
3. Buckberg, G. D., Towers, B., Foglia, D. E., Mulder, D. G., and Maloney, J. V. 1972. Subendocardial ischemia after cardiopulmonary bypass. *J. Thorac. Cardiovasc. Surg.* 64:669–684.
4. De Gasperis, C., Gonzales-Lavin, L., Pellegrini, A., and Ross, D. N. 1971/72. Ultrastructural aspects of human myocardial capillaries during open heart surgery. *Cardiology* 56:333–336.
5. Foglia, R. P., Steed, D. L., Follette, D. M., DeLana, E., and Buckberg, G. D. 1979. Iatrogenic myocardial edema with potassium cardioplegia. *J. Thorac. Cardiovasc. Surg.* 78:217–222.
6. Laks, H., Standeven, J., Blair, D., Hahn, J., Jellinek, M., and Willman, V. L. 1977. The effects of cardiopulmonary bypass with crystalloid and colloid hemodilution on myocardial extravascular water. *J. Thorac. Cardiovasc. Surg.* 73:129–138.
7. Leaf, A. 1973. Cell swelling: A factor in ischemic tissue injury. *Circulation* 48:455–458.
8. Mukherjee, A., Buja, L. M., Scales, G. C., Fink, G. C., Templeton, G. H., Platt, M. R., and Willerson, J. T. 1978. Abnormal myocardial fluid retention as an early manifestation of ischemic injury. In: T. Kobayashi, Y. Ito, and G. Rona (eds.), *Recent Advances in Studies on Cardiac Structure and Metabolism.* Vol. 12: *Cardiac Adaptation*, pp. 245–252. University Park Press, Baltimore.
9. Salisbury, P. F., Cross, C. E., and Rieben, P. A. 1960. Distensibility and water content of heart muscle before and after injury. *Circ. Res.* 8:788–793.
10. Sunamori, M., Hatano, R., Suzuki, T., Yamamoto, N., Yamada, T., Kumazawa, T., and Sunaga, T. 1977. No-reflow phenomenon in the myocardium after the cardiopulmonary bypass: A genesis of the subendocardial ischemia. *Jpn. J. Circ.* 41:1–10.
11. Utley, J. R., Michalsky, G. B., Bryant, L. R., Mobin-Uddin, K., and McKean, H. E. 1973. Determinants of myocardial water content during cardiopulmonary bypass. *J. Thorac. Cardiovasc. Surg.* 68:8–16.
12. Wahlen, D. A., Hamilton, D. G., Ganote, C. E., and Jennings, R. B. 1974. Effect of a transient period of ischemia on myocardial cells: 1. Effects on cell volume regulation. *Am. J. Cardiol.* 74:381–397.
13. Willerson, J. T., Watson, J. T., Hutton, I., Templeton, G. H., and Fixler, D. E. 1975. Reduced myocardial reflow and increased coronary vascular resistance following prolonged myocardial ischemia in the dog. *Circ. Res.* 36:771–781.

Serial Changes in Cytosolic, Mitochondrial, and Lysosomal Enzymes and Cardiac Myosin Light Chain II in Plasma following Coronary Ligation in Conscious Closed-Chest Dogs

R. Nagai, C.-C. Chiu, K. Yamaoki, S. Ueda,
Y. Iwasaki, A. Ohkubo, and Y. Yazaki

Cardiovascular Research Unit
The Third Department of Internal Medicine
Faculty of Medicine, University of Tokyo
Tokyo 113, Japan

Abstract. We studied serial changes in various myocardial enzymes and cardiac myosin light chain II (LCII) in plasma following coronary ligation in 14 conscious closed-chest dogs. Cytoplasmic enzymes [creatine phosphokinase (CPK) and supernatant glutamic oxaloacetic transaminase (sGOT)] reached maximum at 12–24 hr and returned to normal at 72–96 hr. The mitochondrial isozyme of GOT (mGOT) began to rise at 6–9 hr, peaked at 12–30 hr (4.8–42.2 IU/liter), and stayed higher at 96 hr than before infarction. Glutamate dehydrogenase (GLDH), another mitochondrial enzyme, began to elevate at 6–16 hr and reached maximum at 24–60 hr (6.2–20.5 U/liter); GLDH also showed higher levels at 96 hr than before infarction. N-Acetyl-β-glucosaminidase (NAG), a lysosomal enzyme, showed a biphasic pattern in every case. The first peak appeared at 3–12 hr, and the second one at 36–72 hr. Myosin LCII began to rise at 3–9 hr, peaked at 30–120 hr (34–136 ng/ml), and remained elevated for 7 to 10 days. Determination of these myocardial enzymes or LCII in plasma is useful for the diagnosis of acute myocardial infarction.

In acute myocardial infarction, many kinds of myocardial enzymes are released into the circulation, and by determining activities of these enzymes in the blood stream, important information can be obtained concerning the degree as well as the process of destruction of myocardial cells and intracellular organelles. In this study, we produced experimental myocardial infarction in conscious closed-chest dogs by acute coronary ligation, and by using this model we studied serial changes in plasma activities of cytosolic, mitochondrial, and lysosomal enzymes of myocardium. We also determined plasma levels of a structural protein, myosin light chain II (LCII).

MATERIAL AND METHODS

Animal Preparation

Fourteen dogs were anesthetized with sodium pentobarbital. A silk snare was placed loosely around the left anterior descending coronary artery

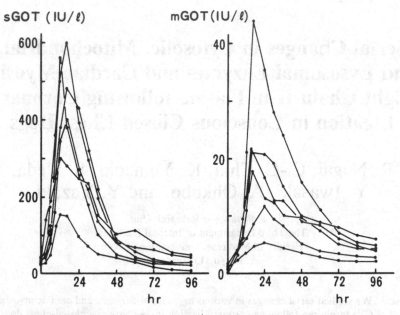

Figure 1.   Serial changes in plasma activities of sGOT and mGOT in six representative cases.

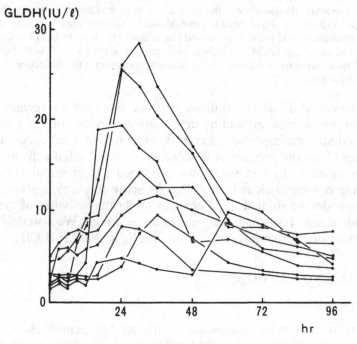

Figure 2.   Serial changes in plasma activities of GLDH in eight representative cases.

(LAD), and dogs were allowed to recover. Seven to 10 days after this operation, the snare was pulled tightly, and the LAD was ligated.

Assays of Myocardial Enzymes and Light Chain II

Blood samples were obtained every 4–6 hr for 72 hr and every 24 hr for 7 days more. Creatine phosphokinase (CPK), cytoplasmic and mitochondrial isozymes of glutamic oxaloacetic transaminase (sGOT and mGOT), glutamate dehydrogenase (GLDH, a mitochondrial enzyme), N-acetyl-β-glucosaminidase (NAG, a lysosomal enzyme), and myosin LCII were measured in cell-free plasma. Activities of CPK, total GOT, and GLDH were measured using reagent kits (Boehringer). Mitochondrial GOT was assayed by the method of Teranishi et al. (6) using sheep red blood cells sensitized with antibody against sGOT (Eiken Chemical). N-Acetyl-β-glucosaminidase activity was measured fluorimetrically by the method of Woollen et al. (9). Myosin LCII was measured by the radioimmunoassay which we have developed (2,3).

Myosin LCII levels and activities of all enzymes in plasma except NAG activity returned to normal levels before coronary ligation; NAG activity before coronary ligation was 6.1 ± 4.3% (mean ± S.D.) higher than before the operation.

RESULTS

Creatine Phosphokinase

Activity of CPK was elevated at 3 hr and was highest at 12–24 hr (4023 ± 2100 IU/liter, mean ± S.D.); CPK activity returned to the level before infarction at 72–96 hr.

Cytoplasmic and Mitochondrial Glutamic Oxaloacetic Transaminase

The sGOT activity was raised at 3–6 hr, reached maximum at 12–24 hr (408 ± 205 IU/liter), and decreased almost to the normal level at 96 hr (28.1 ± 14.9 IU/liter). The mGOT activity began to rise at 6–9 hr, reaching a maximum at 12–30 hr (21.1 ± 11.4 IU/liter); mGOT activity was still higher at 96 hr than before infarction (5.6 ± 2.3 IU/liter vs. 2.8 ± 2.0 IU/liter, $P < 0.025$) (Figure 1).

Glutamate Dehydrogenase

Glutamate dehydrogenase was elevated at (6–16 hr, and peak levels occurred at 24–60 hr (15.6 ± 7.9 U/liter). Changes in GLDH levels were more gradual than those of mGOT. The GLDH activity was also slightly higher at 96 hr than before infarction (5.0 ± 2.2 U/liter vs. 3.7 ± 1.7 U/liter, $P < 0.1$) (Figure 2).

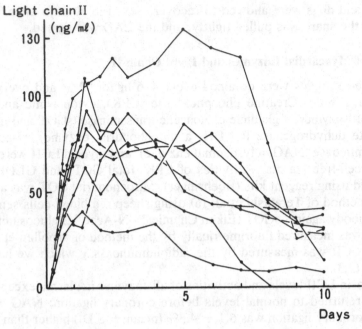

Figure 3. Serial changes in plasma activities of NAG in seven representative cases; NAG activities before coronary ligation were subtracted from all NAG activities after infarction.

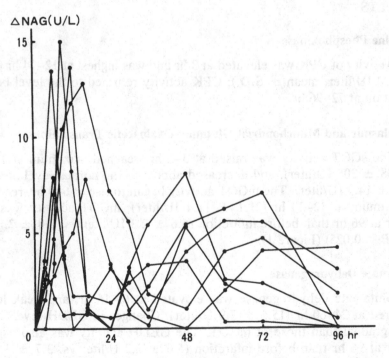

Figure 4. Serial changes in plasma myosin LCII levels in eight representative cases.

N-Acetyl-β-glucosaminidase

The activity of NAG in normal plasma was variable among dogs (14.7 ± 6.4 U/liter). Furthermore, NAG activity before coronary ligation was 6.1 ± 4.3% higher than before the operation; NAG activity after infarction was elevated within 6 hr, reached peak levels at 3–12 hr (21.8 ± 8.5 U/liter), decreased nearly to the level before infarction, and then increased again, reaching the second peak at 36–72 hr (19.2 ± 7.1 U/liter) (Figure 3).

Myosin Light Chain II

Myosin LCII began to rise at 3–9 hr, reached peak levels at 30–120 hr (74.6 ± 29.3 ng/ml), and decreased gradually. Myosin LCII was still elevated at 168 hr in all 14 cases (37.2 ± 30.2 ng/ml) and at 240 hr in 10 cases (18.5 ± 16.7 ng/ml) (Figure 4).

DISCUSSION

Many studies have been reported concerning the clinical significance in acute myocardial infarction of circulating myocardial enzymes such as CPK (5), mGOT (1), and NAG (7,8). However, experimental studies in which a coronary artery is ligated in conscious closed-chest dogs are also important to determine the kinetics of release of cardiac enzymes or other substances in acute myocardial infarction. In our study, cytoplasmic enzymes (CPK and sGOT) showed the most rapid time course. The mitochondrial enzymes (mGOT and GLDH) reached peak levels and returned to normal later than cytosolic enzymes. Lysosomal enzyme (NAG) showed a biphasic pattern. As suggested by the study of Welman et al. (7) in patients with acute myocardial infarction, there may be two phases during which lysosomal enzymes are released: release from myocardial cells and from inflammatory cells. The time course of release of cardiac structural protein (LCII) was the most gradual. Since the disappearance rate of exogenous LCII from the circulation is quite rapid (4), LCII can be liberated continuously for more than 7 days from the infarcted myocardium.

These results show that sensitivity to myocardial ischemia is different among different intracellular structures and that determination of several of these enzymes or LCII can be useful for the diagnosis of acute myocardial infarction at an early stage as well as days after the attack.

ACKNOWLEDGMENT

We are grateful to Yukiko Hatano for her technical assistance.

REFERENCES

1. Inoue, M., Hori, M., Nishimoto, Y., Fukui, S., Abe, H., Wada, H., and Minamino, T. 1978. Immunological determination of serum m-AST activity in patients with acute myocardial infarction. *Br. Heart J.* 50:1251–1256.
2. Nagai, R., Ueda, S., and Yazaki, Y. 1978. Radioimmunoassay of cardiac myosin light chain II in the serum following experimental myocardial infarction. *J. Mol. Cell. Cardiol.* 10:64.
3. Nagai, R., Ueda, S., and Yazaki, Y. 1979. Radioimmunoassay of cardiac myosin light chain II in the serum following experimental myocardial infarction. *Biochem. Biophys. Res. Commun.* 86:683–688.
4. Nagai, R., and Yazaki, Y. 1981. Assessment of myocardial infarct size by serial changes in serum cardiac myosin light chain II in dogs. *Jpn. Circ. J.* 45:661–666.
5. Sobel, B. E., Bresnahan, G. F., Shell, W. E., and Yoder, R. D. 1972. Estimation of infarct size in man and its relation to prognosis. *Circulation* 46:640–648.
6. Teranishi, H., Wada, H., and Sawada, Y. 1978. A simple immunological method for differential determination of serum glutamic–oxaloacetic transaminase isozyme (II) using anti-pig-GOT antibody. *Med. J. Osaka Univ.* 29:191–198.
7. Welman, E., Colbeck, J. F., Selwyn, A. P., Fox, K. M., and Orr, I. 1980. Plasma lysosomal enzyme activity in acute myocardial infarction and the effects of drugs. In: M. Tajuddin, B. Bhatia, H. H. Siddiqui, and G. Rona (eds.), *Advances in Myocardiology*, Vol. 2: *Myocardial Hypoxia, Ischemia, and Infarction*, pp. 359–369. University Park Press, Baltimore.
8. Welman, E., Selwyn, A. P., and Fox, K. M. 1979. Lysosomal and cytosolic enzyme release in acute myocardial infarction: Effects of methylprednisolone. *Circulation* 59:730–733.
9. Woollen, J. W., and Turner, P. 1965. Plasma N-acetyl-β-glucosaminidase and β-glucuronidase in health and disease. *Clin. Chim. Acta* 12:671–683.

Myosin Light Chain Phosphorylation during Regional Myocardial Ischemia

P. Cummins

Molecular Cardiology Unit
Department of Cardiovascular Medicine
University of Birmingham
Birmingham B15 2TH, England

D. M. Yellon and D. J. Hearse

The Rayne Institute
St. Thomas' Hospital
London, England

Abstract. The extent of cardiac myosin light chain phosphorylation was measured during regional myocardial ischemia in the dog. A multiple-projectile cutter was used to sample adjacent biopsies from the normal and ischemic areas of the myocardium in an open-chested dog heart following 30 min of coronary artery ligation. Measurement of metabolite levels and blood flow in the individual biopsies clearly defined the border zone between normal and ischemic myocardium. Myosin light chain phosphorylation was measured after isoelectric focusing of biopsy samples and subsequent densitometric analysis. A 50% increase in phosphorylation was observed in the ischemic zone which may correlate with the reduced contractility which is a feature of the ischemic myocardium.

Following coronary artery ligation, the development of an area of regional ischemia can be seen to be clearly defined from the surrounding normal tissue. Furthermore, it is known that the contractility between these two areas differs considerably, with normal contractile function occurring in the well-perfused areas of the myocardium, whereas in the area of ischemia, the state of contraction is invariably diminished (4,16,20).

The fate of metabolites and blood flow in both of these areas, i.e., the normal and ischemic zones, has been well established (7,22); however, less attention has been centered on the response of the contractile machinery to the onset of severe ischemia, particularly at the level of the contractile proteins.

Although the role of calcium ions in regulating the contraction of striated muscle via troponin and tropomyosin is well established, there is now increasing evidence that phosphorylation of contractile proteins, in particular myosin, may also play a regulatory role (1). The site of phosphorylation is situated on the light chain 2 subunits (15) which are located in the head

479

region of the myosin molecule. As this region is intimately involved in actin binding and ATP hydrolysis, phosphorylation and dephosphorylation of the light chain could modify these processes. In nonmuscle and smooth muscle contractile systems. phosphorylation of myosin appears to be essential for actin activation of myosin ATPase and, consequently, contraction (17). However, in skeletal and cardiac muscle, the effects of myosin phosphorylation appear to be more subtle and have been associated with active tension development in the isolated perfused rat heart (11) and posttetanic potentiation of isometric twitch tension in rat skeletal muscle (18).

Since there have been a number of studies in which impairment of function in the ischemic zone has been related to metabolic disruption, particularly in the measurement of high-energy phosphate (6,12), we were interested to see if there was any way in which impairment of function could be related to the phosphorylation state of cardiac myosin.

Therefore, in the present study we used methods of multiple biopsy retrieval coupled with metabolic and flow analysis to define the interface between normal and ischemic myocardium and subsequently examined the state of myosin light chain phosphorylation in these two zones.

MATERIALS AND METHODS

Ischemic Model and Metabolic Analysis

For these studies we used an open-chested dog heart preparation that had been subjected to 30 min of coronary artery ligation. In order for metabolite and blood flow measurements to be accurately assessed, it is important to take adjacent biopsy samples from the normal tissue through to the center of the ischemic core both rapidly and simply. This has been achieved by using a multiple biopsy cutter (8,21) which allows us to take 40 adjacent biopsies from the core of an area of regional ischemia to the surrounding normal tissue. This cutter consists of a lattice of intersecting blades 30 mm deep which are fused together to form boxlike chambers 4 mm in section. In order for the biopsy cutter to take samples rapidly, it has to be fired from a propulsion unit (8,21). Hence, with the aid of suitable explosive cartridges, the cutter can be propelled at the myocardium at very high velocity.

Thus, following 30 min of ischemia in the open-chest dog heart preparation, radioactive microspheres are injected for use in the determination of blood flow (13), and the gun is positioned above the myocardium and fired. The resistance of the heart is sufficient to force biopsies into the respective chambers of the matrix. Immediately after firing, the cutter is removed from the myocardium and immersed in a freezing mixture ($-135°C$) (22). The whole procedure from the time of firing to that of freezing taking less than 3 sec. The biopsies are then freeze dried in situ in the cutter, and, following a 36-hr lyophilization period, can be easily removed from their grids.

Therefore, with each full-length biopsy intact, we can then remove 3 mm of the epicardial surface and subject it to analysis. Approximately 5 mg dry weight of the tissue is taken for perchloric acid extraction and, using microassay techniques (22), is analyzed for biochemical parameters such as adenosine triphosphate (ATP) and creatine phosphate (CP) using conventional enzyme-linked nicotinamide adenine nucleotide oxidation–reduction reactions measured by ultraviolet spectroscopy. Furthermore, the pellet from the initial perchloric acid precipitation contains all the microspheres in that sample and can thus be taken for radioactive counting and flow determination.

Phosphorylation Determination by Isoelectric Focusing

One milligram freeze-dried weight of canine myocardial biopsy specimen was dissected from each of the individual samples. Each sample was homogenized for 30 sec in 300 µl of 50 mM KH_2PO_4, 70 mM NaF, 5 mM EDTA, 9.0 M urea, and 0.75 M 2-mercaptoethanol, pH 7.0, using a micro-homogenizer. The homogenization buffer was prepared immediately prior to use. After homogenization, the sample was centrifuged at 1000 g for 10 min at 20°C. Aliquots of 100 µl of the supernatant were used for electrophoresis.

Isoelectric focusing was carried out in 4 × 115 mm glass tubes. The method used was similar to that of O'Farrell (14). The final concentrations of reagents in the gel were 4% acrylamide, 0.2% N′N′-methlyenebisacrylamide, 0.05% ammonium persulfate, 0.07% N,N,N′,N′-tetramethylenediamine, 9.2 M urea, 2.0% nonidet P-40, and 1.6% Ampholine carrier ampholytes of pH range 4–6, and 0.4% Ampholines of pH range 3.5–10. The lower gel buffer was 0.01 M phosphoric acid, and the upper gel buffer was 0.02 M sodium hydroxide. Gels were prerun before sample application at 200 V for 15 min, then at 300 V for 30 min, and finally at 400 V for 30 min. After application, samples were overlaid with 8 M urea. Electrophoresis was carried out at 300 V for 19 hr and then at 400 V for 2 hr.

Densitometry

After staining, gels were densitometered at 600 nm using a Gilford Model 2400 recording spectrophotometer fitted with a Gilford Model 2410 gel-scanning attachment. Areas of the individually scanned protein bands were quantitated using an image analyzer.

RESULTS

Following analysis of the biopsies for the flow and metabolic variables, we were able to clearly demonstrate the severely ischemic core from the surrounding normal tissue (22). Figure 1 shows the results obtained for the

	1	2	3	4	5	6	7	8
A	2.0	5.5	7.1	30.3	20.0	24.5	1.3	33.3
B	5.8	3.8	missing	12.9	29.5	23.7	27.4	35.6
C	2.1	3.0	3.6	6.0	9.7	24.7	25.6	31.8
D	4.3	1.0	2.8	14.7	29.8	29.8	30.8	25.9
E	missing	2.7	1.0	6.9	29.3	27.8	40.8	23.0

ISCHEMIC   NORMAL

Figure 1.   Creatine phosphate levels during regional myocardial ischemia. Creatine phosphate levels in individual biopsy samples were determined as described in Materials and Methods and expressed as μmol/g dry weight tissue. The zone demarcating normal and ischemic tissue is outlined.

creatine phosphate content of the heart following 30 min of regional ischemia. From this figure, it can be seen that the values of the normal and ischemic tissue can be separated from each other by a line of maximum change, thereby clearly demarcating the tissue into two well-defined areas. Although not shown in Figure 1, the results from all of the other variables measured, including blood flow, followed precisely the same pattern as that for creatine phosphate.

The extent of myosin light chain phosphorylation was estimated by densitometrically scanning the individually focused myosin light chain components. Under the isoelectric focusing conditions used in this study, the VLC-1 and VLC-2 components of cardiac myosin are clearly resolved in whole-muscle specimens (Figure 2) (3). In addition to the phosphorylated VLC-2P and dephosphorylated VLC-2 forms of myosin LC-2, additional species of altered charge of both of these forms were seen in focused samples. These were designated VLC-2P* and VLC-2*, respectively, and have previously been described by Frearson and Perry (5) and Cummins et al. (3). The modification responsible for the formation of these additional species has not been established, but as it appears to affect the VLC-2 and VLC-2P forms to the same extent, the degree of phosphorylation was calculated as the amount of VLC-2P + VLC-2P* relative to VLC-2 + VLC-2* after quantitation.

In the initial study, 1 mg of freeze-dried myocardial biopsy was ho-mogenized in 300 μl of 9.0 M urea plus 0.75 M 2-mercaptoethanol. Under these conditions, it was assumed that the myosin light chain kinase and phosphatase enzymes, which have been shown to be present in cardiac muscle (9), would be inactivated and that the phosphorylation state of the myosin light chain would be chemically frozen.

Under these conditions, little or no light chain phosphorylation was observed in any of the 40 biopsies studied (Figure 2a). However, Stull et al. (18) have recently suggested that the myosin light chain phosphatase may exhibit significant activity in 8 M urea. They found that frozen hearts ho-mogenized in 8 M urea, 50 mM Tris, pH 8.0, with added [^{32}P]light chain demonstrated a time-dependent loss of radioactivity that could be precipi-tated by trichloroacetic acid. This loss was inhibited by the inclusion of 50 mM potassium phosphate into the buffer system, suggesting the presence of significant phosphatase activity.

For this reason, homogenization of biopsy specimens was carried out in the additional presence of 50 mM KH$_2$PO$_4$, 70 mM NaF, and 5 mM EDTA. Under these conditions, Holroyde et al. (9) have shown that not only is the

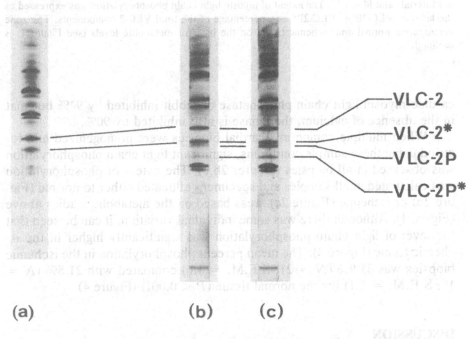

VLC-2
VLC-2*
VLC-2P
VLC-2P*

(a)   (b)   (c)

Figure 2.   Isoelectric focusing of canine myocardial biopsy specimens. Isoelectric focusing of samples was carried out as described in Materials and Methods. (a) Sample homogenized in 9.0 M urea plus 0.75 M 2-mercaptoethanol. Normal and ischemic samples are identical. (b) Sample homogenized in 9.0 M urea, 0.75 M 2-mercaptoethanol, 50 mM KH$_2$PO$_4$, 70 mM NaF, 5 mM EDTA, pH 7.0. Normal tissue. (c) Sample of ischemic tissue homogenized as in (b).

	1	2	3	4	5	6	7	8
A	29	39	21	17	24	29	29	19
B	41	29	48	20	20	29	21	17
C	39	32	37	28	25	14	25	17
D	33	40	31	24	23	21	25	16
E	24	28	33	39	27	29	20	21

ISCHEMIC   NORMAL

Figure 3. Extent of myosin light chain phosphorylation during regional myocardial ischemia. Biopsy samples were homogenized, focused, and densitometrically quantitated as described in Materials and Methods. The extent of myosin light chain phosphorylation was expressed as the level of VLC-2P + VLC-2P* as a percentage of the total VLC-2 components. The zone demarcating normal and ischemic tissue on the basis of metabolite levels (see Figure 1) is outlined.

cardiac myosin light chain phosphatase of rabbit inhibited by 94% but that in the absence of calcium, the kinase is also inhibited by 90%.

When multiple canine myocardial biopsies were homogenized and focused using these sample conditions, significant light chain phosphorylation was observed in all biopsies (Figures 2b,c). The extent of phosphorylation was calculated in all samples and specimens allocated either to normal (Figure 2b) or ischemic (Figure 2c) areas based on the metabolic studies above (Figure 1). Although there was some individual variation, it can be seen that the level of light chain phosphorylation was significantly higher in the ischemic tissue (Figure 3). The mean percent phosphorylation in the ischemic biopsies was 31.9% (N = 21, S.E.M. = 1.6) compared with 21.8% (N = 19, S.E.M. = 1.1) for the normal tissue ($P < 0.001$) (Figure 4).

DISCUSSION

From these preliminary results, it can be seen that with our method for clearly defining normal and ischemic tissue, we have been able to show that during regional myocardial ischemia, the extent of myosin light chain phosphorylation in the ischemic zone differs significantly from that of the normal tissue, being approximately 50% higher in the ischemic area.

Although the precise role of myosin phosphorylation in striated muscles has yet to be established, there are indications that in certain circumstances, phosphorylation of myosin light chains is associated with increased tension development and tetanic contraction. Kopp and Barany (11), using the isolated perfused rat heart, demonstrated a direct correlation between the extent of [^{32}P]phosphate incorporation into myosin light chains and active tension development as a result of isoproterenol or high calcium ion concentration perfusion. Jeacocke and England (10) and Holroyde et al. (9), however, found no change in myosin phosphorylation after perfusion with epinephrine. In isolated frog skeletal muscles (2), the extent of light chain

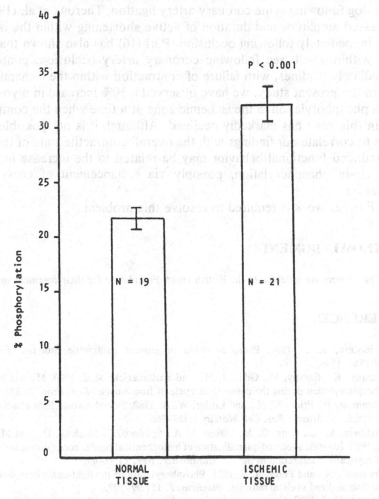

Figure 4.   Phosphorylation of canine myosin light chain during regional myocardial ischemia. Percentage phosphorylation in individual biopsies is expressed as described in Figure 3.

phosphorylation has been shown to depend on duration of tetanic stimulus, being maximal after prolonged tetanic contractions (20–30 sec) or caffeine contractures (20 min). After short tetani, dephosphorylation of light chains approximately followed relaxation, whereas after longer tetani, dephosphorylation lagged behind relaxation. In the intact fast-twitch extensor digitorum longus of the rat (18), myosin was not found to be phosphorylated during 1 sec of tetany but did increase markedly from 0.1 mol PO_4 per mol light chain 2 to 0.70 mol/mol during the subsequent period in which the muscle relaxed, suggesting a relationship between phosphate content and posttetanic potentiation of isometric twitch tension.

The situation with regard to phosphorylation studies in the ischemic myocardium has not been examined. The contractility of the ishemic myocardium is generally considered to be reduced (4,16,19,20). In the open-chest dog following acute coronary artery ligation, Theroux et al. (19) found decreased amplitude and duration of active shortening within the ischemic zone immediately following occlusion. Puri (16) has also shown that in the dog, within 15–30 sec following coronary artery occlusion, contractility immediately declines, with failure of contraction within the ischemic zone.

In the present study, we have observed a 50% increase in myosin light chain phosphorylation in the ischemic zone at a time when the contractility within this zone has markedly declined. Although it is not possible at this stage to correlate our findings with the overall contractile state of the heart, the reduced functional behavior may be related to the increase in myosin light chain phosphorylation, possibly via enhancement of cross bridge formation.

Further work is required to resolve this problem.

ACKNOWLEDGMENT

The authors are indebted to the British Heart Foundation for their continual support.

REFERENCES

1. Adelstein, R. S. 1980. Phosphorylation of muscle contractile proteins. *Fed. Proc.* 39:1544–1546.
2. Barany, K., Barany, M., Gillis, J. M., and Kushmerick, M. J. 1980. Myosin light chain phosphorylation during the contraction cycle of frog muscle. *Fed. Proc.* 39:1547–1551.
3. Cummins, P., Price, K. M., and Littler, W. A. 1980. Foetal myosin light chain in human ventricle. *J. Muscle Res. Cell Motility* 1:357–366.
4. Fishbein, M. C., Hare, C. A., Gissen, S. A., Spadoro, J., Maclean, D., and Maroko, P. R. 1980. Identification and quantification of histochemical border zones during the evolution of myocardial infarction in the rat. *Cardiovasc. Res.* 14:41–49.
5. Frearson, N., and Perry, S. V. 1975. Phosphorylation of the light-chain components from cardiac and red skeletal muscles. *Biochem. J.* 151:99–107.
6. Hearse, D. J. 1980. Oxygen deprivation and early myocardial contractile failure. A reassessment of the possible role of adenosine triphosphate. *Am. J. Cardiol.* 44:1115–1119.

7. Hearse, D. J., Opie, L., Katzeff, I. E., Lubbe, W. F., Van der Werff, T. J., Peisach, M., and Boulle, G. 1977. Characterization of the 'border zone' in acute regional ischemia in the dog. *Am. J. Cardiol.* 40:716–726.
8. Hearse, D. J., Yellon, D. M., Chappell, D. A., Wyse, R. K. H., and Ball, G. A. 1981. A high velocity impact device for obtaining multiple, contiguous myocardial biopsies. *J. Mol. Cell. Cardiol.* 13:197–206.
9. Holroyde, M. J., Small, D. A. P., Howe, E., and Solaro, R. J. 1979. Isolation of cardiac myofibrils and myosin light chains with in vivo levels of light chain phosphorylation. *Biochim. Biophys. Acta* 587:628–637.
10. Jeacocke, S. A., and England, P. J. 1980. Phosphorylation of myosin light chains in perfused rat heart. *Biochem, J.* 188:763–768.
11. Kopp, S. J., and Barany, M. 1979. Phosphorylation of the 19,000-dalton light chain of myosin in perfused rat heart under the influence of negative and positive inotropic agents. *J. Biol. Chem.* 254:12007–12012.
12. Kubler, W., and Katz, A. M. 1977. Mechanism of early pump failure of the ischaemic heart: Possible role of adenosine triphosphate depletion and energic phosphate accumulation. *Am J. Cardiol.* 40:467–471.
13. Lubbe, W. F., Peisach, M., Pretorius, R., Brugreel, K. J. J., and Opie, L. H. 1974. Distribution of myocardial blood flow before and after coronary artery ligation in the baboon. Relation to early ventricular fibrillation. *Cardiovasc. Res.* 8:478–487.
14. O'Farrell, P. H. 1975. High resolution two-dimensional electrophoresis of proteins. *J. Biol. Chem.* 250:4007–4021.
15. Perrie, W. T., Smillie, L. B., and Perry, S. V. 1973. A phosphorylated light-chain component of myosin from skeletal muscle. *Biochem. J.* 135:151–164.
16. Puri, P. S. 1974. Modification of experimental myocardial infarct size by cardiac drugs. *Am. J. Cardiol.* 33:521–528.
17. Small, J. V., and Sobieszek, A. 1977. Ca-regulation of mammalian smooth muscle actomyosin via a kinase–phosphatase dependent phosphorylation and dephosphorylation of the 20,000 M light chain of myosin. *Eur. J. Biochem.* 76:521–530.
18. Stull, J. T., Manning, D. R., High, C. W., and Blumenthal, D. K. 1980. Phosphorylation of contractile proteins in heart and skeletal muscle. *Fed. Proc.* 39:1552–1557.
19. Theroux, P., Franklin, D., Ross, J., Jr., and Kemper, W. S. 1974. Regional myocardial function during acute coronary artery occlusion and its modification by pharmacologic agents in the dog. *Circ. Res.* 35:896–908.
20. Vatner, S. F. 1980. Correlation between acute reductions in myocardial blood flow and function in conscious dog. *Circ. Res.* 47:201–207.
21. Yellon, D. M. 1979. A multiple biopsy gun for the study of three-dimensional metabolic geometry. *J. Physiol.* 293:5–6.
22. Yellon, D. M., Hearse, D. J., Crewe, R., Grannell, J., and Wyse, R. K. H. 1980. Characterization of the interface between normal and ischemic tissue during acute myocardial infarction. *Am. J. Cardiol.* 47:1233–1239.

Myocardial Infarct Size from Serum Cardiac Myosin Light Chain

Clinical and Experimental Studies

Y. Yazaki, R. Nagai, K. Yamaoki, and S. Ueda

Cardiovascular Research Unit
The Third Department of Internal Medicine
Faculty of Medicine, University of Tokyo
Tokyo 113, Japan

Abstract. The relationship between myocardial infarct size and serum cardiac light chain (LC) levels was studied in experimental and clinical myocardial infarction. In dogs with left anterior descending coronary artery occlusion, regression analysis showed good correlation between infarct size and LC II release, but CPK-MB release failed to correlate with infarct size because of a decreasing value of cumulative CPK with larger sized infarctions. In patients with acute myocardial infarction, Peak LC I levels correlated well with CPK release, since the phenomenon of the decreased CPK release in larger sized infarction was not so distinctive in human cases. Thus, LC determination may better qauntitate the extent of myocardial damage as well as provide a specific and sensitive method for diagnosis of acute myocardial infarction.

The serial CPK technique has now been widely used for noninvasive estimation of infarct size as well as the diagnosis of acute myocardial infarction. However, variability of CPK serum release with infarct size has recently been reported in dog coronary ligation experiments (1). Since measurement of a structural protein released into the circulation from damaged myocardial cells may provide a more direct estimate of the extent of myocardial infarction, we have developed a sensitive radioimmunoassay for the smaller subunit of cardiac myosin, light chain (LC).

In this study, we determined by this assay LC levels in the serum of dogs with coronary occlusion and patients with acute myocardial infarction and then compared total amounts of LC release and CPK release as an estimate of the extent of myocardial damage.

MATERIALS AND METHODS

Animal Preparations

Mongrel dogs weighing 7–10 kg were anesthetized with pentobarital sodium. A left thoracotomy was performed, and the left anterior descending coronary artery was dissected free from adjacent tissues and occluded by a silk suture in 15 dogs. In four sham-operated dogs, the left anterior descending artery was dissected but not occluded. Blood samples were obtained every 6 hr for 72 hr and then once daily for 7 days for serial determinations of LC and CPK in the serum.

Human Samples

Twenty-four patients with acute myocardial infarction admitted to the coronary care unit within 12 hr after the onset of attack were examined for serial determinations of LC and CPK. Blood samples were obtained every 4 to 6 hr for 96 hr after admission and then once daily for 2 weeks.

Radioimmunoassay Procedures

Cardiac myosin light chains were prepared from dog and human left ventricles by dilution technique and guanidine denaturation (6). The two species of LCs with molecular weights of 28,000 and 20,000 were individually fractionated by preparative gel electrophoresis (5). Antisera to each LC were prepared by immunizing guinea pigs with the protein emulsified in complete Freund's adjuvant. The radioimmunoassay was carried out in phosphate buffer saline (0.05 M potassium phosphate buffer, pH 7.4, 0.15 M NaCl, 1% bovine serum albumin) using ^{125}I-labeled LC according to the method developed in our laboratory (2). In dogs, we determined LC II (smaller LC) levels, since the antiserum to LC II was more senstive for the radioimmunoassay than that to LC I. On the other hand, a more sensitive radioimmunoassay was obtained for LC I (larger LC) than LC II in humans.

Determination of Infarct Size in Dogs with Coronary Occlusion

Dogs were sacrificed 7 days after coronary ligation. The heart was removed, and the left ventricle was sliced at 5-mm intervals from base to apex. The infarct area of heart muscle was determined by gross inspection and then excised, weighed, and related to 100 g of left ventricle.

Determination of Creatine Phosphokinase

Serum CPK concentrations were determined by the modified Rosalki method (4). Isoenzyme fractionation of CPK (CPK-MB) was performed by electrophoresis (3).

RESULTS

Serum Light Chain II Levels in Dogs after Coronary Occlusion

Serum LC II levels in 40 normal dogs were 2.70 ± 0.71 ng/ml (mean ± S.E.). The serum LC II levels after coronary occlusion in 8 of 15 dogs are summarized in Figure 1. Serum LC II levels began to rise within 6 hr

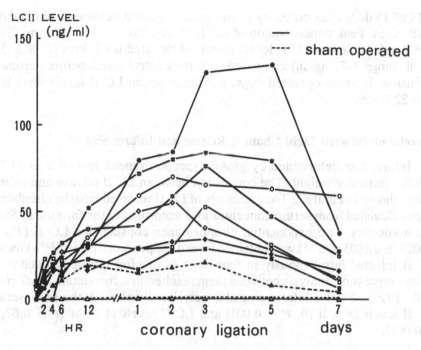

Figure 1.   The time-course study of LC II levels in the serum of dogs with left anterior coronary artery occlusion.

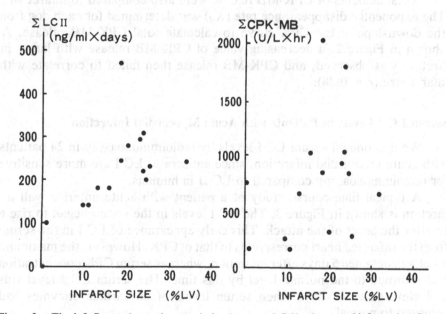

Figure 2.   The left figure shows the correlation between LC II release and infarct size. Serum LC II levels over 7 days were used for the calculation of LC II release. The right figure shows the correlation between CPK-MB release and infarct size.

in 13 of 15 dogs after coronary occlusion and peaked between 2 and 5 days in all cases. Peak concentration of LC II ranged from 27 to 136 ng/ml (59.2 ± 8.9 ng/ml). Serum LC II levels remained elevated for 7 days (27.8 ± 3.7 ng/ml, range 9–70 ng/ml) compared with the control levels before coronary occlusion. In sham-operated dogs, maximum serum LC II levels were less than 22 ng/ml.

Correlation between Light Chain II Release and Infarct Size

Infarct size determined by gross inspection ranged from 0.3 to 33.7% of left ventricular weight. The correlation between LC II release and infarct size is shown in Figure 2. Total amounts of LC II released into the circulation were calculated from serum concentrations according to the formula of Shell and associates. The exponential disappearance constant for LC II (K_d = 0.0023 ± 0.0003 min^{-1}) was obtained from disappearance rate of ^{125}I-labeled LC II injected intravenously in four dogs 48 hr after coronary occlusion. Linear regression analysis between them resulted in a correlation coefficient of 0.72 ($P < 0.001$). Infarct size also correlated well with the peak serum LC II levels ($r = 0.70$, $P < 0.001$) and LC II levels at 24 hr ($r = 0.67$, $P < 0.001$).

Correlation between CPK-MB Release and Infarct Size

Total amounts of CPK-MB release were also compared to infarct size. The exponential disappearance rate (K_d) was determined for each dog from the downslope of the CPK curve to calculate total CPK-MB release. As shown in Figure 2, a decreasing value of CPK-MB release with larger infarction was observed, and CPK-MB release then failed to correlate with infarct size ($r = 0.28$).

Serum LC I Levels in Patients with Acute Myocardial Infarction

We determined serum LC I levels by radioimmunoassay in 24 patients with acute myocardial infarction, since antisera to LC I are more sensitive for radioimmunoassay compared to LC II in humans.

A typical time-course study of a patient with acute anterior wall infarction is shown in Figure 3. The LC I levels in the serum began to rise 6 hr after the onset of the attack. This early appearance of LC I in the serum from the infarcted heart corresponds to that of CPK. However, the maximum level was obtained 5 days after infarction, whereas serum CPK concentration had returned to the normal level by this time. The serum LC I level was still elevated at 14 days when serum levels of all cardiac enzymes had returned to normal.

In most patients, LC I from the infarcted heart first appeared in the serum within 6 hr after the onset of infarction or on admission, reached peak

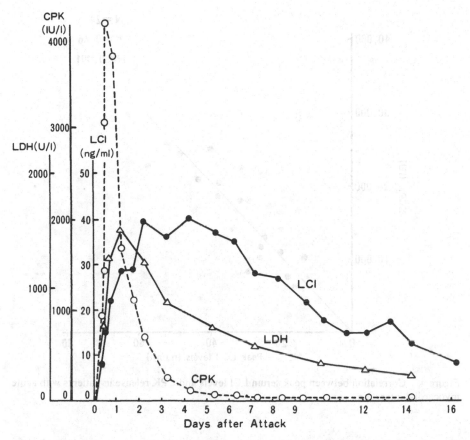

Figure 3.   A typical time course of serum levels of LC I and cardiac enzymes in a patient with acute myocardial infarction.

levels between 3 and 7 days (39.8 ± 13.6 ng/ml, range 18 to 78 ng/ml), and remained elevated for more than 10 days. The mean LC I concentration in 35 normal human sera was 3.7 ± 0.9 ng/ml. This pattern of appearance of LC I in the serum after acute myocardial infarction closely parallels that observed for dog LC II after coronary occlusion.

Correlation between Peak Light Chain I Levels and CPK Release

Peak LC I levels after acute myocardial infarction were compared with cumulative CPK release. As shown in Figure 4, peak LC I levels correlated well with CPK release. The regression coefficient was 0.76 ($P < 0.001$). A given increment of infarct size appears to produce a smaller increment of cumulative CPK than of peak LC I. However, the extent of the decrease in cumulative CPK release with larger-sized infarction was not so distinctive in humans when compared to that in the dog coronary ligation model.

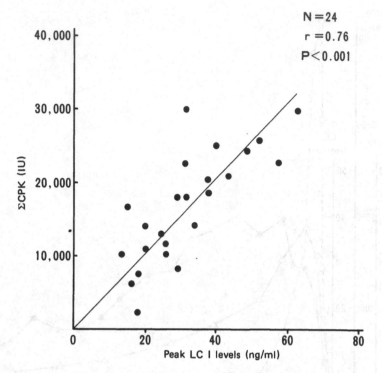

Figure 4.   Correlation between peak serum LCI levels and CPK release in patients with acute myocardial infarction.

DISCUSSION

In this study, serial determinations of serum LC and CPK were compared as an estimate of the extent of myocardial infarction.

Serum LC II levels rose rapidly and remained elevated for a prolonged period in dogs after coronary occlusion. This distinctive pattern of appearance of LC II in the serum has not been observed in time-course studies of many enzymes and myoglobin. Since exogenous LC injected intravenously disappeared rapidly from the circulation with a half-time of disappearance of about 4 hr, this prolonged elevation of LC II can not be attributed to accumulation but reflects the continuous liberation of LC II from damaged myofibrils within the infarcted myocardium.

Light chain II release correlated well with infarct size determined by gross inspection. However, release of CPK-MB into the circulation failed to correlate with infarct size, since a given increment of infarct size would produce a lesser increment of CPK release. Cairns et al. have also proposed that the larger a zone of infarction, the lower would be the fractional escape of CPK from its center (1). Light chain II release from the infarcted myocardium into the serum remained elevated for a longer period, whereas CPK release was more abrupt and shorter. Thus, serum LC II levels seem to be less influenced by changes in the myocardial blood flow in the ischemic area after coronary occlusion than those of CPK.

The pattern of apparence of LC I in the serum of patients with acute myocardial infarction closely parallels that observed in dog LC II after coronary occlusion. However, the phenomenon of decreasing value of cumulative CPK with larger sized infarction was not so distinctive in humans. It is possible that we examined patients with smaller infarct sizes with which survival is possible. On the other hand, human infarction may not be analogous to single ligation.

In conclusion, determinations of serum LC appear to be useful in the quantification of infarct size as well as in providing the specific diagnosis of acute myocardial infarction.

ACKNOWLEDGMENTS

This study was supported by Grant-in-Aid for Special Project Research (Nos. 422004 and 521105) and Grant-in-Aid for Scientific Research (Nos. 457234 and 557209) from the Ministry of Education, Science and Culture.

REFERENCES

1. Cairns, J. A., Missirlis, E., and Fallen, E. L. 1978. Myocardial infarction size from serial CPK: Variability of serum entry ratio with size and model of infarction. *Circulation* 58:1143–1153.
2. Nagai, R., Ueda, S., and Yazaki, Y. 1979. Radioimmunoassay of cardiac myosin light chain II in the serum following experimental myocardial infarction. *Biochem. Biophys. Res. Commun.* 86:683–688.
3. Roe, C. R., Limbird, L. E., Wagner, G. S., and Nerenberg, S. T. 1972. Combined isoenzyme analysis in the diagnosis of myocardial injury: Application of electrophoretic methods for the detection and quantification of the creatine phosphokinase MB isoenzyme. *J. Lab. Clin. Med.* 80:577–590.
4. Rosalki, S. B. 1967. An improved procedure for serum creatine phosphokinase determination. *J. Lab. Clin. Med.* 69:696–705.
5. Yazaki, Y., Mochinaga, S., and Raben, M. S. 1973. Fractionation of the light chains from rat and rabbit cardiac myosin. *Biochim. Biophys. Acta* 328:464–469.
6. Yazaki, Y., and Raben, M. S. 1975. Effect of the thyroid state of the enzymatic characteristics of cardiac myosin. *Circ. Res.* 63:208–215.

Biopsy Assessment of Preservation during Open-Heart Surgery with Cold Cardioplegic Arrest

S. Čanković-Darracott and
M. V. Braimbridge

Department of Heart Research (Surgical Cytochemistry)
The Rayne Institute
St. Thomas' Hospital
London SE1, England

J. Chayen

Division of Cellular Biology
Kennedy Institute of Rheumatology
London, England

Abstract. The efficacy of cold cardioplegic arrest as a method of myocardial preservation has been evaluated by cytochemical and biophysical assessments made on needle biopsies taken from 150 patients undergoing open-heart surgery (e.g., aortic valve replacement, aortic and mitral valve replacement, mitral valve replacement, coronary artery bypass graft, repair of atrial or ventricular septal defects). Comparison of endo- and epicardial preservation showed improved endocardial preservation with cardioplegia compared with that achieved with the previous method used—continuous coronary perfusion at 32°C; however, care had to be taken to ensure adequate cooling of the epicardium. Biopsies also showed the need for repeated infusions of cardioplegic solution if the aorta was occluded for more than 70 min. Preservation of right and left ventricle has also been compared.

During the past 14 years, biopsies have been studied from 680 patients undergoing open-heart surgery to correct various lesions (e.g., aortic and mitral valve disease, coronary artery disease, ventricular or atrial septal defects) using several perfusion techniques (4). Cytochemical and biophysical measurements have been used to evaluate myocardial protection during the period of aortic occlusion. Results obtained from biopsies of patients operated with cold cardioplegic arrest with the St. Thomas' cardioplegic solution (2) have assisted the surgeon in attaining improved clinical protection with this technique.

MATERIALS AND METHODS

Full-thickness left ventricular biopsies approximately 1.5 mm in diameter were taken from the apex of the left ventricle immediately after the

497

aorta was clamped, and comparative biopsies were taken on completion of the corrective surgical procedure and 15 min after removal of the aortic clamp prior to removal of the left ventricular vent.

If the biopsies were of sufficient length, they were bisected into endo- and epicardial halves prior to chilling to $-70°C$ in hexane in order to assess whether preservation was uniform throughout the thickness of the region of ventricle biopsied.

The biopsies were sectioned at 8 μm in a cryostat, usually on the day of sampling. Three chromogenic cytochemical tests were done (5) on serial sections to demonstrate succinate dehydrogenase and myosin adenosine triphosphatase activity. The presence of unsaturated fatty acids of phospholipids was demonstrated by the acid hematein reaction. Any changes in disposition of the colored reaction products of these tests during the period of aortic occlusion were graded semiquantitatively as described by the authors previously (1,4).

Biophysical measurements of changes in birefringence of the myocardial fibers, measured as a change in optical path difference, in response to the addition of buffer containing ATP (2 mM) and calcium (0.036 M) (the incremental birefringence) were made rapidly and simply on a freshly cut section mounted on a microscope slide examined under a quantitative polarizing microscope fitted with a Brace–Köhler λ/30 rotating calibrated compensator (4). Thus, any changes in the ability of the myocardial fibers to respond to the ATP and calcium buffer after the period of aortic occlusion could be measured quantitatively.

RESULTS

Validation of Methods: Correlation with Physiological Assessment at Cardiac Catheterization

In addition to the patients studied during open-heart surgery, a series of patients undergoing cardiac catheterization was fully investigated both by physiological measurements and by cytochemical and quantitative birefringence studies made on sections of left ventricular endomyocardial biopsies obtained during cardiac catheterization. The physiological criteria of Kolettis et al. (6) were used to assess myocardial function. On the basis of eight physiological measurements (left ventricular end-diastolic volume and pressure; cardiac index; ejection rate and fraction; peak ventricular circumferential fiber shortening; KV_{max} postectopic KV_{max}), it was possible to assign each patient to one of three grades, grade 1 being normal and grade 3 highly abnormal. The incremental birefringence in sections of the myocardium from eight grade-1 and 21 grade-3 patients was assessed. The amount of change (nm) in optical path difference induced by the ATP–calcium buffer showed that the mean change ($\pm$ S.E.M.) of the grade-1 myocardium was 4.22 ± 0.10, whereas that of the grade-3 specimens was 3.29 ± 0.16

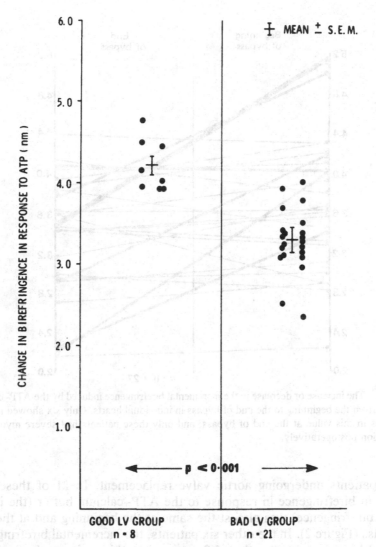

Figure 1. The relationship between the change in birefringence induced by the ATP–calcium medium and the physiological assessment of myocardial function. The difference between the group with good left ventricular (LV) function and the group with bad LV function is highly significant $P < 0.001$ (Student's t test).

(Figure 1). The difference was highly significant ($P < 0.001$; Student's t-test).

Use of Quantitative Birefringence Measurements in Assessing Myocardial Preservation during Open-Heart Surgery

The value of the quantitative measurement of change in birefringence induced by the ATP–calcium buffer was illustrated by a pilot study made

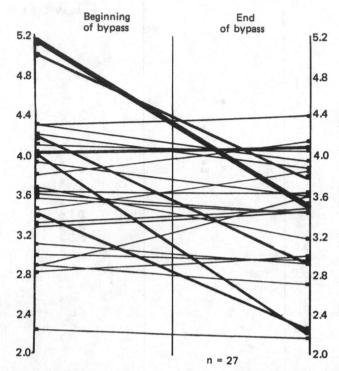

Figure 2.   The increase or decrease in the incremental birefringence induced by the ATP–calcium medium from the beginning to the end of bypass in individual hearts. Only six showed marked decreases in this value at the end of bypass, and only these patients had severe myocardial dysfunction postoperatively.

on 27 patients undergoing aortic valve replacement. In 21 of these, the change in birefringence in response to the ATP–calcium buffer (the incremental birefringence) was almost the same at the beginning and at the end of bypass (Figure 2). In the other six patients, the incremental birefringence declined by values greater than 1.2 nm, and in this series, only these six patients showed a low cardiac output or severe dysrhythmias postoperatively. From such experience, and from the results of obtained subsequently from 653 patients, a decline in the incremental birefringence greater than 0.4 nm during the bypass period has been shown to represent significant myocardial damage (1).

Evaluation of Optimal Perfusion Conditions during Bypass

Effect of Single and Multiple Infusions of Cardioplegic Solution.   When cold cardioplegic arrest was adopted at St. Thomas' Hospital in 1975, a single infusion of the solution was made into the coronary arteries regardless of the duration of the aortic occlusion. Cytochemical and birefringence assessments made on serial biopsies from patients undergoing aortic valve replacement with a mean aortic occlusion time of 90 ± 2.3 min indicated that the myocardium was well protected in 86% during the bypass period. In contrast, of six patients undergoing aortic and mitral valve replacement, 50% deteriorated during the bypass period, and 33% had a low cardiac output postoperatively (Figure 3). In view of the prolonged aortic occlusion time with a single infusion of the cardioplegic solution in these patients (129 ± 0.4 min), it was decided to repeat the infusion at hourly intervals. In the next 11 patients, there was no myocardial deterioration, nor was there low cardiac output postoperatively.

   Comparison of Endo- and Epimyocardial Preservation.   Cytochemical and birefringence measurements have also allowed comparisons to be made of preservation in different areas of the heart. Sixteen patients undergoing aortic valve replacement with continuous blood coronary perfusion of a

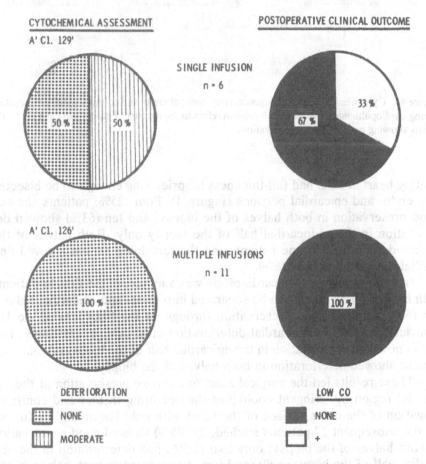

Figure 3. Myocardial preservation in patients undergoing aortic and mitral valve replacements. Combined cytochemical and birefringence assessment of preservation during the bypass period is compared with the postoperative clinical outcome of the same patients.

502   S. Čanković-Darracott et al.

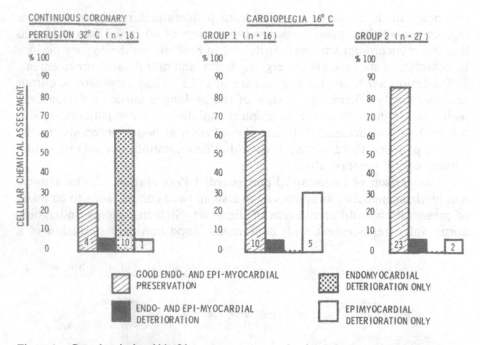

Figure 4. Cytochemical and birefringence assessment of endo- and epimyocardial preservation during cardiopulmonary bypass. Each column refers to the number of patients in each particular group showing good or poor preservation.

beating heart at 32°C had full-thickness biopsies long enough to be bisected into endo- and epicardial portions (Figure 4). Four (25%) patients showed good preservation in both halves of the biopsy, and ten (63%) showed deterioration in the endocardial half of the biopsy only. Both halves of the biopsy deteriorated in one patient, and the remaining patient showed epicardial deterioration only (6%).

In contrast, when cold cardioplegia was adopted, of the first 16 patients with biopsies long enough to be separated into endo- and epicardial halves, ten (63%) showed good preservation throughout the thickness of the left ventricle; none had endocardial deterioration only; and, interestingly, five (31%) now had deterioration in the epicardial half of the biopsy. Again, one patient showed deterioration in both halves of the biopsy.

These results led the surgical team to improve preservation of the epicardial region by stringent cooling of the operating theater and continual irrigation of the outer surface of the heart with cold Hartmann's solution. Of the subsequent 27 patients studied, 23 (85%) showed good preservation in both halves of the biopsy; only two (8.5%) had deterioration in the epicardial half of the biopsy only, and two deteriorated in both halves of the biopsy (one of these was inadvertently infused with warm cardioplegic solution).

DISCUSSION

Cytochemical and biophysical assessments of biopsies taken at surgery have proved of value to the surgeon in predicting postoperative low cardiac output. The results showed that it is patients who deteriorated during cardiopulmonary bypass, regardless of their preoperative myocardial function, who developed postoperative low cardiac output. The assessments were independent of correction of the cardiac defect, and the fact that such assessments are available within 3 hr of the end of bypass makes it possible to monitor with extra care the course of patients in whom the myocardium has shown intraoperative deterioration.

The rapid availability of results means that if a pattern of deterioration occurs over several operations it can be quickly detected and the effect of any corrective action rapidly assessed. When cardioplegia was first used at St. Thomas,' biopsy results clearly indicated that a single infusion of cardioplegic solution at the onset of bypass afforded insufficient protection when the period of aortic occlusion was prolonged, e.g., during multiple valve replacements. When the solution was infused hourly, preservation was enhanced, and this technique became adopted routinely for all open-heart procedures.

When it was possible to do separate estimations of preservation in the endo- and epicardial halves of the biopsies in patients protected by cardioplegia and by continuous coronary perfusion, cold cardioplegia proved more effective in maintaining the integrity of the myocardium as a whole. It was markedly better in preserving the endomyocardial region even though the heart had been kept beating throughout the procedure in the coronary perfusion group (3). The increased incidence of epicardial damage as a result of inefficient cooling of the outer surface of the heart was noted early from biopsy evidence and effectively corrected.

ACKNOWLEDGMENTS

We are grateful to the British Heart Foundation and to St. Thomas' Hospital Endowments Fund for grants to do this work.

REFERENCES

1. Braimbridge, M. V., and Čanković-Darracott, S. 1979. Quantitative polarisation microscopy and cytochemistry in assessing myocardial function. In: J. R. Pattison, L. Bitensky, and J. Chayen (eds.), *Quantitative Cytochemistry and its Applications*, pp. 221–230. Academic Press, New York, London.
2. Braimbridge, M. V., Chayen, J., Bitensky, L., Hearse, D. J., Jynge, P., and Čanković-Darracott, S. 1977. Cold cardioplegia or continuous coronary perfusion? *J. Thorac. Cardiovasc. Surg.* 74:900–906.

3. Buckberg, G. 1972. Subendocardial ischemia after cardiopulmonary bypass. *J. Thorac. Cardiovasc. Surg.* 64:669–684.
4. Čanković-Darracott, S., Braimbridge, M. V., Williams, B. T., Bitensky, L., and Chayen, J. 1977. Myocardial preservation during aortic valve surgery. Assessment of five techniques by cellular chemical and biophysical methods. *J. Thorac. Cardiovasc. Surg.* 73:699–706.
5. Chayen, J., Bitensky, L., and Butcher, R. G. (eds.) 1973. *Practical Histochemistry*, pp. 85–192. John Wiley & Sons, New York.
6. Kolettis, M., Jenkins, B. S., and Webb-Peploe, M. M. 1976. Assessment of left ventricular function by indices derived from aortic flow velocity. *Br. Heart J.* 38:18–31.

Calcium Antagonistic Activity and Myocardial Ischemic Protection by Both Stereoisomers of Verapamil

M. Raschack and K. Engelmann

Department of Pharmacology
Knoll AG
Ludwigshafen, Federal Republic of Germany

Abstract. The effects of the optical isomers of verapamil were compared on intact and partially ischemic pig hearts as well as on vascular smooth muscle of rabbits and rats. In K^+-depolarized strips of rabbit mesenteric artery, both isomers shifted calcium dose–response curves (tension development) in a qualitatively similar manner to the right, with threshold concentrations of 10^{-8} M ($-$)verapamil and 10^{-7} M ($+$)verapamil. In K^+-depolarized rat aortic strips, the calcium antagonistic activity was quantified. ($+$)Verapamil was at least as potent as several other coronary drugs [($\pm$)verapamil = 1]: perhexiline 0.02, prenylamine 0.05, fendiline 0.05, diltiazem 0.15, ($+$)verapamil 0.15, ($-$)verapamil 1.5. The optical isomers of D600 showed a considerably greater difference in calcium antagonistic potency (about a factor of 60) as compared to verapamil (factor of 10). In the pig heart, reversible and reproducible ischemia reactions were provoked by repeated occlusions (3 min) of a branch of the LAD followed by reperfusion for 15 min. In the tested range of 0.4–2.0 mg/kg i.v., ($+$)verapamil dose-dependently reduced ischemic ST elevations in four epicardial leads. At an intermediate dose of 1 mg/kg, ($+$)verapamil diminished ST-elevations by 32% (occlusion 11 min p.i.). Results not statistically different were obtained with 0.1 mg/kg ($-$)verapamil (28%) and 0.2 mg/kg ($\pm$)verapamil (40%). No qualitative differences between the isomers could be observed with regard to hemodynamic parameters with equieffective reduction of the ischemia reaction: slight decrease in heart rate; prolongation of PQ duration with only minimal and insignificant effect of ($+$)verapamil; decrease of systolic and diastolic blood pressure, left ventricular pressure, and LV dp/dt_{max}. In contrast to optically active and racemic verapamil, nifedipine in a hypotensive dose (0.05 mg/kg i.v.) increased heart rate and diminished ischemic ST elevations only moderately (13%). The results obtained on vascular smooth muscle and ischemic pig heart clearly show that there are no remarkable qualitative differences between verapamil enantiomers. It can be concluded that ($+$)verapamil, by its calcium antagonistic properties, contributes to the therapeutic efficacy of the racemic drug.

Verapamil and D600 were first characterized as calcium antagonists by Fleckenstein and co-workers (4). Like several other calcium antagonists or beta blockers, they are racemic drugs. The purpose of this study was to further elucidate whether the optical isomers of verapamil show only quantitative or actual qualitative differences, as was assumed by Bayer et al. from experiments on cat papillary muscle. Surprisingly, these authors attributed quite specific inhibitory effects on the fast Na^+ inward current to the dextrorotatory isomers of verapamil and D600, at least in ventricular myocardium (1). On the other hand, later investigations on cat papillary muscles revealed only quantitative differences between verapamil enantiomers. (7)

Therefore, it seemed to be of interest to compare the optical isomers on the intact, partially ischemic heart as well as on vascular smooth muscle (see also ref. 9).

MATERIALS AND METHODS

Calcium Antagonistic Effects in Arterial Smooth Muscle

Calcium Dose–Response Curves.   Experiments were performed on spiral strips (about 6 mm length and 1.5 mm width) of the A. mesenterica of rabbits (chinchilla, 3.5–4.5 kg body weight) which had been sacrificed by a blow on the neck and bleeding from the A. carotis. Preload was 1.5 g; relaxation was achieved during 1 hr in Tyrode solution at 37°C bubbled with a mixture of 95% O_2 and 5% CO_2. The strips were rinsed three times for 5 min in Ca-free Tyrode solution containing 0.2 mM NaEDTA. The Ca-free strips were depolarized by replacing 100 mM Na^+ by K^+. In the presence of Tris buffer (pH 7.3–7.4), a cumulative calcium dose–response curve was established by adding $CaCl_2$ solution every 10 min until maxium tension had developed. After washing (six times, 10 min) with Tyrode solution, the procedure was repeated. Drugs were injected 15 min before establishing a second calcium dose–reponse curve by adding $CaCl_2$ solution up to the limit of solubility. Tension was recorded isometrically (Harvard transducer 363; Heath-Schlumberger recorder SR-255B) and expressed as percentage of the maximum of the first calcium dose–response curve.

Calcium Antagonistic Activity.   Two calcium test contractions were provoked in K^+-depolarized spiral strips (20 mm length, 2 mm width) of the aorta of Sprague–Dawley rats (250–300 g body weight) which had been anesthetized with ether. Preload was 1 g; relaxation was achieved within about 1 hr in Tyrode solution at 37°C bubbled with a mixture of 95% O_2 and 5% CO_2 (pH 7.3–7.4). Strips were rinsed three times for 5 min in Ca-free Tyrode solution containing 0.2 mM NaEDTA. The Ca-free strips were depolarized using Tyrode solution in which 100 mM Na^+ had been replaced by K^+. After 10 min, a first calcium contraction was provoked by 0.5 mM Ca^{2+}. Fifteen minutes later, strips were washed for 10 min with Ca-free Tyrode solution containing 0.2 mM NaEDTA and again depolarized. Drugs were added 15 min before the second calcium test contraction (0.5 mM). Tension was recorded isometrically (Harvard transducer 363; Heath-Schlumberger recorder SR-255B). The percentage inhibition of the calcium contraction in the presence of different drug concentrations was evaluated. From the linear part of concentration–response curves, linear regressions were calculated. Relative potencies were estimated from the distance of these linear regression lines.

Myocardial Ischemia in Pigs

The investigations were performed in white land-race pigs of 25–30 kg body weight under azaperone–metomidate–nitrous oxide anesthesia (2 mg/kg Stresnil® i.m.; after 15 min, 4 mg/kg Hypnodil® i.v.). Hexacarbacholine bromide in a dose of 0.03 mg/kg (Imbetril®) was given intravenously as a muscle relaxant. This application was repeated within 4 hr if required. Artificial ventilation was performed via an endotracheal tube with a mixture of 75% O_2 and 25% N_2O at a rate of 15–20 per min and an inspiration pressure of 15–20 cm H_2O by a Bird–Mark 8 respirator (Bird Corporation, Palm Springs). The expiratory CO_2 was controlled by means of a CO_2-test apparatus (E. Jaeger, Wuerzburg) and kept constant by varying inspiration pressure and ventilation rate. Body temperature was controlled via a rectal thermistor probe (43 TF, Yellow Springs Instruments, Ohio). For intravenous injection, a catheter was inserted into the left V. jugularis. Left ventricular pressure and aortic pressure were measured by a catheter-tip manometer (PC 780, Millar Instruments, Houston). Heart rate was determined from the ECG (lead II).

After left-side thoracotomy in the fifth intercostal space, the pericardium was opened. To avoid atrial arrhythmias caused by surgical intervention, lidocaine was applied prophylactically onto the left atrium (0.5 ml of a 1% Xylocain® solution). Ischemia was produced by reversible ligature of the first major branch of the left descending coronary artery (LAD) by means of polyethylene tube. Four epicardial leads from the ischemic area were obtained by gold electrodes fixed in pairs into perforations of two elastic rubber strips. The strips were pasted into the epicardium with tissue adhesive (Histoacryl®), thus guaranteeing a thorough and steady contact. After preparation, 2500 I.U. of heparin (Liquemin®) was administered per animal intravenously.

Occlusion time was 3 min, followed by a reperfusion phase of 15 min. Thus, at 18-min intervals, eight occlusions were performed. Drugs or physiological saline (control group) were injected in a volume of 0.5 ml/kg within 2 min starting 5 min after the end of the third occlusion. In this manner, the first drug effect on ischemic ST elevation was evaluated at the end of the fourth occlusion, that is, 11 min after injection.

Subject to assessment was the mean ST elevation (ΣST/N) in the ischemic area at the end of the occlusions. Leads showing elevated ST segments (more than 3 mV) from the start or no clear-cut ST elevation at the first three occlusions (increase of less than 2 mV) were not evaluated.

The following seven experimental series were performed: (+)verapamil, 0.4, 1.0, 2.0 mg/kg; (−)verapamil, 0.1 mg/kg; (±)verapamil, 0.2 mg/kg; nifedipine, 0.05 mg/kg; control, 0.5 ml/kg of 0.9% saline. Each series consisted of six animals. Mean values were compared using Wilcoxon or Kruskal–Wallis tests at the 5% level. Drugs used included verapamil enantiomers and racemate (Knoll, Ludwigshafen), diltiazem (Tanabe Seiyaku, Osaka), fendiline (Dr. Thiemann, Lunen), perhexiline (Merrell Pharma, Gross-

Gerau), prenylamine (Hoechst, Frankfurt/M.), and tiapamil (Hoffmann-La Roche, Basel) as water-soluble salts; doses refer to the bases. Nifedipine (Bayer, Leverkusen) was used as aqueous solution containing 15% ethanol and 15% polyethylene glycol 400 (Lutrol 9®); preparation of the solution and in vitro experiments were done under sodium light.

RESULTS

Calcium Antagonistic Effects in Arterial Smooth Muscle

Qualitative Effects on Calcium Dose–Response Curves.   In the presence of racemic verapamil, calcium dose–response curves on K^+-depolarized strips of rabbit mesenteric artery were shifted to the right in a concentration-dependent manner. At high concentrations (10^{-6} M) the maximum tension obtainable was markedly depressed as well. Similar results were obtained when testing the optical isomers. (+)Verapamil in a dose range of 10^{-7} to 10^{-5} M shifted the calcium dose–response curves in a manner qualitatively equal to (−)verapamil in the range of 10^{-8} to 10^{-6} M.

Calcium Antagonistic Activity. In K^+-depolarized rat aortic strips, (+)verapamil, like several other calcium antagonistic coronary drugs, dose-dependently reduced calcium contractions (Table 1). (+)Verapamil showed one-tenth the activity of its enantiomer and 15% of the potency of the racemic drug. (+)Verapamil was at least as active as several other calcium antagonistic coronary drugs such as perhexiline, fendiline, and prenylamine and exerted nearly the same potency as diltiazem and the verapamil derivative Ro 11-1781 (tiapamil). The optical isomers of D600 showed a considerably greater difference in calcium antagonistic efficacy: they differ by a factor of nearly 60 as compared to a factor of 10 with the verapamil isomers. Whereas (−)D600 was three times more potent than (−)verapamil, (+)D600 showed only half the activity of (+)verapamil. This difference was statistically significant.

Myocardial Ischemia Protection in Pigs

Under control conditions, a 3-min occlusion of a major branch of the left anterior descending coronary artery provoked pronounced and nearly

Table 1.   Calcium Antagonistic Potencies in K^+-Depolarized Rat Aortic Strips

(±)Verapamil	1	Tiapamil	0.17
(+)Verapamil	0.15	Diltiazem	0.15
(−)Verapamil	1.5	Nifedipine	7.5
(±)D600	2.5	Prenylamine	0.05
(+)D600	0.08	Fendiline	0.05
(−)D600	4.5	Perhexiline	0.02

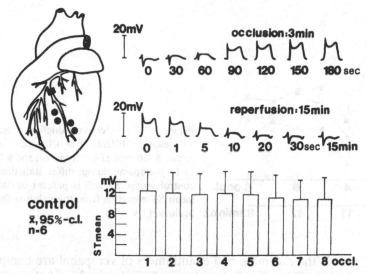

Figure 1.   Ischemic ST elevation in pig hearts. Top left side: ■, site of occlusion; ●, electrode position; top right side: one lead. Bottom: mean ST elevation (four leads) in the control group.

constant ST elevations in four epicardial leads. An example of the time course of the development of the ischemic ST elevation in one lead is given in Figure 1. On reperfusion, these changes were quickly reversible so that, separated by intervals of 15 min, the occlusion could be repeated several times. The lower part of Figure 1 shows the behavior of the mean ischemic ST elevation in the control group: eight consecutive occlusions caused nearly constant ischemia reactions.

With a threshold dose or 0.4 mg/kg of (+)verapamil, the ST elevations at the fourth and fifth occlusions were reduced by 15% and 12% as compared to the value before drug injection at the third occlusion. These effects as well as the differences from the control group were significant. With 1 mg/kg, the maximum effect as well as the duration of action increased. A dose increase to 2 mg/kg further enhanced the maximum effect (Figure 2).

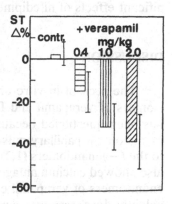

Figure 2.   (+)Verapamil dose-dependently decreases mean ischemic ST elevation. Shown are maximal effects at first occlusion after injection (fourth occlusion). ST Δ% is percent deviation of mean ST elevation from the value at the third occlusion; contr. is control group; bars show 95% confidence limit around mean ($N = 6$).

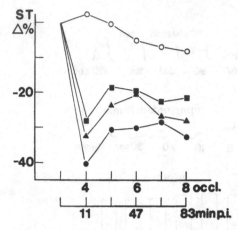

Figure 3.   Equieffective reduction of ischemic ST elevation. Effects of ■ 0.1 mg/kg (−)verapamil, ▲ 1.0 mg/kg (+)verapamil, and ● 0.2 mg/kg (+)verapamil do not differ statistically; ○, control group. ST Δ% is percent deviation of mean ST elevation from the value at the third occlusion ($N = 6$).

In Figure 3, the racemate and enantiomers of verapamil are compared, and control group behavior is also shown. The depression of the ischemic ST elevations after 0.1 mg/kg (−)verapamil, 1.0 mg/kg (+)verapamil, and 0.2 mg/kg (±)verapamil did not differ statistically. Hence, in the pig heart, too, the dose ratio was 10 between the enantiomers and about 5 between (+)verapamil and the racemic compound.

No qualitative differences between the isomers could be observed with respect to hemodynamic parameters at equieffective reduction of ischemia reaction (fourth occlusion, compare Figure 3). At a 32% reduction of the ischemic ST elevation, (+)verapamil caused the following cardiovascular changes: slight decrease in heart rate (− 11%) and insignificant prolongation of PQ duration (+ 8.5%); decrease of systolic (− 14%) and diastolic (− 27%) blood pressure, left ventricular systolic pressure (− 13%), and LV dp/dt_{max} (− 23%); LVEDP remained constant (+ 0.2 mm Hg).

In contrast to optically active and racemic verapamil, nifedipine in a hypotensive dose (0.05 mg/kg) increased heart rate and reduced ischemic ST elevations only moderately: the maximum reduction was 14% at the fourth occlusion (11 min p.i.). The next four occlusions did not reveal significant effects of nifedipine.

DISCUSSION

The present in vitro and in vivo results demonstrate that both optical isomers of verapamil and D600 exert calcium antagonistic properties; this has been questioned because of assumptions drawn from previous experiments on cat papillary muscle, attributing calcium antagonistic effects only to the (−)enantiomers (1,2). In our own studies, the dextrorotatory isomers also showed calcium antagonistic effects in a dose-dependent manner. Both enantiomers of verapamil caused a qualitatively similar shift to the right of calcium dose–response curves obtained in K^+-depolarized strips of rabbit mesenteric artery, the only difference being a ten times higher concentration of (+)verapamil. The same potency ratio was found in K^+-depolarized rat aortic strips against single test contractions produced by a fixed calcium dose. Isomers and racemates of verapamil and D600 revealed parallel concentration–response curves, so that relative potencies could be calculated (see Table 1). It seems noteworthy that (+)verapamil was more potent than several other coronary therapeutics which are described as acting by calcium antagonistic mechanisms. (+)Verapamil showed calcium antagonistic activity comparable to that of diltiazem and tiapamil (Ro 11-1781), a recently described verapamil derivative.

Our finding that (+)verapamil has remarkable calcium antagonistic potency in arterial muscle is in accordance with the latest results of other investigators comparing vascular effects of verapamil enantiomers in vitro as well as in the whole animal. When injected into the septal arteries of the atrioventricular node preparation of the dog, (−)verapamil was only three times as potent as (+)verapamil in increasing blood flow (10). In the intact dog, the difference between the isomers was even smaller; when injected intravenously, (+)verapamil was nearly equipotent with the (−)isomer in increasing coronary sinus outflow (11).

The calcium antagonistic effects of (+)verapamil found in isolated organs led us to the question of whether it would be possible to influence myocardial ischemia with this enantiomer alone. The dose-dependent reduction of ischemic ST elevation in the pig heart by (+)verapamil was a clear-cut result (see Figure 2). Furthermore, other cardiovascular parameters such as left ventricular *dp/dt* and blood pressure were influenced by (+)verapamil as could be expected from results with the racemic compound. When verapamil isomers were compared with respect to hemodynamic changes at equipotent reduction of ischemic ST elevation, no qualitative differences could be detected, but atrioventricular conduction seemed to be influenced by (+)verapamil to a lesser degree. In the dog heart, too, the dose–response relationship for the increase in AV conduction time seems to be steeper with (−)verapamil than with (+)verapamil (11). The question of whether (+)verapamil really has less negative dromotropic effects at equipotent calcium antagonistic actions on myocardium and arterial vessels needs further experimental clarification.

Another noteworthy finding from the present experiments is that with nifedipine, despite its high calcium antagonistic potency in isolated muscle (compare Table 1), only moderate and short-lasting reduction of ischemic ST-elevation occurred in the pig as compared to racemic and optically active verapamil. This applies even to a high dose of nifedipine (0.05 mg/kg) which is hemodynamically active in this model in, for example, lowering blood pressure and increasing heart rate. In contrast, after injection of racemic or optically active verapamil, no augmentation of heart rate occurred. This difference might be caused by the lack of antiarrhythmic properties of nifedipine and might account for its comparably small effects on ischemic ST elevation.

The results on vascular smooth muscle and ischemic heart as well as results of other investigations in different experimental models (3–6,10,11) including subcellular preparations (8) demonstrate that there is no remarkable qualitative difference between the stereoisomers of verapamil.

It can be concluded that (+)verapamil, by its calcium antagonistic properties, contributes to the therapeutic efficacy of the racemic drug.

ACKNOWLEDGMENTS

We thank Mrs. A. Moniac, Miss S. Goeck, Mr. R. Bock, and Mr. G. Schaefer for their excellent technical assistance.

REFERENCES

1. Bayer, R., Kalusche, D., Kaufmann, R., and Mannhold, R. 1975. Inotropic and electrophysiological actions of verapamil and D 600 in mammalian myocardium. III. Effects of the optical isomers on transmembrane action potentials. Naunyn Schmiedebergs Arch. Pharmacol. 290:81–97.
2. Bayer, R., Kaufmann, R., and Mannhold, R. 1975. Inotropic and electrophysiological actions of verapamil and D 600 in mammalian myocardium. II. Pattern of inotropic effects of the optical isomers. Naunyn Schmiedebergs Arch. Pharmacol. 290:69–80.
3. Chiba, S., Kobayashi, M., and Furukawa, Y. 1978. Effects of optical isomers of verapamil on SA nodal pacemaker activity and contractility of the isolated dog heart. Jpn. Heart J. 19:409–414.
4. Fleckenstein, A. 1971. Specific inhibitors and promoters of calcium action in the excitation–contraction coupling of heart muscle and their role in the prevention or production of myocardial lesions. In: P. Harris and L. Opie (eds.), Calcium and the Heart, pp. 135–188. Academic Press, New York.
5. Kaumann, A. J., and Serur, J. R. 1975. Optical isomers of verapamil on canine heart. Prevention of ventricular fibrillation induced by coronary artery occlusion, impaired atrioventricular conductance and negative inotropic and chronotropic effects. Naunyn Schmiedebergs Arch. Pharmacol. 291:347–358.
6. Ludwig, C., and Nawrath, H. 1977. Effects of D 600 and its optical isomers on force of contraction in cat papillary muscles and guinea-pig articles. Br. J. Pharmacol. 59:411–417.
7. Nawrath, H., Blei, J., Gegner, R., Ludwig, C., and Zong, X. 1981. No stereospecific effects of the optical isomers of verapamil and D-600 on the heart. In: A. Zanchetti and D. M. Krikler (eds.), Calcium Antagonism in Cardiovascular Therapy, Experience with Verapamil. Internat. Symposium, Florence. 2nd-4th October, 1980, pp. 52–63, Excerpta Medica, Amsterdam-Oxford-Princeton.
8. Nayler, W. G., Mas-Oliva, J., and Williams, A. J. 1980. Cardiovascular receptors and calcium. Circ. Res. 46(Suppl. 1):161–166.
9. Raschack, M., and Engelmann, K. 1980. Calcium-antagonistic activity and myocardial ischemia protection by both stereoisomers of verapamil. J. Mol. Cell. Cardiol. 12(Suppl. 1):132.
10. Satoh, K., Yanagisawa, T., and Taira, N. 1979. Effects of atrioventricular conduction and blood flow of enantiomers of verapamil and of tetrodotoxin injected into the posterior and the anterior septal artery of the atrioventricular node preparation of the dog. Naunyn Schmiedebergs Arch. Pharmacol. 308:89–98.
11. Satoh, K., Yanagisawa, T., and Taira, N. 1980. Coronary vasodilator and cardiac effects of optical isomers of Verapamil in the dog. J. Cardiovasc. Pharmacol. 2:309–318.

The Effects of β Blockade and Partial Agonist Activity during Myocardial Ischemia

A. S. Manning, J. M. Keogh, D. J. Coltart, and D. J. Hearse

The Myocardial Metabolism and Cardiac Pharmacology Units
The Rayne Institute
St. Thomas' Hospital
London SE1, England

Abstract. In this study, we have investigated the importance of partial agonist activity during myocardial ischemia by comparing the effects of equiblocking doses of oxprenolol, which possesses partial agonist activity, to propranolol which does not. In the isolated, globally ischemic (low-flow) rat heart, when propranolol or oxprenolol was added alone during the ischemic period, only propranolol reduced enzyme leakage relative to control. However, when the hearts were perfused (10 min) prior to ischemia with these drugs, both β blockers caused a significant reduction in enzyme leakage. Under conditions of enhanced sympathetic drive (in the presence of 0.01 μM isoproterenol), both β blockers reduced enzyme leakage to differing extents. In hearts with low sympathetic drive (reserpine pretreatment), enzyme leakage was unaffected by propranolol and exacerbated by oxprenolol. The results of this study suggest that oxprenolol and propranolol influence ischemic damage to differing extents and that this difference is due to partial agonist activity. Also, the protective action of all β-blocking compounds depends greatly on the background level of sympathetic drive.

At present there are a number of β-blocking compounds such as oxprenolol, acebutolol, and pindolol that also possess varying degrees of β-agonist activity. This property removes from the compound the ability to completely antagonize the action of catecholamines, and therefore, they may cause comparatively smaller changes in cardiac function than compounds without this property. The effect is most likely to be seen under conditions of greatly reduced sympathetic support. The role of partial agonist activity during ischemia is controversial, and it has not been established whether this property aids or hinders protection of the ischemic myocardium. Studies (9) in the anesthetized dog with coronary artery ligation suggest that compounds with partial agonist activity are more beneficial than propranolol, whereas in the isolated heart model, compounds with partial agonist activity have been suggested to increase tissue damage compared with control (1,10).

We have therefore undertaken a study aimed at investigating the importance of partial agonist activity during myocardial ischemia. In this study, we have compared the effects of equiblocking doses of oxprenolol (which possesses partial agonist activity) to propranolol which does not. Neither of these compounds is cardioselective, and both possess membrane-stabilizing activity. Thus, in terms of their major subsidiary properties, they differ solely in the possession of partial agonist activity by oxyprenolol. In any study of partial agonist activity, it is clearly important to relate the amount of partial agonist activity inherent in the β-blocking compound to the level of sympathetic drive in the experimental model used, particularly in isolated heart preparations where there is no sustained exogenous drive. Therefore, we have examined the role of partial agonist activity on ischemic injury under various levels of catecholamine drive: near zero levels (animals pretreated with reserpine), under standard perfusion conditions (with only endogenous catecholamine drive), and with enhanced catecholamine drive (isoproterenol added to the perfusion medium).

MATERIALS AND METHODS

Experimental Animals and Drug Pretreatment

Male rats (230–300 g body wt.) of Wistar strain, maintained on a standard diet, were used. In the reserpine-pretreated animals, a single dose (5 mg/kg body wt. i.p.) was administered 24 hr before sacrifice.

Perfusion Techniques

Rats were lightly anethetized with diethyl ether, the right femoral vein was exposed, and 200 I.U. heparin was injected intravenously. Approximately 1 min later, the heart was excised and placed in ice-cold perfusion medium until contraction had ceased (approximately 30 sec). The aorta was cannulated, and the heart perfused in the Langendorff mode at a hydrostatic pressure of 100 cm. Under these conditions, coronary flow was approximately 8 ml/min per g wet wt. After a 10-min aerobic control period, the hearts were made ischemic by perfusing with a controlled, reduced coronary flow of 0.25 ml/min using an infusion pump. In order to insure that the low-flow infusion was delivered to the heart at 37°C, a water-jacketed cannula was used (7).

Although ischemia was induced in this model by a reduction in coronary flow, the residual flow was fully oxygenated ($PO_2 > 600$ mm Hg) through the use of a hollow-fiber oxygenator system (7) which was in line with the aortic cannula. This oxygenator consisted of a length of ultrathin-walled silicone rubber tubing through which the perfusate passed. The tubing facilitated gaseous exchange without fluid loss. The fiber was encased in a column through which passed a countercurrent of 95% O_2, 5% CO_2.

Perfusion Media

Bicarbonate buffer, pH 7.4 (3,6) was the standard solution for all perfusion fluids. During both the control and ischemic period, 11.1 mM glucose and 5 μM ascorbate (to prevent the oxidation of isoproterenol) were added to the perfusion fluid which was gassed with 95% O_2 and 5% CO_2 ($PO_2 >$ 600 mm Hg). Prior to use, all perfusion fluids were filtered through a 5-μm cellulose acetate filter. When β-adrenergic agonists or antagonists were added to the perfusion fluid, the following final concentrations were used: 7 μM propranolol, 10 μM oxprenolol, and 0.01 μM isoproterenol. This dose of isoproterenol produced submaximal increases in heart rate and dP/dt_{max}. In terms of β-blocking potency, these concentrations of propranolol and oxprenolol produced equivalent shifts in response to isoproterenol challenge in the isolated heart and were therefore considered to be equipotent β-blocking doses.

In studies in which contractile activity was abolished by the use of a high-potassium perfusion medium, the potassium concentration was raised to 16 mM, and the sodium concentration approximately lowered.

Assessment of Tissue Injury

Ischemic damage was assessed by the leakage of creatine kinase (CK; ATP–creatine phosphotransferase, E.C. 2.7.3.2). This was collected at intervals of 30 min throughout the entire ischemic period and was assayed by the method of Oliver (11).

RESULTS

Addition of β-Blocking Compounds before and during Ischemia

Perfusion with β blockers for 10 min at normal flow before the onset of ischemia and also throughout the ischemic period reduced the total enzyme released (Figure 1). However, the reduction in enzyme release was greater with propranolol than with oxprenolol. Propranolol reduced enzyme leakage by about 75%, and oxprenolol by approximately 50%.

Addition of β-Blocking Compounds during Ischemia Only

The results for cumulative enzyme leakage during the ischemic period are shown in Figure 2. Propranolol significantly reduced (or delayed) release of enzyme. However, this reduction was not as great as when hearts were preperfused with propranolol. Oxprenolol, when added at the onset of the ischemic period, had no significant effect on enzyme leakage.

Addition of Drugs to the Catecholamine-Depleted Heart

The mean values for creatine kinase release from the hearts of animals pretreated with reserpine were lower than control values, although this

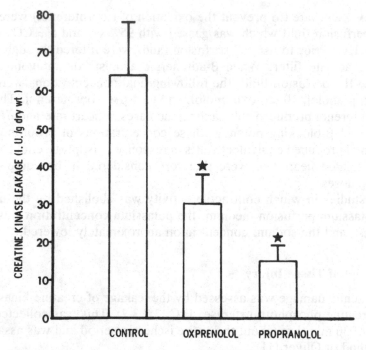

Figure 1. The cumulative total creatine kinase released from the isolated ischemic rat heart with β-blocking compounds preperfused before ischemia and administered throughout the ischemic period. Each value represents the mean of 6–13 hearts, and the bars represent the S.E.M. *$P < 0.05$.

decrease was not statistically significant (Figure 2). Pretreatment and inclusion throughout the ischemic period of oxprenolol exacerbated enzyme leakage, whereas propranolol had no effect.

Effect of Exogenous Catecholamine Addition

Figure 3 shows the cumulative enzyme release during a 6-hr period of ischemia. The addition of isoproterenol resulted in a greater increase in tissue damage against which both oxprenolol and propranolol were able to protect (in contrast to the absence of isoproterenol) to varying extents. Propranolol released approximately 20% of enzyme released by the control group, compared with oxprenolol which released approximately 50% of enzyme released by the control group. In spite of these large differences in enzyme release, no significant difference could be shown in total lactate release during the ischemic period.

In the K^+-arrested heart (zero contractile activity) in the presence of isoproterenol, neither oxprenolol nor propranolol significantly altered enzyme release from control during the ischemic period (Figure 3).

DISCUSSION

There is considerable evidence that treatment with propranolol will reduce the extent of myocardial ischemic injury. This has been demonstrated histologically (5,12) and using enzyme leakage (8). However, in the isolated heart model, there is disagreement over the protective ability of propranolol: claims for a protective effect (5,14) and disputing a protective effect have been made (3,13). Because of this discrepancy in results, we have studied the role of acute β blockade under several different conditions of catechol-amine drive in an attempt to define conditions in which this may influence the degree of myocardial damage.

In our study, the addition of propranolol reduced enzyme release when the drug was added at the onset of ischemia, added before and during is-chemia, and administered in the presence of isoproterenol. The greatest reduction in enzyme leakage produced by propranolol was in the presence of isoproterenol. Thus, in the ischemic, isolated heart, propranolol reduces or delays tissue damage. In the potassium-arrested heart (in the presence of isoproterenol), propranolol had no effect on enzyme release. This is

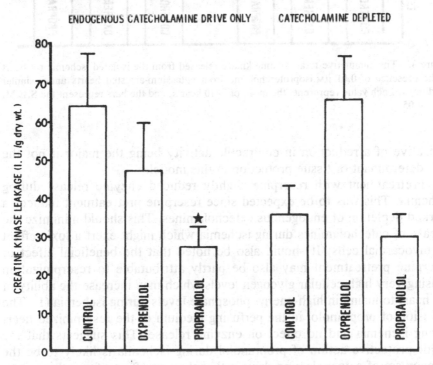

Figure 2. The cumulative total creatine kinase released from the untreated isolated ischemic rat heart and from the reserpinized isolated ischemic rat heart. Each value represents the mean of 6–13 hearts, and the bars represent the S.E.M. *P < 0.05.

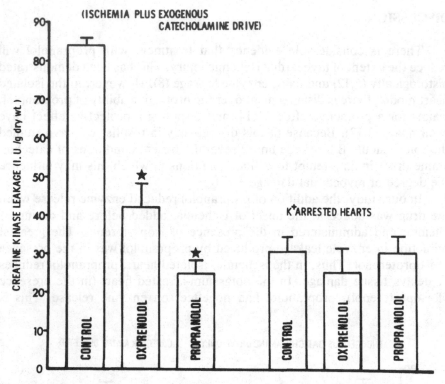

Figure 3.   The cumulative total creatine kinase released from the isolated ischemic rat heart in the presence of 0.01 μM isoproterenol and from potassium-arrested hearts under similar conditions. Each value represents the mean of 5–10 hearts, and the bars represent the S.E.M. *P < 0.05.

indicative of a reduction in contractile activity being the major if not the sole determinant of tissue protection in this model.

Pretreatment with reserpine slightly reduced enzyme release during ischemia. This was to be expected since reserpine pretreatment induces a marked depletion of endogenous catecholamines. This should minimize the release of catecholamines during ischemia which might exert a toxic effect on myocardial cells. It should also be noted that the beneficial effect of reserpine pretreatment may also be partly attributable to reserpinization causing very high cellular glycogen levels which may increase the ability of the heart to maintain high-energy phosphate levels during ischemia (1). The inclusion of propranolol in the perfusing medium of the reserpinized heart during ischemia had no effect on enzyme release. This suggests that the major protective action of propranolol during ischemia is likely to be the antagonism of catecholamine drive rather than an effect of membrane-stabilizing activity or blockade of calcium ion entry (2).

The protection afforded by oxprenolol against enzyme leakage in this model would appear to be more complex. Oxprenolol possesses membrane-stabilizing activity and partial agonist activity as well as being a β-blocking agent. In the reserpinized heart, where catecholamine drive is very low, the β-blocking property of oxprenolol is masked, and its action as a partial agonist becomes evident as an exacerbation of tissue damage which is then greater than control. When oxprenolol was added to the normal heart at the onset of ischemia, no significant protection or exacerbation was seen. However, a significant protection was observed when the hearts were preperfused with oxprenolol. Under conditions of enhanced catecholamine drive (isoproterenol added to the perfusate), the β-blocking action of oxprenolol becomes dominant over its partial agonist activity, and a reduction in enzyme release is observed. This reduction is, however, not equivalent to that produced by propranolol. Again, a major part of the reduction in tissue damage is probably through a diminution in contractile activity, since the removal of this component with potassium arrest eliminates any protective effect of oxprenolol.

Figure 4 summarizes these results, relates the background level of catecholamine drive to the eventual degree of ischemic damage, and shows how β blockade and partial agonist activity may affect these functions. At near zero catecholamine drive, propranolol had very little effect, whereas oxprenolol showed a small increase in tissue damage. At more normal levels, propranolol significantly reduced enzyme leakage, whereas oxprenolol only reduced tissue damage when added before the onset of ischemia. With en-

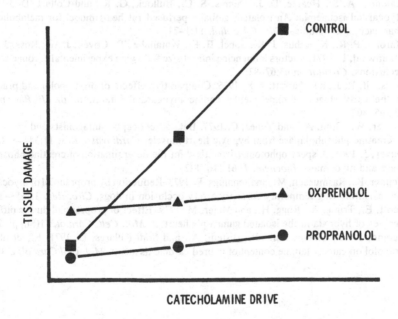

Figure 4. A theoretical summary of the previous results.

hanced catecholamine drive, which normally occurs during myocardial ischemia in vivo, both oxprenolol and propranolol reduced ischemic damage.

In conclusion, the final choice of β blocker may rest on the relative importance of preserving pump function (especially in conditions of borderline left ventricular failure) or reducing ischemic injury.

ACKNOWLEDGMENTS

This work was carried out with the aid of grants from St. Thomas' Hospital Research Endowments Fund and the British Heart Foundation.

REFERENCES

1. De Leiris, J., Peyrot, M., and Feuvray, D. 1978. Pharmacological reduction of ischaemia-induced enzyme release from isolated rat hearts. *J. Mol. Med.* 3:111–121.
2. Dhalla, N. S., Lee, S. L., Anand, M. B., and Chauhan, M. S. 1977. Effects of acebutolol, practolol and propranolol on the rat heart sarcolemma. *Biochem. Pharmacol.* 26:2055–2060.
3. Hearse, D. J., Garlick, P. B., Humphrey, S. M., and Shillingford, J. P. 1978. The effect of drugs on enzyme release from the hypoxic myocardium. *Eur. J. Cardiol.* 7:421–436.
4. Hearse, D. J., Humphrey, S. M., and Bullock, G. R. 1978. The oxygen paradox and the calcium paradox: Two facets of the same problem? *J. Mol. Cel. Cardiol.* 10:641–668.
5. Kloner, R., Fishbein, M., Braunwald, E., and Maroko, P. 1977. Effect of propranolol on mitochondrial morphology during acute myocardial ischemia. *Am. J. Cardiol.* 55:872–886.
6. Krebs, H. A., and Henseleit, K. 1932. Untersuchungen über die Harnstoffbildung im Tierkörper. *Hoppe Seylers Z. Physiol. Chem.* 210:33–66.
7. Manning, A. S., Hearse, D. J., Dennis, S. C., Bullock, G. R., and Coltart, D. J. 1980. Myocardial ischaemia: An isolated, globally perfused rat heart model for metabolic and pharmacological studies. *Eur. J. Cardiol.* 11:1–21.
8. Maroko, P. R., Kjekshus, J. K., Sobel, B. E., Watanabe, T., Covell, J. W., Ross, J., and Braunwald, E. 1971. Factors influencing infarct size following experimental coronary artery occlusions. *Circulation* 43:67–82.
9. Marshall, R. J., and Parratt, J. R. 1976. Comparative effects of propranolol and practolol in the early stages of experimental canine myocardial infarction. *Br. J. Pharmacol.* 57:295–303.
10. Nayler, W., Grau, A., and Yepez, C. 1977. Beta-adrenoceptor antagonists and the release of creatine phosphokinase from hypoxic heart muscle. *Cardiovasc. Res.* 11:344–352.
11. Oliver, J. 1965. A spectrophotometric method for the determination of creatine phosphokinase and myokinase. *Biochem. J.* 61:116–122.
12. Reimer, K., Rasmussen, M., and Jennings, R. 1973. Reduction by propranolol of myocardial necrosis following temporary coronary artery occlusion in dogs. *Circ. Res.* 33:353–363.
13. Scott, E., Truog, A., Rogg, H., and Meier, M. 1979. Effect of propranolol during different degrees of hypoxia in the isolated guinea-pig heart. *J. Mol. Cell. Cardiol.* 11(Suppl. 2):54.
14. Serano, P. A., Chavez-Lara, B., Bisteni, A., and Sodi-Pallares, D. 1971. Effect of propranolol on catecholamine content of injured cardiac tissue. *J. Mol. Cell Cardiol.* 2:91–97.

Cyclic Nucleotides and Changes in Protein Kinase Activity Ratio in the Ischemic and Nonischemic Myocardium

E.-G. Krause, S. Bartel, P. Karczewski, and K.-F. Lindenau

Division of Cellular and Molecular Cardiology
Central Institute of Heart and Circulation Research
Academy of Sciences of the GDR
1115 Berlin–Buch
and
Surgical Clinic
Faculty of Medicine (Charité) of Humboldt University at Berlin
1040 Berlin, German Democratic Republic

Abstract. Following coronary artery ligation (CAL), levels of cAMP and the activity ratio of cAMP-dependent protein kinase, of phosphorylase kinase, and of phosphorylase are significantly elevated in both ischemic and nonischemic areas of the canine left ventricle. The aerobic level of cAMP was found to be 0.4 to 0.6 pmol/mg myocardium only after a precooled clamp or a cryobiopsy device was employed to guarantee tissue freezing in situ. Maximal changes in response to ischemia are observed within 2 min in both parts of the heart. Twenty minutes after the onset of ischemia, different responses have been found in the nonischemic and ischemic tissue. Whereas the levels of cAMP and the activity ratio of protein kinase, of phosphorylase kinase, and of phosphorylase returned to aerobic values in the nonischemic area, these parameters remained elevated in the ischemic area. The changes in the levels of myocardial cAMP and in the cAMP-dependent protein kinase activity ratio following CAL could be prevented by propranolol.

Inasmuch as the cyclic nucleotides play a part in the neural–hormonal regulation of the heart and to the extent that the tissue levels of cAMP and cGMP reflect, directly or indirectly, the intensity of adrenergic and cholinergic input respectively, it is instructive to know these levels in myocardial response to acute ischemia (see 12). The effects of cAMP and cGMP within the cell are thought in almost all cases to be a result of the stimulation of cyclic-nucleotide-dependent protein kinases (8,17). These enzymes, together with Ca^{2+}-dependent protein kinases, phosphorylate a variety of cellular proteins and enzymes, leading in one or more additional steps to the physiological response. Whereas the activity of cAMP-dependent protein kinases has not been examined systematically in the ischemic myocardium up to now, and elevation in the levels of cAMP has been observed in the acute ischemic myocardium by several groups including our laboratory (4,13,24).

521

More recently, however, such a rise in cAMP was questioned (21). The present work deals with changes in cyclic nucleotide levels and the activation of cAMP-dependent protein kinases and some of subsequent metabolic events in both the ischemic and nonischemic parts of the canine left ventricular muscle after CAL. Furthermore a new method—the so-called push–freeze–drill technique (10)—for freezing myocardial tissue samples in situ was employed in determining the levels of cAMP in the aerobic heart muscle.

MATERIALS AND METHODS

Dogs (20–30 kg) were anesthetized with α-chloralose/urethane (50 mg/ 400 mg per kg body weight) and maintained on artificial respiration. After thoracotomy, the left coronary artery was ligated. In experiments in which dogs were pretreated with propranolol (2 mg per kg body weight), the drug was given i.v. 2 min before ligation. If not otherwise indicated, tissue samples were taken simultaneously from both the ischemic and nonischemic areas of the left ventricle with Wollenberger clamps precooled in liquid N_2 at 0, 2, and 20 min after CAL.

Cyclic AMP was measured in the trichloroacetic acid extracts of cardiac tissue by the protein binding assay according to Gilman (5). Prior to the assay, the nucleotide was purified by alumina and Dowex® 1 × 2 chromatography. Cyclic GMP was estimated by a radioimmunoassay according to Harper and Brooker (6). (The antibody was kindly provided by Dr. G. Schulz, Heidelberg.) ATP was enzymatically measured with a Boehringer kit (15979 TAAC).

The determination of cAMP-dependent protein kinse activity was performed in a modification of the procedure of Dobson (3) and Keely and Corbin (8). The enzyme activity is expressed as the protein kinase activity ratio, i.e., the ratio of kinase activity in the absence of added cAMP to that in the presence of cAMP. Measurements of phosphorylase kinase activity (expressed as the activity ratio pH 6.8/pH 8.2) and the phosphorylase activity (expressed as the activity ratio without 5'AMP/with 5'AMP) were performed according to Kres et al. (14) and Illingworth and Cori (7), respectively.

RESULTS

Cyclic AMP Levels

Partly confirming earlier results (13), cAMP was found to increase significantly in ischemic and nonischemic myocardium within 2 min after CAL (Figure 1). Twenty minutes after CAL, cAMP in the nonischemic area had returned to aerobic control. Values for the latter levels averaged 0.60 pmol/ mg wet weight, in agreement with results obtained with hearts of rats and

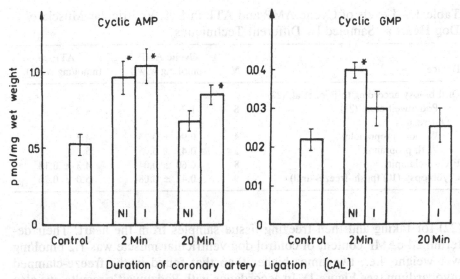

Figure 1.   Changes in the levels of cyclic nucleotides in the nonischemic (NI) and ischemic (I) areas of the left ventricle of dogs following coronary artery ligation (CAL). Means ± S.E.M. ($N = 5$ to 8) are given. Stars indicate changes significantly different from controls ($P < 0.05$).

other animals. The rise in myocardial levels of cAMP in the nonischemic (Figure 2) as well as in ischemic (not shown) tissue following CAL could be prevented by 2 mg/kg racemic propranolol, although (+)-propranolol was ineffective.

Contrary to these and other (2,4) results, Podzuweit et al. (21) did not find an elevation of cAMP in ventricular myocardial biopsies taken from dog and baboon immediately after CAL. From their results, they questioned whether cAMP plays a part in the adjustment of cardiac metabolism to sudden anaerobiosis. However, these authors used a drill biopsy technique

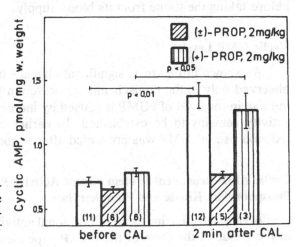

Figure 2.   Influence of propranolol on the levels of cAMP in the nonischemic area of left ventricular muscle before and 2 min after CAL.

Table 1.   Levels of Cyclic AMP and ATP in Left Ventricular Muscle of Dog Heart as Sampled by Different Techniques

Device	N	Cyclic AMP (pmol/mg w.w.)	ATP (nmol/mg w.w.)
Drill biopsy according to Pool et al. (22)			
Podzuweit et al. (21)	8	1.2	4.9
Our results			
Without propranolol	4	0.96 ± 0.23	4.7
With propranolol	2	0.45 ± 0.05	5.2
Freeze-clamping	8	0.60 ± 0.04	4.3 ± 0.18
Cryobiopsy (10) (push–freeze–drill)	9	0.42 ± 0.08	5.0 ± 0.26

(22) for taking and then freezing tissue samples from the heart. Their determined cAMP content of control dog ventricular muscle was 1.2 pmol/mg wet weight, i.e., two times higher than that found in the freeze-clamped myocardium (see Figure 1). In accordance with Podzuweit's results, we also obtained such high levels of cAMP in tissue samples taken from aerobic myocardium by the drill biopsy technique (see Table 1); however, pretreatment of animals with propranolol lowered by one-half this control level of cAMP, which is in sharp contrast to the absence of any effect of propranolol in the freeze-clamped tissue (see Figure 2). Thus, an uncontrolled, probably catecholamine-induced elevation in levels of cAMP occurs during tissue sampling by the drill biopsy technique and overwhelms any rapid rises in cAMP in the myocardium. There were no differences among the levels of ATP in the myocardial tissues sampled by the enumerated procedures.

A value of cAMP of 0.42 pmol/mg myocardium was found in aerobic canine left ventricular muscle employing a new cryobiopsy technique which combines some advantages of the drill procedure with the necessity of freezing the tissue sample in situ to terminate neural and metabolic activities before taking the tissue from its blood supply.

Cyclic GMP Levels

As shown in Figure 1, significant changes in the levels of cGMP were observed only in the nonischemic myocardium 2 min after CAL. Whether the rise in the level of cGMP is caused by increased parasympathetic nerve activity remains to be established. In earlier experiments, the ischemia-induced rise in cGMP was prevented after vagotomy (13).

Cyclic AMP-Dependent Protein Kinase Activity Ratio and Activation of Phosphorylase Kinase and Phosphorylase

A very sensitive indicator of hormonal activity exerted via cAMP exists in the tissue in the form of the cAMP-dependent protein kinase (8). From the subcellular distribution of this enzyme in the dog heart, the particulate form was found to constitute approximately 30% of the total activity. The enzyme exists in two types (isoenzyme type I and type II) in both the cytosolic and in the particulate fraction (Figure 3). Isoenzyme type II predominates in the canine myocardium in agreement with the findings of Matsushita et al. (16).

The value of the activity ratio of the protein kinases extracted from the aerobic myocardium without and with added 250 mM sodium chloride was found to be 0.11 and 0.25, respectively. As shown in Figure 4, the activity ratio of the kinase significantly increases within 2 min after CAL in the nonischemic as well as in the ischemic zone. Pretreatment of the animals with propranolol abolished the activation of the protein kinase. This is in concordance with the unchanged myocardial levels of cAMP under these conditions.

In addition to the elevation in the extent of protein kinase activation, the total activity of the soluble protein kinase was significantly increased

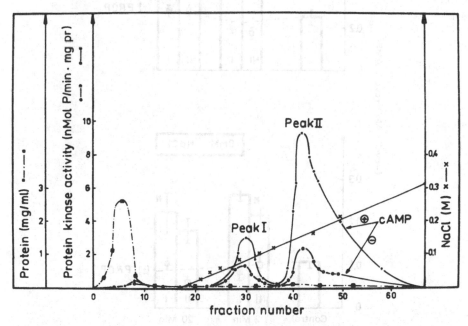

Figure 3.   DEAE-cellulose chromatography of cAMP-dependent protein kinase activity from canine myocardium. Extract was prepared by homogenizing frozen tissue in cold 10 mM potassium phosphate (4 ml/g), pH 6.8, containing 1 mM EDTA and 0.5 mM 1-methyl-3-isobutylxanthine. After centrifugation for 15 min at 27,000 × g, 2 ml of supernatant was applied to a DEAE-cellulose column (4 × 1 cm) equilibrated with the same buffer solution. After washing with 50 ml buffer, a linear gradient (0 to 0.4 M NaCl) was started. Fraction volume was 2 ml (flow rate = 2 ml/5 min). After dialysis, the protein kinase activity was measured in the absence and in the presence of 2 × 10^{-6} M cAMP (Peak I, isoenzyme type I; peak II, isoenzyme type II).

in the nonischemic and ischemic areas of the myocardium 2 min after CAL (data not shown). The fraction of phosphorylase kinase and phosphorylase present in the activated form increases to nearly the same extent at the end of the second and 20th minute after CAL in the ischemic zone. In the nonischemic area, a statistically significant increase was observed only at 2 min after CAL, as was shown for the protein kinase activity ratio in this particulate part of the left ventricle. In agreement with data reported by Dobson and Mayer (4), a cAMP-independent activation of phosphorylase

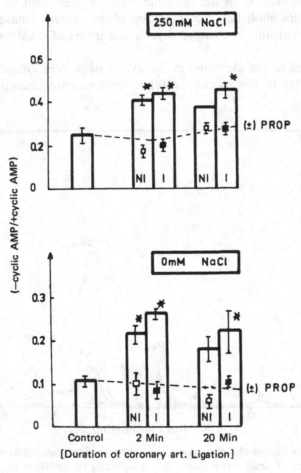

Figure 4. Activity ratio of cAMP-dependent protein kinase in the myocardium before and after coronary artery ligation. Tissues from the heart were homogenized in a buffer solution (1:50 wet wt/vol) containing 10 mM potassium phosphate (pH 6.8), 10 mM EDTA, and 0.5 mM 3-isobutyl-1-methylxanthine with and without 250 mM NaCl. Protein kinase activity was assayed immediately after homogenization by Ultra Turrax for 3 sec. NI, nonischemic area; I, ischemic part of the ventricle. Data (■, □) after pretreatment of animals with propranolol are connected by broken lines. Stars indicate changes significantly different from control ($P < 0.05$).

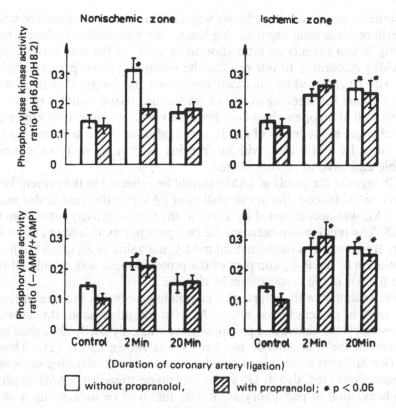

Figure 5. Changes in activities of phosphorylase kinase and phosphorylase in the nonischemic and ischemic areas of dog heart after CAL. Stars indicate changes significantly different from controls ($P \leq 0.05$).

was found in our experiments 2 min after CAL in the nonischemic and ischemic areas of the left ventricle and at 20 min in the latter. Nevertheless, a rise in the extent of phosphorylase kinase activation seems also to occur under these conditions (Figure 5).

DISCUSSION

The present results clearly reaffirm earlier data (2,4,13,24) that the levels of cAMP are elevated in the ischemic as well as nonischemic (2,13) part of the left ventricular muscle after CAL or otherwise-induced hypoxia. The rise in the myocardial levels of cAMP following CAL was completely prevented by the presence of propranolol, supporting the hypothesis that the increase in myocardial cAMP is the result of a stimulation of myocardial β-adrenoceptors and of adenylate cyclase coupled to them. This stimulation is best explained as resulting from release of endogenous cardiac norepinephrine (19) both by a direct effect of tissue ischemia and by increased sympathetic nerve activity (15). As was obvious in the comparative studies concerning tissue sampling from dog heart, only a procedure including tissue freezing in situ permits an estimation to be made of the true aerobic levels of cAMP. According to our results, the commonly used precooled clamp need only be replaced by the newly developed cryobiopsy technique which really permits the freezing in situ of transmural tissue samples of the ventricular wall of an open-chest dog. From this point of view, data concerning rapid changes in the levels of cAMP obtained from tissue samples that have been taken by a drill (i.e., without freezing in situ) are more or less questionable and have to be reestimated.

Changes in the levels of cAMP should be reflected in the protein kinase activity ratio. Indeed, the accumulation of cAMP in the ventricular muscle after CAL was accompanied by a rise in the kinase activity ratio from 0.11 to 0.28. The relationship between the two parameters was found to be non-linear. By means of a mathematical model, the value of K_d of cAMP for the dissociation of the R_2C_2 complex of the protein kinase was calculated to be 0.2 to 0.4 μM in the myocardium in vivo (9).

Pretreatment with propranolol completely prevents the rise in the activity ratio of protein kinase after CAL. On the other hand, the activation of phosphorylase kinase and phosphorylase was only partly abolished in the presence of the β-adrenergic blocker as was shown earlier (11). Thus, at least two different mechanisms may be operative in accelerating myocardial glycogenolysis (see also 4: (1) a catecholamine-triggered, cAMP-mediated phosphorylation of phosphorylase kinase followed by an activation of glycogen phosphorylase and (2) a catecholamine-independent, probably Ca^{2+}-triggered activation of nonactivated phosphorylase kinase, which probably leads to an autophosphorylation of this enzyme (1), followed again by an activation of phosphorylase. The adrenergic-triggered, cAMP-mediated temporary acceleration of glycogenolysis immediately after CAL serves a useful purpose. To some extent, this can also be said of the increase in contractile strength of the well-perfused regions of the heart, an effect that may also be mediated by cAMP (20,23), which ordinarily assists the nonischemic part of the heart to carry an additional work load in compensation for the loss of contractility in the ischemic and infarcted zone.

The temporary increase in the levels of cGMP in the nonischemic part of the heart after CAL suggests that an increase in parasympathetic nerve activity may occur. The feedback loops between AMP and cGMP concerning an acceleration and/or attenuation of metabolic events and of cation movements into and out of the myocardial cell, especially that of Ca^{2+} ions, have not been well understood until now. From the pathophysiological point of view, it seems of interest that the first burst in cAMP, which had been observed at least 5 sec after CAL (24), can be followed by a second one which leads to a rise in cAMP levels up to three to four times over the aerobic value (7). Such a tremendously high level of cAMP, probably in connection with a loss in energy-rich phosphates and other alterations, especially at the level of membrane structure and function, provokes or takes part in the occurrence of cardiac arrhythmias and ventricular fibrillation (18).

REFERENCES

1. Cohen, P. 1973. The subunit structure of rabbit skeletal muscle phosphorylase kinase and the molecular basis of its activation reactions. *Eur. J. Biochem.* 34:1–14.
2. Corr, P. B., Witkowski, F. X., and Sobel, B. E. 1978. Mechanism contributing to malignant dysrhythmias induced by ischemia in the cat. *J. Clin. Invest.* 61:109–119.
3. Dobson, J. G. 1978. Protein kinase regulation of cardiac phosphorylase activity and contractility. *Am. J. Physiol.* 234:H638–H648.
4. Dobson, J. G., and Mayer, S. E. 1973. Mechanisms of activation of cardiac glycogen phosphorylase in ischemia and anoxia. *Circ. Res.* 33:412–420.
5. Gilman, A. 1970. A protein binding assay for adenosine 3′,5′-cyclic monophosphate. *Proc. Natl. Acad. Sci. U.S.A.* 67:305–312.
6. Harper, J. R. and Brooker, G. 1975. Femtomole sensitive radioimmunoassay for cyclic AMP and cyclic GMP after 2′0 acetylation by acetic anhydride in aqueous solution. *J. Cyclic Nucleotide Res.* 1:207–218.
7. Illingworth, B., and Cori, G. T. 1953. Crystalline muscle phosphorylase. *Biochem. Prep.* 3:1–9.
8. Keely, S. L., and Corbin, J. D. 1977. Involvement of cAMP-dependent protein kinase in the regulation of heart contractile force. *Am. J. Physiol.* 2:H269–H275.
9. Krause, E.-G., Bartel, S., Reich, J.-G., and Winkler, J. 1981. On the activation of protein kinase by cAMP in the myocardium *in vivo. Biochem. Soc. Trans.* 9:241P.
10. Krause, E.-G., and Hosenfelder, W. 1981. Probennehmer zur tiefgekühlten Gewebsentnahme aus biologischen Material. Patentschrift 149464, Amt für Erfindungs- und Patentwesen der DDR, Berlin.
11. Krause, E.-G. and Wollenberger, A. 1967. Aktivierung der Phosphorylase-*b*-kinase im akut ischämischen Myokard. *Acta Biol. Med. Germ.* 19:381–386.
12. Krause, E.-G., and Wollenberger, A. 1980. Cyclic nucleotides in heart in acute myocardial ischemia and hypoxia. *Adv. Cyclic Nucleotide Res.* 12:51–61.
13. Krause, E.-G., Ziegelhöffer, A., Fedelesova, M., Styk, J., Kostolansky, S., Gabauer, I., Blasig, I., and Wollenberger, A. 1978. Myocardial cyclic nucleotide levels following coronary artery ligation. *Adv. Cardiol.* 25:119–129.
14. Krebs, E. G., Graves, J. G., and Fischer, E. H. 1959. Factors affecting the activity of muscle phosphorylase *b* kinase. *J. Biol. Chem.* 234:2867–2873.
15. Malliani, A., Schwartz, P. J., and Zanchetti, A. 1969. A sympathetic reflex elicited by experimental coronary occlusion. *Am. J. Physiol.* 217:703–709.
16. Matsushita, S., Shinawaga, T., Sukai, M., Moroki, N., Karamato, K., and Murakami, M. 1978. Comparison of adenosine 3′:5′ monophosphate dependent protein kinase from various cardiac muscle. In: *VIII. World Congress on Cardiology, Tokyo*, p. 560.
17. Nimmo, M. G., and Cohen, P. 1977. Hormonal control of protein phosphorylation. *Adv. Cyclic Nucleotide Res.* 8:146–266.
18. Opie, L. H., Nathan, D., and Lubbe, W. F. 1979. Biochemical aspects of arrhythmogenesis and ventricular fibrillation. *Am. J. Cardiol.* 43:131–148.
19. Shahab, L., Haase, M., Schiller, U., and Wollenberger, A. 1969. Noradrenalinabgabe aus dem Hundeherzen nach vorübergehender Okklusion einer Koronararterie. *Acta Biol. Med. Germ.* 22:135–143.
20. Tsien, R. W. 1977. Cyclic AMP and contractile activity in heart. *Adv. Cyclic Nucleotide Res.* 8:364–420.

21. Podzuweit, T., Dalby, A. J., Cherry, G. W., and Opie, L. H. 1978. Cyclic AMP levels in ischemic and nonischemic myocardium following coronary artery ligation: Relation to ventricular fibrillation. *J. Mol. Cell. Cardiol.* 10:81–94.
22. Pool, P. E., Norris, G. F., Levis, R. M., and Covell, J. W. 1968. A biopsy-drill permitting rapid freezing. *J. Appl. Physiol.* 24:832–833.
23. Wollenberger, A. 1975. The role of cyclic AMP in the adrenergic control of myocardium. In: W. G. Nayler (ed.), *Contraction and Relaxation of the Heart*, pp. 113–190. Academic Press, London.
24. Wollenberger, A., Krause, E.-G., and Heier, G. 1969. Stimulation of 3′,5′-cyclic AMP formation in dog myocardium following arrest of blood flow. *Biochem. Biophys. Res. Commun.* 36:664–670.

Myocardial Biosynthesis of Prostaglandins with Special Consideration of Prostacyclin and the Influence of Dipyridamole and Propranolol

P. Mentz, K. E. Blass, P. Hoffmann, and W. Förster

Department of Pharmacology and Toxicology
Faculty of Medicine
Martin Luther University, Halle–Wittenberg
Halle, German Democratic Republic

Abstract. Experiments with isolated perfused hearts of guinea pigs and rats showed that cardiac action is linked to formation of prostaglandinlike substances (PLS) and prostacyclin (PGI_2). Perfusion of the hearts with arachidonic acid or pretreatment with a linoleic-acid-supplemented diet significantly increased the content of PLS and PGI_2 and exerted an economizing effect on the heart performance. Dipyridamole induced a marked increase in the coronary flow and PGI_2 formation of the hearts but decreased the enhanced myocardial PGI_2 biosynthesis after perfusion with arachidonic acid. Propranolol also caused a rise in PGI_2 efflux but did not show any influence on PGI_2 formation after arachidonic acid. Dipyridamole and propranolol prevent decreased PGI_2 formation after acetylsalicylic acid, supporting the view that a combination of these drugs exerts a preventive effect in patients with angina pectoris and heart infarction.

Prostaglandins have potent cardiovascular effects and may participate in the regulation of cardiac action and coronary blood flow (6,21). Of this group of substances, prostacyclin (PGI_2) is a major metabolite of arachidonic acid in vascular tissue and the heart and is of outstanding importance because of its vasodilating effect and its inhibiting effect on platelet aggregation (9,20). However, little was known about the influence of unsaturated fatty acids and cardiovascular active drugs on myocardial biosynthesis of prostacyclin and its significance for the heart action. The objectives of this study were (1) to determine the myocardial biosynthesis of prostaglandins, especially prostacyclin, and (2) to demonstrate the influence of arachidonic and linoleic acid and the cardiovascular active drugs dipyridamole and propranolol.

MATERIALS AND METHODS

Experiments were carried out in the hearts of guinea pigs and rats ranging in weight from 300 to 500 g and 200 to 300 g, respectively. Different groups of rats were fed a linoleic acid (LA)-supplemented diet (56% LA)

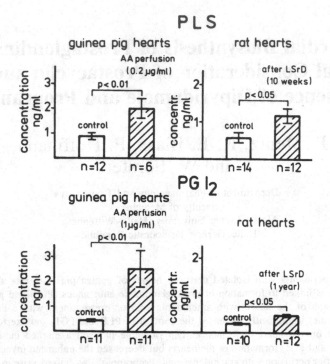

Figure 1.   Concentration of prostaglandinlike substances (PLS) and prostacyclin (PGI₂) in the perfusate of isolated hearts of guinea pigs and rats after perfusion with arachidonic acid (AA) or application of a linoleic-acid-rich diet (LArD)

and a standard pellet diet for 10 weeks. The isolated heart preparations were perfused with Tyrode solution at 37°C, 8 kPa, and gassed with oxygen according to the Langendorff technique. Heart contractions were recorded by strain gauge transducers, and coronary flow by photoelectric drop counting. Prostaglandinlike substances (PLS) in the perfusate were bioassayed by the superfusion technique of isolated rat stomach strips and rat colon strips using PGE_1 as standard.

The PGI_2 content of the perfusates was determined by an inhibition of ADP-induced platelet aggregation in comparison with a PGI_2 standard. Platelet-rich plasma (PRP) was prepared from fresh human venous blood. Nine volumes of blood were mixed with one volume of 3.13% trisodium citrate followed by centrifugation at 2000 rpm at 0°C for 4 min. The aggregation was measured with a Spekol photometer G 315 and thermo-regulated equipment (EK 5, VEB Carl Zeiss, Jena). The perfusates (20 ml) were collected with 0.2 ml 1 N NaOH and cooled to +5°C. Prostacyclin was separated by extraction with redistilled ether twice at pH 10.0 and then after acidification in a very quick step to pH 5.6 at 5°C. The residue was redissolved in 0.2 ml carbonate–NaCl solution (pH 8.9).

RESULTS

Under these conditions, the heart preparations of guinea pigs show a constant release of prostaglandinlike substances (PLS) (0.82 ng/ml) and prostacyclin (PGI$_2$) (0.22 ng/ml). These concentrations could be markedly (two- to tenfold) increased by continuous perfusion with arachidonic acid (0.2 and 1 µg/ml). The average formation rates amounted to 0.2–0.6%. Simultaneously, investigations in isolated Langendorff hearts of rats proved that a linoleic-acid-rich diet induced an increase of PLS (0.52 to 1.15 ng/ml) and PGI$_2$ (0.26 to 0.47 ng/ml) in comparison with control animals ($P < 0.05$) (Figure 1). Furthermore, these findings seem to be associated with simultaneous changes in cardiac action with an enhancement of contraction force (10%), a rise in coronary flow (24%), and a decrease in heart rate (14%) which often parallel the rising PG synthesis (19).

A single injection of 30 µg of dipyridamole caused an increase in the coronary flow (38%, $P < 0.01$) and in PGI$_2$ efflux from 0.56 to 1.71 ng/min ($P < 0.05$). Accordingly, constant perfusion with 1 µg/ml dipyridamole stimulated coronary flow (19%, $P < 0.05$) and the PGI$_2$ release from the heart (1.27 to 2.31 ng/min). In both cases, the heart rate remained unchanged, and

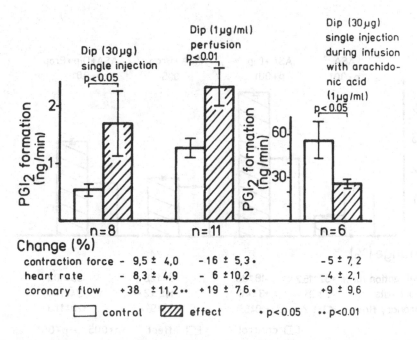

Figure 2.   Influence of dipyridamole (Dip) on the prostacyclin (PGI$_2$) formation in isolated perfused hearts of guinea pigs ($N = 6$–11)

534   P. Mentz et al.

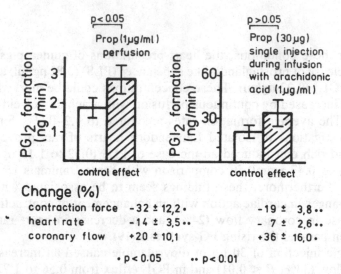

Change (%)

contraction force	−32 ± 12,2 •	−19 ± 3,8 ••
heart rate	−14 ± 3,5 ••	− 7 ± 2,6 ••
coronary flow	+20 ± 10,1 •	+36 ± 16,0 •

• p< 0.05   •• p< 0.01

Figure 3.   Influence of propranolol (Prop) on prostacyclin (PGI₂) formation in isolated perfused hearts of guinea pigs ($N = 8$)

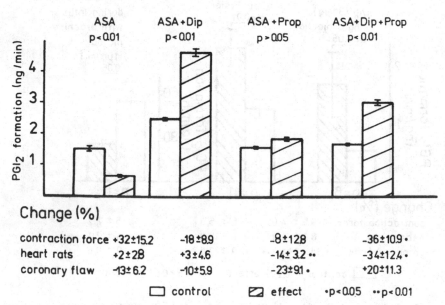

Change (%)

	ASA	ASA+Dip	ASA+Prop	ASA+Dip+Prop
contraction force	+32±15.2	−18±8.9	−8±12.8	−36±10.9 •
heart rats	+2±2.8	+3±4.6	−14± 3.2 ••	−34±12.4 •
coronary flaw	−13± 6.2	−10±5.9	−23±9.1 •	+20±11.3

☐ control   ▨ effect   •p<0.05 ••p<0.01

Figure 4.   Influence of acetylsalicylic acid (ASA, 1 μg/ml) in combination with dipyridamole (Dip, 1 μg/ml) and proporanolol (Prop, 1 μg/ml) on prostacyclin (PGI₂) formation in isolated perfused hearts of guinea pigs ($N = 8$–11)

contractility significantly decreased (10% and 16%, $P < 0.05$) after application of the substance. Arachidonic acid perfusion (1 µg/ml) of the isolated guinea pig hearts induced an increase in coronary flow (26%) and PGI_2 content from 1.5 to 55.6 ng/min ($P < 0.01$). Under these conditions, application of 30 µg dipyridamole caused a decrease in PGI_2 formation from 55.6 to 25.7 ng/min ($P < 0.05$) without changes in cardiac action or the coronary flow (Figure 2).

Propranolol perfusion (1 µg/ml) of isolated hearts of guinea pigs increased the PGI_2 release (52%, $P < 0.05$) and decreased the force of contraction (32%, $P < 0.05$) and heart rate (14%, $P < 0.01$). On the other hand, propranolol (30 µg) did not show any influence on the enhanced PGI_2 efflux after arachidonic acid (20.7 and 34.3 ng/min) but merely exerted a cardiodepressive effect (19%, $P < 0.01$) and caused a rise in the coronary flow (36%, $P < 0.05$) (Figure 3).

Acetylsalicylic acid (ASA) (1 µg/ml) decreased the efflux of PGI_2 from 1.59 to 0.63 ng/min ($P < 0.01$) without changing the cardiac action. Propranolol and dipyridamole antagonize this inhibitory effect. In combination with propranolol, aspirin did not affect PGI_2 synthesis. Additional application of dipyridamole caused a significant increase in PGI_2 in the perfusate in comparison with controls ($P < 0.01$). Combined treatment with propranolol showed a cardiodepressive effect (Figure 4).

DISCUSSION

The findings in the present study indicate that cardiac action is related to formation of prostaglandins. Prostacyclin especially is a very important substance for the heart and coronary vessels. It is a potent inhibitor of platelet aggregation and a vasodilator, increasing myocardial energy supply and reducing myocardial energy demand (6,21). Perfusion with arachidonic acid or pretreatment with a linoleic-acid-supplemented diet significantly increased the content of prostaglandins and prostacyclin and exerted an economizing effect on the heart performance (5,19,26). These results seem to help to explain the preventive effect of a diet rich in polyunsaturated acids in patients with heart infarction (2,19,25).

Dipyridamole and propranolol induce a marked increase in PGI_2 formation in the heart, possibly in association with the mechanism of some drug actions. Obviously, the cardiocirculatory effect of dipyridamole, including coronary dilation (3,16,24) and inhibition of platelet aggregation and thrombus formation (7,10,13,22), seem to be closely related to changes in PG metabolism. The results are consistent with earlier findings in other organs (1,11,12). Thus, dipyridamole has been described as a strong stimulator of PGI_2 biosynthesis in homogenates of rat stomach fundus and isolated perfused rabbit hearts. Dipyridamole and propranolol induce an enhanced conversion of PGH_2 to 6-oxo-$PGF_{1\alpha}$ by pig aortic microsomes, indicating a specific increase of the activity of PGI_2 synthetase. On the other hand, the turnover of high arachidonic acid concentrations is inhibited by dipyridamole, which suggests a dual influence of the drug on the enzymes of PGI_2 formation.

Aspirin has been shown to inhibit platelet aggregation and concomitantly reduce evidence of ischemia. By inhibiting cyclooxygenase, aspirin blocks the synthesis of prostaglandins with vasodilator influence as well as prostaglandins and thromboxanes that favor vasoconstriction and platelet aggregation (6,18). Thus, the net influence of aspirin on tissue perfusion may depend on the relative activity of prostaglandin synthetic pathways within the tissue (4,15,23). Dipyridamole and propranolol prevent the decrease of PGI_2 formation after aspirin. On the other hand, a combined therapy with these drugs decreases platelet aggregability and improves both coronary blood flow and the balance between supply and demand of energy by the myocardium. Combinations of the drugs have been used as antithrombotic agents and are at present under trial for prophylactic use in preventing arterial thrombosis, ischemic heart disease, and infarction in man (8,14,17).

ACKNOWLEDGMENTS

The authors are grateful to Mrs. I. Zobel and Mrs. M. Voigt for expert technical assistance.

REFERENCES

1. Blass, K. E., Block, H. U., Förster, W., and Pönicke, K. 1980. Dipyridamole, a specific stimulator of prostacyclin (PGI_2) biosynthesis. Br. J. Pharmacol. 68:71–73.
2. Boldingh, J. 1975. Lipid metabolism in relation to human health. Chem. Indus. 6:984–993.
3. Bretschneider, H. J., Frank, A., Bernard, U., Kochsiek, K., and Scheler, F. 1959. Die Wirkung eines Pyrimido-pyrimidin-Derivates auf die Sauerstoffversorgung des Herzmuskels. Arzneim. Forsch. 9:49–59.
4. Burch, J. W., Stanford, N., and Majerus, P. W. 1978. Inhibition of platelet prostaglandin synthetase by oral aspirin. J. Clin. Invest. 61:314–319.
5. De Deckere, E. A. M., Nugteren, D. H., and Ten Hoor, F. 1979. Influence of type of dietary fat on the prostaglandin release from isolated rabbit and rat hearts and from rat aortas. Prostaglandins 17:947–954.
6. De Deckere, E. A. M., and Ten Hoor, F. 1980. The role of prostaglandins in the regulation of the spontaneous frequency, coronary flow rate and left ventricular work in the isolated rat heart. Some comparisons with the isolated guinea pig heart. In: W. Förster, B. Sarembe, and P. Mentz (eds.), Prostaglandins and Thromboxanes in the Cardiovascular System and in Gynaecology and Obstetrics, pp. 111–116. VEB Gustav Fischer Verlag, Jena.
7. Didisheim, P., and Owen, C. A., Jr. 1970. Effects of dipyridamole and its derivatives on thrombosis and platelet function. Thromb. Diathes. Haemorrhag. 42(Suppl.):267–275.
8. Douglas, A. S., Chalmers, T. C., Klint, C. R., and Stamler, J. 1976. "Persantin"–aspirin reinfarction study. Lancet 2:465–466.
9. Dusting, G. J., Moncada, S., and Vane, J. R. 1977. Prostacyclin is the endogenous metabolite responsible for relaxation of coronary arteries induced by arachidonic acid. Prostaglandins 13:3–15.

10. Emmons, P. R., Harrison, M. J., Honour, A. J., and Mitchell, J. R. A. 1965. Effect of pyrimidopyrimidine derivative on thrombus formation in the rabbit. *Nature* 208:255–257.
11. Förster, W. 1979. Prostaglandine, Thromboxan A$_2$ und Herz-Kreislauf-Pharmaka. In: P. Oehme, H. Löwe, and E. Göres (eds.), *Beiträge zur Wirkstofforschung*, Vol. 6, pp. 26–36. Akademie-Verlag, Berlin.
12. Förster, W. 1980. Significance of prostaglandins and thromboxane A$_2$ for mode of action of cardiovascular drugs. *Adv. Prostaglandin Thromboxane Res.* 7:609–618.
13. Gray, G. R., Wilson, P. A., and Douglas, A. S. S. 1968. The effect of dipyridamole on platelet aggregation and adhesiveness. *Scot. Med. J.* 13:409–415.
14. Honour, A. J., Hockaday, T. D. R., and Mann, J. J. 1977. The synergistic effect of aspirin and dipyridamole upon platelet thrombi in living blood vessels. *Br. J. Exp. Pathol.* 58:268–272.
15. Jaffe, E. A., and Weksler, B. B. 1979. Recovery of endothelial cell prostacyclin production after inhibition by low doses of aspirin. *J. Clin. Invest.* 63:532–535.
16. Kadatz, R., Schröter, H. W., and Weisenberger, H. 1973, 1974. Persantin: Darstellung der pharmakologischen, biochemischen und klinischen Wirkungen. *Herz Kreislauf* 5:519–524, 6:21–31.
17. Keber, J. Jerse, M., Keber, D., and Stegnar, M. 1979. The influence of combined treatment with propranolol and acetylsalicylic acid on platelet aggregation in coronary heart disease. *Br. J. Clin. Pharmacol.* 7:287–291.
18. Korbut, R., and Moncada, S. 1978. Prostacyclin (PGI$_2$) and thromboxane A$_2$ interaction in vivo. Regulation by aspirin and relationship with antithrombotic therapy. *Thromb. Res.* 13:489–500.
19. Mentz, P., Hoffmann, P., Lenken, V., and Förster, W. 1978. Influence of prostaglandins, prostaglandin-precursor and of a linoleic acid rich and free diet on the cardiac effects of isoprenaline and vasodilators. *Acta Biol. Med. Germ.* 37:801–805.
20. Moncada, S., Gryglewski, R. J., Bunting, S., and Vane, J. R. 1976. An enzyme isolated from arteries transformed prostaglandin endoperoxides to an unstable substance that inhibits platelet aggregation. *Nature* 263:653–655.
21. Mullane, K. M., Moncada, S., and Vane, J. R. 1979. Formation and disappearance of prostacyclin in the circulation. In: J. R. Vane and S. Bergström (eds.), *Prostacyclin*, pp. 221–246. Raven Press, New York.
22. Rajah, S. M., Crow, M. J., Penny, A. F., Ahmad, R., and Watson, D. A. 1977. The effect of dipyridamole on platelet function: Correlation with blood levels in man. *Br. J. Clin. Pharmacol.* 4:129–133.
23. Smith, J. B., and Willis, A. L. 1971. Aspirin selectively inhibits prostaglandin production in human platelets. *Nature* (*New Biol.*) 231:235–237.
24. Tamura, K., Honda, T., Muto, N., and Bannai, S. 1975. The effect of dipyridamole on the coronary hemodynamics in man. *Jpn. Heart J.* 66:361–377.
25. Ten Hoor, F. 1980. Cardiovascular effects of dietary linoleic acid. *Nutr. Metab.* 24(Suppl. 1):162–180.
26. Ten Hoor, F., and De Deckere, E. A. M. 1977. The influence of an essential fatty acid (EFA) deficient diet on coronary flow rate and prostacyclin production of the isolated rat heart. *J. Mol. Cell. Cardiol.* 9(Suppl.):55.

Influence of Cardiovascular Drugs on Platelet Aggregation

W. Förster, H.-U. Block, C. Giessler, I. Heinroth,
P. Mentz, K. Pönicke, W. Rettkowski, and U. Zehl

Department of Pharmacology and Toxicology
Faculty of Medicine
Martin Luther University, Halle-Wittenberg
Halle, German Democratic Republic

Abstract. All vasodilatory drugs reported in this chapter possess an antiaggregatory effect on platelets, some of them with a synergistic effect on prostacyclin-induced inhibition of aggregation. Thus, the question seems valid whether the antiaggregatory effect represents one part of their antianginal and antihypertensive action. Some vasodilators stimulate the biosynthesis of prostacyclin and/or other vasodilating prostaglandins. This stimulation could be linked not only to the antiaggregatory but also to the vasodilating action. The influence on prostaglandin biosynthesis, however, is not obligatory for all vasodilators, as nitroglycerin proves. Trapidil inhibits the biosynthesis and the effect of thromboxane A_2, as our own experiments and those by Ohnishi et al. (7) have shown. This effect could be favorable in patients with heart infarction. Lefer et al. (5) have demonstrated a fivefold increase in thromboxane release after experimental ligation of the coronary artery in the cat. Pinane thromboxane, a thromboxane antagonist, almost completely abolished all deleterious consequences of ischemia. Whether trapidil is also able to inhibit thromboxane biosynthesis and activity under clinical conditions of heart infarction will be the topic of further investigations.

Much about the mode of action of antianginal drugs remains to be clarified. Since the discovery of thromboxane and prostacyclin, the involvement of these endogenous substances in the mechanism of action of antianginal drugs has been a focus of discussion, particularly since patients with angina pectoris have an enhanced tendency to platelet aggregation. Recently, a spastic component in the etiology of heart infarction and Prinzmetal's angina has been in question.

Our institute has been dealing for several years with the interrelations between arachidonic acid metabolism and the therapeutic mechanism of cardiovascular drugs. In the following, we give a brief review of some results with dipyridamole, nitroglycerin, and propranolol as well as two lesser known coronary drugs, trapidil (2,9,10), produced in the GDR, and nonachlazine (3,4), produced in the Soviet Union. We also briefly refer to the antihypertensive drug nitroprusside sodium which has a potent antiaggregatory effect and some influence on prostacyclin biosynthesis.

METHODS, RESULTS, AND DISCUSSION

In 1978, at the Seventh International Congress of Pharmacology in Paris, we reported for the first time that dipyridamole, besides having antiaggregatory and antithrombotic actions, also has specific stimulatory effects on prostacyclin synthetase, for example, on the prostacyclin synthetase in rabbit aortic rings. Dipyridamol (10 μg/ml) potentiates the endogenous biosynthesis of PGI_2 when PGH_2 (100 or 200 ng) is added by 82% ($P < 0.01$) and 66% ($P < 0.05$), respectively. Moreover, it also stimulates cyclooxygenase. Propranolol exerts a similar stimulating effect on the specific prostacyclin synthetase in pig aortic microsomes; corresponding to this, 1 μg/ml stimulates prostacyclin release in the guinea pig Langendorff heart preparation from 1.25 to 2.1 ng/10 ml perfusion fluid ($N = 12$, $P < 0.01$). Further studies are needed to show to what extent other effects of propranolol—for example, the proved normalization of increased platelet aggregation in coronary pa-

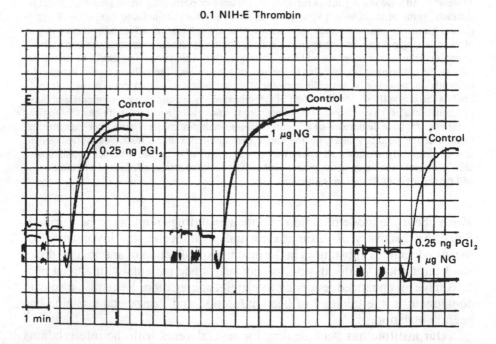

Figure 1. Influence of 0.25 ng PGI_2 and 1 μg nitroglycerin (NG) and a combination of 0.25 ng PGI_2 with 1 μg NG on thrombin-induced rat platelet aggregation. Platelet-rich plasma (PRP) was prepared from fresh rat blood. Nine volumes of blood were mixed with one volume of 3.8% trisodium citrate followed by centrifuging at 2000 r.p.m. for 12 min at 0°C. The PRP (0.2 ml) was incubated at 37°C for 2 min with a 0.9% NaCl solution giving a final volume of 0.6 ml. The drug was diluted in the same NaCl solution. The antiaggregatory effect of drug was expressed as percent change in light transmission after addition of the proaggregatory substance referred to the control change without drug (100%).

tients as demonstrated in 1974 by Frishman et al. (1)—might be explained by stimulation of prostacyclin biosynthesis.

Extensive investigations have dealt with the question of whether there is a connection between the antianginal effect of nitroglycerin and arachidonic acid metabolism. We investigated the influence of nitroglycerin on prostaglandin biosynthesis in various organs of several species in vitro and in vivo and saw—contrary to Morcillo and co-workers (6)—no statistically significant increase in the synthesis of any prostaglandin by sodium nitrite or nitroglycerin. Characteristic results as those from the rabbit Langendorff heart preparation showing an increase in prostacyclin efflux by coronary-dilating doses of adenosine, verapamil, aminophylline, and carbochromen but without any effect of nitroglycerin. There was also no visible influence of nitroglycerin on thromboxane biosynthesis by rabbit spleen homogenate even in high concentrations.

In spite of these negative results, nitroglycerin displayed a dose-dependently increasing antiaggregatory effect on rat platelet-rich plasma in which aggregation was induced by thrombin or ADP. As we demonstrated, it also potentiated, in minute, almost ineffective concentrations, the antiaggregatory action of prostacyclin on rat platelet-rich plasma (Figure 1). There was almost no inhibition of thrombin-induced aggregation by prostacyclin alone (left curve) or nitroglycerin alone (in the middle) in the concentrations used. The combined application of both substances, however, (right curve) induced a complete inhibition of the aggregation. This synergistic potentiation proved to be more potent in rat than in human platelet-rich plasma; therefore, one cannot say at present whether it is of therapeutic significance.

In this regard, the clear synergistic effect of sodium nitroprusside on ADP-induced platelet aggregation in rabbit platelet-rich plasma should be mentioned (Figure 2). On the left side are given the antiaggregatory effects of various concentrations of nitroprusside together with increasing prostacyclin concentrations. On the right side, the isoboles for a 20 and 30% inhibition, respectively, show a clear synergistic effect of the drug combination. Moreover, we could show that nitroprusside sodium increases the prostacyclin synthetized from prostaglandin H_2 by rabbit aortic rings. Thus, the question that emerges is whether the antihypertensive effect of nitroprusside might at least be partially explained by the potentiation of a prostacyclin-induced vasodilation.

The effects of another group of coronary vasodilators seem to result predominantly or partly from inhibition of thromboxane biosynthesis and/or thromboxane effect. This is true for trapidil [5-methyl-7-diethylamino-s-triazolo(1.5-α)-pyrimidine] and seems to be true for nonachlazine. Trapidil (50 μg/ml for 15 min) in vasodilatory concentrations does not influence prostacyclin, prostaglandin E, or prostaglandin $F_{2\alpha}$ release in isolated rabbit Langendorff heart preparations.

Trapidil, compared to other coronary vasodilators, was also investigated

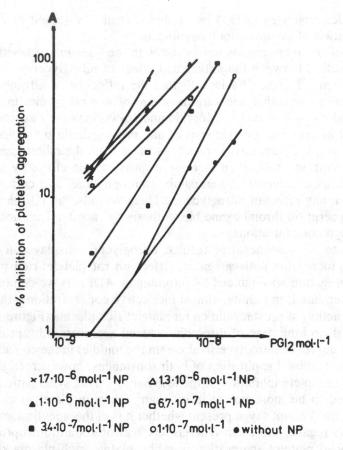

$\times 1.7 \cdot 10^{-6}$ mol·l^{-1} NP $\triangle 1.3 \cdot 10^{-6}$ mol·l^{-1} NP

$\blacktriangle 1 \cdot 10^{-6}$ mol·l^{-1} NP $\square 6.7 \cdot 10^{-7}$ mol·l^{-1} NP

$\blacksquare 34 \cdot 10^{-7}$ mol·l^{-1} NP $\circ 1 \cdot 10^{-7}$ mol·l^{-1} $\bullet$ without NP

Figure 2.   (A) Influence of sodium nitroprusside (SNP) on the dose-dependent antiaggregatory effect of PGI$_2$. (B) Isoboles (20% and 30%) of the aggregation are shown. The effect of SNP and PGI$_2$ on the ADP-induced platelet aggregation was investigated in the platelet-rich plasma (200 µl) of rabbit blood added to Tyrode solution (100 µl) with and without the substances.

with regard to its influence on the formation of malondialdehyde, which is considered by many authors to be an indicator of thromboxane A$_2$ synthesis from arachidonic acid (AA).

In Figure 3, the inhibitory effect of increasing concentrations of trapidil on the formation of malondialdehyde (white columns) with varying concentrations of arachidonic acid compared with nictindole are compared to their antiaggregatory effect (hatched columns). The higher trapidil concentrations of 0.5 and 1 mM are somewhat more inhibitory than the low one of 0.1 mM with regard to malondialdehyde, depending on the concentration of arachidonic acid: with lower concentrations of 0.2 mM being more potent than higher ones of 1 mM. But generally, the inhibition of malondialdehyde by trapidil is relatively weak (no more than 40% in the concentrations inves-

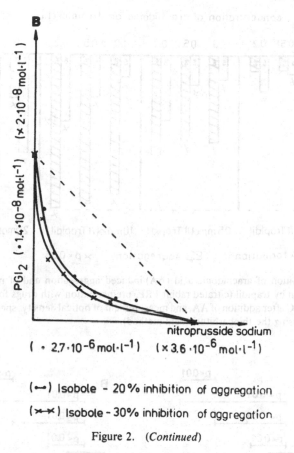

Figure 2. (*Continued*)

tigated) and does not correlate with the inhibitory effect on platelet aggregation by trapidil, this being so potent as to induce a nearly total inhibition of the arachidonic-acid-induced aggregation of rabbit platelet-rich plasma in concentrations of 1 mM. The inhibitory effects on malondialdehyde and platelet aggregation by nictindole, however, run parallel.

Platelet aggregation was also investigated using rat and human platelet-rich plasma. The use of rat platelet-rich plasma, trapidil, in a concentration of 0.1 mM, has a weak but significant effect which is additive with the effect of 1.42 mM prostacyclin. The inhibition is more potent (Figure 4) in ADP- as well as thrombin-induced aggregation with human platelet-rich plasma. Combined with prostacyclin, there is only an additive but no synergistic potentiating effect.

We also investigated the influence of trapidil compared with that of malondialdehyde on thromboxane synthesis in platelets of rabbits (Figure 5). Thromboxane was determined biologically and by gas–liquid chromatography. Both methods gave almost identical results. Trapidil in a concen-

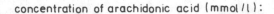

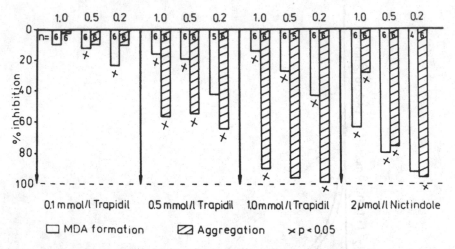

Figure 3.   Inhibition of arachidonic acid (AA)-induced aggregation and of malondialdehyde (MDA) formation by trapidil (citrated rabbit PRP, preincubation with drugs for 3 min, stirring for 1.5 min at 37°C after addition of AA, and measurement of optical density; spectrophotometric assay of MDA using the thiobarbituric acid method).

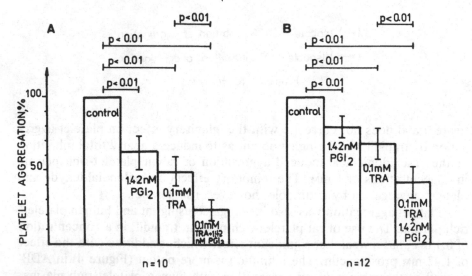

Figure 4.   Influence of 1.42 nM PGI_2 and 0.1 mM trapidil (TRA) and 1.42 nM PGI_2 in combination with 0.1 nM TRA on ADP- (2.12 μM) (A), and thrombin (92 NIH-U/liter) (B)-induced human platelet aggregation. Platelet-rich plasma (PRP) was prepared from fresh human blood. Nine volumes of blood were mixed with one volume of 3.13% trisodium citrate followed by centrifuging at 2000 r.p.m. for 4 min at 0°C. The PRP (0.4 ml) was incubated at 37°C for 2 min with a 0.9% NaCl solution giving a final volume of 0.5 ml. The drug was diluted in the same NaCl solution. The antiaggregatory effect of drugs was expressed as percent change in light transmission after addition of the proaggregatory substance referred to the control change without drug (100%).

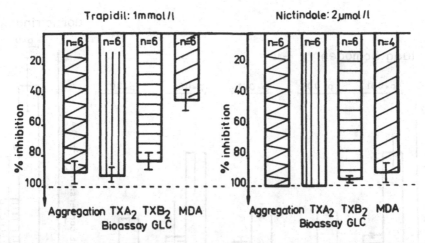

Figure 5. Arachidonic acid (AA)-induced aggregation, thromboxane (TX) and malondialdehyde (MDA) formation and trapidil (Citrated rabbit PRP; AA concentration, 0.2 mm. aggregation product and measurement of MDA as described in Figure 3; simultaneous estimation of the TXA$_2$ level using mesenteric arterial strip of rabbit in presence of a blocking mixture and of TXB$_2$ formation by GLC).

tration of 1 mM inhibited, parallel to its inhibition of platelet aggregation, thromboxane biosynthesis nearly completely. Nictindole, too, inhibited platelet aggregation and thromboxane biosynthesis, but it suppressed in a similar way the production of malondialdehyde.

In contrast to the effects on platelets, there was no influence of trapidil in the rat lung homogenate and aortic rings on prostaglandins (PGI$_2$, F$_{2\alpha}$, E$_2$, D$_2$) and thromboxane A$_2$ formed from [^{3}H]arachidonic acid. Nictindole, used as a standard, inhibited in the same concentration the synthesis of all prostaglandins and of thromboxane A$_2$ with the exception of prostaglandin D$_2$. We have no data to explain whether a difference in potency between nictindole and trapidil or species differences cause the different results or whether trapidil has only an inhibitory effect on thromboxane synthesis in platelets.

Our results are in close agreement with the recently published data of Japanese colleagues [Ohnishi et al. (7)] who found trapidil specifically inhibiting the thromboxane synthetase but competitively inhibiting thromboxane activity as well.

Thus, trapidil represents—as far as has been investigated—the first coronary drug available on the market with a specific inhibitory action on thromboxane synthesis in platelets and on TXA$_2$ effect, thus fulfilling Dr. Vane's demands and those of others (8) for the development of thromboxane inhibitors for the therapy of ischemic heart patients.

In preliminary investigations, which are still continuing, nonachlazine shows an inhibitory effect on the ADP- arachidonic acid-, and thrombin-induced aggregation of rat platelet-rich plasma. Coronary-dilating concen-

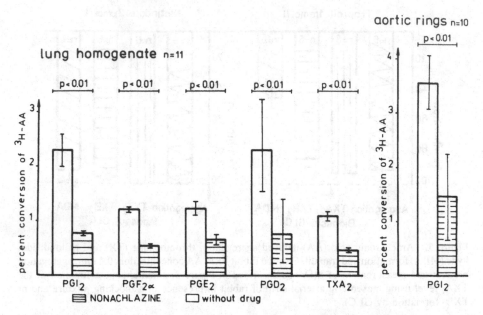

Figure 6.   Influence of nonachlazine (0.75 mM) on the biosynthesis of PGs and TXA$_2$ in lung homogenates and aortic rings of rats. Homogenates of lung (1 part tissue in 10 vol 0.05 M Tris-HCl buffer, pH 8.0, 20 μM EDTA, 100 μl per sample) or aortic rings (1 mg per 100 μl buffer). Preincubation: drug, 3.33 kBq (90 nCi) [³H]-AÁ, 0°C, 10 min. Incubation: 37°C, 30 min; TLC: organic phase of ethylacetate/acetic acid/trimethylpentane/water (110/10/20/100); unsaturated TLC chamber (relative mobilities: 6-oxo-PGF$_{1\alpha}$, 0.24; PGF$_{2\alpha}$, 0.32; TXB$_2$, 0.53; PGE$_2$, 0.58; PGD$_2$, 0.75). TLC plate: Merck Fertigfolien, Kieselgel 60; determination by liquid scintillation counting of the segmented plates.

trations of 0.4 μg/ml did not increase prostacyclin, prostaglandin E, and prostaglandin F$_{2\alpha}$ release from rabbit Langendorff hearts. However, in the concentration of 1 mM, nonachlazine potently inhibited malondialdehyde formation (by 70.0%, $P < 0.05$). This possibly indicates an inhibition of thromboxane synthesis. Further investigations are under way to confirm this by direct methods.

In agreement with this possibility, nonachlazine in rat lung homogenate (Figure 6) significantly inhibited the synthesis of thromboxane from arachidonic acid. The synthesis of all prostaglandins is also inhibited. Similarly, in rat aortic rings (on the right of Figure 6), prostacyclin release is diminished. Further investigations are needed to determine whether this effect of nonachlazine on all products of arachidonic acid metabolism is an expression of cyclooxygenase inhibition.

REFERENCES

1. Frishman, W. H., Weksler, B., Christodoulu, J. P., Smithen, C., and Killin, T. 1974. Reversal of abnormal platelet aggregability and change in patients with angina pectoris following oral propranolol. *Circulation* 50:884–896.

2. Füller, H., Hauschild, F., Modersohn, D., and Thomas, E. 1971. Pharmakologie des 5-Methyl-7-diäthylamino-s-triazolo-(1.5-α)pyrimidin (Trapymin, Rocornal[R]), einer Verbindung mit koronargefäßerweiternder Wirkung. *Pharmazie* 26:554–562.

3. Kaverina, N. V., Arefolow, V. A., Grigorieva, E. K., and Panasynk, L. V. 1976. [The influence of nonachlazine on the uptake and release of noradrenaline.] *Farmakol. Toxikol.* 34:420–424.

4. Kaverina, N. V., Markova, G. A., Chichkanov, G. G., Chumburidze, V. B., and Basaeva, A. J. 1975. [Nonachlasine—a new drug for the treatment of ischaemic heart disease.] *Kardiologiia* 15:43–48.

5. Lefer, A. M., Ogletree, M. L., and Smith, E. F. 1980. Role of prostanoids in acute myocardial ischemia. In: W. Foerster (ed.), *Prostaglandins and Thromboxanes*, pp. 15–20. VEB Gustav Fischer Verlag Jena.

6. Morcillo, E., Reid, P. R., Dubin, N., Ghodgaonkar, R., and Pitt, B. 1980. Myocardial prostaglandin E release by nitroglycerin and modification by indomethacin. *Am. J. Cardiol.* 45:53–57.

7. Ohnishi, H., Kosuzume, H., Yamaguchi, K., Suzuki, Y., and Itho, R. 1979. Experimental studies of trapidil on thromboxane A_2 (TXA_2) induced aggregation of platelet, ischemic changes in heart and synthesis of TXA_2. *Atherosclerosis* 7:407–415.

8. Parratt, J. R., and Coker, S. 1980. The significance of prostaglandin and thromboxane release in acute myocardial ischemia. In: W. Förster (ed.) *Prostaglandins and Thromboxanes*, pp. 21–25. VEB Gustav Fischer Verlag Jena.

9. Schüffler, J., and Frey, J. 1977. Zur Therapie des akuten Myokardinfarktes mit Rocornal. *Medicamentum (Berl.)* 18:11–14.

10. Weser, C., Müller, J. H. A., and Henkel, C. 1972. Zur Anwendung von Rocornal in der dringlichen Medizin. *Dt. Gesundh.-Wesen* 27:830–834.

Effects of L-Carnitine on Tissue Levels of Free Fatty Acid, Acyl CoA, and Acylcarnitine in Ischemic Heart

Y. Suzuki, T. Kamikawa, A. Kobayashi,
and N. Yamazaki

Third Department of Internal Medicine
Hamamatsu University School of Medicine
Hamamatsu, Japan

Abstract. In order to evaluate the protective effects of L-carnitine on ischemic myocardium, its effects on tissue levels of free fatty acid (FFA), acyl CoA, acyl carnitine, and adenosine triphosphate (ATP) were studied in ischemic dog hearts. Myocardial ischemia was induced by the ligation of left anterior descending coronary artery for 15 min. L-Carnitine (100 mg/kg) was administered intravenously prior to coronary ligation. In ischemic myocardium, tissue levels of free carnitine and ATP decreased, whereas long-chain acyl carnitine, long-chain acyl CoA, and FFA increased. Pretreatment of L-carnitine prevented the decrease in free carnitine and ATP and the increase in long-chain acyl carnitine and long-chain acyl CoA. A positive correlation was observed between ATP and free carnitine. On the other hand, a negative correlation was observed not only between ATP and the ratio of long-chain acyl CoA to free carnitine but also between ATP and the ratio of long-chain acyl carnitine to free carnitine. These results suggest that L-carnitine has protective effects on ischemic myocardium, probably by preventing the accumulation of long-chain acyl carnitine and long chain acyl CoA.

Since the accumulation of intermediates subsequent to impaired oxidation of free fatty acids (FFA) had been suggested as a cause of the cellular damage in ischemic myocardium (12), a great deal of attention has been focused on the role of carnitine (4,7) which is essential for the penetration of FFA across the inner mitochondrial membrane. In our previous report (14), a decrease in free carnitine and an increase in FFA were demonstrated in acutely ischemic myocardium, and a positive correlation was observed between free carnitine and adenosine triphosphate (ATP).

The purposes of this study were to observe the changes in tissue levels of carnitine derivatives, acyl CoA, and ATP following myocardial ischemia and to evaluate the effects of exogenous L-carnitine on these metabolic changes. In this study, particular emphasis was directed toward the effects of L-carnitine on the accumulation of long-chain acyl carnitine in ischemic myocardium.

MATERIALS AND METHODS

Seventy mongrel dogs weighing 8–15 kg were anesthetized with intravenous sodium pentobarbital. Ventilation was maintained by means of a Harvard animal respirator with room air. A left thoracotomy was performed through the fourth intercostal space. The pericardium was opened, and the heart was exposed. A short area of the left anterior descending branch of the coronary artery was dissected free from surrounding tissue, and a silk thread was placed around it. The following procedures were performed in three groups: (1) in 23 dogs, the dissected coronary artery was ligated for 15 min; (2) in 24 dogs, 100 mg/kg of L-carnitine (provided by Otsuka Pharmaceutical Factory Inc., Japan) was administered intravenously over 5 min, and after an additional 5 min, the coronary artery was ligated for 15 min; (3) 23 dogs without any interventions were used as normal controls.

After 15 min of coronary occlusion, beating hearts were removed from the animals, and transmural tissues (1–1.5 g) representing the ischemic area (supplied by the ligated artery) and the nonischemic area (supplied by circumflex artery) were rapidly excised. Briefly, the respective tissues were frozen with Wollenberger's clamps cooled to the temperature of liquid nitrogen. These procedures, from removal of the heart until freezing the tissues, were performed within 30 sec. The frozen and pressed samples were cracked into fragments on a block of dry ice and stored at $-70°C$. Extraction and analysis were made on these tissues within 3 days.

Free carnitine was determined enzymatically by the method of Marquis and Fritz (5). Short- and long-chain acyl carnitine were assayed as free carnitine after alkaline hydrolysis (10). Long-chain acyl CoA was extracted according to the method of Williamson and Corkey (16) and determined by the enzymatic cycling method of Veloso and Veech (15). Free fatty acid content was determined by the method of Itaya and Ui (1). ATP was determined by enzyme assay using hexokinase and glucose-6-phosphate dehydrogenase (2).

Values are reported relative to wet tissue weight as mean ± S.D. Statistical analysis was made by paired or nonpaired t-test, as appropriate.

RESULTS

The changes in tissue levels of various metabolites by coronary artery occlusion for 15 min are shown in Figure 1. Compared with the normal control, free carnitine decreased by 40% in the ischemic area and tended to decrease even in the nonischemic area. Short-chain acyl carnitine remained unchanged in both ischemic and nonischemic areas, whereas long-chain acyl carnitine increased 2½ times in the ischemic area and by 80% in the nonischemic area. In spite of the prominent changes in free and long-chain acyl carnitine, no statistical differences were observed in total car-

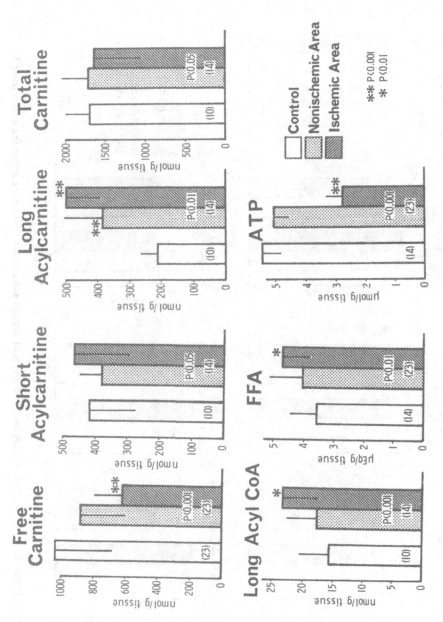

Figure 1. Changes in tissue levels of carnitine derivatives and other metabolites following coronary artery occlusion. Values are expressed per gram wet tissue weight and represented as mean ± S.D. The number of animals is given in parentheses. Asterisks represent a significant difference from the controls; P values represent the difference between ischemic and nonischemic areas.

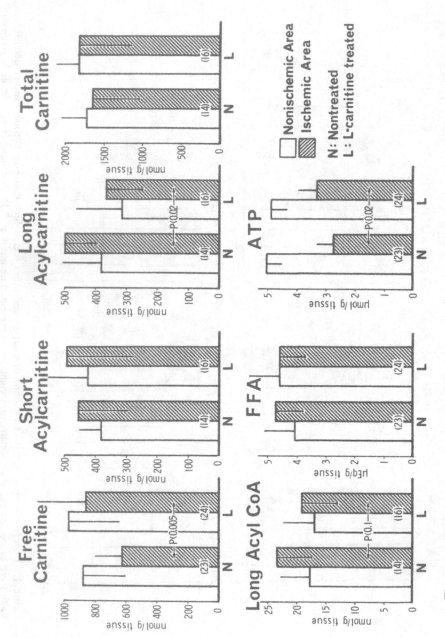

Figure 2. Effects of L-carnitine on tissue levels of various metabolites. Values are expressed as in Figure 1.

nitine. Long-chain acyl CoA increased by 50%, and FFA increased by 30% in the ischemic area. ATP decreased by 50% in the ischemic area. Significant decreases in free carnitine and ATP and increases in short- and long-chain acyl carnitine, long-chain acyl CoA, and FFA were observed in ischemic area relative to the nonischemic area.

The effects of L-carnitine on tissue levels of various metabolites are shown in Figure 2. In the ischemic area, pretreatment with L-carnitine effected a significant increase in free carnitine. Short-chain acyl carnitine remained unchanged, whereas long-chain acyl carnitine decreased. In spite of the administration of exogenous carnitine, no significant increase was observed in the levels of total carnitine. Long-chain acyl CoA tended to decrease, and ATP content significantly increased. However, no decrease in FFA was observed in this study.

The correlations between ATP and various metabolites are shown in Figure 3. A positive correlation between free carnitine and ATP and a negative correlation between long-chain acyl CoA and ATP were observed. The ratio of long-chain acyl carnitine to free carnitine correlated negatively with ATP, as did the ratio of long-chain acyl CoA to free carnitine.

DISCUSSION

The changes in tissue levels of the intermediate metabolites in FFA oxidation following myocardial ischemia and the effects of L-carnitine on the metabolic changes are summarized in Figure 4.

During myocardial ischemia, the amount of oxygen to support oxidative phosphorylation is reduced, and this results in the accumulation of NADH. Accumulated NADH, by inhibiting β-oxidation of fatty acids, increases long-chain acyl CoA and long-chain acyl carnitine levels in the mitochondria. Because high concentrations of long-chain acyl carnitine have been reported to inhibit the carnitine acyl carnitine translocase system (9), long-chain acyl carnitine may increase in the cytosol. In proportion to the increase in long-chain acyl carnitine, free carnitine decreases. The depletion in free carnitine causes the accumulation of long-chain acyl CoA and FFA in the cytosol. Because high levels of long-chain acyl CoA inhibit adenine nucleotide translocase activity (13), ATP production in ischemic myocardium is impaired both by the reduced supply of oxygen and by the accumulation of long-chain acyl CoA.

Pretreatment with L-carnitine prevented the depletion of tissue levels of free carnitine. Increased levels of free carnitine prevent the accumulation of long-chain acyl CoA, probably at first in the cytosol, and may lead to the reduction in inhibition of adenine nucleotide translocase activity. Because reduced inhibition of adenine nucleotide translocase activity increases the removal of ATP from the mitochondrial matrix to the cytosol, the upward metabolic pathways such as the electron transport chain and tricarboxylic

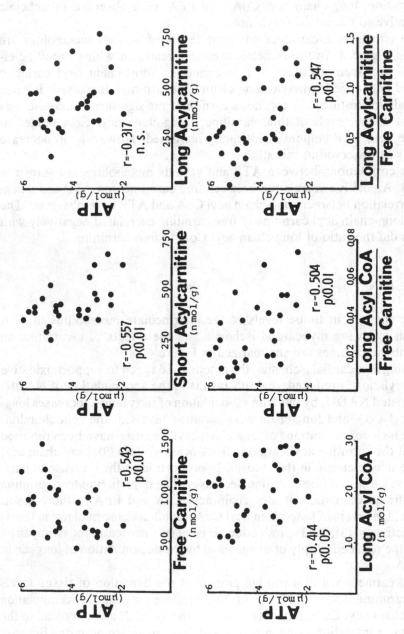

Figure 3.   Correlation between ATP and various metabolites. Samples were obtained from ischemic and nonischemic areas in the dogs untreated with L-carnitine.

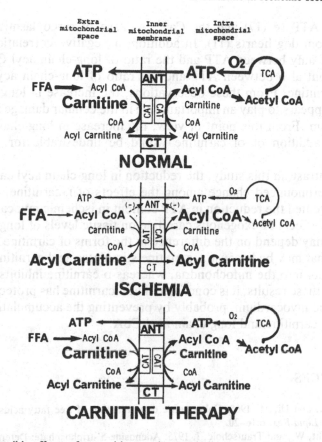

Figure 4. Possible effects of L-carnitine on the metabolic changes in ischemic myocardium. Sizes of letters represent the amounts of metabolites, and thickness of lines represent the activity of the metabolic pathways. Broken lines represent inhibitory effects. Abbreviations: FFA, free fatty acid; TCA, tricarboxylic acid cycle; ATP, adenosine triphosphate; ANT, adenine nucleotide translocase; CAT, carnitine acyl transferase; CT, carnitine acyl carnitine translocase.

acid cycle may be activated and lead to reduced accumulation of long-chain acyl CoA in the mitochondria. Reduction in long-chain acyl CoA in intra- and extramitochondrial space results in the increase in ATP production.

One of the interesting observations in this study was the reduction in long-chain acyl carnitine by treatment with L-carnitine. According to Liedtke et al. (3), 100 mg/kg of DL-carnitine caused a significant increase in long-chain acyl carnitine and failed to increase ATP content in ischemic swine hearts. As an explanation, they suggested that the presence of the D-isomer in DL-carnitine inhibited acyl carnitine transport and resulted in the increase in long-chain acyl carnitine in the cytosol. In ischemic myocardium, as in other studies (6,8), the increase in long-chain acyl carnitine was nearly three times the increase in long-chain acyl CoA. Long-chain acyl carnitine has been also reported to be a powerful inhibitor of the activity of bovine heart

Na^+–K^+ ATPase (17) and the Ca^{2+} ATPase of sarcoplasmic reticulum isolated from dog hearts (11). In addition, a negative correlation was observed not only between ATP and the ratio of long-chain acyl CoA to free carnitine but also between ATP and the ratio of long-chain acyl carnitine to free carnitine. From these observations, the increase in long-chain acyl carnitine appears to play an important role in the cellular damage in ischemic myocardium. From this point of view, the increase in long-chain acyl carnitine by addition of DL-carnitine would be undesirable for myocardial function.

In contrast, in this study, the reduction in long-chain acyl carnitine was the most pronounced change among the effects of L-carnitine. And L-carnitine prevented the reduction in ATP content in ischemic myocardium. The discrepant effects of exogenous carnitine on tissue levels of long-chain acyl carnitine may depend on the difference in the forms of carnitine used in the studies. That may be because L-carnitine stimulates acyl carnitine transport from cytosol into the mitochondria, whereas D-carnitine inhibits it.

From these results, it is concluded that L-carnitine has protective effects on ischemic myocardium, probably by preventing the accumulation of long-chain acyl carnitine and long-chain acyl CoA.

REFERENCES

1. Itaya, K., and Ui, M. 1965. Colorimetric determination of free fatty acids in biological fluids. *J. Lipid Res.* 6:16–20.
2. Lamprecht, W., and Trautschold, I. 1975. Adenosine-5'-triphosphate: Determination with hexokinase and glucose-6-phosphate dehydrogenase. *Methods Enzymat. Anal.* 4:2101–2105.
3. Liedtke, A. J., and Nellis, S. H. 1979. Effects of carnitine in ischemic and fatty acid supplemented swine hearts. *J. Clin. Invest.* 64:440–447.
4. Liedtke, A. J., Nellis, S., and Neely, J. R. 1978. Effects of excess free fatty acids on mechanical and metabolic function in normal and ischemic myocardium in swine. *Circ. Res.* 43:652–661.
5. Marquis, N. R., and Fritz, I. B. 1964. Enzymological determination of free carnitine concentrations in rat tissues. *J. Lipid Res.* 5:184–187.
6. Neely, J. R., Rovetto, M. J., and Whitmer, J. T. 1976. Rate-limiting steps of carbohydrate and fatty acid metabolism in ischemic hearts. *Acta Med. Scand [Suppl.]* 587:9–15.
7. Opie, L. H. 1979. Role of carnitine in fatty acid metabolism of normal and ischemic myocardium. *Am. Heart J.* 97:375–388.
8. Oram, J. F., Bennetch, S. L., and Neely, J. R. 1973. Regulation of fatty acid utilization in isolated perfused rat hearts. *J. Biol. Chem.* 248:5299–5309.
9. Pande, S. V. 1975. A mitochondrial carnitine acylcarnitine translocase system. *Proc. Natl. Acad. Sci. U.S.A.* 72:883–887.
10. Pearson, D. J., Chase, J. F. A., and Tubbs, P. K. 1969. The assay of (−)-carnitine and its o-acyl derivatives. *Methods Enzymol.* 14:612–622.
11. Pitts, B. J. R., Tate, C. A., Von Winkle, W. B., Wood, J. M., and Entman, M. L. 1978. Palmitylcarnitine inhibition of calcium pump in sarcoplasmic reticulum: A possible role in myocardial ischemia. *Life Sci.* 23:391–402.
12. Shrago, E., Shug, A. L., Sul, H., Bittar, N., and Folts, J. D. 1976. Control of energy production in myocardial ischemia. *Circ. Res.* 38(Suppl. 1):75–79.

13. Shug, A. L., Shrago, E., Bittar, N., Folts, J. D., and Koke, J. R. 1975. Acyl-CoA inhibition of adenine nucleotide translocation in ischemic myocardium. *Am. J. Physiol.* 228:689–692.
14. Suzuki, Y., Kamikawa, T., and Yamazaki, N. 1980. Protective effects of L-carnitine on ischemic heart. In: R. A. Frenkel and J. D. McGarry (eds.), *Carnitine Biosynthesis, Metabolism, and Functions*, pp. 341–352. Academic Press, New York.
15. Veloso, D., and Veech, R. L. 1974. Stoichiometric hydrolysis of long chain acyl-CoA and measurement of the CoA formed with an enzymatic cycling method. *Anal. Biochem.* 62:449–450.
16. Williamson, J. R., and Corkey, B. E. 1969. Assays of intermediates of the citric acid cycle and related compounds by fluometric enzyme methods. *Methods Enzymol.* 13:437–440.
17. Wood, J. M., Bush, B., Pitts, B. J. R., and Schwartz, A. 1977. Inhibition of bovine heart Na^+, K^+-ATPase by palmitylcarnitine and palmityl-CoA. *Biochem. Biophys. Res. Commun.* 74:677–684.

Effect of Coenzyme Q$_{10}$ on Hypertrophied Ischemic Myocardium during Aortic Cross Clamping for 2 hr, from the Aspect of Energy Metabolism

F. Okamoto, K. Karino, K. Ohori, T. Abe, and S. Komatsu

Department of Thoracic and Cardiovascular Surgery
Sapporo Medical College
Sapporo 060, Japan

Abstract. In order to perform intracardiac repair safely during aortic cross clamping, we designed this study to evaluate the protective effect of coenzyme Q$_{10}$ (CoQ$_{10}$) on hypertrophied ischemic myocardium from the aspect of energy metabolism. Six to nine months preceding the study, aortic bandings were carried out on 14 puppies to produce left ventricular hypertrophy (LVH). These dogs with LVH were then subjected to total cardiopulmonary bypass and were evenly divided into control and CoQ$_{10}$-treated groups (10 mg/kg of intravenous administration plus 1 mg/kg per hr of intracoronary injection). Myocardial ischemia was induced by aortic cross clamping for 2 hr under moderate systemic hypothermia. The results indicated that the administration of CoQ$_{10}$ had a protective effect on hypertrophied ischemic myocardium, since depletion of high-energy phosphate (HEP) was uniformly prevented, and accumulation of lactate was simultaneously decreased during the 2 hr of aortic cross clamping. On the other hand, there were marked exhaustion of HEP and rapid increase in lactate following the 2 hr of ischemia in the control group, these being much more predominant in the subendocardial layer.

Although a motionless and bloodless operative field for performing precise intracardiac repair can be easily obtained by aortic cross clamping, irreversible changes may develop in the myocardium with a prolonged period of ischemia (2,8). Accordingly, a great deal of research concerning myocardial protection has been accomplished in the last few years with the availability of cold cardioplegia, which has insured security in open-heart surgery (1,4,8,11). However, although the effect of regional hypothermia is now well established, the detailed composition of chemical cardioplegia remains controversial and uncertain (1,11).

The subendocardial layer, because of its anatomic and hemodynamic background, has been found to be more susceptible to ischemia than the subepicardial layer, especially in cases of LVH (7,9). It has been also reported that the state of so-called "stone heart" might be encountered more often in severe LVH following ischemia and that irreversible changes might progress from the subendocardium (2,7).

From these points of view, and with the utilization of a hypertrophied model heart and attention to transmural differences, we attempted to clarify the protective effect of CoQ_{10} on hypertrophied ischemic myocardium in terms of energy metabolism.

MATERIALS AND METHODS

Six to nine months preceding this study, banding procedures at the root of the ascending aorta were carried out on 14 puppies weighing 3 to 5 kg in order to produce LVH, with the animals thereafter being observed for any signs of cardiac failure. These dogs having developed LVH and weighing 5.5 to 10.5 kg, were subjects of the study and were evenly divided into control and CoQ_{10}-treated groups. The CoQ_{10}-treated group was given 10 mg/kg of CoQ_{10} intravenously 1 hr before aortic cross clamping, and an additional 1 mg/kg of 10% diluted CoQ_{10} was injected into the coronary arteries just after and 1 hr after the beginning of ischemia.

The experimental animals were anesthetized with sodium pentobarbital (25 mg/kg, i.v.), were placed in a supine position on the operating table, and were ventilated with a Harvard respirator. According to the routine technique of open-heart surgery, the extracorporeal circulation was provided with a bubble oxygenator (All-In-One® type, Senko Med. Ind.), a roller pump (T.D.O. pump, Mizuho Med. Ind.), and a disposable heat exchanger (Travenol, 5MO338). The left ventricle was vented through the left atrium, and myocardial temperature during the experiment was continuously monitored with a thumbtack-shaped thermistor probe placed on the left apex.

Total cardiopulmonary bypass was performed with more than 60 ml/kg per min of perfusion flow, and global myocardial ischemia was induced by aortic cross clamping for 2 hr under moderate systemic hypothermia (at a rectal temperature of 30°C). Coronary circulation was then restored by the release of cross clamping with gradual systemic rewarming, and, at the same time, the heart was electrically defibrillated.

Myocardial tissue biopsies for metabolic analysis were transmurally obtained from the free wall of the left ventricle just before the onset of ischemia, 1 and 2 hr after the aortic cross clamping, and 30 min after coronary reflow. The myocardial specimens were then immediately separated into subendo- and subepicardial layers and plunged into liquid nitrogen with stainless steel tongs. After serial procedures, involving homogenization with perchloric acid and centrifugation, extract samples were obtained, and the levels of adenosine triphosphate (ATP), adenosine diphosphate (ADP), adenosine monophosphate (AMP), creatine phosphate (CP), and lactate were finally quantified by the enzymatic methods of Bücher, Jaworek, Takahashi, and Gutmann, respectively. Statistical analyses by means of Student's t-test were performed among the subendo- and the subepicardial layers of the two groups as well as between the two layers in each group.

RESULTS

The hearts of dogs used in this study exhibited obvious LVH with a value of 1.81 ± 0.05 for the LV/RV ratio (that ratio in normal hearts was 1.43 ± 0.05). During aortic cross clamping, the myocardial temperature was strictly controlled to maintain a temperature around 25°C under moderate systemic hypothermia, with no significant difference being observed between the two groups (Figure 1).

As shown in Figure 2, the preischemic level of subendocardial ATP was significantly higher than that of the subepicardial layer within the control group. The ATP of both layers in the control group rapidly decreased with the prolonged period of ischemia, whereas that in the CoQ_{10}-treated group was maintained at higher levels, with significant differences existing between the layers of the two groups throughout and after ischemia. The levels of subendo- and subepicardial ATP in the control group decreased from the preischemic levels of 6.97 ± 0.25 μmol/g and 6.03 ± 0.13 μmol/g to 1.08 ± 0.14 μmol/g and 1.46 ± 0.10 μmol/g, respectively, following 2 hr of ischemia. On the other hand, those in the CoQ_{10}-treated group corresponded to values from 6.99 ± 0.31 μmol/g and 6.20 ± 0.15 μmol/g to 3.37 ± 0.27 μmol/g ($P < 0.001$) and 3.18 ± 0.23 μmol/g ($P < 0.001$), respectively. In addition, as shown on the right side of Figure 2, there was a significantly rapid decrease of ATP in the subendocardium as compared to that in the subepicardium within the control group 2 hr after ischemia, whereas the decreases in ATP of both layers were relatively uniform in the CoQ_{10}-treated group.

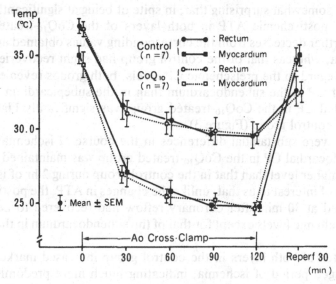

Figure 1.   Time course of temperatures during and after ischemia. The myocardial temperatures in both groups were kept around 25°C during the 2 hr of aortic cross clamping under moderate systemic hypothermia (at a rectal temperature of 30°C).

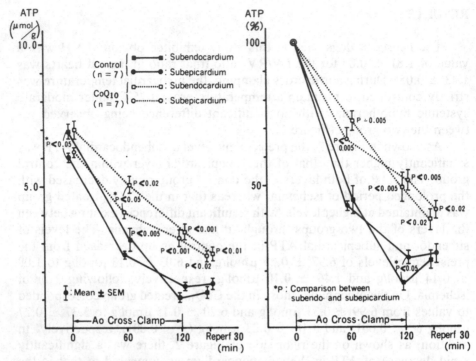

Figure 2. Effects of CoQ$_{10}$ on subendo- and subepicardial ATP level in LVH dog during and after ischemic arrest. Results illustrated on the right side are expressed as a percentage of the ATP level relative to the respective preischemic level.

It was somewhat surprising that, in spite of being at significantly higher levels, the postischemic ATP in both layers of the CoQ$_{10}$-treated group showed further decreases from the corresponding values obtained at the end of ischemia, whereas that of the control group had slight recoveries.

With regard to the preischemic CP levels, both groups revealed higher amounts of CP in the subendocardium than in the subepicardium, and the subepicardial CP in the CoQ$_{10}$-treated group was significantly higher than that in the control group (Figure 3).

There were substaintial differences in the course of ischemia; that is, the subendocardial CP in the CoQ$_{10}$-treated group was maintained at a significantly higher level than that in the control group during 2 hr of ischemia. It was also of interest to us that, unlike the changes in ATP, the postischemic CP obtained at 30 min after coronary reflow had recovered to nearly the same preischemic levels except for that of the subendocardium in the control group.

Lactates of both layers in the control group increased markedly with the prolonged period of ischemia, indicating much more predominance in the subendocardium (Figure 4). On the other hand, those in the CoQ$_{10}$-treated group were significantly lowered at the end of ischemia as compared with the control group. The subendo- and subepicardial lactates in the control group increased from the preischemic levels of 3.0 ± 0.7 μmol/g and 4.1 ± 1.8 μmol/g to 47.4 ± 2.1 μmol/g and 41.2 ± 2.5 μmol/g following 2 hr of ischemia, whereas those in the CoQ_{10}-treated group increased from values of 5.6 ± 1.2 μmol/g and 4.1 ± 1.2 μmol/g to 37.2 ± 1.8 μmol/g ($P < 0.02$) and 33.1 ± 1.6 μmol/g ($P < 0.05$), respectively.

After the restoration of coronary blood flow for 30 min, all of the values, except for that of the subendocardium in the control group, showed rapid decreases towards two- to threefold of their respective preischemic levels.

DISCUSSION

Coenzyme Q_{10} (CoQ_{10}) was first found in the mitochondria of the bovine heart by Crane and his colleagues in 1957 (3) and has been recognized as being located in the electron-transfer system of the mitochondria which is greatly responsible for aerobic energy metabolism (5,6). In addition, several investigations during the last few years have produced evidence that CoQ_{10} might also have protective effects on ischemic organ tissue (5,12,13). In this regard, therefore, we designed our study with the objective of examining

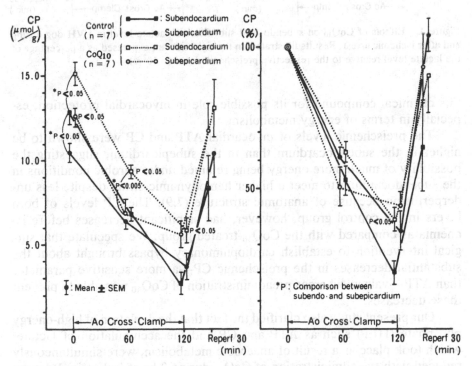

Figure 3. Effects of CoQ_{10} on subendo- and subepicardial CP level in LVH dog during and after ischemic arrest. Results illustrated on the right side are expressed as a percentage of the CP level relative to the respective preischemic level.

564   F. Okamoto et al.

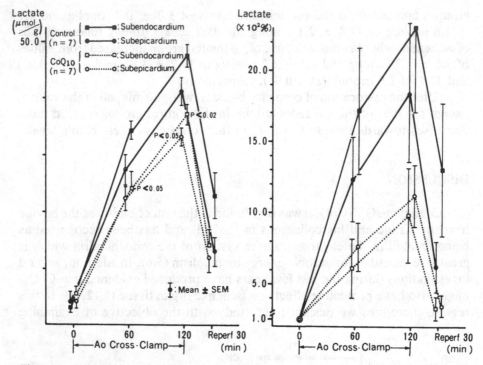

Figure 4.   Effects of CoQ$_{10}$ on subendo- and subepicardial lactate level in LVH dog during and after ischemic arrest. Results illustrated on the right side are expressed as a percentage of the lactate level relative to the respective preischemic level ($\times 10^2$%).

this chemical compound for its possible role in myocardial protection, especially in terms of energy metabolism.

The preischemic levels of myocardial ATP and CP were shown to be higher in the subendocardium than in the subepicardium, suggesting the possibility of much more energy being retained under aerobic conditions in the subendocardium to meet a higher hemodynamic strain despite less underperfusion because of anatomic structure (7,9). The CP levels of both layers in the control group, however, had significant decreases before ischemia as compared with the CoQ$_{10}$-treated group. We speculate that surgical intervention to establish cardiopulmonary bypass brought about the substantial decreases in the preischemic CP—a more sensitive parameter than ATP—values, whereas preadministration of CoQ$_{10}$ was able to prevent these decreases.

Our present study also clarified the fact that the depletion of high-energy phosphate (HEP) such as ATP and CP and the accumulation of lactate, which took place as a result of anaerobic metabolism, were simultaneously reduced with the administration of CoQ$_{10}$ during 2 hr of ischemia. Because CoQ$_{10}$ has an essential role in aerobic metabolism (5,6), this phenomenon seems to be quite unexpected but of great interest. Two possible explanations may account for this phenomenon: one is that CoQ$_{10}$ itself might have reduced the metabolic rate in the ischemic myocardium; and the other is that under conditions of extreme oxygen deprivation, CoQ$_{10}$ might have continued insufficient energy production, utilizing the very small amount of oxygen derived from the so-called, noncoronary collateral flow (1). At present, however, we do not have any distinct evidence to support these hypotheses, which are somewhat speculative.

We could find no explanation for the levels of ATP in the CoQ$_{10}$-treated group showing further decreases after restoration of coronary flow in spite of marked recoveries of the postischemic CP values. There is a possibility that postischemic changes in the myocardial cellular environment, such as magnesium loss, may have altered the kinetic balance of the reaction that existed between ATP and CP, that is, Lohmann's reaction (10), toward CP formation. Consequently, the levels of myocardial CP were greatly restored by the release of cross clamping, whereas newly producted ATP eventually showed a further decrease through consumption in the resumed mechanical activity of the heart.

In addition, it was also observed that depletion of HEP was more marked in the subendocardium than in the subepicardium when no treatment of CoQ$_{10}$ was employed, which suggests the susceptibility of the subendocardium to ischemia, as has been reported in the literature (2,7,9).

REFERENCES

1. Buckberg, G. D. 1979. A proposed "solution" to the cardioplegic controversy, *J. Thorac. Cardiovasc. Surg.* 77:803–815.
2. Cooley, D. A., Reul, G. J., and Wukash, D. C. 1972. Ischemic contracture of the heart: "Stone heart." *Am. J. Cardiol.* 29:575–577.
3. Crane, F. L., Hatefi, Y., Lester, R. L., and Widmer, C. 1957. Isolation of a quinone from beef heart mitochondria. *Biochim. Biophys. Acta* 25:220–221.
4. Engelman, R. M., Rousou, J. H., O'Donoghue, M. J., Longo, F., and Dobbs, W. A. 1980. A comparison of intermittent and continuous arrest for prolonged hypothermic cardioplegia. *Ann. Thorac. Surg.* 29:217–223.
5. Ernster, L. 1977. Facts and ideas about the functions of coenzyme Q$_{10}$ in mitochondria. In: K. Folkers and Y. Yamamura (eds.), *Biomedical and Clinical Aspects of Coenzyme Q*, pp. 15–21. Elsevier, Amsterdam.
6. Folkers, K., Watanabe, T., and Kaji, M. 1977. Critique of coenzyme Q in biochemical and biomedical research and in ten years of clinical research on cardiovascular disease. *J. Mol. Med.* 2:431–460.
7. Guy, C., and Eliot, R. S. 1970. The subendocardium of the left ventricle, a physiologic enigma. *Chest* 58:555–556.
8. Hearse, D. J., Stewart, D. A., and Chain, E.B. 1974. Recovery from cardiac bypass and elective cardiac arrest. The metabolic consequences of various cardioplegic procedures in the isolated rat heart. *Circ. Res.* 35:448–457.
9. Kirk, E. S., and Honig, C. R. 1964. An experimental and theoretical analysis of myocardial tissue pressure. *Am. J. Physiol.* 207:361–367.
10. Kuby, S. A., and Naltman, E. A. 1962. In: P. D. Boyer, H. A. Lardy, and K. Myrbäcck (eds.), *The Enzymes*, Vol. VI, pp. 515–603. Academic Press, New York.

11. Roe, B. B., Hutchinson, J. C., Fishman, N. H., Ullyot, D. J., and Smith, D. L. 1977. Myocardial protection with cold, ischemic, potassium-induced cardioplegia. *J. Thorac. Cardiovasc. Surg.* 73:366–370.
12. Samokhvalov, G. I., Obolnikova, F. A., and Naifakh, S. A. 1977. Biochemical aspects of administration of hexahydroubequinone-4 and derivative of reduced form thereof. In: K. Folkers and Y. Yamamura (eds.), *Biomedical and Clinical Aspects of Coenzyme Q*, pp. 201–217. Elsevier, Amsterdam.
13. Tatsukawa, Y., Dohi, Y., Yamada, K., and Kawasaki, T. 1979. The role of coenzyme Q_{10} for preservation of the rat kidney: An model experiment for kidney transplantation. *Life Sci.* 24:1309–1314.

Preservation of Oxidative Phosphorylation by Lidocaine in Ischemic and Reperfused Myocardium

D. W. Baron, M. Sunamori, and C. E. Harrison

Cardiac Muscle Research Laboratory
Mayo Clinic and Mayo Foundation
Rochester, Minnesota 55905, USA

Abstract. The effect of lidocaine (2 mg/kg bolus, 0.04 mg/kg per min infusion) on ischemic and reperfused myocardial respiration was assessed in 32 dogs, using indices of mitochondrial respiration (ADP:O ratio, state 3 and state 4 respiration, and respiratory control index). Heart rate, left ventricular (LV) pressure, LV dp/dt, cardiac index, epicardial ST segment, and regional myocardial blood flow, using 9 ± 1 μm radiospheres, were measured after 40 min of constriction of the anterior descending coronary artery ($N = 16$) and after 20 min of reperfusion ($N = 16$). Results showed that lidocaine increased state 3 respiration and respiratory control in reperfused myocardium ($P < 0.05$) with both glutamate and succinate–rotenone as substrate. It is concluded that lidocaine improves postischemic mitochondrial oxidative phosphorylation independent of altered hemodynamics or change in myocardial blood flow.

Local anesthetics have marked stabilizing effects on the electrogenic gradient of the cell membrane (18) and may have an important role in the maintenance of cellular integrity during anoxia (9,16). In the presence of large quantities of diffusible ions during postischemic reperfusion, the inability of the cell membrane to regulate intracellular homeostasis may result in ultrastructural damage (8).

Methylprednisolone, a corticosteroid, has a stabilizing effect on biological membranes (14) and reduces the loss of intracellular enzymes during and after ischemia (20). Barbiturates also may protect ischemic brain (2,11,15), and thiopental reduces the loss of creatine kinase from anoxic myocardium (19).

Schaub et al. (17) lent support to the concept that anesthetics may protect myocardium by demonstrating that lidocaine reduced ultrastructural damage during normothermic ischemic arrest in dogs undergoing cardiopulmonary bypass. More recently, lidocaine has been shown to reduce myocardial infarct size (13) and ischemic myocardial injury (3). It has been suggested (1,12,18,21) that local anesthetics might be expected to have important in vivo effects not only on the cell membrane but also on intracellular membrane systems such as the mitochondrion.

MATERIALS AND METHODS

Experimental Preparations

Healthy mongrel dogs weighing 6 to 14 kg (mean 10.2 kg) were anesthetized with sodium pentobarbital, 30 mg/kg intravenously, and ventilated with room air on a Harvard respirator sufficient to maintain normal arterial gas partial pressures and pH. A left thoracotomy was performed, and the heart was loosely suspended in a pericardial sling. The proximal 1 to 2 cm of the anterior descending coronary artery was isolated and snared with a 2-0 silk ligature. Pressures were recorded in the left ventricle, left atrium, and descending aorta, and cardiac output was measured in triplicate using a cardiac output computer.

Regional myocardial blood flow was measured using carbonized plastic 9 ± 1 μm radiospheres labeled with either ^{85}Sr or ^{46}Sc, injected via the left atrium (7). Myocardial blood flow was measured in control and ischemic tissue at the end of 40 min of occlusion of the anterior descending coronary artery and at the end of 20 min of reperfusion. Myocardial blood flow (MBF) was calculated from the formula:

MBF (ml/g per min) = Reference blood flow (ml/min)

   × (corrected 5-min counts/g myocardium)/(5-min reference blood counts)

Mitochondrial Respiratory Function

Mitochondrial respiration was measured in 32 dogs divided into four groups: group 1 ($N = 8$), control group, coronary artery occlusion for 40 min; group 2 ($N = 8$), control group, coronary artery occlusion for 40 min followed by 20 min of reperfusion; group 3 ($N = 8$), lidocaine-treated group, coronary artery occlusion for 40 min; and group 4 ($N = 8$), lidocaine-treated group, coronary artery occlusion for 40 min followed by 20 min of reperfusion. In dogs treated with lidocaine (2 mg/kg bolus, 0.04 mg/kg per min), infusion was commenced 10 min before occlusion and was continued throughout ischemia and reperfusion. The total dose of lidocaine administered was 10.4 ± 0.6 mg/kg for group 3 and 15.0 ± 1.0 mg/kg for group 4. At the end of the experiments, hearts were rapidly excised and rinsed in ice-cold (0 to 4°C) saline. Transmural biopsy specimens of 3 to 4 g were taken from ischemic (or reperfused) and nonischemic myocardia and were divided into endocardial and epicardial specimens. Results are reported for subendocardium.

Mitochondrial isolation was performed using standard techniques (6). Electron microscopy (Phillips HTG 400) was performed on samples from ischemic and nonischemic myocardia to ascertain the purity of the mitochondrial pellet. Cytochrome oxidase activity was measured in both homogenate and mitochondrial specimens to determine mitochondrial yields, according to the method of Cooperstein and Lazarow (5). Optical density of reduced cytochrome c was measured spectrophotometrically at 550 nm at room temperature, and readings were taken at 15-sec intervals for 2 min. The rate of oxidation of reduced cytochrome c was calculated assuming an extinction coefficient at 550 nm (ΔE_{550}) of cytochrome c of 19.6/mM per cm (23).

Oxygen consumption curves were recorded with a Gilson platinum electrode oxygraph using 1.5 ml of 0.15 M sucrose, 10 mM PO_4, 0.10 M Tris, and 10 mM glutamate or 10 mM succinate with 2.5 μg rotenone as substrate at pH 7.4 and a temperature of 29°C. Mitochondrial protein was determined by the method of Lowry et al. (10). Approximately 250 nmol of adenosine diphosphate was added in repeated determinations (average two to three) of oxygen consumption for each mitochondrial suspension.

RESULTS

Effect of Lidocaine on Hemodynamics

Lidocaine did not produce any significant alterations in resting heart rate, LV systolic pressure, LV end-diastolic pressure, LV dp/dt, cardiac index, regional myocardial blood flow, or LV stroke work either at rest or during ischemia (Figure 1). During reperfusion, myocardial blood flow increased from 122 ± 12 ml/100 g per min in control nonischemic tissue to 187 ± 86 ml/100 g per min in ischemic reperfused tissue. In lidocaine-treated myocardium, myocardial blood flow increased from 123 ± 6 ml/100 g per min to 178 ± 100 ml/100 g per min (differences not significant). Plasma lidocaine levels averaged 3.6 ± 0.4 mg/ml.

Mitochondrial Respiration

Compared with that of nonischemic endocardium, state 3 respiration and respiratory control of ischemic tissue were both significantly depressed. During ischemia in lidocaine-treated hearts, state 3 respiration increased by a mean of approximately 33%, although this increase did not obtain significance with either substrate (Table 1). After reperfusion, lidocaine increased state 3 respiration by an average of 40%: 50% for glutamate substrate ($P < 0.05$) and 29% for succinate–rotenone ($P < 0.05$).

Lidocaine increased state 4 respiration of reperfused endocardium by an average of 4.0 natom O/mg protein per min and that of nonischemic tissue by 2.5 natom O/mg protein per min. Respiratory control, however, expressed as the ratio of ischemic (or reperfused) tissue to nonischemic tissue, increased by 22% in both the ischemic and the reperfused, lidocaine-treated tissue. Lidocaine did not significantly alter the ADP:O ratio.

Mitochondrial protein yields averaged 1.7 ± 0.1 mg/g wet tissue in ischemic myocardium and 1.9 ± 0.2 mg/g wet tissue in ischemic, lidocaine-

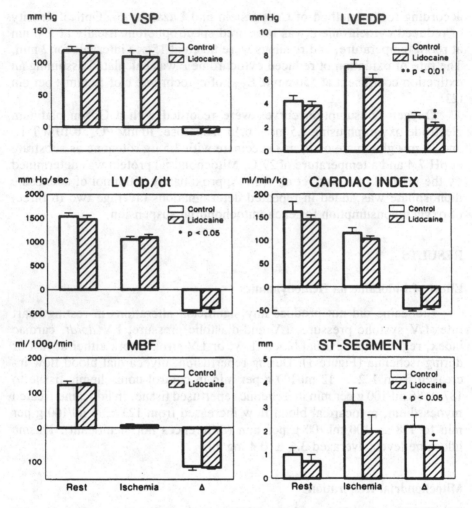

Figure 1.   Left ventricular systolic pressure (LVSP), LV end-diastolic pressure (LVEDP), LV *dp/dt*, cardiac index, myocardial blood flow (MBF), and ST segment at rest, during regional myocardial ischemia, and the differences (Δ) between ischemic and rest values.

treated myocardium. Mitochondrial yields were 5.5% for both ischemic and control myocardia. Electron microscopy revealed virtually pure mitochondrial populations from both ischemic and nonischemic myocardia, with nonmitochondrial cell fragments present only occasionally over many fields.

DISCUSSION

In the present study, mitochondrial state 3 respiration was reduced in ischemic control tissue to approximately 57% that of nonischemic myocardium ($P < 0.05$). However, in lidocaine-treated ischemic myocardium, state

3 respiration was restored to 82% that of nonischemic tissue (not significantly depressed). Respiratory control, a measure of the degree of effectiveness of coupling of oxidation to phosphorylation, of mitochondria isolated from ischemic and reperfused endocardia also was improved in the lidocaine-treated groups. These data using isolated mitochondria are consistent with data found using in vivo nicotinamide adenine dinucleotide fluorescence (1). The improvement in mitochondrial respiratory function was not dependent on increased myocardial blood flow during ischemia or reperfusion and was independent of altered resting hemodynamics. Lidocaine was associated with a reduced LV end-diastolic pressure and epicardial ST-segment elevation during ischemia and with an increased LV dp/dt and a maintained cardiac output. These alterations appear to represent the effect of an altered response to ischemia in the presence of administered lidocaine in vivo and exclude decreased myocardial oxygen consumption as a possible cause for improved mitochondrial respiratory function.

It is interesting to speculate on the mechanism whereby lidocaine may protect myocardium during ischemia. Considerable evidence thus far indicates that ischemia-induced ultrastructural changes result from increased permeability of the cell membrane (22). Defects in cellular and subcellular membranes with an inability to effectively regulate water and electrolyte homeostasis may be important factors, if not the primary events, in the

Table 1.   Effect of Lidocaine on Mitochondrial Respiratory Function in Ischemic and Reperfused Hearts (Means ± S.E.)

	Ischemia		Ischemia and reperfusion	
	Control (N = 8)	Lidocaine (N = 8)	Control (N = 8)	Lidocaine (N = 8)
Glutamate substrate				
ADP:O ratio	2.7 ± 0.1	2.8 ± 0.1	3.0 ± 0.1	3.0 ± 0.0
State 3 respiration (natom O/mg per min)	58.2 ± 10.9	78.1 ± 8.4	78.6 ± 12.1	118.0 ± 10.6[a]
State 4 respiration (natom O/mg per min)	11.9 ± 0.9	11.7 ± 1.4	8.1 ± 0.5	12.2 ± 1.11[a]
Respiratory control index (%)[b]	29.2 ± 6.6	62.2 ± 9.2[a]	57.6 ± 7.3	86.2 ± 7.3[a]
Succinate–rotenone substrate				
ADP:O ratio	1.4 ± 0.1	1.4 ± 0.1	1.4 ± 0.1	1.6 ± 0.0
State 3 respiration (natom O/mg per min)	73.5 ± 8.9	97.4 ± 7.5	95.7 ± 9.3	123.8 ± 8.4[a]
State 4 respiration (natom O/mg per min)	34.5 ± 3.2	40.2 ± 2.9	41.4 ± 2.0	45.1 ± 1.7
Respiratory control index (%)[b]	60.9 ± 5.5	71.4 ± 8.8	67.4 ± 3.9	83.3 ± 6.7[a]

[a] Significant difference from corresponding control value ($P < 0.05$).
[b] Respiratory control index of ischemic or reperfused myocardium expressed as percentage of nonischemic myocardium.

pathogenesis of irreversible ischemic injury to the cell (8). Calcium deposition has been a fundamental component of myocardial cell necrosis, and calcium antagonists such as verapamil reduce the ischemia-induced net influx of intracellular calcium. However, these agents in the dosages reported have additional nonmembrane effects, such as coronary vasodilatation and negative inotropism, which also may influence cell preservation.

It has been predicted that biological membranes should expand in the presence of anesthetics, on the basis that anesthetics penetrate and expand monolayer films of stearic acid, cholesterol, and phospholipid and increase the resistance of erythrocyte ghosts to hypotonic hemolysis (18). Support for a primary effect on cell membranes is based on evidence that synaptic block and action potentials are inhibited by anesthetic concentrations much lower than that required to inhibit metabolism and oxygen consumption.

Johnson and Schwartz (9) postulated that local anesthetics may affect specific membrane sites involved in cation transport. Chance et al. (4) suggested that, in the presence of anesthetics, movement of protons, accompanied by countermovement of monovalent and divalent cations, caused a pH gradient which may be essential for maintaining physiological function. Using isolated mitochondria from rat liver, Scarpa and Lindsay (16) found that dibucaine, a local anesthetic, caused powerful inhibition of phospholipase A_2, resulting in stabilized energy-linked functions and maintenance of membrane phospholipid in aging mitochondria. Ischemia and aging are both known to activate (via calcium and magnesium ions, free fatty acids, and decreased pH) endogenous phospholipases (21) which are specific for subcellular organelles including mitochondria and lysozymes. The addition of dibucaine restored the phospholipid–lysophospholipid balance toward the fully acylated compounds. These data thus provide in vitro evidence supporting the hypothesis that lidocaine protects ischemic myocardium.

ACKNOWLEDGMENT

This investigation was supported in part by Research Grant HL-12997 from the National Institutes of Health, U. S. Public Health Service.

REFERENCES

1. Baron, D. W., Dewey, J. D., and Harrison, C. E. 1980. In vivo NADH fluorescence and its reduction by lidocaine hydrochloride. *J. Mol. Cell. Cardiol.* 12(Suppl. 1):12.
2. Bleyaert, A. L., Nemoto, E. M., Safar, P., Stezoski, S. M., Mickell, J. J., Moossy, J., and Rao, G. R. 1978. Thiopental amelioration of brain damage after global ischemia in monkeys. *Anesthesiology* 49:390–398.
3. Boudoulas, H., Karayannacos, P. E., Lewis, R. P., Kakos, G. S., Kilman, J. W., and Vasko, J. S. 1978. Potential effect of lidocaine on ischemic myocardial injury: Experimental and clinical observations. *J. Surg. Res.* 24:469–476.
4. Chance, B., Mela, L., and Harris, E. J. 1968. Interaction of ion movements and local anesthetics in mitochondrial membranes. *Fed. Proc.* 27:902–906.

5. Cooperstein, S. J., and Lazarow, A. 1951. A microspectrophotometric method for the determination of cytochrome oxidase. *J. Biol. Chem.* 189:665–670.

6. Harrison, C. E., Jr., Cooper, G. IV, Zujko, K. J., and Coleman, H. N. III. 1972. Myocardial and mitochondrial function in potassium depletion cardiomyopathy. *J. Mol. Cell. Cardiol.* 4:633–649.

7. Heymann, M. A., Payne, B. D., Hoffman, J. I., and Rudolph, A. M. 1977. Blood flow measurements with radionuclide-labeled particles. *Prog. Cardiovasc. Dis.* 20:55–79.

8. Jennings, R. B. 1976. Cell volume regulation in acute myocardial ischemic injury. *Acta Med. Scand.* [*Suppl.*] 587:83–92.

9. Johnson, C. L., and Schwartz, A. 1969. Some effects of local anesthetics on isolated mitochondria. *J. Pharmacol. Exp. Ther.* 167:365–373.

10. Lowry, O. H., Rosebrough, N. J., Farr, A. L., and Randall, R. J. 1951. Protein measurement with the folin phenol reagent. *J. Biol. Chem.* 193:265–275.

11. Michenfelder, J. D., Milde, J. H., and Sundt, T. M., Jr. 1976. Cerebral protection by barbiturate anesthesia: Use after middle cerebral artery occlusion in Java monkeys. *Arch. Neurol.* 33:345–350.

12. Mullins, L. J. 1968. From molecules to membranes. *Fed. Proc.* 27:898–901.

13. Nasser, F. N., Walls, J. T., Edwards, W. D., and Harrison, C. E., Jr. 1980. Lidocaine-induced reduction in size of experimental myocardial infarction. *Am. J. Cardiol.* 46:967–975.

14. Okuda, M., Young, K. R., Jr., and Lefer, A. M. 1976. Localization of glucocorticoid uptake in normal and ischemic myocardial tissue of isolated perfused cat hearts. *Circ. Res.* 39:640–646.

15. Safar, P. N. 1978. Brain resuscitation. In: M. H. Weil and R. J. Henning (eds.), *Handbook of Critical Care Medicine*, pp. 435–449. Symposia Specialists, Miami.

16. Scarpa, A., and Lindsay, J. G. 1972. Maintenance of energy-linked functions in rat-liver mitochondria aged in the presence of Nupercaine. *Eur. J. Biochem.* 27:401–407.

17. Schaub, R. G., Stewart, G., Strong, M., Ruotolo, R., and Lemole, G. 1977. Reduction of ischemic myocardial damage in the dog by lidocaine infusion. *Am. J. Pathol.* 87:399–414.

18. Seeman, P. 1972. The membrane actions of anesthetics and tranquilizers. *Pharmacol. Rev.* 24:583–655.

19. Sinclair, D. M., De Moes, D., Boink, A. B. T. J., and Ruigrok, T. J. C. 1980. A protective effect of thiopentone on hypoxic heart muscle. *J. Mol. Cell. Cardiol.* 12:225–227.

20. Spath, J. A., Jr., Lane, D. L., and Lefer, A. M. 1974. Protective action of methylprednisolone on the myocardium during experimental myocardial ischemia in the cat. *Circ. Res.* 35:44–51.

21. Waite, M., and Sisson, P. 1972. Effect of local anesthetics on phospholipases from mitochondria and lysosomes: A probe into the role of the calcium ion in phospholipid hydrolysis. *Biochemistry* 11:3098–3105.

22. Whalen, D. A., Jr., Hamilton, D. G., Ganote, C. E., and Jennings, R. B. 1974. Effect of a transient period of ischemia on myocardial cells. I. Effects on cell volume regulation. *Am. J. Pathol.* 74:381–397.

23. Yonetani, T. 1967. Cytochrome oxidase: Beef heart. *Methods Enzymol.* 10:332–335.

On the Mechanism of Action of the Antianginal Drug Nonachlazine on Ischemic Myocardium

N. V. Kaverina, A. I. Turilova, Yu. B. Rozonov, T. N. Azvolinskaya, and S. A. Kryzhanovsky

Institute of Pharmacology
Academy of Medical Sciences of the USSR
Moscow 125315, USSR

Abstract. The activity of a new antianginal drug, nonachlazine, synthetized in the Institute of Pharmacology, Academy of Medical Sciences of the USSR, has been demonstrated using model myocardial ischemias on anesthetized dogs and conscious cats. Antianginal activity was evaluated by ECG, epicardial electrogram, lactate level, and lactate/pyruvate ratio in the venous blood flowing from the ischemic myocardial area. The study of the cardiotropic effect of nonachlazine provided the following findings: (1) nonachlazine enhances ino- and chronotropic functions of the heart via stimulation of its β-adrenergic receptors; (2) nonachlazine's positive chronotropic effect is substantially less marked than the inotropic one; (3) nonachlazine decreases the intensity of chronotropic reactions of the heart induced by isopreterenol. Biochemical analysis showed that in addition to its activation of oxidative phosphorylation, the ability of nonachlazine to stimulate glycogenolysis is also of importance in the development of its antianginal effect. This conclusion has been suggested by the following: (1) in acute myocardial ischemia, nonachlazine decreased lactate level and increased ATP level up to the norm; (2) at day 3 after ligation of the coronary artery, nonachlazine did not change lactate content, increased ATP and NAD, and decreased $NADH_2$; (3) in experiments on rabbit myocardial mitochondria in vivo and in vitro nonachlazine was found to stimulate oxidative phosphorylation; (4) nonachlazine was found capable of increasing the norepinephrine level and of increasing phosphorylase a activity and the rate of glycogenolysis.

In 1969, A. M. Likhosherstov and L. S. Nazarova of the Institute of Pharmacology, Academy of Medical Sciences of the USSR synthesized a new drug, 10-[β-(1,4-diazabicyclo[4,3,0]nonanyl-4)-propionyl]-2-chlorphenothiazine dihydrochloride, later given the name of nonachlazine. Experimental findings led to its being recommended for clinical use as an antianginal drug. This chapter contains the data that made it possible to recommend nonachlazine as an antianginal drug and also some findings concerning probable mechanisms of its antianginal properties.

RESULTS AND DISCUSSIONS

Antianginal activity of nonachlazine was most convincingly shown on model myocardial ischemia in experiments on anesthetized dogs and conscious cats. Chichkanov and Bogolepov studied the effect of nonachlazine on the functional state of the ischemic area in experiments on anesthetized dogs (2). To create ischemia, they used a model similar to the one described by Szekeres et al. (21). They partially occluded the descending branch of the left coronary artery with a special clamp and, via electrical stimulation of the right atrial auricle, imposed a high rate on the heart. Coronary artery occulsion or the stimulation of the cardiac chronotropic function separately failed to cause ischemic changes. The state of the ischemic area was estimated by epicardial electrogram, the degree of lactate increase, and the lactate/pyruvate ratio in venous blood flowing from the ischemic area. Functionally, this model is similar to the exercise test used in clinics for diagnosing ischemic heart disease (IHD) and for the evaluation of the efficiency of its treatment.

Intravenous administration of 3 mg/kg of nonachlazine was shown to cause a substantial decrease of ST-segment elevation observed when a high rhythm was imposed on the heart, and 5 mg/kg completely eliminated it. Simultaneously, the increase in lactic acid is almost completely prevented, and the lactate/pyruvate ratio in blood flowing from the ischemic area is decreased. These changes are evidence of the positive effects of nonachlazine on the functional state and metabolism of the myocardial ischemic area.

Published data and our observations indicate that drugs used for general anesthesia may change the intensity and even the character of the effect of cardiovascular drugs. Therefore, in a series of experiments, we studied the effect of nonachlazine on conscious animals. The experiments were conducted in the following manner. A cat's thorax was opened under phenobarbital anesthesia, and a special device for producing slow occlusion and reperfusion of the myocardial area supplied with blood from a given artery was fixed to the cardiac tissue. To record electrograms in the thoracic leads, the arterial pressure, and the administration of drugs, electrodes and catheters were implanted in the carotid artery and jugular vein of the animals. The experiments were started 3–4 days after the operation.

Coronary artery occlusion causes ischemic changes on the electrogram which are most often manifested by a shift of the ST segment from the isoline. Intravenous dosing with 3 mg/kg of nonachlazine substantially improved and in some experiments completely normalized the electrocardiograms (Figure 1).

Experimental data indicating an antianginal activity of nonachlazine were confirmed in clinics. A clinical study of nonachlazine carried out in ten institutions in the Soviet Union using blind and double-blind methods with the application of placebo control showed nonachlazine to have a good effect in the treatment of IHD patients of different gravity. Nonachlazine reduces the frequency of or completely eliminates anginal attacks, reduces the number of nitroglycerine administrations, and increases tolerance to exercise. The drug proved effective both in tension and resting angina pectoris (4,11,13,14,23,24).

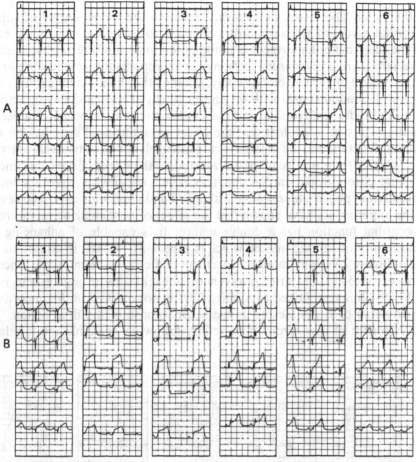

Figure 1. The effect of nonachlazine (3 mg/kg) on the ECG of a conscious cat with partial occlusion of the descending branch of the left coronary artery. (A) Changes of ECG (thoracic leads) during occlusion and reperfusion of the coronary artery: (1), background; (2,3), after the occlusion; (4,5,6), 2, 5, and 10 min after reperfusion. (B) Changes of ECG induced by non-achlazine: (1), backgrounds (2,3), after the occlusion; (4,5), 5 and 15 min after nonachlazine; (6), after reperfusion at nonachlazine background.

The high antianginal activity of nonachlazine served as a basis for a more comprehensive study on its mechanism of action. In our laboratory, experiments were carried out on dogs with a ligated descending branch of the left coronary artery with simultaneous recording of the blood flow in normal and ischemic areas of the heart. These studies have shown nonach-lazine to increase the blood flow in the ischemic area and to have practically no affect on the blood supply of healthy myocardial areas. Thus, the type of effect of nonachlazine on cardiac blood supply is closest to that of the most effective antianginal drugs, nitroglycerin and propranolol.

Myocardial ischemia is known to result, as a rule, in development of the heart failure of which increased end-diastolic pressure in the heart is one of the signs. The latter, in its turn, decreases the blood supply of subendocardial myocardial layers most vulnerable to ischemia. This is the basis for the idea that enhancement of contractile function of the cardiac muscle, especially during myocardial ischemia, is an important factor leading to the improvement of cardiac blood supply. On the other hand, tachycardia, often observed simultaneously with the enhancement of myocardial contractility, is undoubtedly unfavorable for the cardiac muscle, especially under ischemia. Thus, it is evident that the effect an antianginal drug has on myocardial function may be in large part responsible for its antianginal activity.

Starting from this assumption, we studied the effect of nonachlazine on ino- and chronotropic cardiac function. The experiments were conducted on urethane- plus α-chloralose-anesthetized and conscious cats. The results of the experiments have shown that the effect of nonachlazine on inotropic myocardial function has a double nature. It is capable of enhancing the contractility of cardiac muscle which is especially marked in conscious animals (Figure 2A). Maximum enhancement of the cardiac contractile function is observed 5–10 min after intravenous nonachlazine (6 mg/kg) and is 58 ± 17.8%. In anesthetized cats, this effect is not marked in the majority of experiments or is manifested as the second phase of the drug action. The enhancement of myocardial contractility following nonachlazine is related

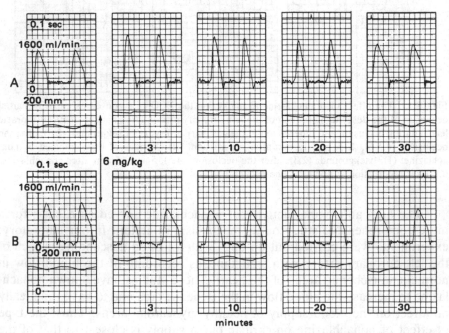

Figure 2.   The effect of nonachlazine (6 mg/kg intravenously) on blood flow in the ascending part of the aortic arch (conscious cat). (A) Intact animal; (B) after practolol (5 mg/kg). A and B from top to bottom: time mark (1 sec), blood flow in the aorta, arterial pressure. From left to right: background, 3, 10, 20, and 30 min after nonachlazine.

to the stimulation of myocardial β_1-adrenoceptors. This conclusion is based on the prevention of this effect by practolol pretreatment (Figure 2B).

In addition to the stimulating effect, nonachlazine has a direct inhibitory influence on the myocardium. This effect is marked in conscious animals with blocked myocardial β-adrenoceptors and also in anesthetized cats. In conscious cats after practolol or propranolol pretreatment, nonachlazine always causes a substantial inhibition of myocardial contractility. Anesthetized animals treated with nonachlazine mostly (nine experiments out of 15) showed only the inhibition of myocardial contractility (27 $\pm$ 5.6%) or 10–20 min duration followed by a recovery. In six experiments, the nonachlazine effect was biphasic. A short-term (13 $\pm$ 3.4%) decrease of cardiac contractility was followed by its enhancement (24 $\pm$ 5.2%) of 10–15 min duration.

Nonachlazine also showed an inhibitory effect in in vitro experiments. According to Senova (18), nonachlazine in 4 $\times$ 10^{-6} to 8 $\times$ 10^{-6} concentrations, in most experiments, decreased the amplitude of the contractions of isolated guinea pig atrial auricle.

We believe our findings on the effect of nonachlazine on myocardial chronotropic function to be of great interest. According to our experiments, nonachlazine increases cardiac inotropic function without causing significant tachycardia. The rate of heart beat after intravenous nonachlazine (6 mg/kg) increased by 8.3 $\pm$ 4.6% on the average, whereas the increase in inotropic function was 58 $\pm$ 17.8%. Nonachlazine in a dose of 3 mg/kg does not cause changes in the heart rate in the majority of experiments, but it enhanced myocardial contractility.

Clinical results are similar. A number of authors report an enhancement of myocardial contractile function during nonachlazine treatment of IHD patients and the absence of changes in the heart rate.

As we have mentioned above, enhancement of cardiac contractility while the heart rate decreases or at least remains unchanged is the most favorable combination of actions of antianginal drugs on the cardiac function. It should be noted that even most effective antianginal drugs such as nitroglycerin and propranolol do not have this combination of effects. Nitroglycerin enhances myocardial inotropic function, but it causes tachycardia which is unfavorable during IHD. Propranolol causes bradycardia, but it also inhibits cardiac inotropic function. The latter effect of propranolol limits its application in patients with heart failure symptoms. As was shown earlier, nonachlazine has advantages in this respect over nitroglycerin and propranolol. It enhances myocardial contractility and does not significantly change the rate of the heart beat. This property of nonachlazine is undoubtedly a positive factor in the development of its antianginal effect.

There is another noteworthy property of nonachlazine which, in our opinion, plays a rather positive role in the development of its antianginal effect. Our experiments on conscious cats have shown nonachlazine to decrease the intensity of cardiac chronotropic reactions induced by isoproterenol (Figure 3). Thus, the positive inotropic action of nonachlazine develops, and its chronotropic reactions which proceed via sympathetic innervation are restricted.

To sum up the abovementioned data, it may be concluded that non-achlazine produces a positive effect on the functional state of the cardiac ischemic area and causes blood redistribution to this area from the normal myocardial regions. It enhances cardiac inotropic function substantially more than it does the chronotropic one, which plays a positive role in the development of its antianginal effect. The combination of cardiostimulating properties of nonachlazine with its ability to decrease the sensitivity of myocardial β-adrenoceptors to isoproterenol is also noteworthy. This combination of effects, named partial β-adrenoblockade (15), gives nonachlazine advantages over the majority of β-adrenoblockers which decrease the sensitivity of cardiac β-adrenoceptors to isoproterenol and at the same time substantially inhibit myocardial contractility.

As will be shown below, a specific feature of the mechanism of action of nonachlazine consists in its promoting the accumulation of norepinephrine in the myocardium and increasing the amount of the transmitter in the sympathetic space with simultaneous blockade of its uptake (7,8).

The data reported indicate that this nonachlazine action has some new elements which distinguish it from the majority of known antianginal drugs applied in clinics. Further investigations on the mechanism of action of nonachlazine necessitated studies to provide answers to the following questions: (1) Which biochemical processes play the main role in nonachlazine-induced improvement of the functional state of the ischemic area? (2) What is the role of these processes in nonachlazine-induced improvement of the cardiac contractile function? (3) What is the role of nonachlazine's adrenergic properties in the development of its positive action?

Myocardial ischemia is known to cause important changes in oxidative and energetic processes, thus leading to substantial alterations of cardiac

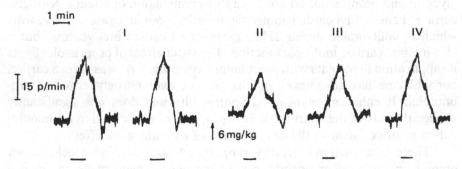

Figure 3. The effect of nonachlazine (6 mg/kg intravenously) on the intensity of cardiac chronotropic reaction induced by isoproterenol. From top to bottom: time mark (1 min), rate of heart beat (p/min), isoproterenol administration mark. From left to right: two control reactions and, 5, 25, 45 min after nonachlazine.

metabolism and function. We have mentioned above that nonachlazine, by improving the blood supply and functional state of myocardial area, causes a simultaneous enhancement of myocardial contractility. Therefore, we have studied the effect of nonachlazine on the content of ATP, ADP, NAD, and $NADH_2$ in the cardiac muscle at various stages of the ischemic process, and we have estimated the lactate level.

The experiments were conducted on cats anesthetized with urethane and chloralose. An ECG was recorded throughout the experiment with standard leads. For biochemical analysis, we used the left ventricle of the cat 30 min and 3 days after the ligation of the left descending branch of the coronary artery in its medial third. Nonachlazine was administered intravenously in a dose of 6 mg/kg. In the first case, it was injected 15 min after the ligation, and in the second one, three times daily. Hearts were excised 15 min after the injection. ATP and ADP were estimated as described by Tsetlin (22), lactate as by Barker and Summerson (1), NAD as by Severin and Tseitlin (19), and $NADH_2$ according to Stollar (20).

Nonachlazine (6 mg/kg intravenously) causes no changes in the content

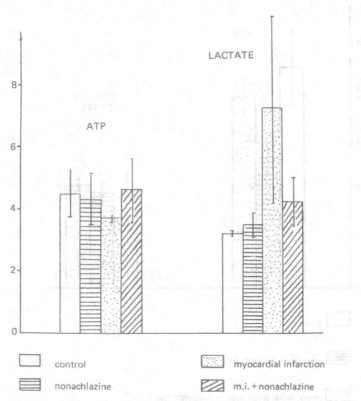

Figure 4.   The effect of nonachlazine on ATP and lactate contents (μmol/g damp tissue mass) in cat myocardium under acute ischemia.

of ATP, ADP, or lactate (Figure 4). Nonachlazine administered during acute myocardial ischemia causes an increase in ATP content to as high as the control level. Moreover, it induces a decrease in the lactic acid content by 42% as compared to its amount in animals with acute ischemia without nonachlazine.

Myocardial ischemia is known to result in a sharp increase in myocardial lactate (because of stimulation of the glycolytic cycle). This is accompanied by an ATP decrease as a result of the inhibition of oxidative phosphorylation; this is followed by an important inhibition of cardiac muscle contractility. Comparison of our data with literature reports of the nonachlazine improvement in the contractile function of ischemic myocardium suggests that the nonachlazine-induced ATP increase under ischemia is related to the drug's ability to stimulate ATP synthesis.

The nonachlazine-induced decrease in lactic acid content under acute myocardial ischemia is unlikely to be caused by its elimination into blood. This is confirmed by the data of Chichkanov et al. (3) in which lactate content in the venous blood flowing from the ischemic myocardial area was

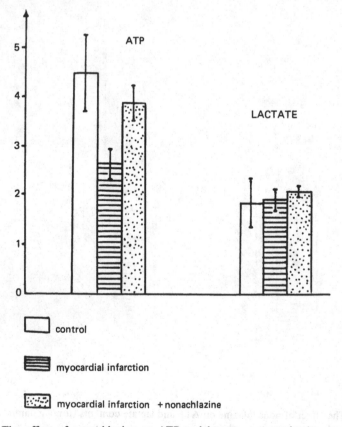

Figure 5.   The effect of nonachlazine on ATP and lactate contents in the myocardium of nonachlazine-treated cats.

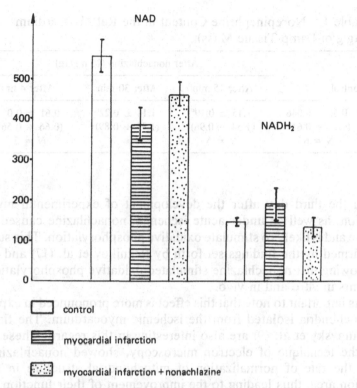

Figure 6. The effect of nonachlazine on NAD and NADH₂ contents in the myocardium of nonachlazine-treated cats.

studied. It was shown that nonachlazine prevented the increase in the lactate content of the venous blood from the ischemic area.

Thus, the nonachlazine-induced decrease of myocardial lactate in ischemia is likely to be a result of the stimulation of oxidative processes. Presently, it is common opinion that an increase in intracellular acidosis is one of the reasons for the decrease of cardiac muscle contractility. This is probably why the nonachlazine-induced decrease of lactate in the ischemic myocardium plays a role in the improvement of contractility of the ischemic heart.

Since maximum inhibition of the activity of glycolytic enzymes, an ATP decrease, and also the most marked changes in the system of nicotinamide coenzymes develop within the first 2 days after myocardial infarction, the second experimental series dealt with the effect of nonachlazine on the content of lactate, ATP, NAD, and NADH₂ on the third day after the development of the infarction. Nonachlazine was injected daily, three times a day, with a total dosage of 18 mg/kg daily. Figure 5 shows that nonachlazine does not significantly change the amount of lactate as compared to the control, but it increases ATP and NAD contents; NAD-H₂ decreases (Figure 6). In this period, according to Kryzhanovsky and Matsievsky (10), nonachlazine improved cardiac contractile function. These observations show

Table 1.   Norepinephrine Content in the Rat Myocardium
(μg/g of Damp Tissue Mass)

| Control | After nonachlazine (10 mg/kg) | | |
	After 15 min	After 30 min	After 4 hr
0.66 ± 0.046	1.15 ± 0.19[a]	1.11 ± 0.22[a]	0.61 ± 0.05[a]
(0.71 ÷ 0.61)	(1.34 ÷ 0.96)	(1.33 ÷ 0.89)	(0.66 ÷ 0.56)
N = 6	N = 5	N = 7	N = 5

[a] $P \leq 0.05$.

that on the third day after the development of experimental myocardial infarction, as well as under acute ischemia, nonachlazine caused an ATP increase and is likely to stimulate oxidative phosphorylation. This suggestion is confirmed by the findings set forth by Reznikov et al. (17) and Pichugin (16) showing that nonachlazine stimulated oxidative phosphorylation in experiments in vitro and in vivo.

It is important to note that this effect is more pronounced in experiments on mitochondria isolated from the ischemic myocardium. The findings of Kryzhanovsky et al. (9) are also interesting in this regard. These authors, using the technique of electron microscopy, showed nonachlazine to increase the rate of normalization of mitochondrial structure in the peri-infarction area, thus leading to the improvement of their function. All that has been mentioned indicates that the ability of nonachlazine to stimulate oxidative phosphorylation is of great importance for the development of its antianginal effect, namely, the improvement of the functional state of the ischemic area and myocardial contractility.

We have mentioned above that nonachlazine is capable of stimulating myocardial β-adrenoceptors. A question arises whether this effect is related to a direct action of nonachlazine on β-adrenoceptors or is mediated by the transmitter. To provide an answer, two experimental series were carried out. The first studied the effect of nonachlazine on norepinephrine and epinephrine levels in rat myocardium. Nonachlazine was injected intravenously in the dose of 10 mg/kg. Catecholamines were estimated as described

Table 2.   Percent of Phosphorylase a in Rat Myocardium[a]

Control (saline)	14.41 ± 3.49[b]
Nonachlazine (10 mg/kg)	32.4 ± 5.25[b]
Propranolol (5 mg/kg)	13.00 ± 2.89[b]
Nonachlazine (10 mg/kg) after propranolol pretreatment (5 mg/kg)	17.23 ± 3.30[b]

[a] Samples are taken 15 min after the administration of drug or saline.
[b] $P \leq 0.05$.

by Euler and Lishayko (5) and modified by Menshikov (12). It is seen in Table 1 that norepinephrine content in the rat myocardium increased by 74% within 15 min after nonachlazine, and the epinephrine level remaining unchanged.

In the second experimental series, Kaverina et al. (7) studied the effect of nonachlazine on the uptake of labeled norepinephrine in experiments on isolated rat heart using the techniques of Iversen (6). Nonachlazine appeared capable of blocking norepinephrine uptake and, hence, of accumulating the transmitter in the synaptic space. It was further shown that nonachlazine substantially increased the percentage of phosphorylase a in the rat myocardium (Table 2). This effect does not develop in experiments with β-blocker (propranolol) pretreatment. It is important to note that the nonachlazine-induced increase in norepinephrine content and phosphorylase a activity in the myocardium coincide in time with the increase in cardiac muscle contractility (8). Catecholamines are known to activate adenylate cyclase and to lead to the accumulation of cAMP in the myocardium. Therefore, it may be assumed that nonachlazine increases unbound norepinephrine and activates adenylate cyclase, thus leading to the accumulation of cAMP and development of a positive inotropic effect.

Accumulation of norepinephrine and activation of the phosphorylase are followed by glycogen decomposition. Naturally, these data provoked a question about the importance of this process in the development of the antianginal effect of nonachlazine. Presently, data are available indicating that daily intravenous injection of nonachlazine in the total daily dose of 18 mg/kg causes a substantial increase in glycogenolysis in cat ischemic myocardium.

These data indicate that in addition to the activation of oxidative phosphorylation, nonachlazine's ability to stimulate glycogenolysis is also of importance in the development of its antianginal effect.

It may be suggested that the intensity of the effect of nonachlazine on each of these processes depends on the extent and gravity of the ischemic changes in the myocardium and also on the degree of the utilization of the coronary reserve. Further experimental studies as well as clinical observations will try to reveal these so far unsolved problems.

REFERENCES

1. Barker, J. B., and Summerson, W. H. 1941. The colorimetric determination of lactic acid in biological material. *J. Biol. Chem* 138:535–554.
2. Chichkanov, G. G., and Bogolepov, A. K. 1978. [The effect of nonachlazine and oxyfedrine on myocardial ischemic area.] *Biull. Eksp. Biol. Med.* 12:691–694.
3. Chichkanov, G. G., Bogolepov, A. K., Turilova, A. I., and Shevchenko, T. N. 1978. The effect of nonachlazine and oxyfedrine on the functional state of myocardial ischemic area. In: *Theoretical and Methodical Problems of Molecular Cardiology*, p. 52. USSR Cardiology Research Center, Moscow.

4. Dubova, G. A., Davydova, R. G., and Markova, G. A. 1974. [Nonachlazine treatment of chronic ischemic heart disease patients.] *Klin. Med.* 10:47–49.

5. Euler, U. S. von, and Lishayko, G. 1959. The estimation of catecholamines in urine. *Acta Physiol. Scand.* 45:122–132.

6. Iversen, L. L. 1963. The uptake of noradrenaline by the isolated perfused rat heart. *Br. J. Pharmacol.* 21:523–537.

7. Kaverina, N. V., Arefolov, V. A., Grigorieva, E. K., and Panasiuk, L. V. 1976. [The effect of nonachlazine on uptake and release of noradrenaline.] *Farmakol. Toksikol.* 4:420–425.

8. Kaverina, N. V., Griglevsky, R., Basayeva, A. I., Markova, G. A., and Chumburidze, V. B. 1975. [On the mechanism of action of nonachlazine on the blood supply and heart activity.] *Biull. Eksp. Biol. Med.* 11:48–50.

9. Kryzhanosvky, S. A., Kleimenova, N. N., and Arefolov, V. A. 1980. The effect of nonachlazine on myocardial ultrastructure during myocardial experimental infarction. In: *Actual Problems of the Pharmacology of Circulation*, p. 30. Medical Institute of Gorky, Gorky.

10. Kryzhanovsky, S. A., and Matsievsky, D. D. 1979. The effect of nonachlazine and oxyfedrine on blood supply and heart activity in animals with disturbed myocardium. In: *New Drugs*, p. 39. USSR Ministry of Health, Moscow.

11. Kukes, V. G., Buyanov, V. V., Selyanov, V. N., Abugov, A. M., Borovkov, A. I., and Borisov, V. G. 1976. [On the application of coronary active drugs with β-stimulating effect in ischemic heart disease patients.] *Kardiologiia* 16(4):88–93.

12. Menshikov, V. V. 1963. Fluorimetric estimation of catecholamines in urine and tissues. In: *Studies of the Functional State of Adrenal Cortex and Sympathoadrenal System in Experiment and Clinics. Methods and Equipment*, p. 149. Medical Institute of Moscow, Moscow.

13. Metelitsa, V. I., Chazova, K. V., Grigoryants, R. A., Krol, V. A., Trubetskoy, A. V., Golubykh, V. L., and Yaroshevskaya, F. M. 1977. [The results of the clinical study of β-stimulants in the treatment of chronic ischemic heart disease.] *Ter. Arkh.* 49(4):44–48.

14. Metelitsa, V. I., Matveyeva, L. S., Borisova, G. A., and Lupanov, V. P. 1975. [Cordarone and nonachlazine in the treatment of chronic coronary failure patients.] *Kardiologii* 15(7):48–50.

15. Parratt, J. R. 1974. The haemodynamic effects of prolonged oral administration of oxyfedrine, a partial agonist β-adrenoreceptors: Comparison of propranolol. *Br. J. Pharmacol.* 51:15.

16. Pichugin, V. V. 1979. The effect of nonachlazine on myocardial contractility, collateral coronary circulation and energetic metabolism in the ischemic area. In: *New Drugs*, p. 35. USSR Ministry of Health, Moscow.

17. Reznikov, K. M., Kaverina, M. V., Alabovsky, V. V., Turilova, A. I., and Azvolinskaya, T. N. 1979. The effect of nonachlazine on energetic metabolism in the myocardium under normal and pathological conditions. In: *New Drugs*. p. 33. USSR Ministry of Health, Moscow.

18. Senova, Z. P. 1977. [The effect of nonachlazine on the rate and amplitude of the contractions of isolated atrium.] *Biull. Eksp. Biol. Med.* 3:298–300.

19. Severin, S. E., and Tseitlin, L. A. 1964. [Enzymatic splitting of diphosphopiridine nucleotide (DPN) in homogenates of the cardiac muscle under experimental myocarditis.] *Vopr. Med. Khim.* 10(3): 300–305.

20. Stollar, V. 1960. Studies with phenazine methosulfate: effect on mitochondrian assay for reduced puridine nucleotide coenzymes. *Biochim. Biophys. Acta* 44:245–250.

21. Szekeres, L., Csik, V., and Udvary, E. 1976. Nitroglycerin and dipyridamole on cardiac metabolism and dynamics in a new experimental model of angina pectoris. *J. Pharmacol. Exp. Ther.* 196(1):15–28.

22. Tsetlin, L. A. 1962. Components of adenyl system and creatine phosphate in rabbit cardiac muscle under experimental myocarditis. *Vopro. Med. Khim.* 8(3):279–283.
23. Yaagus, Kh. K. 1980. [On the effect of nonachlazine on echocardiographic indices in patients with postinfarction cardiosclerosis.] *Ter. Arkh.* 5:42–46.
24. Yurenev, A. P., Chumburidze, V. B., and At'kov, O. Yu. 1977. [The effect of nonachlazine on myocardial contractility, cardiac volumes and tolerance to physical exercise in chronic coronary failure patients.] *Klin. Med.* 5:50–53.

Studies on Slow Cardiac Action Potentials Occurring in Potassium-Rich Media as a Simulation of the Early Phase of Myocardial Infarction

Influence of Potassium-Conductance Blockers and Antiarrhythmic Drugs

M. Sebeszta* and E. Coraboeuf

Laboratory of Comparative Physiology
University of Paris XI
Orsay, France

Abstract. In the acute phase of myocardial infarction, a marked intracellular potassium loss and the lack of intact coronary circulation are known to result in extracellular hyperpotassemia partially depolarizing the damaged cells. To simulate these conditions, isolated guinea pig papillary muscles were superfused with K^+-rich Tyrode solution, the minimal norepinephrine concentration required to trigger slow action potentials (SR) was measured, and the characteristics of SR were studied with glass microelectrodes. The threshold norepinephrine concentration was found to be about 1.04×10^{-6} M. This threshold concentration was decreased by substances inhibiting the outward potassium currents (4-aminopyridine, tetraethylammonium, cesium); the SR duration and the maximal rate of depolarization were increased by them. Lidocaine and procainamide have no influence on these parameters. Phenytoin and the Mg^{2+} ion were found to have a marked inhibitor effect by increasing the threshold norepinephrine concentration and decreasing the maximal rate of depolarization of SR.

There are several clinical and experimental observations proving that in the acute phase of myocardial infarction slow action potentials can arise and by their very slow propagation can elicit dangerous arrhythmias (for review, see 4,6,16,17).

In the acute phase of myocardial infarction, the loss of intracellular potassium and the lack of intact coronary circulation result in an extracellular hyperpotassemia. The degree of this hyperpotassemia is about five times the control level (15). This result, obtained by potassium-selective electrodes, demonstrated that extracellular potassium activity is considerably higher than indicated by the traditional technique of coronary vein sampling.

The slow action potentials that occur in potassium-rich media (1,7,12,13), i.e., in partially depolarized fibers, are caused by the activation of the slow

---

* Present address: Second Medical Clinic, Postgraduate Medical School, H-1389 Budapest, Hungary.

channel. However, it is clear that other ionic conductances can interfere with the depolarizing slow inward current and therefore influence slow action potentials.

The aim of the present study was to investigate the participation in slow action potential development of substances altering potassium conductances and antiarrhythmic drugs that are not known for their calcium-blocker properties.

Isolated guinea pig papillary muscles were superfused with potassium-rich (28 mM) Tyrode solution (34°C, pH 7.4) saturated with a 95% O_2, 5% CO_2 gas mixture, which depolarized the membrane to about -40 mV. Transmembrane potentials were recorded through floating microelectrodes. Since the aim of the present study was to investigate the development of propagated slow responses, microelectrodes were impaled at a distance from the stimulating electrode greater than 3 mm which is three times the space constant. To determine the smallest concentration of norepinephrine required to elicit propagated slow responses (the threshold norepinephrine concentration), a perfusion containing a suprathreshold norepinephrine concentration was changed for another perfusion containing half of the previous norepinephrine concentration, and this procedure was repeated until there was suppression of slow responses.

The threshold norepinephrine concentration was found to be 1.04×10^{-6} M. To check to what extent changes in potassium conductances may influence the genesis of slow action potentials, we studied the effects of tetraethylammonium (TEA, 20 mM), 4-aminopyridine (4AP, 5 mM), cesium (Cs^+, 20 mM), and magnesium (Mg^{2+}, 5 mM). 4-Aminopyridine and to a smaller extent TEA reduced the norepinephrine threshold. Cesium was much less efficient, whereas Mg^{2+} exerted the opposite effect and markedly increased the norepinephrine threshold.

Figure 1 shows the effect of the four compounds on the slow action potential duration (SRD) measured at -20 mV and the maximal rate of depolarization ($\dot{V}_{max}$) for two different norepinephrine concentrations corresponding to four and two times the control norepinephrine threshold. Interrupted lines refer to the control values. It may be seen that 4AP markedly increased both SRD and $\dot{V}_{max}$. The effect of TEA is similar to that of 4AP, but it is more marked. Cesium increased SRD slightly and $\dot{V}_{max}$ to a higher degree. Magnesium increased SRD slightly but noticeably decreased $\dot{V}_{max}$.

The abovementioned compounds do not exert similar effects on potassium conductances (3,8–10,14), and, in addition, their degree of specificity as potassium conductance blockers is different. However, they exert facilitatory effects on the slow action potential with the exception of Mg^{2+} which inhibits such responses in spite of the fact that it decreases potassium exchange in the rat ventricle (14). The blocking effect of Mg^{2+}, and therefore its protective effect against slow-response-induced arrhythmias, probably

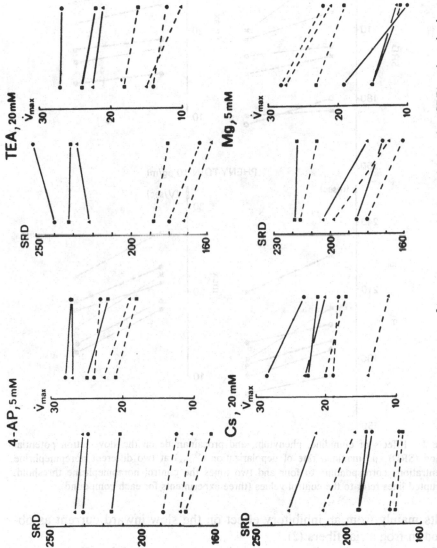

Figure 1. Effects of 4AP, TEA, Cs$^+$, and Mg^{2+} on the slow action potential duration (SRD) and maximal rate of depolarization ($\dot{V}_{max}$) at two different norepinephrine concentrations corresponding to four and two times the control norepinephrine threshold. Interrupted lines refer to the control values (three experiments for each compound).

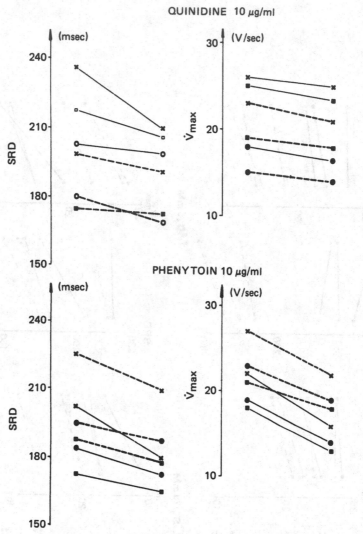

Figure 2. Effects of quinidine, phenytoin, and procainamide on the slow action potential duration (SRD) and maximal rate of depolarization ($\dot{V}_{max}$) at two different norepinephrine concentrations corresponding to four and two times the control norepinephrine threshold. Interrupted lines refer to the control values (three experiments for each compound).

results mainly from an inhibitory effect on the slow inward current as observed in frog atrial fibers (2).

In a second part of the present work, we have studied the effect of some generally used antiarrhythmic agents on the threshold norepinephrine concentration. The concentrations of the drugs were about the clinically effective serum levels: procainamide, 20 µg/ml; quinidine, lidocaine, and phenytoin, 10 µg/ml. Only phenytoin increased the norepinephrine threshold and had an inhibitory effect on slow responses. Quinidine decreased the nor-

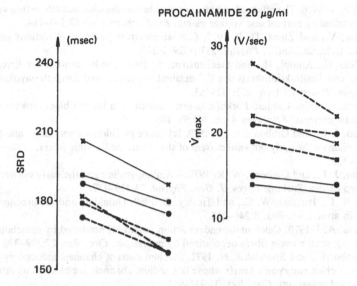

Figure 2.   (Continued)

epinephrine threshold, whereas procainamide tended to decrease it. Lidocaine had no effect on the norepinephrine threshold or on the characteristics of slow action potentials. Procainamide increased SRD. Although it did not increase the norepinephrine threshold, it markedly decreased $\dot{V}_{max}$. Quinidine increased both SRD and $\dot{V}_{max}$. Phenytoin in a clinically effective concentration decreased SRD slightly and $\dot{V}_{max}$ more markedly (Figure 2).

The above results show that (1) slow responses can be triggered by low norepinephrine concentrations that very likely can be reached in the acute phase of myocardial infarction, and (2) slow responses can be influenced by agents and drugs that are not primarily specific for the slow channel and, particularly, can be triggered by potassium conductance blockers. In relation with this observation, drugs like quinidine, which are known to exert some inhibitory effect on potassium conductance (5,11), can facilitate the genesis of propagated slow responses.

REFERENCES

1. Carmeliet, E., and Vereecke, J. 1969. Adrenaline and the plateau phase of cardiac action potential. *Pfluegers Arch.* 313:300–315.
2. Chesnais, J. M., Coraboeuf, E., Sauviat, M. P., and Vassas, M. 1975. Sensitivity to H, Li and Mg ions of the slow inward sodium current in frog atrial fibers. *J. Mol. Cell. Cardiol.* 7:627–642.
3. Coraboeuf, E., and Vassort, G. 1968. Effects of some inhibitors of ionic permeabilities on ventricular action potential and contraction of rat and guinea-pig hearts. *J. Electrocardiol.* 1:19–30.
4. Cranefield, P. F. 1975. *The Conduction of the Cardiac Impulse.* Futura, New York.

5. Ducouret, P. 1976. The effect of quinidine on membrane electrical activity in frog ventricular fibres studied by current and voltage clamp. *Br. J. Pharmacol.* 57:163–184.

6. Elharrar, V., and Zipes, D. P. 1977. Cardiac electrophysiologic alterations during myocardial ischemia. *Am. J. Physiol.* 233:H329–H345.

7. Engtsfeld, G., Antoni, H., and Fleckenstein, A. 1961. Die Restitution der Erregungsfortleitung und Kontraktionskraft des K^+-gelahmten Frosch- und Saugetiermyokards durch Adrenalin. *Pfluegers Arch.* 273:145–163.

8. Isenberg, G. 1976. Cardiac Purkinje fibers: Cesium as a tool to block inward rectifying potassium currents. *Pfluegers Arch.* 365:99–106.

9. Kenyon, J. L., and Gibbons, W. R. 1979. Influence of chloride, potassium and tetraethylammonium on the early outward current of sheep cardiac Purkinje fibers. *J. Gen. Physiol.* 73:117–138.

10. Kenyon, J. L., and Gibbons, W. R. 1979. 4-Aminopyridine and the early outward current of sheep cardiac Purkinje fibres. *J. Gen. Physiol.* 73:139–157.

11. Klein, R. L., Holland, W. C., and Tinsley, B. 1969. Quinidine and unidirectional cation fluxes in atria. *Circ. Res.* 8:246–252.

12. Pappano, A. J. 1970. Calcium dependent action potentials produced by catecholamines in guinea-pig atrial muscle fibers depolarized by potassium. *Circ. Res.* 27:379–390.

13. Shigenobu, K., and Sperelakis, N. 1972. Calcium current channels induced by catecholamines in chick embryonic hearts whose fast sodium channels are blocked by tetrodotoxin or elevated potassium. *Circ. Res.* 31:932–952.

14. Shines, K. I., and Douglas, A. M. 1974. Magnesium effects on ionic exchange and mechanical function in rat ventricle. *Am. J. Physiol.* 227:317–324.

15. Wiegand, V., Guggi, M., Meesmann, W., Kessler, M., and Gritschus, F. 1979. Extracellular potassium activity changes in the canine myocardium after coronary occlusion and the influence of beta-blockade. *Cardiovasc. Res.* 13:297–302.

16. Wit, A. L., and Bigger, J. T. 1977. Possible electrophysiological mechanisms for lethal arrhythmias accompanying myocardial ischemia and infarction. *Circulation* 56(Suppl. III):96–108.

17. Wit, A. L., and Friedman, P. L. 1975. Basis for ventricular arrhythmias accompanying myocardial infarction. *Arch. Intern. Med.* 35:459–472.

Antiischemic Effects of Molsidomine in an Experimental Model of Coronary Artery Stenosis

R.-E. Nitz, A. M. Mogilev, and H. Göbel

Department of Medical and Biological Research
Department of Pharmacology
Cassella AG
Frankfurt/Main, Federal Republic of Germany

Abstract. The effect of molsidomine, a novel antianginal agent, on the epicardial electrographic changes induced by reduced perfusion of the left anterior descending coronary artery (LAD) was investigated in the anesthetized dog. The LAD was cannulated and perfused at a constant volume with blood taken from a carotid artery. The perfusion volume was than reduced by approximately 75%. The sum of the ST-segment changes obtained from six unipolar epicardial leads was taken as a measure of myocardial hypoxia. Simultaneously, heart rate, blood pressure, left ventricular end-diastolic pressure, pulmonary arterial pressure, and heart contractility were also recorded. In control animals, reduction of the perfusion volume of the LAD resulted in a dramatic elevation of the ST segments lasting more than 4 hr. Molsidomine administered after the induction of the ischemia at a dose of 0.05 mg/kg i.v. resulted within 40 min in a complete normalization of the electrographic changes. This effect was evident for over 4 hr in spite of the continuous reduced perfusion of the LAD. The beneficial effect of molsidomine on the electrical changes paralleled the reduction of the left ventricular end-diastolic pressure. It is suggested that the effect of molsidomine on the ischemic electrographic changes is brought about by a reduction of the preload, resulting in a better perfusion of the ischemic zones.

The modern treatment of coronary heart disease consists of an effort to normalize the imbalance between oxygen supply and oxygen demand by reducing the work load of the heart. This goal can be obtained by increasing the capacity of the venous system (venous pooling) which results in a reduced venous return and decreased ventricular volume and ventricular wall-tension. This has as a consequence a reduction in heart work and oxygen demand.

The novel antianginal compound molsidomine, N-ethoxyearbonyl-3-morpholinosydnonimine, has these abovementioned pharmacological characteristics as assessed in man and in the laboratory animal (1–9,11–14, 18–25,29,30,34–39). This compound, which belongs to a new chemical class, was found to reduce the preload without affecting heart rate and contractility (4,5,7,8,13,14,18,22,23,34–36,38,39). This results in reduced cardiac work and oxygen demand as well as in a reduction of the extravascular factors of coronary artery resistance with a better perfusion of the endocardial layers (1,3,4,8,9,14,18,22,29,34,35,38).

In the present study, the effect of molsidomine was investigated on the ST elevation of the epicardial electrogram in an animal model of severe myocardial ischemia. Previous studies (10,15–17,26,27,31) had shown that the elevation of the ST segment is a reflection of the degree of cardiac ischemia and that the effect of a compound on this parameter can be taken as a measure of its antianginal activity. In the present investigation, contrary to previous studies in which a coronary artery was completely occluded (1,4,10,16,26,27,31–36), the coronary flow was only reduced by approximately 70–80% of its original value. With this methodology, a myocardial hypoxia could be induced without altering physiological coronary autoregulation (28).

METHODS

Sixteen mongrel dogs of both sexes were anesthetized with pentobarbitol sodium (40 mg/kg i.v.) and ventilated with a Bird Mark-6 respirator with a mixture of N_2O-O_2 in the ratio 4:1. The expired air CO_2 content was analyzed with a URAS (Hartmann & Braun) and kept between 4 and 5%. The systemic arterial blood pressure (BP) was measured from a femoral artery by means of a pressure transducer (Type P 23 Db, Statham Lab., Harbour Rey, Puerto Rico). The left ventricular pressure (LVP) was recorded with a catheter-tip manometer (type PC-350, Millar Instruments, Houston, Texas) passed retrogradely from a carotid artery into the left ventricle. Heart rate (HR) was determined from the LVP waveform, and the left ventricular end-diastolic pressure (LVEDP) was measured on a high-sensitivity scale. Myocardial contractility was measured as the rate of rise of LVP (dp/dt_{max}). The pulmonary arterial pressure (PAP) and the arterial pressure were recorded with two tip manomters (Millar Instruments, Houston, Texas) passed retrogradely from a jugular vein.

The heart was exposed through a left thoracotomy, and the left descending coronary artery (LAD) was dissected and cannulated just distal to the first diagonal branch. The coronary cannula was connected to a cannula inserted into a carotid artery so that the LAD was autoperfused at a constant volume with the aid of a roller pump (Stöckert, Munich). The perfusion pressure was monitored with a pressure transducer (type P 23 Db, Statham Lab., Harbour Rey, Puerto Rico). Six epicardial electrodes were placed on the heart in such a way that five were lying on the hypoxic zone and one on the border zone (Figure 1). The electrodes were made of gold, of conical form, 2 mm wide and 4 mm long. They were placed in form of a line on the epicardium, and their signal was magnified with a unipolar lead by a universal amplifier (Brush Instruments, Cleveland, Ohio). All recordings were made using two multichannel recorders (type Mark-260, Gould Corp., Brush In-

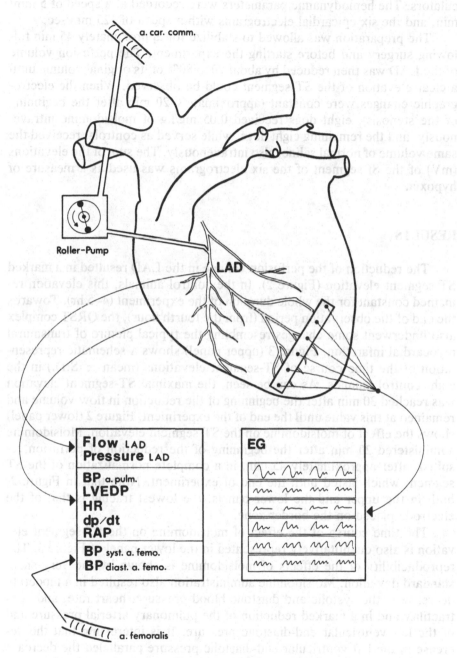

Figure 1.   Scheme of the experimental procedures.

strument Division, Cleveland, Ohio) with appropriate preamplifiers and cal-culators. The hemodynamic parameters were recorded at a speed of 5 mm/min, and the six epicardial electrograms with a speed of 125 mm/sec.

The preparation was allowed to stabilize for approximately 45 min following surgery and before starting the experiment. The perfusion volume of the LAD was then reduced by about 70 to 80% of its original volume until a clear elevation of the ST segment could be observed. When the electrographic changes were constant (approximately 20 min after the beginning of the stenosis), eight dogs received 0.05 mg/kg of molsidomine intravenously, and the remaining eight dogs, while served as controls, received the same volume of normal saline, also intravenously. The sum of the elevations (mV) of the St segment of the six electrograms was used as a measure of hypoxia.

RESULTS

The reduction of the perfusion volume in the LAD resulted in a marked ST-segment elevation (Figure 2). In the control animals, this elevation remained constant for the whole duration of the experiment (4–5 hr). Towards the end of the observation period (from the fourth hour), the QRST complex also underwent some changes resembling the typical picture of transmural myocardial infarction. Figure 3 (upper panel) shows a schematic representation of the time course of ST-segment elevations (mean ± S.D.) in the eight control animals. As can be seen, the maximal ST-segment elevation was reached 30 min after the beginning of the reduction in flow volume and remained at this value until the end of the experiment. Figure 2 (lower panel) shows the effect of molsidomine on the ST-segment elevation. Molsidomine administered 20 min after the beginning of the reduction of perfusion resulted, after approximately 45 min, in a complete normalization of the ST segment which lasted until the end of experiment. Note that in Figure 2, both in the upper and the lower panels, the lowest tracing is that of the electrode placed on the border zone.

The time course of the effect of molsidomine on the ST-segment elevation is also quantitatively represented in the lower panel of Figure 3. The reproducibility of the effects of molsidomine is shown by the very small standard deviation. Molsidomine administration also resulted in a moderate decrease in the systolic and diastolic blood pressure, heart rate, and contractility and in a marked reduction of the pulmonary arterial pressure and of the left ventricular end-diastolic pressure. It is interesting that the decrease in the left ventricular end-diastolic pressure paralleled the decrease of ST-segment elevation. This is shown in Figure 4 where, in the upper panel, we have the effect of molsidomine on the ST-segment elevation in mV and, in the lower panel, the effect of molsidomine on the left ventricular end-diastolic pressure in mm Hg.

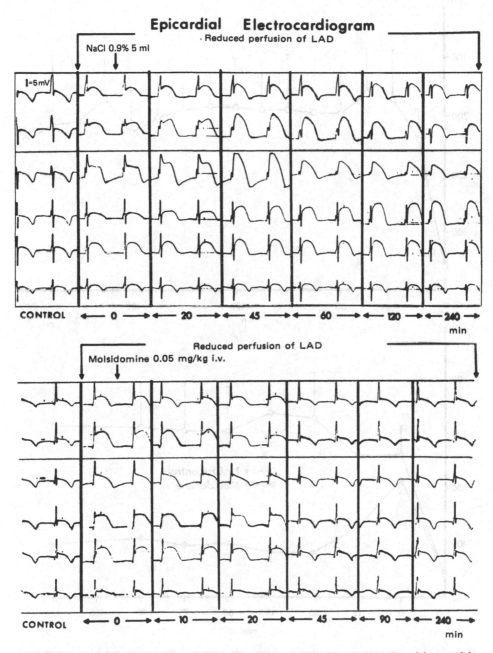

Figure 2.   Example of the epicardial electrogram in a control (upper panel) and in a molsi-domine-treated dog (lower panel).

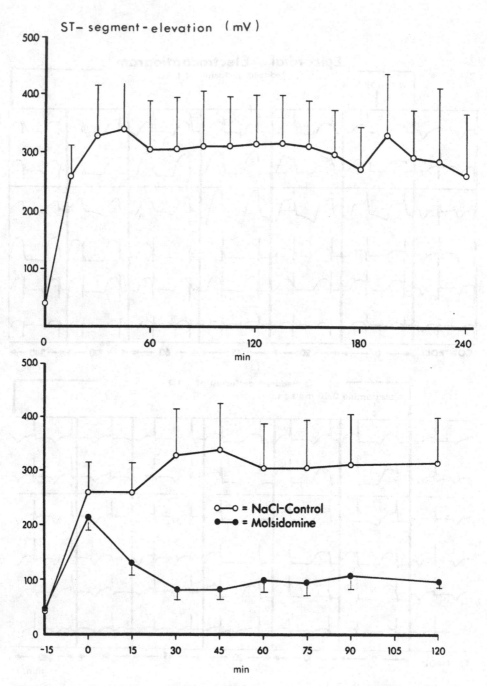

Figure 3. A schematic representation of the time course of changes in the ST segment (in mV). Upper panel, mean values of eight control animals; lower panel, comparison of controls and molsidomine-treated animals.

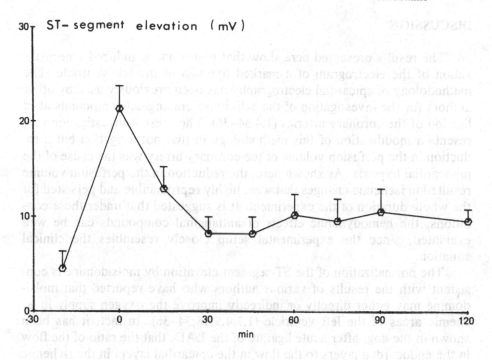

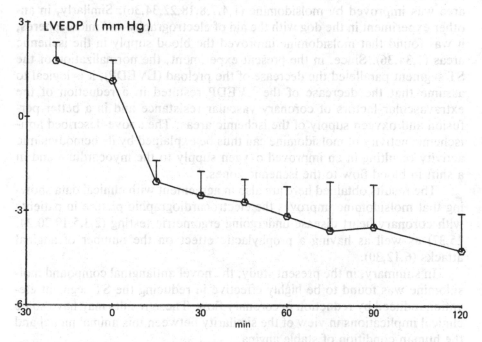

Figure 4.   Schematic representation of the time course of changes induced by molsidomine administration on the sum of ST-segment elevation (mV) (upper panel) and on the left ventricular end-diastolic pressure (mm Hg) (lower panel). Molsidomine was administered at the time 0. The data present the mean ± standard deviation of eight experiments.

DISCUSSION

The results presented here show that molsidomine induced a normalization of the electrogram of a marked hypoxia of the left ventricle. The methodology of epicardial electrography has been previously used by other authors for the investigation of the activity of antianginal compounds after ligation of the coronary arteries (1,4,34–36). The present investigation represents a modification of this methodology in that not a ligation but a reduction in the perfusion volume of the coronary artery was the cause of the myocardial hypoxia. As shown here, the reduction in the perfusion volume resulted in ischemic changes that were highly reproducible and persisted for the whole duration of the experiment. It is suggested that under these conditions, the hemodynamic effects of antianginal compounds can be well evaluated, since the experimental setup closely resembles the clinical situation.

The normalization of the ST-segment elevation by molsidomine is consistent with the results of various authors who have reported that molsidomine may either directly or indirectly improve the oxygen supply in ischemic areas of the left ventricle (1,3,4,9,18,34–36). In fact, it has been shown in the dog, after acute ligature of the LAD, that the ratio of the flow in the endocardial layers to the flow in the epicardial layers in the ischemic area was improved by molsidomine (1,4,7,8,18,22,34,36). Similarly, in another experiment in the dog with the aid of electrography and microspheres, it was found that molsidomine improved the blood supply in the ischemic areas (1,34,36). Since, in the present experiment, the normalization of the ST segment paralleled the decrease of the preload (LVEDP), it is logical to assume that the decrease of the LVEDP resulted in a reduction of the extravascular factors of coronary vascular resistance and in a better perfusion and oxygen supply of the ischemic areas. The above-described antiischemic activity of molsidomine can thus be explained by its hemodynamic activity resulting in an improved oxygen supply to the myocardium and in a shift in blood flow to the ischemic zones.

The results obtained here are also in agreement with clinical data showing that molsidomine improves the electrocardiographic picture in patients with coronary heart disease undergoing ergometric testing (2,3,5,19,20,24,25,37) as well as having a prophylactic effect on the number of anginal attacks (6,12,30).

In summary, in the present study, the novel antianginal compound molsidomine was found to be highly effective in reducing the ST-segment elevation induced by reduction in coronary flow. These results may have some clinical implications in view of the similarity between this animal model and the human condition of stable angina.

ACKNOWLEDGMENTS

The authors thank Mrs. U. Strathmann for her secretarial assistance.

REFERENCES

1. Berdeaux, A., Tato, F., Ho, S., Boissier, J.-R., and Giudicelli, J.-F. 1978. Molsidomine, debit coronaires regionaux et segment ST au niveau du myocarde sain et/ou ischemique chez le chien. *J. Pharmacol.* (*Paris*) 9:219–234.
2. Blazek, G., Gaul, G., and Heeger, H. 1977. Zur Wirkung von Molsidomin auf das Pulmonalarteriendruckverhalten Koronarkranker im ergometrischen Arbeitsversuch. *Herz Kreisl.* 9:478–481.
3. Bussmann, W. D., Neidel, K., and Kaltenbach, M. 1979. Wirkung von Molsidomin auf Hamodynamik und Ischamie bei Patienten mit frischem Herzinfarkt. In: W. Lochner and F. Bender (eds.), *Molsidomin, Neue Aspekte in der Therapie der Ischamischen Herzerkrankung*, pp. 100–104. Urban & Schwarzenberg, Munich, Vienna.
4. Dirschinger, J., Fleck, E., Bierner, M., Redl, A., and Rudolph, W. 1978. Poststenotische Myocarddurchblutung und Linksventrikelfunktion unter Molsidomin. *Z. Kardiol.* 67(Suppl. 5):62.
5. Enke, K. U., Keller, W., and Wagner, J. 1978. Wirksamkeit einer parenteralen Molsidomingabe auf die Hamodynamik des großen und kleinen Kreislaufes in Ruhe und unter Belastung. *Z. Kardiol.* 67(Suppl. 5):63.
6. Fleck, E., Dirschinger, J., and Rudolph, W. 1979. Hamodynamische Wirkungen von Molsidomin bei koronarer Herzerkrankung. *Herz* 4:285–292.
7. Fiedler, V. B. 1978. Behaviour of heart dimensions and other hemodynamic parameters after molsidomine, isosorbide dinitrate, nitroglycerin and nifedipine in dogs. *Trans. Eur. Soc. Cardiol.* 1:85.
8. Fiedler, V. B., and Scholtholt, J. 1978. Haemodynamic effects of molsidomine. *Arzneim. Forsch.* 28:1605–1612.
9. Fiedler, V. B., Scholtholt, J., and Gobel, H. 1978. Molsidomin: Wirkungen auf den myocardialen Sauerstoffverbrauch (MVO$_2$) des Hundes. *Verh. Dtsch. Ges. Kreislaufforsch.* 44:184.
10. Fozzard, H. A., and Dasgupta, D. S. 1976. ST-segment potentials and mapping. *Circulation* 54:533–537.
11. Grund, E., Muller-Rucholtz, E.-R., Lapp, E. R., Losch, H.-M., and Lochner, W. 1978. Comparative study of nitroglycerin and molsidomine. Effects on the integrated systemic venous bed and the arterial pressure in the dog. *Arzneim. Forsch.* 28:1624–1628.
12. Guerchicoff, S., Vasquez, A., Kunik, H., Drajer, S., and Diaz, F. 1978. Acute double blind trial of a new anti-anginal drug: Molsidomine. *Eur. J. Clin. Pharmacol.* 23:247–250.
13. Hashimoto, K., Taira, N., Hirata, M., and Kokubun, M. 1971. The mode of hypotensive action of newly synthetized sydnonimine derivatives. *Arzneim. Forsch.* 21:1329–1332.
14. Hirata, M., and Kikushi, K. 1970. Coronary collateral vasodilatator action of N-ethoxycarbonal-3-morpholino-sydnonimine (SIN-10) in heart with chronic coronary insufficiency in dogs. *Jpn. J. Pharmacol.* 20:187–193.
15. Holland, R. P., and Brooks, H. 1975. ST-segment mapping: Fact and fallacy. *Circulation* 52(Suppl. II):6.
16. Holland, R. P., and Brooks, H. 1975. Precordial and epicardial surface potentials during myocardial ischemia in the pig. A theoretical and experimental analysis of the TQ and ST segments. *Circ. Res.* 73:471–480.
17. Holland, R., Pashkow, F., and Brooks, H. 1974. Atraumatic epicardial electrode and rapid sampling switch for cardiac surface mapping. *J. Appl. Physiol.* 37:424–427.
18. Holtz, J., Bassenge, E., and Kolin, A. 1978. Hemodynamic and myocardial effects of long-lasting venodilation in the conscious dog: Analysis of molsidomine in comparison with nitrates. *Basic Res. Cardiol.* 73:469–481.
19. Jansen, E., and Klepzig, H. 1978. Zum Einfluß von Molsidomin in verschiedener Dosierung auf die Belastungskoronarinsuffizienz. *Med. Klin.* 73:983–986.
20. Karsch, K. R., Rentrop, K. P., Blanke, H., and Kreuzer, H. 1978. Haemodynamic effects of molsidomine. *Eur. J. Clin. Pharmacol.* 13:241–245.

21. Kikuchi, H., Hirata, M., and Nagaoka, A. 1970. Hypotensive action of N-ethoxycarbonyl-3-morpholinosydnonimine, SIN-10. *Jpn. J. Pharmacol.* 20:102–115.
22. Kikuchi, K., Hirata, M., Nagaoka, A., and Aramaki, Y. 1970. Cardiovascular action of mesionic compounds, 3-substituted sydnonimines. *Jpn. J. Pharmacol.* 20:23–42.
23. Lochner, W., Muller-Rucholtz, E.-R., Grund, E., Hauer, F., and Lapp, E. 1978. Integrated systemic venous volume as influenced by antianginal drugs: Effects of beta-blockers, nitroglycerin and molsidomine. In: *Abstracts, VIII World Congress of Cardiology (Tokyo)*, p. 192.
24. Majid, P. A., DeFeyter, P. J. F., van der Wall, E. E., Warden, R., and Roos, J. P. 1980. Molsidomine in the treatment of patients with angina pectoris. Acute hemodynamic effects and clinical efficacy. *N. Engl. J. Med.* 302:1–6.
25. Mannes, G. A., Goebel, G., Kafka, W., and Rudolph, W. 1978. Behandlung der Angina pectoris mit Molsidomin. *Herz* 3:172–184.
26. Maroko, P. R., and Braunwald, W. 1976. Effects of metabolic and pharmacologic interventions on myocardial infarct size following coronary occlusion. *Circulation* 53:162.
27. Maroko, P. R., Kiekshus, R., Sobel, B. E., Watanabe, T., Cowell, J. W., Ross, J., and Braunwald, E. 1971. Factors influencing infarct size following coronary artery occlusion. *Circulation* 43:67–82.
28. Mogilev, A. M., Gobel, H., and Nitz, R. E. 1980. Antiischemic effect of molsidomine on experimental left anterior descending coronary artery stenosis. *Z. Kardiol.* 69:205 (abstr.).
29. Nitz, R.-E. 1979. Zur Pharmakologie von Molsidomin. In: W. Lochner and F. Bender (eds.), *Molsidomin, Neue Aspekte in der Therapie der Ischamischen Herzerkrankung* pp. 6–13. Urban & Schwarzenberg, Munich.
30. Pirzada, A. M., DeFeyter, P. J. F., van der Wall, E. E., Wardeh, R., and Roos, J. P. 1980. Molsidomin in the treatment of patients with angina pectoris. *N. Engl. J. Med.* 302:1–6.
31. Ross, J. 1976. Electrocardiographic ST-segment analysis in the characterization of myocardial ischemic and infarction. *Circulation [Suppl.]* 53:73–81.
32. Schaper, W. 1979. Zur Pathophysiologie der koronaren Herzkrankheit. 1. In: W. Lochner and F. Bender (eds.), *Molsidomin, Neue Aspekte in der Therapie der Ischamischen Herzerkrankung*, pp. 2–5. Urban & Schwarzenberg, Munich.
33. Schaper, W., Flameng, W., Winckler, B., Wusten, B., Turschmann, W., Neugebauer, G., Carl, M., and Pasyk, S. 1976. Quantification of collateral resistance in acute and chronic experimental coronary occlusion in the dog. *Cir. Res.* 39:371–377.
34. Scholtholt, J., Fiedler, V. B., and Keil, M. 1977. Molsidomine, effects on blood flow of normal and ischemic myocardium. In: *Joint Meeting German and Italian Pharmacologists, Venice*, p. 184. Fondazione Cini, Venice.
35. Scholtholt, J., Fiedler, V. B., and Keil, M. 1978. Die Wirkung von Molsidomin auf die regionale Verteilung des Herzminutenvolumens des narkotisierten Hundes. *Arzneim. Forsch.* 28:1612–1619.
36. Scholtholt, J., Fiedler, V. B., and Keil, M. 1978. Die Wirkung von Molsidomin und Nitroglycerin auf die regionale Durchblutung des normalen und akut-ischamischen Myokards. *Arzneim. Forsch.* 28:1619–1624.
37. Slany, J., Mosslacher, H., Schmoliner, R., and Kronik, G. 1976. Einfluß von Molsidomin auf Hamodynamik und Arbeitstoleranz bei Patienten mit Angina pectoris. *Med. Welt* 27:2369–2400.
38. Takenaka, F., Takeya, N., Ishihara, T., Inoue, S., Tsutsumi, E., Nakamura, R. Mitsufuji, Y., and Sumie, M. 1970. Effects of N-ethoxycarbonyl-3-morpholinosydnonimine (SIN-10) on the cardiovascular system. *Jpn. J. Pharmacol.* 20:253–263.
39. Takeshita, A., Nakamura, M., Tajimi, T., Matsuguchi, H., Kuroiwa, A., Tanaka, S., and Kikuchi, Y. 1977. Long-lasting effect of oral molsidomine on exercise performance. A new antianginal agent. *Circulation* 55:401–407.

Effect of Molsidomine on Spontaneous Ventricular Fibrillation following Myocardial Ischemia and Reperfusion in the Dog

P. A. Martorana, A. M. Mogilev, B. Kettenbach, and R.-E. Nitz

Department of Medical and Biological Research
Department of Pharmacology
Cassella AG
Frankfurt/Main, Federal Republic of Germany

Abstract. The effect of the novel antianginal agent molsidomine on the incidence of spontaneous ventricular fibrillation during myocardial ischemia and reperfusion was investigated in the anesthetized dog. Molsidomine was administered as an intravenous bolus at the dose of 0.05 mg/kg. Twenty minutes later, the left anterior descending coronary artery was occluded for 90 min. During the occlusion period, molsidomine was given as a continuous intravenous infusion at the dose of 0.5 µg/kg per ml per min. After release of the occlusion, the animals that survived were monitored for another 30 min. Control animals received saline. In the control animals, coronary occlusion was accompanied by an increase in heart rate, heart contractility, left ventricular end-diastolic pressure, and blood pressure as well as by ventricular arrhythmias. Molsidomine either abolished or reduced both hemodynamic and electrical changes. During the reperfusion period, 10 out of 12 control animals died, and the deaths were from ventricular fibrillation; one out of eight molsidomine-treated animals also died of ventricular fibrillation. It is postulated that the protective effect of molsidomine rests on its hemodynamic effects resulting in a shift in blood flow toward the ischemic zones and, consequently, in an increase in ventricular electrical stability.

Molsidomine, N-ethoxycarbonyl-3-morpholino-sydnonimine,

is a novel therapeutic agent for the treatment of coronary heart disease. In the experimental animal and in man, the activity of molsidomine is brought about by a reduction of the venous return, cardiac output, ventricular work, and myocardial oxygen consumption (1,6–9,11–14,19,22). The effect of molsidomine on the peripheral blood pressure is moderate and is usually not accompanied by reflex tachycardia (6,9,11,19).

Clinical observations suggest that molsidomine, in view of its hemodynamic profile, may be of benefit in acute myocardial infarction (4). However, the effect of this compound on the number of ventricular premature complexes or more serious forms of arrhythmia in acute myocardial infarction is not known. Similarly, the possibility that molsidomine may prevent the occurrence of ventricular arrhythmia and fibrillation after reperfusion of the ischemic myocardium in the experimental animal has not been explored.

In the present study, we investigated the effect of molsidomine on the incidence of spontaneous ventricular fibrillation during myocardial ischemia and reperfusion in the dog.

METHODS

Mongrel dogs of both sexes in the weight range of 20 to 26 kg were used. Anesthesia was induced with thiobutobarbital (30 mg/kg i.v.) and maintained with a chloralose–urethane mixture (20 and 250 mg/kg i.v., respectively) followed by morphine (2 mg/kg s.c.). The animals were ventilated with a Bird Mark 7 respirator using room air. The heart was exposed through a left thoracotomy, and a sling was placed around the left descending coronary artery (LAD) approximately 1 cm below its origin and just distal to the first diagonal branch. The systemic peripheral arterial blood pressure (BP) was measured from a femoral artery by means of a pressure transducer (type P 23 Db, Statham Lab., Habo Rey, Puerto Rico). The left ventricular pressure (LVP) was recorded with a catheter-tip manometer (type PC-350, Millar Instruments, Houston, Texas) passed retrogradely from a carotid artery into the left ventricle. Heart rate (HR) was determined from the LVP waveform, and the left ventricular end-diastolic pressure (LVEDP) was measured on a high-sensitivity scale. Myocardial contractility was measured as the rate of rise of LVP (dp/dt_{max}). The sum of the ST-segment elevations was calculated from five values of the peripheral limbs in ECG lead 2. The pressure–rate index (PRI) served as measure of oxygen consumption.

The preparation was allowed to stabilize for approximately 45 min following surgery and before starting the experiment. Molsidomine was than administered as an intravenous bolus at the dose of 0.05 mg/kg. Twenty minutes later, the left anterior descending coronary artery was occluded for 90 min. This occlusion period was chosen to increase the likelihood of inducing spontaneous ventricular fibrillation on reperfusion. During the occlusion period, molsidomine was given as a continuous intravenous infusion at the dose of 0.5 μg/kg per ml per min. After release of the coronary obstruction, the animals that survived were monitored for another 30 min. The hemodynamic parameters were monitored prior to molsidomine administration, 1 min before the LAD occlusion, at the time of maximal changes during the occlusion period, usually 10 min after the ligature, 1 min before release of the occlusion, and, in the animals that survived, 15 and 30 min after release of the ligature.

Control animals received saline instead of molsidomine; otherwise, the same experimental procedure was followed.

RESULTS

In control animals, occlusion of the LAD resulted in a marked and sustained tachycardia and in a moderate but long-lasting increase in blood pressure (Figure 1). Release of the occlusion dramatically magnified the tachycardia for a short period of time. Thirty minutes after the reperfusion, the heart rate had returned to normal values. Release of the occlusion also induced a further small and short-lasting increase in blood pressure. In the treated animals, molsidomine administration as a bolus resulted in a drop in blood pressure and in a small increase in heart rate (Figure 1). Occlusion of the LAD during molsidomine infusion did not induce an increase in the heart rate and resulted in a modest increase in blood pressure which returned to its original, pretreatment value (Figure 1). Release of the ligature resulted in a short-lasting tachycardia which, however, did not reach the values seen in the control animals. The reperfusion had no effect on the blood pressure in the animals (Figure 1). The rate–pressure product, taken as an index of myocardial oxygen consumption, showed that molsidomine favorably affected this parameter during both the occlusion and the reperfusion (Figure 1).

In the control animals, the left ventricular pressure increased after the LAD occlusion. During the reperfusion, this parameter slowly returned to control values (Figure 2). In the treated animals, molsidomine, as a bolus, reduced the left ventricular pressure. Occlusion under molsidomine infusion increased the ventricular pressure only slightly (Figure 2).

In the control animals, the occlusion of the LAD induced a marked but short-lasting increase of the left ventricular end-diastolic pressure; the reperfusion had no effect on this parameter (Figure 2). Molsidomine, as a bolus, induced a clear decrease in the end-diastolic pressure. In the ischemic period with molsidomine infusion, the end-diastolic pressure continued to decrease. In the reperfusion period, however, there was a clear but short-lived increase in the LVEDP (Figure 2).

In the controls, the ligature of the LAD induced a dramatic and sustained increase in heart contractility. This parameter remained elevated during the early phase of the reperfusion and returned to control values 30 min after the beginning of the reperfusion (Figure 2). Molsidomine offered almost complete protection against these changes.

In the control animals, both the occlusion and the release of the LAD induced electrical derangements in the myocardium. In the occlusion period, there was a multitude of ectopic activity which paralleled the development of myocardial ischemia, here shown as depression of the ST segment and peaking of T waves (Figure 3). After reperfusion, ventricular tachycardia

608   P. A. Martorana et al.

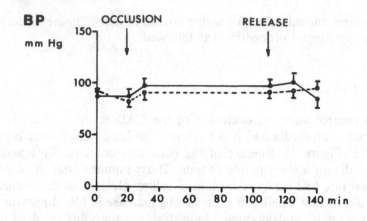

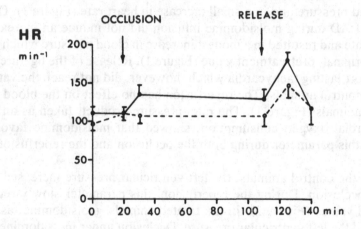

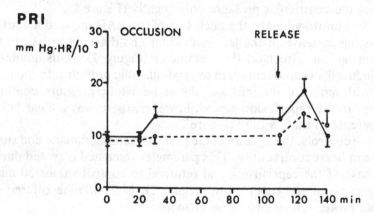

Figure 1. Schematic representation of the time course of changes in blood pressure (BP) (upper panel), heart rate (HR) (middle), and pressure–rate index (PRI) (lower panel) during coronary occlusion and release in the dog. ●——●, Controls (12 animals); ○– –○, molsidomine-treated animals (eight animals).

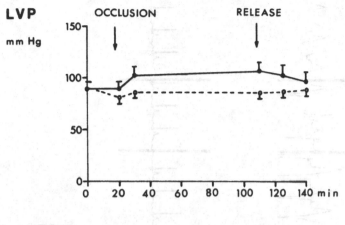

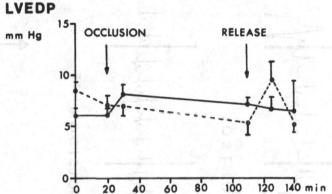

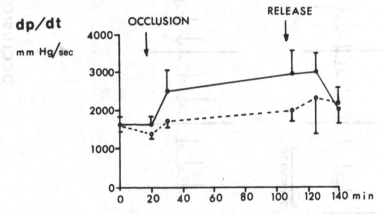

Figure 2. Schematic representation of the time course of changes in left ventricular pressure (LVP) (upper panel), left ventricular end-diastolic pressure (LVEDP) (middle), and heart contractility (dp/dt_{max}) (lower panel) during coronary occlusion and release in the dog. ●——●, Controls (12 animals); ○– –○, molsidomine-treated animals (eight animals).

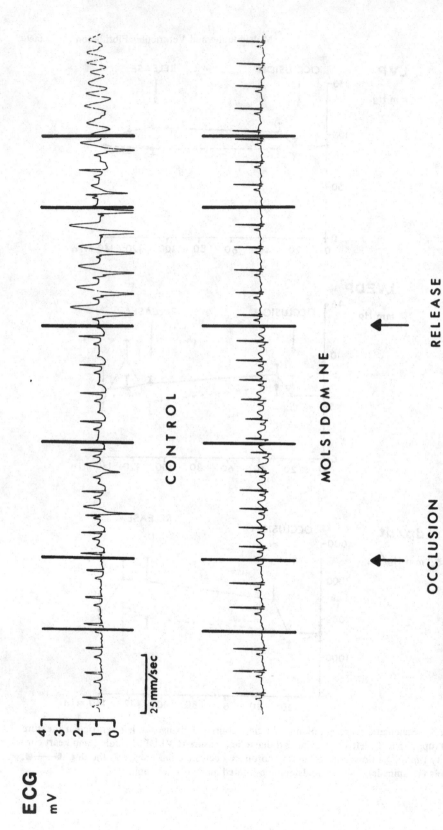

Figure 3. Electrocardiographic changes (ECG) (lead 2) during coronary occlusion and release in a control (upper panel) and a molsidomine-treated (lower panel) dog.

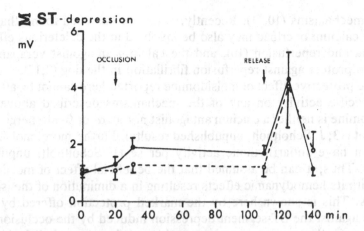

Figure 4. Schematic representation of the time course of changes of the ST segment (electrocardiogram, lead 2) during coronary occlusion and release in the dog. ●——●, Controls (12 animals); O— -O, molsidomine-treated animals (eight animals).

developed which, in most cases, was abruptly followed by ventricular fibrillation (Figure 3). Molsidomine had a favorable effect on the electrical derangements consequent to ischemia as well as on those elicited by the reperfusion (Figure 3). With regard to the ST depression, molsidomine markedly prevented these ischemic changes during the occlusion phase, although there was no difference between the surviving controls and molsidomine-treated animals in the reperfusion phase (Figure 4).

Ten out of 12 control animals died; death was from ventricular fibrillation and always occurred in the reperfusion period. One out of eight molsidomine-treated animals died, and the death was also from ventricular fibrillation in the reperfusion phase.

DISCUSSION

Molsidomine showed a marked protection against spontaneous ventricular fibrillation during reperfusion in this model. The basis of the beneficial electrophysiological activity of molsidomine is only speculative, since the mechanism that precipitates ventricular fibrillation is uncertain. There is evidence to suggest that during the ischemic (occlusion) period a marked cardiocardiac sympathetic activation occurs (3,15), and α- and β-adrenergic blocking agents have been found to block the electrical cardiac derangements induced by coronary occlusion (5). A different mechanism, however, seems to be responsible for the ventricular arrhythmia and fibrillation that follow the abrupt release of the coronary occlusion. A sudden washout of substances (potassium, calcium, lactic acid, cyclic nucleotides) that accumulate in the ischemic area during the occlusion phase as well as alterations in transcellular gradients of hydrogen ions have been suggested as the precipitating mechanisms (10,21). Recently, evidence has been found that intracellular calcium overload may also be involved in the deleterious effects of ischemia and reperfusion (16), and the calcium antagonist verapamil was found to protect against reperfusion fibrillation in the dog (2,17).

The protective effect of molsidomine reported here cannot be attributed to a specific activity on any of the mechanisms described above, since molsidomine is neither a calcium antagonist nor an α- or β-adrenergic blocking agent (13; J. Scholtholt, unpublished results). Furthermore, molsidomine does not have antiarrhythmic activity per se (J. Scholtholt, unpublished results). Thus, it can be assumed that the beneficial effect of molsidomine rests with its hemodynamic effects resulting in a diminution of the ischemic changes. This is shown here by the marked protection offered by molsidomine against the ST-segment depression induced by the occlusion. Molsidomine, in the present experiment, either reduced or abolished the hemodynamic changes consequent to LAD occlusion and possibly related to sympathetic activation (increase in heart rate, contractility, left ventricular end-diastolic pressure, and blood pressure). Consistent with these hemodynamic effects of molsidomine would be a reduction in the extravascular factors of coronary vascular resistance, resulting in an improved ratio of the flow in the endocardial layers to the flow in the epicardial layers in the ischemic area. This has recently been shown in the dog with the help of the radioactive particle distribution technique (1,18). Furthermore, a direct dilating effect of molsidomine on the large coronary arteries resulting in an increased blood flow to myocardial sites supplied by an occluded coronary artery cannot be excluded. In both cases, the shift in blood flow toward the ischemic zones would reduce the disparity between the refractory periods in normal and ischemic areas, resulting in an increased ventricular electrical stability (21).

This may in part or wholly explain the protective effect of molsidomine on spontaneous ventricular fibrillation seen here. This hypothesis is supported by a recent report that nitroglycerin, which has a similar hemodynamic profile, was also effective in this model (20).

Since there is reason to believe that sudden death in man may, in some cases, be caused by reperfusion following release of coronary artery spasm or platelet disaggregation, the present findings may have some clinical implications.

ACKNOWLEDGMENT

The authors thank Mrs. U. Strathmann for her secreterial assistance.

REFERENCES

1. Berdeaux, A., Tato, F., Ho, S., Boissier, J. R., and Giudicelli, J. F. 1978. Molsidomine, debits coronaires regionaux et segment ST au niveau du myocarde sain et/ou ischemique chez le chien. *J. Pharmacol. (Paris)* 9:219–234.

2. Brooks, W. W., Verrier, R. L., and Lown, B. 1980. Protective effect of verapamil on vulnerability to ventricular fibrillation during myocardial ischemia and reperfusion. *Cardiovasc. Res.* 14:295–302.
3. Brown, A. M. 1967. Excitation of cardiac afferent sympathetic nerve fibres during myocardial ischemia. *J. Physiol. (Lond.)* 190:35–53.
4. Bussmann, W. D., Neidel, K., and Kaltenbach, M. 1979. Wirkung von Molsidomin auf Hämodynamik und Ischämie bei Patienten mit frischem Herzinfarkt. In: W. Lochner and F. Bender (eds.), *Molsidomin, Neue Aspekte in der Therapie der ischämischen Herzerkrankung*, pp. 100–104. Urban & Schwarzenberg, Munich.
5. Corbalan, R., Verrier, R. L., and Lown, B. 1976. Differing mechanisms for ventricular vulnerability during coronary artery occlusion and release. *Am. Heart J.* 92:223–230.
6. Fiedler, V. B., and Scholtholt, J. 1978. Hemodynamic effects of molsidomine. *Arzneim. Forsch.* 9:1605–1612.
7. Fleck, E., Dirschinger, J., and Rudolph, W. 1979. Hämodynamische Wirkungen von Molsidomin bei koronarer Herzerkrankung. *Herz* 4:285–292.
8. Grund, E., Müller-Rucholtz, E. R., and Lapp, E. R., Lösch, H. M., and Lochner, W. 1978. Comparative study of nitroglycerin and molsidomine. Effects of the integrated systemic venous bed and the arterial pressure in dogs. *Arzneim. Forsch.* 9:1624–1628.
9. Hashimoto, K., Taira, N., Hirata, M., and Kokubun, M. 1971. The mode of hypotensive action of newly synthesized sydnonimine derivatives. *Arzneim. Forsch.* 21:1329–1332.
10. Hearse, D. J. 1977. Reperfusion of ischemic myocardium. *J. Mol. Cell. Cardiol.* 9:607–616.
11. Holtz, J., Bassenge, E., and Kolin, A. 1978. Hemodynamic and myocardial effects of long lasting venodilatation in the conscious dog: Analysis of molsidomine in comparison with nitrates. *Basic Res. Cardiol.* 73:469–481.
12. Karsch, K. R., Rentrop, K. P., Blanke, H., and Kreuzer, H. 1978. Hemodynamic effects of molsidomine. *Eur. J. Clin. Pharmacol.* 13:241–245.
13. Kikuchi, K., Hirata, M., and Nagaoka, A. 1970. Hypotensive action of N-ethoxycarbonyl-3-morpholinosydnonimine, SIN-10. *Jpn. J. Pharmacol.* 20:102–115.
14. Majid, P. A., DeFeyter, P. J. F., van der Wall, E. E., Warden, R., and Roos, J. P. 1980. Molsidomine in the treatment of patients with angina pectoris. Acute hemodynamic effects and clinical efficacy. *N. Engl. J. Med.* 302:1–6.
15. Malliani, A., Schwartz, P. J., and Zanchetti, A. 1969. A sympathetic reflex elicited by experimental coronary occlusion. *Am. J. Physiol.* 217:703–709.
16. Nayler, W. G. 1980. The pharmacological protection of the ischemic heart. The use of calcium and beta-adrenoceptor antagonists. In: *Abstracts, VII European Congress of Cardiology, Paris*, p. 242.
17. Ribeiro, L. G. T., DeBauche, T. L., Brandon, T. A., Reduto, L. A., Maroko, P. R., and Miller, R. R. 1980. Comparative effects of calcium antagonists on reactive hyperemia and ventricular arrhythmias during coronary artery reperfusion. In: *Abstracts, VII European Congress of Cardiology, Paris*, p. 242.
18. Scholtholt, J., Fiedler, V. B., and Keil, M. 1978. Die Wirkung von Molsidomin und Nitroglycerin auf die regionale Durchblutung des normalen und akutischämischen Myokards. *Arzneim. Forsch.* 28:1619–1624.
19. Scholtholt, J., Fiedler, V. B., and Keil, M. 1978. Die Wirkung von Molsidomin auf die regionale Verteilung des Herzminutenvolumens des narkotisierten Hundes. *Arzneim. Forsch.* 28:1612–1619.
20. Stockman, M. B., Verrier, R. L., and Lown, B. 1979. Effect of nitroglycerin on vulnerability to ventricular fibrillation during myocardial ischemia and reperfusion. *Am. J. Cardiol.* 43:233–238.
21. Surawicz, B. 1971. Ventricular fibrillation. *Am. J. Cardiol.* 28:268–287.
22. Takenaka, F., Takeya, N., Ishihara, T., Inoue, S., Tsutsumi, E., Nakamura, R., Mitsufuji, Y., and Sumie, M. 1970. Effects of N-ethoxycarbonyl-3-morpholinosydnonimine (SIN-10) on cardiovascular system. *Jpn. J. Pharmacol.* 20:253–263.

Contributors

H. ABE, Department of Radiology, Nihon University School of Medicine, Tokyo, 173, Japan

T. ABE, The Department of Thoracic and Cardiovascular Surgery, Sapporo Medical College, Sapporo 060, Japan

F. L. ABEL, Department of Physiology, USC School of Medicine, Columbia, South Carolina 29208, USA

J. AMANO, Department of Cardiothoracic Surgery, Juntendo University School of Medicine, Tokyo, Japan

I. S. ANAND, Department of Cardiology, Postgraduate Institute of Medical Education and Research, Chandigarh 160012, India

Z. ANTALÓCZY, Second Medical Clinic of Postgraduate Medical School, H-1389 Budapest, Hungary

J. AUSSEDAT, Laboratory of Animal Physiology, Scientific and Medical University of Grenoble, 38041 Grenoble Cedex, France

T. N. AZVOLINSKAYA, Institute of Pharmacology, Academy of Medical Sciences of the USSR, Moscow 125315, USSR

M. BALLAK, Laboratory of Pathobiology, Clinical Research Institute of Montreal; and Department of Pathology, University of Montreal and Hôtel-Dieu of Montreal, Montreal, Quebec H2W 1R7, Canada

D. W. BARON, Cardiac Muscle Research Laboratory, Mayo Clinic and Mayo Foundation, Rochester, Minnesota 55905, USA

S. BARTEL, Division of Cellular and Molecular Cardiology, Central Institute of Heart and Circulation Research, Academy of Sciences of the GDR, 1115 Berlin–Buch; and Surgical Clinic, Faculty of Medicine (Charité) of Humboldt University at Berlin, 1040 Berlin, German Democratic Republic

J. BEUZERON-MANGINA, Laboratory of Pathobiology, Clinical Research Institute of Montreal; and Department of Pathology, University of Montreal and Hôtel-Dieu of Montreal, Montreal, Quebec H2W 1R7, Canada

P. S. BIDWAI, Department of Cardiology, Postgraduate Institute of Medical Education and Research, Chandigarh 160012, India

K. E. BLASS, Department of Pharmacology and Toxicology, Faculty of Medicine, Martin Luther University, Halle-Wittenberg, Halle, German Democratic Republic

H.-U. BLOCK, Department of Pharmacology and Toxicology, Faculty of Medicine, Martin Luther University, Halle-Wittenberg, Halle, German Democratic Republic

615

T. K. BORG, Department of Pathology, USC School of Medicine, Columbia, South Carolina 29208, USA

M. BOUTET, Department of Pathology, McGill University, Montreal, Quebec H3A 2B4, Canada

A. BOYLETT, The Rayne Institute, St. Thomas' Hospital, London, England

M. V. BRAIMBRIDGE, Department of Heart Research (Surgical Cytochemistry), The Rayne Institute, St. Thomas' Hospital, London SE1, England

S. ČANKOVIĆ-DARRACOTT, Department of Heart Research (Surgical Cyto-chemistry), the Rayne Institute, St. Thomas' Hospital, London, England

M. CANTIN, Laboratory of Pathobiology, Clinical Research Institute of Montreal; and Department of Pathology, University of Montreal and Hôtel-Dieu of Montreal, Montreal, Quebec H2W 1R7, Canada

J. B. CAULFIELD, Department of Pathology, USC School of Medicine, Columbia, South Carolina 29208, USA

J. ČERNÝ, Institute of Pathological Physiology, Faculty of Medicine, IInd Surgical Clinic, University of J. E. Purkinje; and Research Center for Heart Support and Total Heart Substitution, Regional Institute of National Health, Brno, Czechoslovakia

R. N. CHAKRAVARTI, Department of Experimental Medicine, Postgraduate In-stitute of Medical Education and Research, Chandigarh 160012, India

J. CHAYEN, Division of Cellular Biology, Kennedy Institute of Rheumatology, London, England

A. M. CHERNUKH, Institute of General Pathology and Pathological Physiology, Academy of Medical Sciences of the USSR, Moscow, USSR

C.-C. CHIU, Cardiovascular Research Unit, The Third Department of Internal Medicine, Faculty of Medicine, University of Tokyo, Tokyo 113, Japan

B. CHUA, Department of Physiology, The Milton S. Hershey Medical Center, The Pennsylvania State University, Hershey, Pennsylvania 17033, USA

D. J. COLTART, The Myocardial Metabolism and Cardiac Pharmacology Units, The Rayne Institute, St. Thomas' Hospital, London, England

E. CORABOEUF, Laboratory of Comparative Physiology, University of Paris XI, Orsay, France

J. S. CRIE, Pauline and Adolph Weinberger Laboratory for Cardiopulmonary Re-search, Department of Physiology, The University of Texas Health Science Center at Dallas, Dallas, Texas 75235, USA

P. CUMMINS, Molecular Cardiology Unit, Department of Cardiovascular Medicine, University of Birmingham, Birmingham B15 2TH, England

U. DELABAR, Department of Pharmacology, Faculty of Medicine, University of Tübingen, D-7400 Tübingen, Federal Republic of Germany

M. R. de LEVAL, Department of Paediatric Cardiology, Institute of Child Health, London WC1N 3EH, England; present address: Thoracic Unit, The Hospital for Sick Children, London WC1N 3JH, England

S. C. DENNIS, The Rayne Institute, St. Thomas' Hospital, London, England; present address: The Likoff Cardiovascular Institute. The Hahnemann Medical College, Philadelphia, Pennsylvania 19102, USA

J. W. de JONG, Cardiochemical Laboratory, Thoraxcenter, Erasmus University Rotterdam, Rotterdam, The Netherlands

P. P. de TOMBE, Cardiochemical Laboratory, Thoraxcenter, Erasmus University Rotterdam, Rotterdam, The Netherlands

M. DOSTÁL, Institute of Pathological Physiology, Faculty of Medicine, IInd Surgical Clinic, University of J. E. Purkinke; and Research Center for Heart Support and Total Health Substitution, Regional Institute of National Health, Brno, Czechoslovakia

K. EBISAWA, The Fourth Department of Internal Medicine, Faculty of Medicine, The University of Tokyo, Tokyo, Japan

G. EBRECHT, Physiological Institute (II), University of Tubingen, Federal Republic of Germany

K. ENGELMANN, Department of Pharmacology, Knoll AG, Ludwigshafen, Federal Republic of Germany

D. FEUVRAY, Laboratory of Comparative Physiology, University of Paris-Sud, 91405 Orsay, France

W. FÖRSTER, Department of Pharmacology and Toxicology, Faculty of Medicine, Martin Luther University, Halle-Wittenberg, Halle, German Democratic Republic

E. O. FULLER, Department of Physiology, The Milton S. Hershey Medical Center, The Pennsylvania State University, Hershey, Pennsylvania, 17033, USA

N. K. GANGULY, Department of Parasitology, Postgraduate Institute of Medical Education and Research, Chandigarh 160012, India

C. E. GANOTE, Department of Pathology, Northwestern University Medical School, Chicago, Illinois 60611, USA

P. GASTINEAU, I.N.S.E.R.M. U2, Hôpital Léon Bernard, 94450 Limeil-Brévannes, France

C. GIESSLER, Department of Pharmacology and Toxicology, Faculty of Medicine, Martin Luther University, Halle-Wittenberg, Halle, German Democratic Republic

H. GÖBEL, Department of Pharmacology, Cassella AG, Frankfurt/Main, Federal Republic of Germany

O. A. GOMAZKOV, Institute of General Pathology and Pathological Physiology, Academy of Medical Sciences of the USSR, Moscow, USSR

Z. GREGOR, Institute of Pathological Physiology, Faculty of Medicine, IInd Surgical Clinic, University of J. E. Purkinje; and Research Center for Heart Support and Total Heart Substitution, Regional Institute of National Health, Brno, Czechoslovakia

I. GREGOROVÁ, Third Medical Department and Laboratory for Endocrinology and Metabolism, Faculty of Medicine, Charles University, Prague, Czechoslovakia

M. GREGOROVÁ, Institute of Pathological Physiology, Faculty of Medicine, IInd Surgical Clinic, University of J. E. Purkinje; and Research Center for Heart Support and Total Heart Substitution, Regional Institute of National Health, Brno, Czechoslovakia

P. GUBA, Institute of Pathological Physiology, Faculty of Medicine, IInd Surgical Clinic, University of J. E. Purkinje; and Research Center for Heart Support and Total Heart Substitution, Regional Institute of National Health, Brno, Czechoslovakia

P. HANZELKA, Institute of Pathological Physiology, Faculty of Medicine, IInd Surgical Clinic, University of J. E. Purkinje; and Research Center for Heart Support and Total Heart Substitution, Regional Institute of National Health, Brno, Czechoslovakia

E. HARMSEN, Cardiochemical Laboratory, Thoraxcenter, Erasmus University Rotterdam, Rotterdam, The Netherlands

C. E. HARRISON, Cardiac Muscle Research Laboratory, Mayo Clinic and Mayo Foundation, Rochester, Minnesota 55905, USA

B. HARTMANNOVÁ, Institute of Pathological Physiology, Faculty of Medicine, IInd Surgical Clinic, University of J. E. Purkinje; and Research Center for Heart Support and Total Heart Substitution, Regional Institute of National Health, Brno, Czechoslovakia

P. Y. HATT, I.N.S.E.R.M. U2, Hôpital Léon Bernard, 94450 Limeil-Brévannes, France

D. J. HEARSE, The Rayne Institute, St. Thomas' Hospital, London, England

I. HEINROTH, Department of Pharmacology and Toxicology, Faculty of Medicine, Martin Luther University, Halle-Wittenberg, Halle, German Democratic Republic

M. L. HILL, Department of Pathology, Duke University Medical Center, Durham, North Carolina 27710, USA

P. HOFFMANN, Department of Pharmacology and Toxicology, Faculty of Medicine, Martin Luther University, Halle-Wittenberg, Halle, German Democratic Republic

C. HOLUBARSCH, Physiologiscal Institute (II), University of Tubingen, Tubingen, Federal Republic of Germany

A. R. HORAK, MRC Ischaemic Heart Disease Research Unit, Department of Medicine, University of Cape Town and Groote Schuur Hospital, Cape Town, South Africa

I. HÜTTNER, Department of Pathology, McGill University, Montreal, Quebec H3A 2B4, Canada

H. IJICHI, Second Department of Medicine, Kyoto Prefectural University of Medicine, Kyoto 602, Japan

Y. ITO, Sanraku Hospital, Tokyo 101, Japan

V. E. IVANOV, Department of Experimental Cardiology, USSR Cardiology Research Center, Academy of Medical Sciences, Moscow 101837, USSR

Y. IWASAKI, Cardiovascular Research Unit, The Third Department of Internal Medicine, Faculty of Medicine, University of Tokyo, Tokyo 113, Japan

R. JACOB, Physiological Institute (II), University of Tubingen, Tubingen, Federal Republic of Germany

H. JANEČKOVÁ, Institute of Pathological Physiology, Faculty of Medicine, IInd Surgical Clinic, University of J. E. Purkinje; and Research Center for Heart Support and Total Heart Substitution, Regional Institute of National Health, Brno, Czechoslovakia

G. JASMIN, Department of Pathology, Faculty of Medicine, University of Montreal, Montreal, Quebec H3C 3J7, Canada

R. B. JENNINGS, Department of Pathology, Duke University Medical Center, Durham, North Carolina 27710, USA

S. K. JOHRI, Faculty of Medicine, Aligarh Muslim University, Aligarh, India

M. JONES, Department of Paediatric Cardiology, Institute of Child Health, London WC1N 3EH, England; present address: Surgery Branch, National Heart, Lung and Blood Institute, National Institutes of Health, Bethesda, Maryland 20205, USA

L. KAIJSER, Department of Clinical Physiology, Huddinge Hospital, Karolinska Hospital; and St. Erik's Hospital, Stockholm, Sweden; and Department of Pharmacology, Catholic University, Rome, Italy

J. P. KALTENBACH, Department of Pathology, Northwestern University Medical School, Chicago, Illinois 60611, USA

T. KAMEDA, Department of Cardiothoracic Surgery, Juntendo University School of Medicine, Tokyo, Japan

T. KAMIKAWA, Third Department of Internal Medicine, Hamamatsu University School of Medicine, Hamamatsu, Japan

V. I. KAPELKO, Department of Experimental Cardiology, USSR Cardiology Research Center, Academy of Medical Sciences, Moscow 101837, USSR

P. KARCZEWSKI, Division of Cellular and Molecular Cardiology, Central Institute of Heart and Circulation Research, Academy of Sciences of the GDR, 1115 Berlin–Buch; and Surgical Clinic, Faculty of Medicine (Charité) of Humboldt University at Berlin, 1040 Berlin, German Democratic Republic

K. KARINO, The Department of Thoracic and Cardiovascular Surgery, Sapporo Medical College, Sapporo 060, Japan

P. KÁRPÁTI, Second Medical Clinic of Postgraduate Medical School, H-1389 Budapest, Hungary

Y. KASHIWAKURA, Department of Cardiology, Urawa City Hospital, Urawa, Japan

T. KATAGIRI, The Third Department of Internal Medicine, Showa University School of Medicine, Tokyo 142, Japan

N. V. KAVERINA, Institute of Pharmacology, Academy of Medical Sciences of the USSR, Moscow 125315, USSR

E. KEIJZER, Cardiochemical Laboratory, Thoraxcenter, Erasmus University Rotterdam, Rotterdam, The Netherlands

J. M. KEOGH, The Myocardial Metabolism and Cardiac Pharmacology Units, The Rayne Institute, St. Thomas' Hospital, London, England

B. KETTENBACH, Department of Pharmacology, Cassella AG, Frankfurt/Main, Federal Republic of Germany

A. K. KHANNA, Department of Cardiology, Postgraduate Institute of Medical Education and Research, Chandigarh 160012, India

I. KIMURA, Second Department of Medicine, Prefectural University of Medicine, Kyoto 602, Japan

Y. KIRA, The Fourth Department of Internal Medicine, Faculty of Medicine, The University of Tokyo, Tokyo, Japan

G. KISSLING, Physiological Institute (II), University of Tubingen, Tubingen, Federal Republic of Germany

A. KIZU, Second Department of Medicine, Kyoto Prefectural University of Medicine, Kyoto 602, Japan

A. KOBAYASHI, Third Department of Internal Medicine, Hamamatsu University, School of Medicine, Hamamatsu, Japan

Y. KOBAYASHI, The Third Department of Internal Medicine, Showa University School of Medicine, Tokyo 142, Japan

T. KOIZUMI, The Fourth Department of Internal Medicine, Faculty of Medicine, The University of Tokyo, Tokyo, Japan

F. KÖLBEL, Third Medical Department and Laboratory for Endocrinology and Metabolism, Faculty of Medicine, Charles University, Prague, Czechoslovakia

S. KOMATSU, The Department of Thoracic and Cardiovascular Surgery, Sapporo Medical College, Sapporo 060, Japan

E.-G. KRAUSE, Division of Cellular and Molecular Cardiology, Central Institute of Heart and Circulation Research, Academy of Sciences of the GDR, 1115 Berlin–Buch; and Surgical Clinic, Faculty of Medicine (Charité) of Humboldt University at Berlin, 1040 Berlin, German Democratic Republic

L. KRČEK, Institute of Pathological Physiology, Faculty of Medicine, IInd Surgical Clinic, University of J. E. Purkinje; and Research Center for Heart Support and Total Heart Substitution, Regional Institute of National Health, Brno, Czechoslovakia

V. KRČMA, Institute of Pathological Physiology, Faculty of Medicine, IInd Surgical Clinic, University of J. E. Purkinje; and Research Center for Heart Support and Total Heart Substitution, Regional Institute of National Health, Brno, Czechoslovakia

S. A. KRYZHANOVSKY, Institute of Pharmacology, Academy of Medical Sciences of the USSR, Moscow 125315, USSR

B. KWIATKOWSKA-PATZER, Department of Medicine, University of Chicago, Chicago, Illinois 60637, USA; present address: Academy of Medicine, Warsaw, Poland

K. LAUSTIOLA, Department of Biomedical Sciences, University of Tampere, 33101 Tampere 10, Finland

Y. LECARPENTIER, I.N.S.E.R.M. U2, Hôpital Léon Bernard, 94450 Limeil-Brévannes, France

K.-F. LINDENAU, Division of Cellular and Molecular Cardiology, Central Institute of Heart and Circulation Research, Academy of Sciences of the GDR, 1115 Berlin–Buch; and Surgical Clinic, Faculty of Medicine (Charité) of Humboldt University at Berlin, 1040 Berlin, German Democratic Republic

S. Y. LIU, Department of Pathology, Northwestern University Medical School, Chicago, Illinois 60611, USA

A. S. MANNING, The Myocardial Metabolism and Cardiac Pharmacology Units, The Rayne Institute, St. Thomas' Hospital, London, England

J. L. MARTIN, E.N.S.T.A., Ecole Polytechnique, 91120 Palaiseau, France

P. A. MARTORANA, Department of Pharmacology, Cassella AG, Frankfurt/Main, Federal Republic of Germany

S. MATSUMOTO, The Fourth Department of Internal Medicine, Faculty of Medicine, The University of Tokyo, Tokyo, Japan

I. MEDUGORAC, Physiologiscal Institute (II), University of Tubingen, Tubingen, Federal Republic of Germany

F. Z. MEERSON, Institute of General Pathology and Pathologic Physiology, USSR Academy of Medical Sciences, Moscow, USSR

P. MENTZ, Department of Pharmacology and Toxicology, Faculty of Mcdicine, Martin Luther University, Halle-Wittenberg, Halle, German Democratic Republic

T. METSÄ-KETELÄ, Department of Biomedical Sciences, University of Tampere, 33101 Tampere 10, Finland

T. MINAGA, Second Department of Medicine, Kyoto Prefectural University of Medicine, Kyoto 602, Japan

H. MINATOGUCHI, The Third Department of Internal Medicine, Showa University School of Medicine, Tokyo 142, Japan

K. MIYATA, Department of Internal Medicine, Josai Dental University, Saitama, Japan

A. M. MOGILEV, Department of Pharmacology, Cassella AG, Frankfurt/Main, Federal Republic of Germany

H. E. MORGAN, Department of Physiology, The Milton S. Hershey Medical Center, The Pennsylvania State University, Hershey, Pennsylvania 17033, USA

R. NAGAI, Cardiovascular Research Unit, The Third Department of Internal Medicine, Faculty of Medicine, University of Tokyo, Tokyo 113, Japan

N. NAKAMURA, The Third Department of Internal Medicine, Showa University School of Medicine, Tokyo 142, Japan

K. NAKAMURA, Second Department of Medicine, Kyoto Prefectural University of Medicine, Kyoto 602, Japan

H. NIITANI, The Third Department of Internal Medicine, Showa University School of Medicine, Tokyo 142, Japan

R.-E. NITZ, Department of Medical and Biological Research, Cassella AG, Frankfurt/Main, Federal Republic of Germany

J. NOWAK, Department of Clinical Physiology, Huddinge Hospital, Karolinska Hospital; and St. Erik's Hospital, Stockholm, Sweden; and Department of Pharmacology, Catholic University, Rome, Italy

E. OGATA, The Fourth Department of Internal Medicine, Faculty of Medicine, The University of Tokyo, Tokyo, Japan

A. OHKUBO, Cardiovascular Research Unit, The Third Department of Internal Medicine, Faculty of Medicine, University of Tokyo, Tokyo 113, Japan

K. OHORI, The Department of Thoracic and Cardiovascular Surgery, Sapporo Medical College, Sapporo 060, Japan

F. OKAMOTO, The Department of Thoracic and Cardiovascular Surgery, Sapporo Medical College, Sapporo 060, Japan

T. OKAMURA, Department of Cardiothoracic Surgery, Juntendo University School of Medicine, Tokyo, Japan

J. OLIVARES, Laboratory of Animal Physiology, Scientific and Medical University of Grenoble, 38041 Grenoble Cedex, France

L. H. OPIE, MRC Ischaemic Heart Disease Research Unit, Department of Medicine, University of Cape Town and Groote Schuur Hospital, Cape Town, South Africa

J. M. ORD, Pauline and Adolph Weinberger Laboratory for Cardiopulmonary Research, Department of Physiology, The University of Texas Health Science Center at Dallas, Dallas, Texas 75235, USA

K. OZAWA, The Third Department of Internal Medicine, Showa University School of Medicine, Tokyo 142, Japan

C. PATRONO, Department of Clinical Physiology, Huddinge Hospital, Karolinska Hospital; and St. Erik's Hospital, Stockholm, Sweden; and Department of Pharmacology, Catholic University, Rome, Italy

V. PAVLÍČEK, Institute of Pathological Physiology, Faculty of Medicine, IInd Surgical Clinic, University of J. E. Purkinje; and Research Center for Heart Support and Total Heart Substitution, Regional Institute of National Health, Brno, Czechoslovakia

O. I. PISARENKO, Department of Experimental Cardiology, USSR Cardiology Research Center, Academy of Medical Sciences, Moscow 101837, USSR

K. PÖNICKE, Department of Pharmacology and Toxicology, Faculty of Medicine, Martin Luther University, Halle-Wittenberg, Halle, German Democratic Republic

I. PRÉDA, Second Medical Clinic of Postgraduate Medical School, H-1389 Budapest, Hungary

T. PŘIBYL, Third Medical Department and Laboratory for Endocrinology and Metabolism, Faculty of Medicine, Charles University, Prague, Czechoslovakia

G. PRIOR, Department of Medicine, University of Chicago, Chicago, Illinois 60637, USA

L. PROSCHEK, Department of Pathology, Faculty of Medicine, University of Montreal, Montreal, Quebec H3C 3J7, Canada

V. RAM, Faculty of Medicine, Aligarh Muslim University, Aligarh, India

M. RASCHACK, Department of Pharmacology, Knoll AG, Ludwigshafen, Federal Republic of Germany

A. RAY, Laboratory of Animal Physiology, Scientific and Medical University of Grenoble, 38041 Grenoble Cedex, France

K. A. REIMER, Department of Pathology, Duke University Medical Center, Durham, North Carolina 27710, USA

W. RETTKOWSKI, Department of Pharmacology and Toxicology, Faculty of Medicine, Martin Luther University, Halle-Wittenberg, Halle, German Democratic Republic

T. L. RICH, Department of Biochemistry and Biophysics, University of Pennsylvania School of Medicine, Philadelphia, Pennsylvania, 19104, USA; present address: Cardiovascular Research Laboratory, Department of Physiology, UCLA Medical Center, Los Angeles, California 90024, USA

G. RONA, Department of Pathology, McGill University, Montreal, Quebec H3A 2B4, Canada

A. ROSSI, Laboratory of Animal Physiology, Scientific and Medical University of Grenoble, 38041 Grenoble Cedex, France

Yu. B. ROZONOV, Institute of Pharmacology, Academy of Medical Sciences of the USSR, Moscow 125315, USSR

P. P. RUMYANTSEV, Institute of Cytology of the Academy of Sciences of the USSR, Leningrad 190121, USSR

H. RUPP, Physiological Institut (II), University of Tubingen, Tubingen, Federal Republic of Germany

S. SAFAVI, Department of Pathology, Northwestern University Medical School, Chicago, Illinois 60611, USA

Y. SASAI, The Third Department of Internal Medicine, Showa University School of Medicine, Tokyo 142, Japan

E. SCHRAVEN, Department of Medical and Biological Research, Cassella AG, Frankfurt/Main, Federal Republic of Germany

V. SCHREIBER, Third Medical Department and Laboratory for Endocrinology and Metabolism, Faculty of Medicine, Charles University, Prague, Czechoslovakia

M. SEBESZTA, Laboratory of Comparative Physiology, University of Paris XI, Orsay, France; present address: Second Medical Clinic of Postgraduate Medical School, H-1389 Budapest, Hungary

H. J. SEIFART, Department of Pharmacology, Faculty of Medicine, University of Tübingen, D-7400 Tübingen, Federal Republic of Germany

D. L. SIEHL, Department of Physiology, The Milton S. Hershey Medical Center, The Pennsylvania State University, Hershey, Pennsylvania 17033, USA

M. SIESS, Department of Pharmacology, Faculty of Medicine, University of Tübingen, D-7400 Tübingen, Federal Republic of Germany

E. D. SILOVE, Department of Paediatric Cardiology, Institute of Child Health, London WC1N 3EH, England; present address: The Children's Hospital, Ladywood Middleway, Birmingham, England

T. SLÁDEK, Institute of Pathological Physiology, Faculty of Medicine, IInd Surgical Clinic, University of J. E. Purkinje; and Research Center for Heart Support and Total Heart Substitution, Regional Institute of National Health, Brno, Czechoslovakia

V. N. SMIRNOV, Department of Experimental Cardiology, USSR Cardiology Research Center, Academy of Medical Sciences, Moscow 101837, USSR

E. S. SOLOMATINA, Department of Experimental Cardiology, USSR Cardiology Research Center, Academy of Medical Sciences, Moscow 101837, USSR

E. ŠOTÁKOVÁ, Institute of Pathological Physiology, Faculty of Medicine, IInd Surgical Clinic, University of J. E. Purkinje; and Research Center for Heart Support and Total Heart Substitution, Regional Institute of National Health, Brno, Czechoslovakia

O. ŠOTOLOVÁ, Institute of Pathological Physiology, Faculty of Medicine, IInd Surgical Clinic, University of J. E. Purkinje; and Research Center for Heart Support and Total Heart Substitution, Regional Institute of National Health, Brno, Czechoslovakia

J. ŠTĚPÁN, Third Medical Department and Laboratory for Endocrinology and Metabolism, Faculty of Medicine, Charles University, Prague, Czechoslovakia

I. M. STUDNEVA, Department of Experimental Cardiology, USSR Cardiology Research Center, Academy of Medical Sciences, Moscow 101837, USSR

M. SUNAMORI, Cardiac Muscle Research Laboratory, Mayo Clinic and Mayo Foundation, Rochester, Minnesota 55905, USA

A. SUZUKI, Department of Cardiothoracic Surgery, Juntendo University School of Medicine, Tokyo, Japan

Y. SUZUKI, Third Department of Internal Medicine, Hamamatsu University School of Medicine, Hamamatsu, Japan

M. R. TAJUDDIN, Faculty of Medicine, Aligarh Muslim University, Aligarh, India

Y. TAKEYAMA, The Third Department of Internal Medicine, Showa University School of Medicine, Tokyo 142, Japan

K. K. TALWAR, Department of Cardiology, Postgraduate Institute of Medical Education and Research, Chandigarh 160012, India

M. TARIQ, Faculty of Medicine, Aligarh Muslim University, Aligarh, India

C. TAUTU, Laboratory of Pathobiology, Clinical Research Institute of Montreal; and Department of Pathology, University of Montreal and Hôtel-Dieu of Montreal, Montreal, Quebec H2W 1R7, Canada

A. TOLEIKIS, Laboratory of Metabolism, Institute for Cardiovascular Research, Kaunas, Lithuanian SSR, USSR

D. TROTTNOW, Department of Medical and Biological Research, Cassella AG, Frankfurt/Main, Federal Republic of Germany

A. I. TURILOVA, Institute of Pharmacology, Academy of Medical Sciences of the USSR, Moscow 125315, USSR

S. UEDA, Cardiovascular Research Unit, The Third Department of Internal Medicine, Faculty of Medicine, University of Tokyo, Tokyo 113, Japan

E. URBÁNEK, Institute of Pathological Physiology, Faculty of Medicine, IInd Surgical Clinic, University of J. E. Purkinje; and Research Center for Heart Support and Total Heart Substitution, Regional Institute of National Health, Brno, Czechoslovakia

P. URBÁNEK, Institute of Pathological Physiology, Faculty of Medicine, IInd Surgical Clinic, University of J. E. Purkinje; and Research Center for Heart Support and Total Heart Substitution, Regional Institute of National Health, Brno, Czechoslovakia

H. VAPAATALO, Department of Biomedical Sciences, University of Tampere, 33101 Tampere 10, Finland

J[aromír] VAŠKŮ, Institute of Pathological Physiology, Faculty of Medicine, IInd Surgical Clinic, University of J. E. Purkinje; and Research Center for Heart Support and Total Heart Substitution, Regional Institute of National Health, Brno, Czechoslovakia

J[an] VAŠKŮ, Institute of Pathological Physiology, Faculty of Medicine, IInd Surgical Clinic, University of J. E. Purkinje; and Research Center for Heart Support and Total Heart Substitution, Regional Institute of National Health, Brno, Czechoslovakia

P. L. WAHI, Department of Cardiology, Postgraduate Institute of Medical Education and Research, Chandigarh 160012, India

J. R. WAKELAND, Pauline and Adolph Weinberger Laboratory for Cardiopulmonary Research, Department of Internal Medicine, The University of Texas Health Science Center at Dallas, Dallas, Texas, 75235, USA

K. C. WELHAM, Department of Paediatric Cardiology, Institute of Child Health, London WC1N 3EH, England; present address: Department of Molecular and Life Sciences, Dundee College of Technology, Dundee, Scotland

P. WENDSCHE, Institute of Pathological Physiology, Faculty of Medicine, IInd Surgical Clinic, University of J. E. Purkinje; and Research Center for Heart Support and Total Heart Substitution, Regional Institute of National Health, Brno, Czechoslovakia

A. WENNMALM, Department of Clinical Physiology, Huddinge Hospital, Karolinska Hospital; and St. Erik's Hospital, Stockholm, Sweden; and Department of Pharmacology, Catholic University, Rome, Italy

K. WILDENTHAL, Pauline and Adolph Weinberger Laboratory for Cardiopulmonary Research, Departments of Physiology and Internal Medicine, The University of Texas Health Science Center at Dallas, Dallas, Texas 75235, USA

J. R. WILLIAMSON, Department of Biochemistry and Biophysics, University of Pennsylvania School of Medicine, Philadelphia, Pennsylvania 19104, USA

R. K. H. WYSE, Department of Paediatric Cardiology, Institute of Child Health, London WC1N 3EH, England

Y. YABE, Cardiovascular Diagnostic Laboratory Center, Toho University School of Medicine, Tokyo, Japan

T. YAMADA, Department of Internal Medicine, Josai Dental University, Saitama, Japan

K. YAMAOKI, Cardiovascular Research Unit, The Third Department of Internal Medicine, Faculty of Medicine, University of Tokyo, Tokyo 113, Japan

N. YAMAZAKI, Third Department of Internal Medicine, Hamamatsu University, School of Medicine, Hamamatsu, Japan

M. YASUMI, Second Department of Medicine, Kyoto Prefectural University of Medicine, Kyoto 602, Japan

Y. YAZAKI, Cardiovascular Research Unit, The Third Department of Internal Medicine, Faculty of Medicine, University of Tokyo, Tokyo 113, Japan

D. M. YELLON, The Rayne Institute, St. Thomas' Hospital, London, England

M. YOKOYAMA, The Third Department of Internal Medicine, Showa University School of Medicine, Tokyo 142, Japan

A. YOSHIDA, Department of Internal Medicine, Josai Dental University, Saitama, Japan

R. ZAK, Department of Medicine, University of Chicago, Chicago, Illinois 60637, USA

U. ZEHL, Department of Pharmacology and Toxicology, Faculty of Medicine, Martin Luther University, Halle-Wittenberg, Halle, German Democratic Republic

Index

627